Fertility Preservation in Male Cancer Patients

Fertility Preservation in Male Cancer Patients

Editor-in-Chief
John P. Mulhall
Director, Male Sexual and Reproductive Medicine Program,
Urology Service, Department of Surgery,
Memorial Sloan–Kettering Cancer Center,
New York, NY, USA

Associate Editors
Linda D. Applegarth
Associate Professor of Psychology, Perlman Cohen Center
for Reproductive Medicine and Infertility,
Weill Cornell Medical College,
New York, NY, USA

Robert D. Oates
Professor of Urology, Boston University Medical Center,
Boston, MA, USA

Peter N. Schlegel
Professor and Chairman, Department of Urology,
Weill Cornell Medical College,
New York, NY, USA

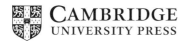

CAMBRIDGE UNIVERSITY PRESS
Cambridge, New York, Melbourne, Madrid, Cape Town,
Singapore, São Paulo, Delhi, Mexico City

Cambridge University Press
The Edinburgh Building, Cambridge CB2 8RU, UK

Published in the United States of America by Cambridge University
Press, New York

www.cambridge.org
Information on this title: www.cambridge.org/
9781107012127

First published 2013

Printed and bound in the United Kingdom by the MPG Books Group

*A catalog record for this publication is available from the British
Library*

Library of Congress Cataloging in Publication data
Fertility preservation in male cancer patients / editor-in-chief, John
P. Mulhall ; associate editors, Linda D. Applegarth, Robert D. Oates,
Peter N. Schlegel V.
    p. ; cm.
Includes bibliographical references and index.
ISBN 978-1-107-01212-7 (hardback)
I. Mulhall, John P.
[DNLM: 1. Infertility, Male – chemically induced.   2. Infertility,
Male – prevention & control.   3. Antineoplastic Agents – adverse
effects.   4. Fertility Preservation – methods.   5. Neoplasms –
complications.   6. Radiotherapy – adverse effects.   WJ   709]
616.6′921 – dc23   2012021049

ISBN 978-1-107-01212-7 Hardback

Contents

Section 5 – Post-therapy considerations

Color figures are to be found between pp. 230 and 231.

Contributors

Ashok Agarwal, PhD
Center for Reproductive Medicine, Cleveland Clinic, Cleveland, OH, USA

Linda D. Applegarth, EdD
Associate Professor of Psychology, Perlman Cohen Center for Reproductive Medicine and Infertility, Weill Cornell Medical College, New York, NY, USA

Nelson E. Bennett Jr., MD
Department of Urology, Lahey Clinic, Burlington, MA, USA

Nancy L. Brackett, PhD
Department of Urology, University of Miami Miller School of Medicine, Miami, FL, USA

Melissa B. Brisman, Esq. BS, JD
One Paragon Drive, Suite 158, Montvale, NJ

Mark F. H. Brougham, MD, MRCPCH
Consultant Paediatric Oncologist, Department of Paediatric Haematology and Oncology, Royal Hospital for Sick Children, Edinburgh, UK

Cara B. Cimmino, MD
Department of Urology, Lahey Clinic, Burlington, MA, USA

Owen K. Davis, MD, FACOG
Associate Director, IVF Program, The Center for Reproductive Medicine and Infertility, Weill Cornell Medical College, New York, NY, USA

Rian J. Dickstein, MD
Department of Urology, The University of Texas M. D. Anderson Cancer Center, Houston, TX, USA

Michael L. Eisenberg, MD
Assistant Professor, Department of Urology, Stanford University School of Medicine, Stanford, CA, USA

Mikkel Fode, MD
Department of Urology, Herlev Hospital, Herlev, Denmark

Gretchen A. Gignac, MD
Assistant Professor, Department of Medicine, Section of Hematology and Oncology, Boston University/ Boston Medical Center, Boston, MA, USA

Bruce R. Gilbert, MD, PhD
Director, Reproductive and Sexual Medicine, The Arthur Smith Institute for Urology, North Shore Long Island Jewish Health System, New Hyde Park, NY, USA

Ellen R. Goldmark, MD
Division of Urology, University of Maryland, Baltimore, MD, USA

Marc Goldstein, MD, Dsc(hon), FACS
Matthew P. Hardy Distinguished Professor of Reproductive Medicine and Urology; Surgeon-in-Chief, Male Reproductive Medicine and Surgery, Weill Cornell Medical College, New York Presbyterian Hospital, New York, NY, USA

Wayne J. G. Hellstrom, MD, FACS
Professor of Urology, Chief, Section of Andrology, Tulane University Health Sciences Center, Department of Urology, New Orleans, LA, USA

Wayland Hsiao, MD
Assistant Professor of Urology, Emory University, Atlanta, GA, USA

Jack Huang
The Center for Reproductive Medicine and Infertility, Weill Cornell Medical College, New York, NY, USA

Kathleen Hwang, MD
Associate Faculty Member, Department of
Molecular and Cellular Biology, Scott Department
of Urology, Baylor College of Medicine, Houston,
TX, USA

Ann A. Jakubowski, MD, PhD
Clinical Director, Adult Bone Marrow
Transplantation Outpatient Unit, Memorial
Sloan–Kettering Cancer Center, Professor of
Medicine, Weill Cornell Medical College, New York,
NY, USA

Keith Jarvi, MD, FRCSC
Professor, Division of Urology, Department of
Surgery, University of Toronto; Director, Murray
Koffler Urologic Wellness Center, Mount Sinai
Hospital, Toronto, Canada

Loren Jones, MD
Department of Urology, University of Illinois at
Chicago, Chicago, IL, USA

Hey-Joo Kang, MD
The Center for Reproductive Medicine and Infertility,
Weill Cornell Medical College, New York, NY,
USA

Joanne Frankel Kelvin, MSN
Clinical Nurse Specialist, Memorial Sloan–Kettering
Cancer Center, New York, NY, USA

Mohit Khera, MD, MBA, MPH
Assistant Professor of Urology, Division of Male
Reproductive Medicine and Surgery, Baylor College
of Medicine, Houston, TX, USA

Thomas F. Kolon, MD
Associate Professor of Urology, Perelman School of
Medicine at the University of Pennsylvania, Pediatric
Urology Fellowship Program Director, Children's
Hospital of Philadelphia, Philadelphia, PA,
USA

Kate H. Kraft, MD
Pediatric Urology Fellow, Perelman School of
Medicine at the University of Pennsylvania,
Children's Hospital of Philadelphia, Philadelphia, PA,
USA

Andrew C. Kramer, MD
Division of Urology, University of Maryland,
Baltimore, MD, USA

Dolores J. Lamb, PhD
Lester and Sue Smith Chair in Urologic Research,
Professor of Urology and Molecular and Cellular
Biology, Scott Department of Urology, Baylor College
of Medicine, Houston, TX, USA

Andrew B. Lassman, MD
Department of Neurology and Brain Tumor Center,
Memorial Sloan–Kettering Cancer Center, New York,
NY, USA

Helen R. Levey, DO, MPH
The Arthur Smith Institute for Urology, North Shore
Long Island Jewish Health System, New Hyde Park,
NY, USA

Larry I. Lipshultz, MD
Professor of Urology; Lester and Sue Smith Chair in
Reproductive Medicine; Chief, Division of Male
Reproductive Medicine and Surgery, Scott
Department of Urology, Baylor College of Medicine,
Houston, TX, USA

Charles M. Lynne, MD
The Miami Project to Cure Paralysis, University of
Miami Miller School of Medicine, Miami, FL, USA

Akanksha Mehta, MD
Fellow in Male Reproductive Medicine and
Microsurgery, Department of Urology, Weill Cornell
Medical College, New York, NY, USA

Marvin L. Meistrich, PhD
Department of Experimental Radiation Oncology,
The University of Texas M. D. Anderson Cancer
Center, Houston, TX, USA

Gregory C. Mitchell, MD
Tulane University Health Sciences Center,
Department of Urology, New Orleans, LA, USA

Mark A. Moyad, MD, MPH
Jenkins/Pokempner Director of Preventive and
Alternative Medicine, Department of Urology,
University of Michigan Medical Center, Ann Arbor,
MI, USA

John P. Mulhall, MD
Director, Male Sexual and Reproductive Medicine
Program, Urology Service, Department of Surgery,
Memorial Sloan–Kettering Cancer Center, New York,
NY, USA

Lauren Murray, Esq. BA, JD
One Paragon Drive, Suite 158, Montvale, NJ

Craig Niederberger, MD
Clarence C. Saelhof Professor and Head, Department of Urology, University of Illinois at Chicago College of Medicine; Professor, Department of Bioengineering, University of Illinois at Chicago College of Engineering, Chicago, IL, USA

Ariella Noy, MD
Associate Member and Attending Physician, Lymphoma Working Group Chair, Hematology Division, Lymphoma Service, AIDS Malignancy Consortium, Memorial Sloan–Kettering Cancer Center, New York, NY, USA

Robert D. Oates, MD
Professor of Urology, Boston University School of Medicine, Boston, MA, USA

Dana A. Ohl, MD
Department of Urology, University of Michigan Medical Center, Ann Arbor, MI, USA

Kutluk Oktay, MD, FACOG
Institute of Fertility Preservation, Department of Obstetrics and Gynecology, New York Medical College, Valhalla, NY, USA

Ndidiamaka Onwubalili, MD
Division of Reproductive Endocrinology and Infertility, Department of Obstetrics, Gynecology and Women's Health, UMDNJ-New Jersey Medical School, Newark, NJ, USA

Fabio Firmbach Pasqualatto, MD, PhD
Institute of Biotechnology, University of Caxias do Sul; CONCEPTION – Center for Human Reproduction, Caxias do Sul, RS, Brazil

Elena Pentsova, MD
Department of Neurology and Brain Tumor Center, Memorial Sloan–Kettering Cancer Center, New York, NY, USA

Susanne A. Quallich, ANP-BC
Department of Urology, University of Michigan Medical Center, Ann Arbor, MI, USA

Gwendolyn P. Quinn, PhD
Associate Member, Moffitt Cancer Center, Associate Professor, College of Medicine, University of South Florida

Alex Ridgeway, MS
Department of Molecular and Cellular Biology, Scott Department of Urology, Baylor College of Medicine, Houston, TX, USA

Matthew T. Roberts, MD, MEd, FRCSC
Assistant Professor, Division of Urology, Department of Surgery, University of Ottawa, Canada

Kenny A. Rodriguez-Wallberg, MD, PhD
Karolinska Institute, Department of Clinical Science, Intervention and Technology, Division of Obstetrics and Gynecology; Karolinska University Hospital Huddinge, Fertility Unit, Stockholm, Sweden

Allison B. Rosen, PhD
Adjunct Assistant Professor, Department of Obstetrics and Gynecology, New York Medical College, Valhalla, NY, USA

Lisa Rosenzweig, PhD
Postdoctoral Psychology Fellow, Department of Pain Medicine and Palliative Care, Beth Israel Medical Center, New York, NY, USA

Edmund S. Sabanegh Jr., MD
Glickman Urological and Kidney Institute, Cleveland Clinic Foundation, Cleveland, OH, USA

Hossein Sadeghi-Nejad, MD, FACS
Professor of Surgery in Urology, UMDNJ-New Jersey Medical School, Newark, NJ; Chief of Urology, VA NJ Health Care System, Center for Male Reproductive Medicine, Hackensack University Medical Center, Hackensack, NJ, USA

Mary K. Samplaski, MD
Glickman Urological and Kidney Institute, Cleveland Clinic Foundation, Cleveland, OH, USA

Jay I. Sandlow, MD
Professor and Vice-Chair, Department of Urology, Medical College of Wisconsin, Milwaukee, WI, USA

Peter N. Schlegel, MD
Professor and Chairman, Department of Urology,
Weill Cornell Medical College, New York, NY, USA

Gunapala Shetty, PhD
Department of Experimental Radiation Oncology,
The University of Texas M. D. Anderson Cancer
Center, Houston, TX, USA

Mark Sigman, MD
Krishanmurthi Professor of Surgery (Urology) and
Chief of Urology Alpert Medical School of Brown
University; Chief of Urology The Rhode Island and
Miriam Hospitals, Providence, RI, USA

Jens Sønksen, MD, DMSci
Department of Urology, Herlev Hospital, Herlev,
Denmark

Peter J. Stahl, MD
Assistant Professor of Urology, Columbia University
College of Physicians & Surgeons, New York, NY,
USA

Eytan Stein, MD
Lymphoma Division, Memorial Sloan–Kettering
Cancer Center, New York, NY, USA

Doron S. Stember, MD
Department of Urology, Beth Israel Medical Center,
New York, NY, USA

Raanan Tal, MD
Male Sexual and Reproductive Medicine Program,
Department of Urology, Beilinson Hospital,
Rabin Medical Center, Petah Tikva, Israel

Susan T. Vadaparampil, PhD, MPH
Associate Member, Moffitt Cancer Center, Associate
Professor, College of Medicine, University of South
Florida

W. Hamish B. Wallace, MD, FRCP, MRCPCH
Department of Paediatric Haematology and
Oncology, Royal Hospital for Sick Children,
Edinburgh, UK

Leonard H. Wexler, MD
Associate Attending Physician, Department of
Pediatrics, Memorial Sloan–Kettering Cancer Center,
New York, NY, USA

Daniel H. Williams IV, MD
Assistant Professor, Department of Urology,
University of Wisconsin School of Medicine and
Public Health, Madison, WI, USA

Chapter

1

Functional anatomy of the hypothalamic–pituitary–gonadal axis and the male reproductive tract

Nelson E. Bennett Jr.

Anatomy of reproductive function

The reproductive functional axis of the male can be divided into three major subdivisions: (1) the hypothalamus, (2) the pituitary gland, and (3) the testis. Each level elaborates a signal, or transmitter molecule, that stimulates or inhibits the subsequent level of the axis. The end result is the production and expulsion of semen that contains spermatozoa. This chapter examines the hypothalamic–pituitary–gonadal (HPG) axis, and reviews the functional anatomy of the testis, epididymis, vas deferens, seminal vesicles, prostate, and penis.

Hypothalamus and anterior pituitary gland

The control of male sexual and reproductive function begins with secretion of gonadotropin-releasing hormone (GnRH) by the hypothalamus (Fig. 1.1). This hormone in turn stimulates the anterior pituitary gland to secrete two downstream hormones (termed gonadotropins). These hormones are luteinizing hormone (LH) and follicle-stimulating hormone (FSH). LH is the primary stimulus for the testicular secretion of testosterone, while FSH mainly stimulates spermatogenesis.

Gonadotropin-releasing hormone (GnRH)

The neuronal cells of the arcuate nuclei of the hypothalamus secrete GnRH, a 10-amino-acid peptide. The endings of these neurons terminate in the median eminence of the hypothalamus, where they release GnRH into the hypothalamic–hypophysial portal vascular system. The GnRH is transported to the anterior pituitary gland via the hypophysial portal blood

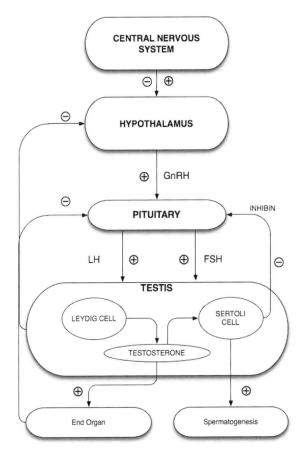

Figure 1.1. Feedback regulation of the hypothalamic–pituitary–gonadal (HPG) axis in males. Positive (stimulatory) effects are shown by + and inhibitory (negative feedback) effects by –. GnRH, gonadotropin-releasing hormone; LH, luteinizing hormone; FSH, follicle-stimulating hormone.

and stimulates the release of the two gonadotropins, LH and FSH [1]. The output of GnRH is influenced by three types of rhythmicity: seasonal, on a timescale of

Fertility Preservation in Male Cancer Patients, ed. John P. Mulhall, Linda D. Applegarth, Robert D. Oates and Peter N. Schlegel.
Published by Cambridge University Press. © Cambridge University Press 2013.

months and peaking in the spring; circadian, resulting in highest testosterone levels during the early morning hours; and pulsatile, with peaks occurring every 90–120 minutes on average [2]. The intensity of this hormone's stimulus is determined (1) by the frequency of the cycles of secretion and (2) by the quantity of GnRH released with each cycle. LH secretion by the anterior pituitary gland is also cyclical. LH follows the pulsatile release of GnRH. On the other hand, FSH secretion changes slowly with the fluctuation of GnRH secretion over a period of many hours.

Gonadotropic hormones: LH and FSH

Luteinizing hormone and follicle-stimulating hormone are glycoproteins that are secreted by gonadotropic cells in the anterior pituitary gland. In the absence of GnRH secretion from the hypothalamus, the gonadotropes in the pituitary gland secrete essentially no LH or FSH. They exert their effects on their target tissues in the testes via the cyclic adenosine monophosphate (cAMP) second messenger system. This, in turn, activates specific enzyme systems in the respective target cells.

Testosterone and LH

Testosterone is secreted by the Leydig cells in the interstitium of the testes in response to stimulation by LH from the anterior pituitary gland. The quantity of testosterone secreted is nearly directly proportional to the level of LH stimulation. Mature Leydig cells are normally found in a child's testes for a few weeks after birth, but then involute until puberty. The secretion of LH at puberty causes testicular interstitial cells that look like fibroblasts to evolve into functional Leydig cells.

Negative feedback of testosterone

The testosterone secreted by the testes in response to LH inhibits the secretion of LH from the anterior pituitary. The bulk of this inhibition is most likely from the direct effect of testosterone on the hypothalamus to decrease the secretion of GnRH. A decrease in GnRH secretion results in a parallel decrease in secretion of both LH and FSH by the anterior pituitary. This decrease in LH, in turn, decreases the secretion of testosterone by the testes. Hence, whenever serum level of testosterone exceeds the body's preset homeostatic level, the automatic negative feedback

effect, operating through the hypothalamus and anterior pituitary gland, reduces the testosterone secretion back toward the desired operating level (see Chapter 30). On the contrary, a testosterone-poor environment allows the hypothalamus to secrete large amounts of GnRH, with a corresponding increase in LH and FSH from the anterior pituitary and an increase in testicular testosterone secretion.

Testosterone and FSH

In the seminiferous tubules, both FSH and testosterone are necessary for the maintenance of spermatogenesis. Specific FSH-dedicated receptors on the Sertoli cells induce Sertoli cell growth and elaboration of various spermatogenic substances. Simultaneously, the paracrine action of testosterone and dihydrotestosterone from the interstitial Leydig cells stimulates and supports spermatogenesis in the seminiferous tubule.

Inhibin

Inhibin is a glycoprotein, like both LH and FSH. It has a molecular weight of 36 000 daltons. Inhibin is dimeric in structure, and the two monomers are linked together by a single disulfide bond. The monomers are termed α and β subunits. The α subunit is conserved in the different types of inhibin, but the β subunit varies. In humans, the Sertoli cells secrete inhibin B ($\alpha\beta_B$). Inhibin B selectively suppresses FSH secretion in the anterior pituitary gland by inhibiting transcription of the gene encoding the β subunit of FSH [3]. Additionally, inhibin has a slight effect on the hypothalamus to inhibit secretion of GnRH. Inhibin is released from the Sertoli cells in response to robust, rapid spermatogenesis. The end result is to diminish the pituitary secretion of FSH. Conversely, when the seminiferous tubules fail to produce sperm, inhibin production diminishes, resulting in a marked increase in FSH secretion. This potent inhibitory feedback effect on the anterior pituitary gland provides an important negative feedback mechanism for control of spermatogenesis, operating simultaneously with and in parallel to the negative feedback mechanism for control of testosterone secretion.

Testis

Embryologically, the testes develop at the urogenital ridge and descend into the scrotum via the inguinal canal at birth. These two paired organs are suspended

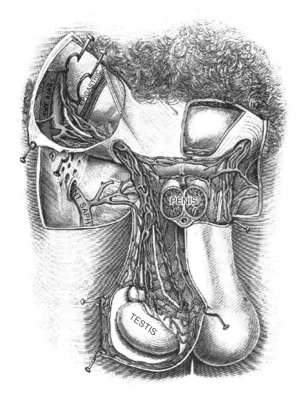

Figure 1.2. Vascular anatomy of the spermatic cord and testis. (Reproduced from Gray H. *Anatomy of the Human Body.* Philadelphia, PA: Lea & Febiger, 1918; Bartleby.com, 2000.) *See color plate section.*

on the spermatic cords and are covered by numerous layers of tissue. Upon emerging from the inguinal ring in utero, they are covered by the tunica vaginalis, internal spermatic fascia, cremasteric muscle, external spermatic fascia, dartos fascia, and skin.

Arterial and venous supply

The arterial supply of the testis is derived from three different sources (Fig. 1.2). The testicular artery arises from the aorta. The artery of the vas deferens (vasal artery) originates from the internal iliac artery. Lastly, the cremasteric artery (external spermatic artery) arises from the inferior epigastric artery [4].

The testicular artery becomes part of the countercurrent exchange phenomenon when it associates with a network of veins known as the pampiniform plexus. Several veins (pampiniform plexus) surround the convoluted testicular artery. The surrounding venous blood cools down arterial blood arriving at the testis. The accepted explanation for the

pampiniform plexus is that it functions to efficiently maintain the optimal temperature for spermatogenesis, which is below body temperature. Skandhan and Rajahariprasad hypothesized that the process of spermatogenesis results in a large amount of heat, which has to be regulated [5]. The pampiniform plexus and the human scrotal skin act as a radiator for the robust heat generation. The scrotal skin is devoid of subcutaneous fat, and the presence of high sweat-gland density enables heat transmission. Upon exposure to cold temperatures, the scrotal surface is minimized by contraction, preventing temperature loss, and cremaster muscles retract the testes closer to the abdomen, for temperature maintenance.

The rich anastomoses between the testicular (internal spermatic) and vasal arteries allow maintenance of testicular viability if the internal spermatic artery is transected. In the testis, the artery gives rise to centrifugal arteries that pierce the testicular parenchyma. Further branches divide into arterioles that bring in blood to peritubular and intertubular capillaries [6]. In some men, up to 90% of testicular blood supply derives from the testicular artery.

Testicular venous drainage is through the pampiniform plexus, which in the region of the internal inguinal ring gives origin to the testicular vein [7]. The left testicular vein discharges into the left renal vein at a right angle, whereas the right testicular vein discharges directly into the inferior vena cava at an oblique angle. All testicular veins have valves. In the region of the fourth lumbar vertebra the testicular veins divide into two trunks, one lateral and one medial [7,8]. The lateral trunk is anastomosed with retroperitoneal veins, mainly colonic and renal capsular veins, and the medial trunk is anastomosed with ureteral veins [7,8].

Testicular organization

The interior of the testis can be divided into compartments (Fig. 1.3). Within each compartment, are seminiferous tubules and interstitial tissue. The seminiferous tubules are long, looped structures that house spermatozoa production. The length of the uncoiled seminiferous tubules is approximately 240 meters (800 feet) [9,10]. The seminiferous tubules drain into the rete testis. Before draining into the epididymis, the tubules of the rete testis unite into 6–12 ductuli efferentes.

3

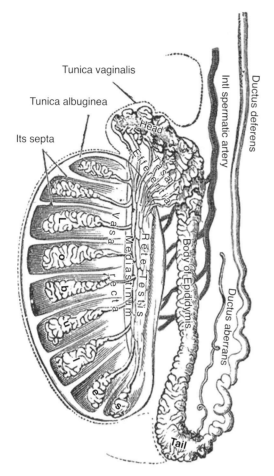

Figure 1.3. Internal structure of the testis and epididymis. (Reproduced from Gray H. *Anatomy of the Human Body.* Philadelphia, PA: Lea & Febiger, 1918; Bartleby.com, 2000.) *See color plate section.*

The seminiferous tubules contain two types of cells, spermatogenic cells and Sertoli cells, which have several functions in support of spermatogenesis. Stem cells (spermatogonia) develop from primordial germ cells that arise from the yolk sac and enter the testes during the fifth week of development (see Chapter 2). In the embryonic testes, the primordial germ cells differentiate into spermatogonia, which remain dormant during childhood and actively begin producing sperm at puberty. Toward the lumen of the seminiferous tubule are layers of progressively more mature cells. In order of advancing maturity, these are primary spermatocytes, secondary spermatocytes, spermatids, and spermatozoa. After a spermatozoon has formed, it is released into the lumen of the seminiferous tubule.

Large Sertoli cells are embedded among the spermatogenic cells in the seminiferous tubules. These "sustentacular cells" extend from the basement membrane to the lumen of the tubule. Internal to the basement membrane and spermatogonia, tight junctions join neighboring Sertoli cells to one another. These junctions form the blood–testis barrier. This barrier isolates the developing gametes from the blood and prevents an immune response against the spermatogenic cell's surface antigens, which are recognized as alien by the immune system.

Sertoli cells support and protect developing spermatogenic cells in several ways. They (1) nourish spermatocytes, spermatids, and sperm, (2) phagocytize excess spermatid cytoplasm, (3) control movements of spermatogenic cells and the release of sperm into the lumen of the seminiferous tubule, and (4) produce fluid for sperm transport, secrete inhibin, and regulate the effects of testosterone and FSH.

Spermatogenesis

In humans, spermatogenesis takes 74 days. It begins with the spermatogonia, which contain the diploid ($2n$) number of chromosomes. Spermatogonia are a variety of stem cell; when they undergo mitosis, some spermatogonia remain near the basement membrane of the seminiferous tubule in an undifferentiated state to serve as a reservoir of cells for future cell division and subsequent sperm production. The rest of the spermatogonia lose contact with the basement membrane, squeeze through the tight junctions of the blood–testis barrier, undergo developmental changes, and differentiate into primary spermatocytes. Primary spermatocytes are diploid ($2n$) and have 46 chromosomes. Shortly after it forms, the primary spermatocyte replicates its DNA in preparation for meiosis. The two cells formed by meiosis I are secondary spermatocytes. Each secondary spermatocyte is haploid (n) and has 23 chromosomes. Each chromosome within a secondary spermatocyte has two chromatids (two copies of DNA). Next, the secondary spermatocytes undergo meiosis II. In meiosis II, the two chromatids of each chromosome separate. The four haploid cells resulting from meiosis II are called spermatids. Thus, a single primary spermatocyte produces four spermatids via two rounds of cell division (meiosis I and meiosis II).

As spermatogenic cells proliferate, they fail to complete cytoplasmic separation (cytokinesis). The cells remain in contact via cytoplasmic bridges through their entire development. This allows for the synchronized production of sperm in any given area of seminiferous tubule. The final stage of spermatogenesis is called spermiogenesis. It is the transformation of spermatids (*n*) into sperm. In spermiogenesis, no cell division occurs. The spermatid becomes a single spermatozoon. During this process, spherical spermatids are transformed into elongated, slender sperm. During this time, mitochondria multiply, and an acrosome and a flagellum develop. Sertoli cells dispose of the excess cytoplasm. Lastly, spermatozoa enter into the lumen of the seminiferous tubule as they are released from their connections to Sertoli cells in a process called spermiation. Fluid secreted by Sertoli cells pushes sperm toward the ducts of the testes. At this point, sperm are immobile and will complete maturation in the epididymis.

Epididymis

The epididymis is a tightly coiled structure, which when unfurled can be 6 meters long. Anatomically, the epididymis can be divided into three regions: the head (caput), the body (corpus), and the tail (cauda). The epididymal head consists of 8–12 efferent ducts and the initial segment of the ductus epididymis. As we move from the head to the tail of the epididymis, the lumen of the epididymis is first large and asymmetrical. It then narrows as the body of the epididymis is approached. When the tail of the epididymis is encountered, the lumen enlarges significantly (Fig. 1.3).

The epididymis is lined with pseudostratified columnar epithelium and encircled by layers of smooth muscle [11]. The free surfaces of the columnar cells contain stereocilia that increase the surface area for the reabsorption of degenerated sperm. Around the caput epididymis, a wispy layer of contractile cells encircles the tubule. In the cauda epididymis, smooth muscle cells can be seen organized in three distinct layers. Connective tissue around the muscle layers attaches the loops of the ductus epididymis and carries blood vessels and nerves.

Innervation

The innervation of the human epididymis is a product of the pelvic plexus and the hypogastric plexus. These give rise to the inferior and intermediate spermatic nerves [12]. The density of the nerve fibers increases proportionally along the length of the epididymis,

similar to the increase in density of smooth muscle cells [11,13,14]. Van De Velde and Risely postulated that the peristaltic activity of the epididymis could be associated with the increasing density of smooth muscle cells and nerve fibers [15].

Arterial and venous supply

The testicular artery divides into the superior and inferior epididymal branches, which delivers blood to the head and body of the epididymis [16]. The blood supply to the epididymal tail (cauda) is derived from the deferential artery (artery of the vas). As in the testis, the epididymis enjoys a rich anastamotic system through the deferential, cremasteric, and testicular arteries to ensure collateral blood flow.

In his seminal 1954 publication, MacMillan described the vessels draining blood from the body and tail of the epididymis as joining to form the vena marginalis of Haberer. This vein unites with the pampiniform plexus, the cremasteric vein, or the deferential vein [16].

Lymphatic drainage of the caput and corpus epididymis follows the internal spermatic vein and terminates in the preaortic nodes. The lymph from the cauda epididymis drains into the external iliac nodes.

Epididymal function

The function of the epididymis can be divided into three broad categories: (1) sperm storage, (2) sperm maturation, and (3) sperm transport.

Storage of sperm

The two testes of the human adult form up to 120 million sperm each day. An average of 215 million spermatozoa are stored in each epididymis [17]. Approximately half of the total number of epididymal spermatozoa is stored in the caudal region. They can remain stored, maintaining their fertility, for at least a month. During this time, they are kept in a deeply suppressed inactive state by multiple inhibitory substances in the secretions of the ducts. Conversely, with a high level of sexual activity and ejaculations, storage may be no longer than a few days [18]. After ejaculation, the sperm become motile, and they also become capable of fertilizing the ovum. The Sertoli cells and the epithelium of the epididymis secrete a special nutrient fluid that is ejaculated along with the sperm. This fluid contains hormones (including both testosterone and estrogens), enzymes, and special nutrients that are essential for sperm maturation.

Maturation of sperm

After formation in the seminiferous tubules, the sperm require several days to pass through the 6-meter-long tubule of the epididymis. Sperm removed from the seminiferous tubules and from the early portions of the epididymis are non-motile, and they cannot fertilize an ovum [19]. However, after the sperm have been in the epididymis for some 18–24 hours they develop the capability of motility, even though several inhibitory proteins in the epididymal fluid still prevent final motility until after ejaculation [20–23].

The normal motile, fertile sperm are capable of flagellated movement though the fluid medium at velocities of 1–4 mm/min. The activity of sperm is greatly enhanced in a neutral and slightly alkaline medium, as exists in the ejaculated semen, but it is greatly depressed in a mildly acidic medium. A strong acidic medium can cause rapid death of sperm. The activity of sperm increases markedly with increasing temperature, but so does the rate of metabolism, causing the life of the sperm to be considerably shortened. Although sperm can live for many weeks in the suppressed state in the genital ducts of the testes, life expectancy of ejaculated sperm in the female genital tract is only 1–2 days.

Transport of sperm

Sperm transport from the caput epididymis to the cauda epididymis takes between 2 and 12 days [17,24]. Transit of sperm through the cauda can be variable, and it is affected by sexual activity [25]. Movement of the sperm through the epididymis is influenced by motile cilia and the muscular contraction of the ductuli efferentes. As previously mentioned, the density of smooth muscle cells increases proportionally along the length of the epididymis, which is responsible for the spontaneous rhythmic contractions of the epididymis.

Vas deferens and ejaculatory duct

In its caudal portion, the epididymis becomes less convoluted, and its outer diameter increases to 2–3 mm (inner diameter 300–500 μm). Beyond this point, the duct is known as the vas deferens or ductus deferens. The ductus deferens is 45 cm long and travels within the spermatic cord towards the pelvis. In the pelvis it runs superior to the ureter at the level of the bladder

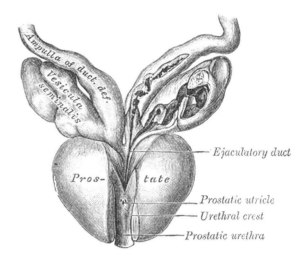

Figure 1.4. Prostate, seminal vesicles, vas deferens and ejaculatory ducts and prostatic urethra. (Reproduced from Gray H. *Anatomy of the Human Body*. Philadelphia, PA: Lea & Febiger, 1918; Bartleby. com, 2000.)

and travels in an inferior medial direction to enter the superior-posterior surface of the prostate. The ejaculatory duct then continues within the prostate gland.

The blood supply of the vas deferens is derived from the inferior vesicle artery via the deferential artery [26]. The vas deferens has both parasympathetic and sympathetic input. However, the dominant source of innervation is from the sympathetic adrenergic system.

The mucosa of the vas deferens consists of pseudostratified columnar epithelium and lamina propria [27]. The vas deferens is composed of three layers of smooth muscle: an inner and outer longitudinal layer, and a middle circular layer.

The primary function of the vas deferens and ejaculatory duct is to transport mature sperm to the prostatic urethra. Similar to the epididymis, the vas deferens exhibits a sperm storage capacity for several months.

Seminal vesicles

The seminal vesicles lie posterior to the base of the urinary bladder and anterior to the rectum (Fig. 1.4). The arterial supply of the seminal vesicles is derived from the inferior vesical artery and the middle rectal artery. Venous drainage is through the inferior vesical and middle rectal veins. Lymphatic drainage is directed to the internal iliac lymph nodes.

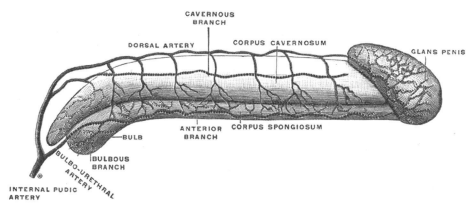

Figure 1.5. Arterial anatomy of the penis. (Reproduced from Gray H. *Anatomy of the Human Body.* Philadelphia, PA: Lea & Febiger, 1918; Bartleby.com, 2000.) *See color plate section.*

The embryonic origin of the seminal vesicles is the Wolffian duct. Its convoluted structure houses a secretory epithelial lining. Fluid secreted by the seminal vesicles normally constitutes about 80% of the volume of semen. The fluid is an alkaline, viscous fluid that contains fructose, prostaglandins, and clotting proteins. The alkaline nature of the seminal fluid helps to neutralize the acidic secretions of the female reproductive tract that otherwise would inactivate and kill sperm. The fructose is an important energy source for the sperm. Prostaglandins may contribute to sperm motility and viability [28]. The clotting proteins help semen coagulate after ejaculation, but the semen is subsequently liquefied by prostatic proteases.

Prostate

The prostate is a walnut-sized gland that lies at the base of the bladder (Fig. 1.4). It measures about 4 × 3 × 2 cm. The arterial supply of the prostate is derived from branches of the internal iliac artery: the inferior vesical artery, the internal pudendal artery, and the middle rectal artery. The prostatic venous plexus drains into the internal iliac veins. Lymphatic vessels terminate mainly in the internal iliac nodes.

Prostatic secretions constitute approximately 25–30% of the fluid volume of the ejaculate. The fluid is a milky, slightly acidic fluid that contains several substances such as citric acid, prostate-specific antigen, pepsinogen, lysozyme, amylase, hyaluronidase, and acid phosphatase. These substances are presumed to contribute to sperm motility and viability.

Bulbourethral glands

The bulbourethral glands (sometimes called Cowper's glands) are about the size of peas. They lie posterolateral to the membranous urethra within the muscles of the pelvic floor. Their ducts open into the spongy urethra. During sexual arousal, these glands secrete a fluid that acts to lubricate the urethra and the penile glans. The fluid is slightly alkaline and plays a role in neutralizing residual urethral urine.

Penis

The functional unit of the penis consists of the corpora cavernosa. These dual cylindrical erectile bodies form the basis of the erection. They are connected to each other for the distal two-thirds of their length. There are robust fenestrations within the corpora cavernosa that allow cross-talk between the corpora. Proximally, they are connected to the undersurface of the inferior pubic rami. A thick fibrous covering called the tunica albuginea surrounds each corpus cavernosum. As a result of cavernous nerve signals, the spongy sinusoidal spaces fill with blood and expand against the tunica albuginea, compressing the subtunical venous plexuses, decreasing venous outflow. The sinusoidal spaces (lacunar spaces) are lined by vascular endothelium. The walls of these spaces are referred to as trabeculae and are composed of smooth muscle and collagen.

Arterial and venous supply

The internal iliac artery supplies vascular inflow to the corpus cavernosum (Fig. 1.5). This artery splits into the

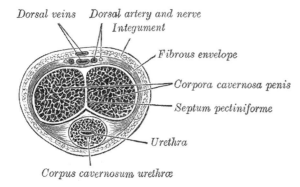

Figure 1.6. Cross-section of the penis. (Reproduced from Gray H. *Anatomy of the Human Body.* Philadelphia, PA: Lea & Febiger, 1918; Bartleby.com, 2000.) *See color plate section.*

inferior gluteal and the internal pudendal artery just proximal to the coccygeus muscle. The internal pudendal runs beneath the sacrospinous ligament and over the sacrotuberous ligament where it enters Alcock's canal. As the artery exits the canal, it gives off the perineal artery before piercing the urogenital diaphragm. The perineal artery continues its course anteriorly and superiorly to deliver blood to the ischiocavernosus muscle, aspects of the bulbospongiosus muscle, and the posterior surface of the scrotum.

After the internal pudendal artery emerges from Alcock's canal, it is referred to as the common penile artery. The common penile artery then branches into the artery of the penile bulb, urethral artery, dorsal penile artery, and the deep artery of the penis (cavernosal artery). The paired cavernosal arteries enter the tunica albuginea at the base of the penis. They travel centrally within each corpus, sprouting helicine arteries at regular intervals. These small serpentine vessels terminate directly into the sinusoidal spaces. Neuromediated relaxation of the trabeculae (walls of the sinusoidal spaces) allows expansion of these sinusoids and the subsequent initiation and maintenance of erection (Fig. 1.6).

Venous drainage of the penis loosely mirrors the arterial supply. Blood leaves the penis via three paths: deep, middle, and superficial venous system. The deep system drains the proximal third of the penis. Emissary veins emerge from this region of the penis and link with the cavernosal, bulbar, and crural veins. Blood from this region drains into the internal pudendal vein.

The middle drainage system receives blood from the glans and corpus spongiosum, as well as the distal two-thirds of the penile shaft. Blood draining the sinusoidal (lacunar) spaces is directed into a rich network of subtunical veins called the subtunical plexus. This plexus sends emissary veins through the tunica albuginea, where they anastamose with circumflex veins. The circumflex veins drain into the deep dorsal vein and then the retrocoronal venous plexus before continuing to the dorsal venous complex in the pelvis.

The superficial drainage system is largely composed of the paired superficial penile veins. They accept blood from numerous surface veins. Blood from this system ultimately ends up in the saphenous system.

Neuroanatomy

Innervation from the sacral parasympathetic (pelvic), thoracolumbar sympathetic, and somatic (pudendal) nerves is required for the generation of erection and ensuing detumescence [29–33]. Parasympathetic neurons originate in the sacral spinal cord (S2–S4). They provide the major excitatory input to the penis. Excitatory signals leave the intermediolateral nuclei and travel via the pelvic nerve (or nervi erigentes) to the pelvic plexus. Here, the preganglionic fibers relay their information to the short, postganglionic cavernosal nerve. The cavernosal nerve courses along the posterolateral aspect of the prostate before exiting the pelvis [34]. As the nerves leave the pelvis, they are intimately related to the urethra. Before entering the corpus cavernosum at the crus, the cavernous nerve sends branches to the corpus spongiosum [29,34].

Sympathetic innervation of the penis originates in the intermediolateral columns of the thoracolumbar spinal cord. Fibers pass through in the sympathetic chain before descending to the inferior mesenteric and superior hypogastric plexuses. The nerve fibers then coalesce to form the hypogastric nerve en route to the pelvic plexus. From there, the sympathetic fibers reach the penis via the cavernous nerves. Additionally, sympathetic input may be accomplished through the pelvic nerve and the pudendal nerve [35].

Additionally, sympathetic innervation is responsible for ejaculation. This reflex is initiated by stimulation of the postganglionic fibers of the lumbar spinal cord and results in the contraction of the bladder neck with simultaneous contraction of the ejaculatory duct. Prior to ejaculation, emission occurs. During emission, the epididymis, vas deferens, seminal vesicles, and prostate contract to force semen into the posterior urethra. Somatic contractions of the bulbospongiosus, ischiocavernosus, and superficial transverse perineus muscles assist in semen propulsion.

The third component of penile neuroanatomy is the somatic system [29,30,36]. The afferent fibers transmit tactile information from the genitalia to the central nervous system [29]. Efferent fibers carry impulses to skeletal muscles [36]. The pudendal nerve conveys motor and sensory impulses. The cell bodies originate in the spinal segments S2–S4. The nerve courses through Alcock's canal before giving off inferior rectal, perineal, and posterior scrotal nerves. The last branch of the pudendal nerve is the dorsal nerve of the penis. It provides motor innervation for the ischiocavernosus and bulbospongiosus muscle. In the penis, this paired nerve runs laterally to the dorsal artery and communicates sensory information from the glans penis and the penile shaft to the sacral cord.

Erection and detumescence: cavernosal smooth muscle physiology

Relaxation of the cavernosal smooth muscle cell is the biological event responsible for the erection [37–39]. As previously mentioned, the trabeculae between the lacunar spaces are occupied by smooth muscle and collagen, in a ratio of 1 : 1 [37,39,40]. The smooth muscle cells are composed of thin, intermediate, and thick filaments [40–42]. The most important of these are the thin (actin) and thick (myosin) filaments [41,42].

The cavernous nerve releases nitric oxide that stimulates the conversion of guanosine triphosphate (GTP) to cyclic guanosine monophosphate (cGMP). cGMP and cAMP cause the potassium channels to open, resulting in cellular hyperpolarization. The calcium channels close, causing the endoplasmic reticulum to sequester intracellular calcium, leaving a Ca^{2+}-poor microenvironment [43]. The calcium–calmodulin complex (which is bound to myosin light chain kinase [MLCK] in the contractile state) disassociates, causing decoupling of the myosin–actin cross-bridges [41,42]. Smooth muscle relaxation ensues, resulting in filling of sinusoidal spaces and penile rigidity [40,43].

Sympathetic-mediated release of norepinephrine and epinephrine sets a second messenger system in motion that increases intracellular concentration of calcium ions. The higher Ca^{2+} stimulates the formation of a calcium–calmodulin complex that binds to and activates MLCK, allowing the chain reaction for smooth muscle contraction to occur, leading to detumescence after orgasm.

References

1. de Kretser DM, Meinhardt A, Meehan T, *et al.* The roles of inhibin and related peptides in gonadal function. *Mol Cell Endocrinol* 2000; 161: 43–6.

2. Wein AJ, Kavoussi LR, Novick AC, Partin AW, Peters CA. *Campbell–Walsh Urology*, 9th edn. Philadelphia, PA: Saunders, 2007.

3. Clarke IJ, Rao A, Fallest PC, Shupnik MA. Transcription rate of the follicle stimulating hormone (FSH) beta subunit gene is reduced by inhibin in sheep but this does not fully explain the decrease in mRNA. *Mol Cell Endocrinol* 1993; 91: 211–16.

4. Harrison RG, Barclay AE. The distribution of the testicular artery (internal spermatic artery) to the human testis. *Br J Urol* 1948; 20: 57–66.

5. Skandhan KP, Rajahariprasad A. The process of spermatogenesis liberates significant heat and the scrotum has a role in body thermoregulation. *Med Hypotheses* 2007; 68: 303–7.

6. Muller I. [Architectonic of the canals and capillaries of rat testes]. *Z Zellforsch Mikrosk Anat* 1957; 45: 522–37.

7. Wishahi MM. Detailed anatomy of the internal spermatic vein and the ovarian vein. Human cadaver study and operative spermatic venography: clinical aspects. *J Urol* 1991; 145: 780–4.

8. Sofikitis N, Dritsas K, Miyagawa I, Koutselinis A. Anatomical characteristics of the left testicular venous system in man. *Arch Androl* 1993; 30: 79–85.

9. Lennox B, Ahmad KN. The total length of tubules in the human testis. *J Anat* 1970; 107: 191.

10. Lennox B, Ahmad KN, Mack WS. The total length of tubules in normal and atrophic testes. *J Pathol* 1970; 100: P3–4.

11. Baumgarten HG, Holstein AF. [Direct adrenergic innervation of Leydig cells in the vertebrate testis]. *J Neurovisc Relat* 1971; 0 (Suppl 10): 563–72.

12. Mitchell GA. The innervation of the kidney, ureter, testicle and epididymis. *J Anat* 1935; 70: 10–32.

13. Baumgarten HG, Holstein AF. [Catecholamine-containing nerve fivers in the testis of man]. *Z Zellforsch Mikrosk Anat* 1967; 79: 389–95.

14. Baumgarten HG, Falck B, Holstein AF, Owman C, Owman T. [Adrenergic innervation of the human

testis, epididymis, ductus deferens and prostate: a fluorescence microscopic and fluorimetric study]. *Z Zellforsch Mikrosk Anat* 1968; 90: 81–95.

15. Van De Velde RL, Risley PL. The origin and development of smooth muscle and contractility in the ductus epididymidis of the rat. *J Embryol Exp Morphol* 1963; 11: 369–82.

16. Macmillan EW. The blood supply of the epididymis in man. *Br J Urol* 1954; 26: 60–71.

17. Johnson L, Varner DD. Effect of daily spermatozoan production but not age on transit time of spermatozoa through the human epididymis. *Biol Reprod* 1988; 39: 812–17.

18. Amann RP, Howards SS. Daily spermatozoal production and epididymal spermatozoal reserves of the human male. *J Urol* 1980; 124: 211–15.

19. Moore HD, Hartman TD, Pryor JP. Development of the oocyte-penetrating capacity of spermatozoa in the human epididymis. *Int J Androl* 1983; 6: 310–18.

20. Schoysman RJ, Bedford JM. The role of the human epididymis in sperm maturation and sperm storage as reflected in the consequences of epididymovasostomy. *Fertil Steril* 1986; 46: 293–9.

21. Jardin A, Izard V, Benoit G, *et al.* [In vivo and in vitro fertilizing ability of immature human epididymal spermatozoa]. *Reprod Nutr Dev* 1988; 28: 1375–85.

22. Matthews GJ, Schlegel PN, Goldstein M. Patency following microsurgical vasoepididymostomy and vasovasostomy: temporal considerations. *J Urol* 1995; 154: 2070–3.

23. Silber SJ. Results of microsurgical vasoepididymostomy: role of epididymis in sperm maturation. *Hum Reprod* 1989; 4: 298–303.

24. Rowley MJ, Teshima F, Heller CG. Duration of transit of spermatozoa through the human male ductular system. *Fertil Steril* 1970; 21: 390–6.

25. Silber SJ. Role of epididymis in sperm maturation. *Urology* 1989; 33: 47–51.

26. Harrison RG. The distribution of the vasal and cremasteric arteries to the testis and their functional importance. *J Anat* 1949; 83: 267–82.

27. Paniagua R, Regadera J, Nistal M, Abaurrea MA. Histological, histochemical and ultrastructural variations along the length of the human vas deferens before and after puberty. *Acta Anat (Basel)* 1982; 111: 190–203.

28. White IG, Goh P, Voglmayr JK. Effect of male reproductive tract fluids and proteins on the metabolism and motility of ram spermatozoa. *Arch Androl* 1987; 19: 115–25.

29. Steers WD. Neural pathways and central sites involved in penile erection: neuroanatomy and clinical implications. *Neurosci Biobehav Rev* 2000; 24: 507–16.

30. Everaert K, de Waard WI, Van Hoof T, *et al.* Neuroanatomy and neurophysiology related to sexual dysfunction in male neurogenic patients with lesions to the spinal cord or peripheral nerves. *Spinal Cord* 2010; 48: 182–91.

31. Akman Y, Liu W, Li YW, Baskin LS. Penile anatomy under the pubic arch: reconstructive implications. *J Urol* 2001; 166: 225–30.

32. Lue TF, Zeineh SJ, Schmidt RA, Tanagho EA. Neuroanatomy of penile erection: its relevance to iatrogenic impotence. *J Urol* 1984; 131: 273–80.

33. Lue TF, Schmidt RA, Tanagho EA. Electrostimulation and penile erection. *Urol Int* 1985; 40: 60–4.

34. Lepor H, Gregerman M, Crosby R, Mostofi FK, Walsh PC. Precise localization of the autonomic nerves from the pelvic plexus to the corpora cavernosa: a detailed anatomical study of the adult male pelvis. *J Urol* 1985; 133: 207–12.

35. Giuliano F, Rampin O. Neural control of erection. *Physiol Behav* 2004; 83: 189–201.

36. Yang CC, Jiang X. Clinical autonomic neurophysiology and the male sexual response: an overview. *J Sex Med* 2009; 6 (Suppl 3): 221–8.

37. Goldstein AM, Padma-Nathan H. The microarchitecture of the intracavernosal smooth muscle and the cavernosal fibrous skeleton. *J Urol* 1990; 144: 1144–6.

38. Jiang J, He Y, Jiang R. Ultrastructural changes of penile cavernous tissue in multiple sclerotic rats. *J Sex Med* 2009; 6: 2206–14.

39. Murat N, Soner BC, Demir O, Esen A, Gidener S. Contractility of diabetic human corpus cavernosum smooth muscle in response to serotonin mediated via Rho-kinase. *Pharmacology* 2009; 84: 24–8.

40. Gratzke C, Angulo J, Chitaley K, *et al.* Anatomy, physiology, and pathophysiology of erectile dysfunction. *J Sex Med* 2010; 7: 445–75.

41. Somlyo AP, Somlyo AV. Signal transduction and regulation in smooth muscle. *Nature* 1994; 372: 231–6.

42. Walsh MP. Regulation of vascular smooth muscle tone. *Can J Physiol Pharmacol* 1994; 72: 919–36.

43. Lue TF. Erectile dysfunction. *N Engl J Med* 2000; 342: 1802–13.

Spermatogenesis

Kathleen Hwang, Alex Ridgeway, and Dolores J. Lamb

Introduction

Spermatogenesis refers to the process by which the production and development of the spermatozoa, the mature male gamete of most sexually reproducing species, occurs. This chapter will review both the macroscopic and microscopic anatomy of the testis, and the endocrine and paracrine regulation of testicular function and spermatogenesis.

Macroscopic testicular anatomy

From physical examination, the testis size during development is easily assessed. The ovoid testis in a young healthy male measures 15–25 mL in volume and has a longitudinal length of 4.5–5.1 cm [1]. A capsule made up of three distinct layers surrounds the parenchyma of the testis: the tunica vaginalis, the tunica albuginea (which provides a tough protective layer), and the tunica vasculosa. The testes receive their blood supply from the testicular arteries, the cremasteric arteries, and the deferential arteries, and proper control of blood flow is required for normal spermatogenesis. The testicular artery arises from the abdominal aorta just below the renal artery and becomes a component of the spermatic cord above the internal inguinal ring as well as being intimately associated with a network of anastomotic veins, which eventually form the pampiniform plexus, a key structure required for normal spermatogenesis. Countercurrent heat exchange in the spermatic cord provides blood to the testis that is 2–4 °C lower than rectal temperature in a normal male. The testicular arteries penetrate the tunica albuginea and then travel inferiorly along the posterior surface of the testis and eventually ascend onto the anterior surface, with several branches that course into the parenchyma. The location of these vessels should be noted, as they may be injured during biopsy or orchidopexy. The medial and lateral aspects of the superior pole have a lower density of superficial vessels compared with the inferior and anterior portions of the testis.

The testis is divided into compartments by septa, which are projections of the tunica albuginea. Each septum separates the seminiferous tubules, as well as the interstitial tissue, which is composed of Leydig cells, blood vessels, lymphatics, mast cells, nerves, and macrophages. The seminiferous tubules are the site of germ cell mitosis, meiosis, and differentiation. The seminiferous tubules are looped tubules continuous at their ends with the rete testis, a network of collecting tubes that eventually coalesce to form efferent ducts that provide a conduit for collecting and distributing the testicular fluid and spermatozoa to the caput epididymis. The seminiferous tubule is composed of Sertoli cells, germ cells, and peritubular myoid cells.

The epididymis

Spermatozoa acquire the capacity to become fully motile as well as the ability to recognize and fertilize an egg during maturation in the epididymis. The development of sperm motility and capacity for fertilization in the epididymis are both androgen-dependent processes. The loss of androgens results in the loss of epididymal weight, as well as changes in the components of the epididymal fluid secretions [2]. The epididymis, derived from the Wolffian (mesonephric) duct, is an organ consisting of a single highly convoluted duct, which the testicular sperm must traverse. It is attached to the superior and inferior pole of the testis and is closely applied to the posterior aspect. The epididymis is divided into three major regions: caput (head), corpus (body), and cauda (tail). The caput epididymis

Fertility Preservation in Male Cancer Patients, ed. John P. Mulhall, Linda D. Applegarth, Robert D. Oates and Peter N. Schlegel.
Published by Cambridge University Press. © Cambridge University Press 2013.

overlies the superior pole of the testis and the cauda overlies the inferior pole. The intervening region is referred to as the corpus.

The visceral layer of the tunica vaginalis surrounds the epididymis, except over the posterior aspect, which is attached to the scrotum and spermatic cord by fibro-fatty connective tissue. Approximately 10–15 ductuli efferentes (efferent ducts) arise from the rete testis and eventually coalesce to form the epididymal duct. In humans, the epididymal tubule is approximately 3–4 meters in length [3]. The vascular supply to the epididymis is from two sources. The caput and corpus are supplied from the superior and inferior epididymal branches of the testicular artery. The cauda is supplied from the branches of the deferential artery. This blood supply is characterized by tortuosity of the vessels as well as a large number of anastomotic communications [4]. While the venous drainage of the epididymis may vary, the veins of the caput and proximal corpus communicate directly with the pampiniform plexus. The veins arising form the cauda and distal corpus eventually communicate with the deferential or cremasteric veins.

The three primary functions of the epididymis are sperm maturation, sperm transport, and sperm storage. Maturational changes allow sperm to become motile and able to fertilize as they transit from the testis, through the epididymis to the vas deferens. As human spermatozoa migrate through the epididymis they acquire increased motility. In comparison to the caput epididymis, the more distal portions of the epididymis house a higher percentage of spermatozoa capable of efficient motility [5]. While the exact mechanisms of sperm maturation are not fully understood, the consensus is that these processes are potentiated through interaction with the epididymis during migration into more distal regions of the duct.

The transit time of the sperm in the human epididymis averages 12 days but is highly variable, with some sperm moving ahead through the epididymis in as few as 2 days [6,7]. Transport through the proximal epididymal duct is principally due to spontaneous, peristaltic contractions of the smooth muscle that surrounds the epididymal duct. Other contributing factors that aid in the transport of sperm include motile cilia as well as the flow of the secreted testicular fluid. Sperm transport time through the epididymis varies with age and sexual activity – with a direct correlation to the differences in daily rate of sperm production [8].

In humans the major storage site of spermatozoa is the cauda epididymis, where approximately half of the total number of spermatozoa are stored [9]. Preservation of sperm viability and motility may not be as efficient in humans as in other species [10]. While there are numerous studies on this topic using experimental animals, the fate of non-ejaculated sperm remains unknown.

The vas deferens

The vas deferens is a thick muscular tube that measures approximately 30–40 cm from the cauda epididymis to the point of fusion with the seminal vesicle and ejaculatory ducts. Five portions have been described: epididymal, scrotal, inguinal, pelvic, and ampulla. The vas deferens, like the epididymis and seminal vesicle, is derived from the Wolffian duct. The ability to propel sperm forcefully is dependent on a three-layered muscular coat, with an inner and outer longitudinal layer and a middle circular layer. While the vas deferens receives nerve fibers from both sympathetic and parasympathetic nervous system, the rich supply of adrenergic fibers contributes to the efficiency of sperm transport. The vas deferens receives its blood supply from the deferential artery via the inferior vesical artery, and the deferential vein accompanies it.

Microscopic anatomy

The Leydig cell

Leydig cells can be identified by their location in the interstitium of the testis. They are distinguished by the presence of a round nucleus, prominent nucleolus, and Reinke crystals in the cytoplasm. Numerous gap junctions allow direct communications between Leydig cells. The Leydig cell is responsible for the majority of steroid production in the testis. The potency of the steroid hormones secreted by Leydig cells is reflected by the small percentage of the human testis occupied by Leydig cells [11]. Circulating levels of testosterone in the serum dramatically fluctuate in a life cycle, as well as during a 24-hour period. Testosterone secretion is maximal in the morning and declines during the day. The maximal concentration of testosterone is reached during the second and third decade of life, reaching a plateau and then proceeding to decline thereafter. Pituitary hormones (specifically luteinizing hormone, LH) and paracrine factors secreted by cells within the seminiferous tubules, as well as autoregulatory factors, regulate Leydig cell function.

The Sertoli cell

The Sertoli cell is a non-dividing somatic cell of epithelial origin that rests on the basement membrane and forms the wall of the tubule. An irregularly shaped nucleus, prominent tripartite nucleolus, voluminous cytoplasm, low mitotic index, and Sertoli–germ cell connections, as well as unique tight junctional complexes between adjacent Sertoli cell membranes, characterize this unique cell. Surface processes from the Sertoli cells extend outward to surround germ cells and provide an arrangement such that each germ cell is supported by a number of adjacent Sertoli cells [12]. The Sertoli cell has several distinct functions that facilitate the maturation of the germ cells. First, it provides a physical scaffold upon which the germ cells develop and migrate towards the lumen of the tubule. Second, the specialized tight junctions between the Sertoli cells form the blood–testis barrier. Third, Sertoli cells create the focused microenvironment essential for germ cell maturation. These distinctive functions also encompass phagocytosis, fluid secretion, and production of a variety of molecules. Finally, the Sertoli cell mediates the actions of testosterone and follicle-stimulating hormone (FSH) on spermatogenesis, as these hormones do not act directly on the germ cells.

The quest for a Sertoli cell product as a marker of Sertoli cell function that is helpful in the evaluation of an infertile patient has yet to be elucidated. Inhibin is a glycoprotein hormone secreted primarily by the Sertoli cells that suppresses FSH secretion. Some have proposed that inhibin could possibly be an independent marker of impaired testicular function, as well as a predictor of the presence of sperm in the testes of infertile men [13].

The blood–testis barrier

Within the testis there exists a functional blood–testis barrier. This barrier, made up of specialized junctions between adjacent Sertoli cells, creates a division in the seminiferous epithelium to form a basal compartment, containing the spermatogonia, and an adluminal compartment [14]. The basal compartment is accessible to blood-borne substances via the extracellular spaces. However, due to the occluding nature of the barrier, these substances are prevented from directly reaching the adluminal compartment. The adluminal compartments contain mature germ cells, while the basal compartment contains spermatogonia and young spermatocytes. The different functional components of the blood–testis barrier include the tight junctional complexes between Sertoli cells, peritubular myoid cells, and endothelial cells in the nearby capillaries [15]. The clinical significance of this barrier is demonstrated in postpubertal testicular insults and the development of anti-sperm antibodies.

Spermatogenesis

Spermatogenesis is the process of sperm cell development (Fig. 2.1). Germ cells undergo successive mitotic and meiotic divisions (spermatocytogenesis) and a metamorphic change (spermiogenesis) to produce spermatozoa. Spermatogenesis can be characterized by three specific functional phases: proliferation, meiosis, and metamorphosis. In the proliferation phase, spermatogonia undergo several mitotic divisions to form spermatocytes, which undergo two meiotic divisions to form haploid spermatids. The latter develop into spermatozoa as a result of a complicated metamorphosis involving dramatic structural modifications to the shape of their nucleus, compaction of their nuclear chromatin, formation of an acrosome, and establishment of a flagellum eventually permitting motility. Spermatogenesis occurs in the seminiferous epithelium of the testis, which consists of Sertoli cells (non-germinal somatic cells) and several types of germ cells [16]. These germ cell types are spermatogonia (progenitor A_{dark}-spermatogonia, progenitor A_{pale}-spermatogonia, committed A_{pale}-spermatogonia, B-spermatogonia), spermatocytes (pre-leptotene, leptotene, zygotene, pachytene, diplotene, and secondary spermatocytes), spermatids, and spermatozoa.

Germ cells are organized in a well-defined manner and form concentric layers with immature germ cells, the spermatogonia, residing at the base of the epithelium adjacent to the limiting membrane and more advanced germ cells generally occupying successive layers (spermatocytes, early and late spermatids) situated closer to the tubular lumen. These concentric layers are known as "generations," and they can be further divided into six consistent cellular associations [17]. In adults, germ cells develop to a fixed timescale with little biological variation. At isolated positions within individual seminiferous tubules, A_{pale}-spermatogonia become committed and

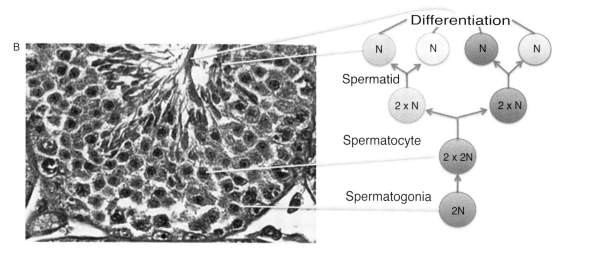

A **Abnormal Spermatogenesis**

ALF	DAZL	SDHA
AP1	MSY2	SOX8
ATM	NLRP14	XRCC1
ATMAC	POLG	XPD
DAX1	PRM1/2	YBX2

Oligozoospermia

ACT	HOMG4	SDHA
ATPase6	KLH10	TSSK4
FASL	PRM1&2	UBE2B
H19&MEST	SHBG	VASA

Acrosome/Fertilization
ERP57

DNA Damage/Infertility

PRM1	GSTM1	IL1
TSSK4	KIT/KITLG	AR USP26
OAZ3	TSPY	MSY2

Azoospermia

ERCC1	RBMY1	APOB
ERCC2	RBMYA1	ACT
FASL	SPATA16	RBMY1F
ACSBGR	FKBP6	SYCP1
ART3	HNRNP	SYCP3
ATM	HSFY TAF7L	TGIFLX
BOULE	KLH10	TSPY
BPY2	MBOAT1	TSSK4
BRCA2	MEI1	UTY
CDY1	MLH1 XPD	XPC
CFTR	MLH3	XRCC1
CREM	MSY2	UBE2B
DAZ	MTR	UPS9Y
DDX25	NYD-SP12	USP26
DDX3Y(DBY)	NLRP14	UTP14c
DRFFY	RBMX YCP1	YBX2
RBMXL9	ZNF230	

Asthenozoospermia

AKAP3	GP130	SNBP
AKAP4	GNA12	SPAG16
CATSPER2	HILS1	POLG
DNMT3b	mtDNA	T mt DNA Haplotypes
DHAH5	MTHFR	TEKT1
DNAH11	ND4	TEKT2
DNAI1	PP1	TPN1
DYN	PRKAR1	TPN2
SHBG	TXNDC3	

Teratozoospermia

AURKC	SPATA16	
NECTIN-2	PRM1	SP1

Oligoasthenozoospermia
JUND mt-ND4   NALP14

Figure 2.1. (A) Genetic basis of human male infertility defects: spermatogenesis and sperm function. Single nuclear polymorphisms (SNP) shown in blue. (B) Seminiferous tubule, demonstrating spermatogenesis and meiosis. *See color plate section.*

enter spermatogenesis at intervals of about 16 days. Progenitor A_{dark}-spermatogonia are thought of as progenitor spermatogonia cells due to their location, infrequent division, and the ability to produce progenitor A_{pale}-spermatogonia through an unknown stimulus. Progenitor and committed A_{pale}-spermatogonia look alike, but the latter divide to produce B-spermatogonia.

Continuous production of spermatozoa throughout life depends on the ability of spermatogonia to replenish themselves. This self-renewal is dependent upon a subgroup of spermatogonia, known as spermatogonial stem cells. These stem cells are defined by their functional characteristics including proliferation, self-renewal, and ability to produce differentiated progeny. Characterization and identification of these stem cells is of crucial importance, as the preservation and expansion of these stem cells can potentially allow restoration of fertility following gonadotoxic treatment and exposure. Although the presence of stem cells was first described by Huckins in 1971, spermatogonial stem cell transplantation was introduced in the mouse in 1994 by Brinster [18] as an assay for stem cell function. These studies serve as stepping stones for research in male germline stem cells, and provide hope for future translation to humans.

There are two major models for the pattern of division of A_{pale}-spermatogonia. In the first model, each member of a pair of committed A_{pale}-spermatogonia undergoes only one division, to provide two

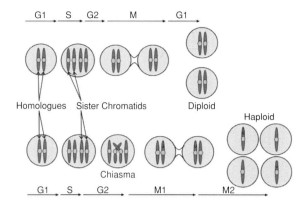

Figure 2.2. Diagrammatic representation of mitosis and meiosis. *See color plate section.*

B-spermatogonia [16,19]. The alternative model has one member of a pair of committed A_{pale}-spermatogonia dividing to provide a new pair of committed A_{pale}-spermatogonia, while the other member of the original pair undergoes a division to provide two daughter A_{pale}-spermatogonia which, in turn, divide to produce B-spermatogonia [19]. Whichever model is accurate, eight pre-leptotene spermatocytes are produced per original pair of A_{pale}-spermatogonia. It is still unclear when B-spermatogonia are formed or divide, with studies by Clermont indicating their formation at the transition from cellular association VI to I and the forming of pre-leptotene spermatocytes at association II [20]. This is in contradiction to another study, which concluded that the formation of B-spermatogonia occurs sometime during cellular association V and remains present through cellular association II [21].

Meiosis

Meiosis is a specialized type of cell division that ultimately produces two haploid gametes from a single diploid parental cell. The meiotic process involves a reduction in the chromosomal number due to a single round of DNA replication followed by two rounds of chromosome segregation. Fusion of two gametes during sexual reproduction restores the diploid chromosomal complement. Contrastingly, mitosis produces daughter cells with a chromosomal complement that is identical to that of the parental cell. The stages of meiosis consist of a single S phase, followed by G2 and two rounds of chromosomal segregation, meiosis I and meiosis II (Fig. 2.2).

The decision for a cell to enter meiosis occurs in response to extrinsic cues from surrounding cells that can control the differentiation of germline stem cells. However, the molecular mechanism that mediates this change is still largely unknown [22]. The decision to enter meiosis is made in the G1 phase, which ultimately affects how the G1–S transition is controlled. Commitment to undergo meiosis begins with pre-meiotic S phase, when DNA replication is triggered by S-phase cyclin-dependent kinases (CDKs) such as CDK2 as well as cyclin A and E [23]. In many respects pre-meiotic DNA replication is similar to that of pre-mitotic S phase through the use of the same replicative machinery and regulators [24]. However, pre-meiotic S phase is substantially longer [25]. This lengthening of S phase may be necessary for initiation of important interactions between sister chromatids. These interactions include: meiotic recombination, the formation of the synaptonemal complex (SC), and the pairing of sister homologs. Cohesin, a protein complex that holds sister chromatids together, is important for the completion of these interactions and transition into meiotic G2 [25,26].

The meiotic G2 phase is defined by the presence of low CDK activity. The linkages formed here between the sister homologs are used to ensure their alignment on the spindle in preparation for meiosis I. This linkage is brought about by at least one chiasma, a so-called "obligatory chiasma," generated by meiotic recombination between homologous chromosomes. The distribution of chiasmata along the chromosome is seen to be non-random, although chiasmata can occur at different positions along each pair of homologs in different meiotic nuclei [27].

Homologous recombination (Fig. 2.3) is initiated through the introduction of double stranded breaks (DSBs) into the DNA by Spo11 [28]. These DSBs are processed in order to allow the generation of two stable species in which sequences from the broken chromatid are joined to corresponding sequences on a homologous chromatid. This can lead to two types of recombination products, either a crossover (CO) or a non-crossover (NCO) product. Only COs lead to homologous pair linkage, which is important in the correct segregation of homologous pairs during meiosis I. What determines if a DSB will mature into a CO as opposed to an NCO is that COs and NCOs form via alternative modes of resolution of a common precursor, the Holliday junction [29]. Meiotic recombination causes a great amount of DNA damage, and

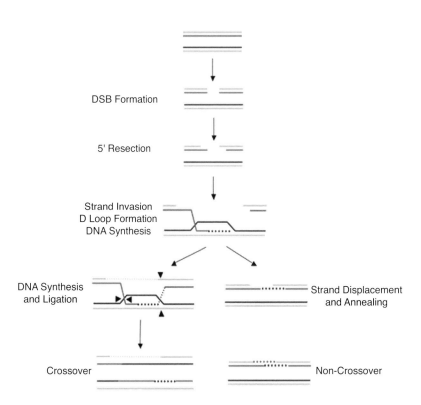

Figure 2.3. Diagrammatic representation of homologous recombination. DSB, double strand break. *See color plate section.*

DSB Formation

5' Resection

Strand Invasion
D Loop Formation
DNA Synthesis

DNA Synthesis
and Ligation

Strand Displacement
and Annealing

Crossover

Non-Crossover

cells that either fail to complete the process or repair the DNA damage are prevented from undergoing meiotic nuclear division by the pachytene checkpoint [30]. The pachytene checkpoint prevents chromosomal missegregation and formation of aneuploid gametes by inhibition of meiotic CDKs that mediate entry into meiosis I.

Upon successful completion of recombination, cells enter meiosis I and undergo the first round of meiotic divisions. Unlike what happens in mitosis (and meiosis II), it is the homologous pairs that segregate apart rather than the sister chromatids. In order to perform this specialized division and yet leave in place the machinery needed in order to undergo meiosis II, the chromosome-segregation machinery is modified. These modifications involve: (a) linked homologous pairs, (b) cohesion between sister chromatids maintained post meiosis I, and (c) sister chromatids attached to microtubules that originate from the spindle poles.

Sister chromatids generated in S phase are held together by cohesin, a protein complex that is thought to form a ring around duplicated DNA [31]. These cohesins are cleaved by the protease, separase, in order

to allow separation during anaphase. Separase is held inactive until the onset of anaphase through its binding to a protein inhibitor, securin. Securin is targeted for proteosomal degradation by the anaphase-promoting complex/cyclosome (APC/C) and Cdc20 [32,33]. During meiosis and its two consecutive rounds of segregation the cohesin binding between sister chromatids is broken down in a stepwise manner. During meiosis I cohesion is lost on the chromosomal arms, allowing for separation of homologous pairs to opposite poles. Cohesion between sister chromatids, however, is maintained at the centromeric region. A meiotic-specific cohesin subunit, Rec8, is believed to play a role in this stepwise separation. Rec8 is selectively lost from chromosomal arms during meiosis I but retained around the centromere until meiosis II [34]. Since separase is believed to control the loss of cohesions in both meiosis I and meiosis II, this may suggest that the cohesin complexes located at the centromeres are protected from separase activity during meiosis I. This protection could come via Rec8 dependence on Cdc5 for its cleavage and its possible inhibition around the centromeric regions [35] during meiosis I. Another additional protective factor may be Sgo1, which is seen to associate with kinetochores during G2 and may prevent premature cleavage of Rec8 around the centromere [36].

Kinetochores are a large complex of proteins at the chromosomal centromeres that help mediate the attachment of chromosomes to microtubules. In meiosis I and II the kinetochores of sister chromatids attach to microtubules from opposite poles in order to segregate. During meiosis I, sister kinetochores attach in a synthetic fashion and are mono-oriented [37]. It may be that the kinetochores in meiosis I are modified to allow for co-orientation of sister chromatids, and this modification is undone to allow bi-orientation during meiosis II [38]. The linkages at the chiasmata may create the required tension at the kinetochore in order not to engage the spindle checkpoint or aurora-B, two regulatory factors in mitosis that regulate M phase [39,40].

The meiosis I to meiosis II transition has the unique attribute of lacking a DNA replication phase by prevention of formation of pre-replicative complexes (high CDK activity) while maintaining the conditions necessary to trigger meiotic spindle disassembly (low CDK activity). The two seemingly opposite conditions seem to be resolved by the retention of an intermediate level of CDK activity when transitioning from meiosis I to II [41]. Overall, however, CDK down-regulation seems to be critical for the disassembly of meiosis I spindle [42].

Meiosis II chromosomal segregation closely resembles that of mitosis. How CDKs are re-activated to allow entry into meiosis II is not yet known. Sister kinetochores are bi-oriented, and the centromeric cohesin that remained after meiosis I prevents premature separation of sister chromatids before anaphase II. At the onset of anaphase II, separase once again becomes active and is now able to cleave the remaining Rec8 at chromosomal centromeres and allow the segregation of sister chromatids. This ultimately leads to the generation of four haploid gametes from each meiotic cell.

Spermatids were initially thought to develop via a series of 12 steps consisting of subtle changes in acrosome morphology and gradual changes in nucleus shape [43]. This was later narrowed down to eight steps as described by Holstein [44]. Six types of spermatids (Sa, Sb1, Sb2, Sc, Sd1, and Sd2) [20] (or seven if distinguishing Sa1 and Sa2 spermatids) are generally defined. Spermatids Sa and Sd1 or Sd2 are found in cellular associations I and II, whereas cellular associations III–V contain primary spermatocytes (pre-leptotene, leptotene, or zygotene + pachytene or diplotene). In humans, the duration of spermatogenesis probably does not change. Testis descent is completed years before initial commitment of A_{pale}-spermatogonia to form B-spermatogonia. A single cycle of the seminiferous epithelium requires about 16 days with a total of approximately 4.6 cycles to complete the process [45], resulting in a total time of ∼74 days.

The round spermatids occupy the most central region of the seminiferous tubules and are incapable of further division. They have a spherical nucleus with dispersed chromatin and absence of nucleoli [46]. By a complex set of changes during the process of spermiogenesis, the round, haploid spermatid differentiates into a hydrodynamically shaped spermatozoon with a head containing the condensed nucleus and acrosome, the mid-piece, and the principal piece. It is during this phase that several cellular organelles (nucleus, endoplasmic reticulum, Golgi apparatus, mitochondria, centriole, etc.) undergo structural and biochemical changes. All of these changes require a series of shape alterations from round to elongate, as the spermatid metamorphoses into a developing spermatozoon [46,47]. At the end of this period, the sperm plasma membrane has differentiated into specialized areas of function and organization. The nucleus compacts and elongates, chromatin condenses, and the nucleus shifts toward the cell surface. At this point, spermatozoal proteins rich in arginine and cysteine replace testis-specific histones. Similarly, the mitochondria also elongate and migrate from the peripheral cytoplasm, where they are positioned into a helical arrangement along the mid-piece of the forming tail.

In addition, new structures such as the axoneme, cytoskeletal elements, and acrosome are formed from cytoplasmic organelles (e.g., centrioles, endoplasmic reticulum, and Golgi apparatus) and take positions in the developing spermatozoa. The elongation of the spermatid begins in the late stages of spermiogenesis when the sperm cell flattens as the chromatin condenses and the acrosome becomes compact. A thin rim of cytoplasm encounters the nucleus, whereas the bulk of the cytoplasm is within the cytoplasmic lobe that detaches from the late spermatid to yield the residual body, leaving behind a small mass referred to as the cytoplasmic droplet. The spermatids are in close association with the Sertoli cells until spermatozoa are fully differentiated, when they detach from the Sertoli cells and intercellular bridges connecting them and are released into the lumen of the seminiferous tubule [48].

At this point, the spermatozoon becomes an isolated cell characterized on the basis of its electron-dense nucleus and a fully developed acrosome. The sperm cells continue to evolve during passage through the epididymal duct, gaining forward motility and fertilizing ability, a process termed epididymal maturation [49]. The epididymal duct is connected to the testis via the ductuli efferentes. The mammalian epididymis provides a specific intraluminal environment in which functionally immature testicular spermatozoa undergo morphological and biochemical modifications. During epididymal maturation, many intra-acrosomal and sperm plasma membrane molecules are modified [49]. These modifications are an essential part of the maturation process resulting in the production of a self-propelled functionally competent spermatozoon. The precise region of the epididymis where the spermatozoa become functionally mature varies from species to species. However, most agree that spermatozoa from the distal corpus region of several species are usually functional.

The spermatozoon is the final product of spermatogenesis and spermiation. The events preceding its differentiation result in the extensive remodeling of the spermatid into a mature sperm with an acrosome, a flagellum, minimal cytoplasm, and a condensed nucleus. The two main components of the sperm are the head and the flagellum, which are joined together through the connecting piece. The sperm is about 60 μm in length and > 1 μm in diameter at the connecting piece, tapering towards the end of the flagellum. Contained in the head region are the nucleus, acrosome, cytoskeletal structures, and minimal cytoplasm.

The acrosome, a membrane-enclosed cytoplasmic vesicle containing hydrolytic enzymes, sits on the anterior of the nucleus. Multiple lysosomal enzymes are present as well as enzymes specific to the sperm cell, giving it both lysosomal and secretory vesicle-like characteristics [50]. The contents of the acrosome are released via calcium-mediated exocytosis and allow penetration of the zona pellucida surrounding the egg [51]. The best-studied constituent of the acrosome is acrosin, a serine protease unique to the sperm cell [52]. Its synthesis occurs predominately in the round spermatid but can also be detected as early as pachytene [53]. The sperm nucleus houses tightly packed chromatin with a volume much reduced from that of a somatic cell. The two meiotic divisions during the process of spermatogenesis result in each sperm being haploid. The major proteins associated with the mammalian sperm nucleus are the highly basic protamines, rich in arginine and cysteine [54]. Both genes encoding the protamines in humans are transcribed from the haploid genome in round spermatids, with translation being delayed until elongation has taken place [55]. Protamines are essential for nuclear formation and DNA stability, and therefore for fertility [56].

Like that of somatic cells, the sperm nucleus is also enclosed by a nuclear envelope. The sperm nucleus differs, however, in lacking nuclear pores and possessing smaller distances between the inner and outer membranes over much of its surface [57]. Caudal to the posterior ring, in an area known as the "redundant nuclear envelope," sperm nuclear pores are present and arranged in a hexagonal pattern. The purpose of this spatial separation of the nuclear pores is unknown.

The head of the sperm has three major cytoskeletal regions. The subacrosomal region is located between the acrosome and the nucleus. The postacrosomal region lies between the nucleus and the plasma membrane, posterior to the acrosome. The para-acrosomal region is located between the anterior tip and convex surface of the acrosome and the plasma membrane. The composition of the sperm head cytoskeleton plays an important role during the series of biochemical modifications within the female reproductive tract known as capacitation. Only those sperm that are capacitated can undergo the acrosome reaction upon binding of the egg's zona pellucida and achieve fertilization [58].

From the connecting piece to the tip of the flagellum, the flagellum is divided into three regions, the mid-piece, the principal piece, and the end-piece region. The mid-piece houses a tightly wrapped helix of mitochondria known as the mitochondrial sheath, which itself encompasses the axoneme, a central complex of microtubules and dense fibers. The majority of the flagellum is accounted for by the principal piece; however, the elongated shape and accessory cytoskeletal organelles in the tail, novel to sperm flagella in higher vertebrates, may have evolved with the development of internal fertilization [59]. Both the flagellum and the head are tightly enclosed by the plasma membrane.

The main components of the connecting piece are the capitulum and the segmented columns [60]. The capitulum is a dense fibrous plate-like structure that forms a basal plate responsible for attaching the capitulum of the connecting piece to the head [61]. Extending posteriorly from the capitulum are the segmented columns, of which there are two major and five minor. Both the major and minor segmented columns fuse to the outer dense fibers extending throughout the flagellum as well as cross-striated, giving structural support and assisting in motility [62].

Regulation of spermatogensis: the hypothalamic–pituitary–gonadal (HPG) axis

The male hypothalamic–pituitary–gonadal (HPG) axis is a finely tuned system whose role is to promote spermatogenesis and androgen biosynthesis. Maintenance of normal reproductive function is dependent on the coordinated release of hormones in the hypothalamic–pituitary–testis cascade. Gonadotropin-releasing hormone (GnRH) is released periodically into the pituitary portal blood system from neuroendocrine cells in the basal hypothalamus and acts to stimulate gonadotropes in the anterior pituitary to synthesize and release two peptide hormones, follicle-stimulating hormone (FSH) and luteinizing hormone (LH), into the circulation. Once in the bloodstream these hormones reach the testis, where LH stimulates testosterone production by the Leydig cells in the interstitium while FSH supports spermatogenesis in the seminiferous epithelium by stimulation of the Sertoli cells. Focused networks of negative feedback relationships finesse testosterone secretion and sperm production. This cascade is maintained by steroid and peptide feedback within the testis as well the hypothalamus and pituitary gland.

Testosterone applies negative-feedback suppression to the release of GnRH through androgen receptors in the pituitary and hypothalamic neurons. Testosterone is also readily metabolized to dihydrotestosterone and estradiol by 5α-reductase and aromatase, respectively, in the testis and peripheral tissues. Both testosterone and estrogen play important roles in the regulation of reproductive function at the cellular and tissue levels. This can be demonstrated clinically by individuals with genetic mutations resulting in partial or complete loss of function in androgen and estrogen receptors with increased pituitary release of LH [63].

Stimulation of the Sertoli cell by FSH results in production of inhibin, a glycoprotein hormone, which suppresses FSH secretion by gonadotropes. Inhibin, a heterodimeric protein that belongs to the transforming growth factor (TGF)-β family of glycoproteins, acts to decrease secretion of gonadotropins. Inhibin feeds back directly on the pituitary to inhibit transcription of the gene encoding the β subunit of FSH [64]. Regulation of gonadotropin secretion exists for different steroids. While the negative effect of testosterone on LH secretion is primarily mediated by the androgen itself, the effect of testosterone on FSH secretion is mediated by estradiol [65].

FSH from the pituitary and testosterone from the Leydig cells act upon the Sertoli cell to promote maturation of spermatogenic cells. Tight internal control of the secretion of FSH and testosterone as well as high levels of both FSH and testosterone are essential if spermatogenesis is to progress and complete in an efficient manner [66].

Endocrine control of the spermatogenic process is relatively well understood, and the role played by LH, FSH, and testosterone in spermatogenesis has been studied extensively. However, regulation of spermatogenesis seems to be affected on many other levels, such as paracrine regulators including cytokines and growth factors. Paracrine regulators of Sertoli and testis function include interleukins 1 and 6, leukemic inhibitory factory, tumor necrosis factor, and interferon-γ (reviewed in [67]). One of the first demonstrations of a true role for growth factors in spermatogenesis was the discovery of the c-kit ligand and receptor. The fact that the presence of the c-kit ligand and receptor was found to be required for the survival and proliferation of primordial germ cells was highlighted in mutant mouse models [68]. These regulators, among others, contribute to the local communication within the testis that allows the complex coordination between Sertoli cells and germ cells.

Conclusion

Spermatogenesis is a fascinating biological process whereby billions of sperm are produced over a lifetime with a high degree of accuracy. However, there is a fine balance that is easily disturbed by environmental exposures, gonadotoxic treatment, genetic errors, changes in the hormonal milieu, or physiological insults. Understanding the intricate dynamics of spermatogenesis is the correct approach to the diagnosis and treatment of disorders of the male reproductive system, particularly in the preservation of fertility.

Acknowledgments

This study was supported in part by the Eunice Kennedy Shriver National Institute of Child Health and Human Development P01HD36289 to DJL, and by the National Institute of Kidney and Digestive Diseases 1K12DK083014 Multidisciplinary K12 Urology Research Career Development Program at Baylor (DJL and KH).

References

1. Winter JS, Faiman C. Pituitary–gonadal relations in male children and adolescents. *Pediatr Res* 1972; 6: 126–35.

2. Cohen J, Ooms MP, Vreeburg JT. Reduction of fertilizing capacity of epididymal spermatozoa by 5 alpha-steroid reductase inhibitors. *Experientia* 1981; 37: 1031–2.

3. Turner TT, D'Addario D, Howards SS. Further observations on the initiation of sperm motility. *Biol Reprod* 1978; 19: 1095–101.

4. Macmillan EW. The blood supply of the epididymis in man. *Br J Urol* 1954; 26: 60–71.

5. Bedford JM, Calvin H, Cooper GW. The maturation of spermatozoa in the human epididymis. *J Reprod Fertil Suppl* 1973; 18: 199–213.

6. Johnson L, Varner DD. Effect of daily spermatozoan production but not age on transit time of spermatozoa through the human epididymis. *Biol Reprod* 1988; 39: 812–17.

7. Rowley MJ, Teshima F, Heller CG. Duration of transit of spermatozoa through the human male ductular system. *Fertil Steril* 1970; 21: 390–6.

8. Curtis SK, Amann RP. Testicular development and establishment of spermatogenesis in Holstein bulls. *J Anim Sci* 1981; 53: 1645–57.

9. Amann RP, Howards SS. Daily spermatozoal production and epididymal spermatozoal reserves of the human male. *J Urol* 1980; 124: 211–15.

10. Bedford JM. The status and the state of the human epididymis. *Hum Reprod* 1994; 9: 2187–99.

11. Kaler LW, Neaves WB. Attrition of the human Leydig cell population with advancing age. *Anat Rec* 1978; 192: 513–18.

12. Nagano T. [Some observations on the fine structure of the Sertoli cell in the human testis]. *Z Zellforsch Mikrosk Anat* 1966; 73: 89–106.

13. von Eckardstein S, Simoni M, Bergmann M, *et al.* Serum inhibin B in combination with serum follicle-stimulating hormone (FSH) is a more sensitive marker than serum FSH alone for impaired spermatogenesis in men, but cannot predict the presence of sperm in testicular tissue samples. *J Clin Endocrinol Metab* 1999; 84: 2496–501.

14. Fawcett DW. Observations on the organization of the interstitial tissue of the testis and on the occluding cell junctions in the seminiferous epithelium. *Adv Biosci* 1973; 10: 83–99.

15. Dym M, Fawcett DW. The blood-testis barrier in the rat and the physiological compartmentation of the seminiferous epithelium. *Biol Reprod* 1970; 3: 308–26.

16. Clermont Y. Kinetics of spermatogenesis in mammals: seminiferous epithelium cycle and spermatogonial renewal. *Physiol Rev* 1972; 52: 198–236.

17. Roosen-Runge EC. Kinetics of spermatogenesis in mammals. *Ann N Y Acad Sci* 1952; 55: 574–84.

18. Brinster RL, Avarbock MR. Germline transmission of donor haplotype following spermatogonial transplantation. *Proc Natl Acad Sci U S A* 1994; 91: 11303–7.

19. Ehmcke J, Schlatt S. A revised model for spermatogonial expansion in man: lessons from non-human primates. *Reproduction* 2006; 132: 673–80.

20. Clermont Y. Spermatogenesis in man: a study of the spermatogonial population. *Fertil Steril* 1966; 17: 705–21.

21. Rowley MJ, Heller CG. [Quantitation of the cells of the seminiferous epithelium of the human testis employing the sertoli cell as a constant]. *Z Zellforsch Mikrosk Anat* 1971; 115: 461–72.

22. Geijsen N, Horoschak M, Kim K, *et al.* Derivation of embryonic germ cells and male gametes from embryonic stem cells. *Nature* 2004; 427: 148–54.

23. Koepp DM, Harper JW, Elledge SJ. How the cyclin became a cyclin: regulated proteolysis in the cell cycle. *Cell* 1999; 97: 431–4.

24. Collins I, Newlon CS. Chromosomal DNA replication initiates at the same origins in meiosis and mitosis. *Mol Cell Biol* 1994; 14: 3524–34.

25. Cha RS, Weiner BM, Keeney S, Dekker J, Kleckner N. Progression of meiotic DNA replication is modulated by interchromosomal interaction proteins, negatively by Spo11p and positively by Rec8p. *Genes Dev* 2000; 14: 493–503.

26. Parisi S, McKay MJ, Molnar M, *et al.* Rec8p, a meiotic recombination and sister chromatid cohesion phosphoprotein of the Rad21p family conserved from fission yeast to humans. *Mol Cell Biol* May 1999; 19: 3515–28.

27. Lynn A, Koehler KE, Judis L, *et al.* Covariation of synaptonemal complex length and mammalian meiotic exchange rates. *Science* 2002; 296: 2222–5.

28. Keeney S, Giroux CN, Kleckner N. Meiosis-specific DNA double-strand breaks are catalyzed by Spo11, a member of a widely conserved protein family. *Cell* 1997; 88: 375–84.

29. Holliday R, Whitehouse HL. The wrong way to think about gene conversion? *Mol Gen Genet* 1970; 107: 85–93.

30. Roeder GS, Bailis JM. The pachytene checkpoint. *Trends Genet* 2000; 16: 395–403.

31. Gruber S, Haering CH, Nasmyth K. Chromosomal cohesin forms a ring. *Cell* 2003; 112: 765–77.

32. Cohen-Fix O, Peters JM, Kirschner MW, Koshland D. Anaphase initiation in *Saccharomyces cerevisiae* is controlled by the APC-dependent degradation of the anaphase inhibitor Pds1p. *Genes Dev* 1996; 10: 3081–93.

33. Ciosk R, Zachariae W, Michaelis C, *et al.* An ESP1/PDS1 complex regulates loss of sister chromatid cohesion at the metaphase to anaphase transition in yeast. *Cell* 1998; 93: 1067–76.

34. Lee J, Iwai T, Yokota T, Yamashita M. Temporally and spatially selective loss of Rec8 protein from meiotic chromosomes during mammalian meiosis. *J Cell Sci* 2003; 116: 2781–90.

35. Lee BH, Amon A. Role of Polo-like kinase CDC5 in programming meiosis I chromosome segregation. *Science* 2003; 300: 482–6.

36. Kitajima TS, Kawashima SA, Watanabe Y. The conserved kinetochore protein shugoshin protects centromeric cohesion during meiosis. *Nature* 2004; 427: 510–17.

37. Nasmyth K. Disseminating the genome: joining, resolving, and separating sister chromatids during mitosis and meiosis. *Annu Rev Genet* 2001; 35: 673–745.

38. Suja JA, de la Torre J, Gimenez-Abian JF, Garcia de la Vega C, Rufas JS. Meiotic chromosome structure: kinetochores and chromatid cores in standard and B chromosomes of *Arcyptera fusca* (Orthoptera) revealed by silver staining. *Genome* 1991; 34: 19–27.

39. Dewar H, Tanaka K, Nasmyth K, Tanaka TU. Tension between two kinetochores suffices for their bi-orientation on the mitotic spindle. *Nature* 2004; 428: 93–7.

40. Shonn MA, Murray AL, Murray AW. Spindle checkpoint component Mad2 contributes to biorientation of homologous chromosomes. *Curr Biol* 2003; 13: 1979–84.

41. Furuno N, Nishizawa M, Okazaki K, *et al.* Suppression of DNA replication via Mos function during meiotic divisions in Xenopus oocytes. *Embo J* 1994; 13: 2399–410.

42. Marston AL, Lee BH, Amon A. The Cdc14 phosphatase and the FEAR network control meiotic spindle disassembly and chromosome segregation. *Dev Cell* 2003; 4: 711–26.

43. Clermont Y, Leblond CP. Spermiogenesis of man, monkey, ram and other mammals as shown by the periodic acid-Schiff technique. *Am J Anat* 1955; 96: 229–53.

44. Holstein AF. Ultrastructural observations on the differentiation of spermatids in man. *Andrologia* 1976; 8: 157–65.

45. Heller CG, Clermont Y. Spermatogenesis in man: an estimate of its duration. *Science* 1963; 140: 184–6.

46. Hermo L, Pelletier RM, Cyr DG, Smith CE. Surfing the wave, cycle, life history, and genes/proteins expressed by testicular germ cells. Part 2: changes in spermatid organelles associated with development of spermatozoa. *Microsc Res Tech* 2010; 73: 279–319.

47. Hermo L, Pelletier RM, Cyr DG, Smith CE. Surfing the wave, cycle, life history, and genes/proteins expressed by testicular germ cells. Part 1: background to spermatogenesis, spermatogonia, and spermatocytes. *Microsc Res Tech* 2010; 73: 241–278.

48. de Kretser DM, Loveland KL, Meinhardt A, Simorangkir D, Wreford N. Spermatogenesis. *Hum Reprod* 1998; 13 (Suppl 1): 1–8.

49. Tulsiani DR, Orgebin-Crist MC, Skudlarek MD. Role of luminal fluid glycosyltransferases and glycosidases in the modification of rat sperm plasma membrane glycoproteins during epididymal maturation. *J Reprod Fertil Suppl* 1998; 53: 85–97.

50. Allison AC, Hartree EF. Lysosomal enzymes in the acrosome and their possible role in fertilization. *J Reprod Fertil* 1970; 21: 501–15.

51. Beyler SA, Zaneveld LJ. Inhibition of in-vitro fertilization of mouse gametes by proteinase inhibitors. *J Reprod Fertil* 1982; 66: 425–31.

52. Klemm U, Maier WM, Tsaousidou S, *et al.* Mouse preproacrosin: cDNA sequence, primary structure and postmeiotic expression in spermatogenesis. *Differentiation* 1990; 42: 160–6.

53. Escalier D, Gallo JM, Albert M, *et al.* Human acrosome biogenesis: immunodetection of proacrosin in primary spermatocytes and of its partitioning pattern during meiosis. *Development* 1991; 113: 779–88.

54. Bellve AR, Anderson E, Hanley Bowdoin L. Synthesis and amino acid composition of basic proteins in mammalian sperm nuclei. *Dev Biol* 1975; 47: 349–65.

55. Steger K, Klonisch T, Gavenis K, *et al.* Expression of mRNA and protein of nucleoproteins during human spermiogenesis. *Mol Hum Reprod* 1998; 4: 939–45.

56. Balhorn R. A model for the structure of chromatin in mammalian sperm. *J Cell Biol* 1982; 93: 298–305.

57. Fawcett DW. The mammalian spermatozoon. *Dev Biol* 1975; 44: 394–436.

58. Breitbart H, Cohen G, Rubinstein S. Role of actin cytoskeleton in mammalian sperm capacitation and the acrosome reaction. *Reproduction* 2005; 129: 263–8.

59. Baccetti B. Evolutionary trends in sperm structure. *Comp Biochem Physiol A Comp Physiol* 1986; 85: 29–36.

60. Toshimori K. Maturation of mammalian spermatozoa: modifications of the acrosome and plasma membrane leading to fertilization. *Cell Tissue Res* 1998; 293: 177–87.

61. Stackpole CW, Devorkin D. Membrane organization in mouse spermatozoa revealed by freeze-etching. *J Ultrastruct Res* 1974; 49: 167–87.

62. Fawcett DW, Phillips DM. The fine structure and development of the neck region of the mammalian spermatozoon. *Anat Rec* 1969; 165: 153–64.

63. Shupnik MA, Schreihofer DA. Molecular aspects of steroid hormone action in the male reproductive axis. *J Androl* 1997; 18: 341–4.

64. O'Donnell L, Meachem S, Stanton P. Endocrine regulation of spermatogenesis. In Knobil E, Neill JD, eds., *The Physiology of Reproduction*. New York, NY: Raven Press, 1994; pp. 1017–69.

65. Hayes FJ, Pitteloud N, DeCruz S, Crowley WF, Boepple PA. Importance of inhibin B in the regulation of FSH secretion in the human male. *J Clin Endocrinol Metab* 2001; 86: 5541–6.

66. Kumar TR. What have we learned about gonadotropin function from gonadotropin subunit and receptor knockout mice? *Reproduction* 2005; 130: 293–302.

67. Cheng CY, Wong EW, Yan HH, Mruk DD. Regulation of spermatogenesis in the microenvironment of the seminiferous epithelium: new insights and advances. *Mol Cell Endocrinol* 2010; 315: 49–56.

68. Witte ON. Steel locus defines new multipotent growth factor. *Cell* 1990; 63: 5–6.

Chapter

3

The semen analysis

Mary K. Samplaski and Edmund S. Sabanegh Jr.

Introduction

Spermatozoa were first described by Leeuwenhoek in the seventeenth century, but it was not until 1928 that a link between sperm count and fertility potential was discovered. Years later, in 1951 MacLeod and Gold reported differences in sperm characteristics between fertile and infertile men. Subsequent innovators included Freund (1966), Eliasson (1971), and Hellinga (1976), who refined the techniques of, and scientific basis for, the modern semen analysis (SA). Since then, a multitude of reports have emerged confirming differences in the SA of infertile men and redefining values for "normal" semen parameters (Table 3.1). With time our understanding of each of the semen parameters has progressed, fueled by the hope that each will provide some predictive value for conception.

The SA evaluates sperm production by the testes, patency of the reproductive tract, activity of accessory glands, and the capability for ejaculation. In addition to its now well-established significance in the evaluation of male infertility, the SA is also used in diagnosing genital infections, the adverse effects of chemicals and environmental exposures, non-sexual diseases affecting men's fertility, as well as a de facto assessment of endocrine status. Some studies suggest that men with systemic malignancies have abnormal SA and impaired fertility potential even prior to treatment [1], but the SA is far from being a marker for malignancy. In the meantime, cancer treatments are well established as gonadotoxic, and men are encouraged to bank semen for cryopreservation prior to treatment.

The SA can provide valuable information in evaluating the subfertile male, but it is important to realize that it is not a direct measure of fertility, and there is

Table 3.1. Standard criteria for a normal semen analysis

Volume	≥ 1.5 mL
pH	≥ 7.2
Sperm concentration	≥ 15 million spermatozoa/mL
Total sperm count	≥ 39 million spermatozoa/ejaculate
Progressive motility	≥ 32%
Total (progressive + non-progressive) motility	≥ 40%
Morphology	≥ 4% normal forms
Vitality	≥ 58% living spermatozoa

substantial overlap in SA characteristics between fertile and infertile men [2]. However, while imperfect, the SA is helpful in determining the etiology of infertility in many men (Table 3.2). Individual components of the SA, specifically sperm concentration, morphology, and motility, have prognostic value for natural conception as well as assisted reproductive technology (ART) success [3–4]. It remains unclear which of the semen parameters are most predictive of fertility, and while each of these has been shown to be predictive of pregnancy in some studies [2,5], others have shown little or no correlation [4].

One reason for the discrepancy in correlation may be the inherent heterogeneity of human semen. Conventional parameters may vary significantly between countries, regions, individuals, and even consecutive samples obtained from the same man. For example, as much as a threefold difference has been seen in the semen parameters of men from Thailand and France, and substantial variation has been seen between major American cities [6]. Some of this variability may be due to differing social and environmental exposures or customs, including alcohol consumption, cigarette

Fertility Preservation in Male Cancer Patients, ed. John P. Mulhall, Linda D. Applegarth, Robert D. Oates and Peter N. Schlegel. Published by Cambridge University Press. © Cambridge University Press 2013.

Table 3.2. Semen analysis parameters and their clinical significance

Parameter	Normal value	Abnormalities	Clinical significance
Appearance	Gray-opalescent	Clear Brown Yellow	Low sperm concentration Hematospermia Jaundice Urine contamination Pyridium
pH	7.2–7.8	Acidic Basic	Ejaculatory duct obstruction Congenital absence of the vas deferens Seminal vesicle or vasal agenesis or occlusion Prostatitis leading to decreased production of prostatic secretions
Coagulation/ liquefaction	Semen coagulates upon ejaculation and liquefies within 25 minutes	No coagulation Excessive coagulation	Congenital absence of the seminal vesicles Deficiency in prostatic enzyme secretions Prostatitis Ejaculatory duct obstruction Anti-sperm antibodies
Viscosity	4 mm threading	> 6 mm, no threading	Congenital absence of vas deferens Ejaculatory duct obstruction Poor prostatic secretions Hypofunction of seminal vesicles
Volume	2–4 mL	0 (azoospermia) < 2 mL (oligospermia) > 6 mL	Retrograde ejaculation Obstruction (congenital or acquired) No sperm production Incomplete collection Partial retrograde ejaculation Short duration of sexual abstinence Absence or obstruction of the seminal vesicles Androgen deficiency Recent febrile illness Accessory gland overproduction Seminal vesicle dysfunction Varicocele Prolonged sexual abstinence
Count	20–250 million sperm/mL	Polyspermia	Prostate or seminal vesicle dysfunction
Morphology		Immature forms Teratospermia	Epididymal dysfunction Frequent ejaculations A variety of structural defects
Other cell types		Immature spermatogenic cells Leukocytes Red blood cells	Pathology with spermatogenesis Premature release of immature sperm forms Underlying genital infection Inflammatory condition Infection Genital tract tumors Ductal obstruction Vascular malformation
Motility	32% progressive and 40% total motile sperm	Asthenospermia	Improper sample collection, transport, or analysis Ultrastructural defect Necrospermia Varicocele Anti-sperm antibodies Genital infections

smoking, or geographically related illnesses [7]. Heterogeneity within a single individual was dramatically highlighted in a classic graph from the 1987 and 1999 WHO manuals of 60 consecutive samples from one man over 120 weeks, where sperm count in one sample peaked at 170 million/mL but on several other occasions fell below 20 million/mL, findings which have been confirmed by others [8].

In order to establish uniformity in laboratory procedures, the World Health Organization (WHO) publishes a laboratory manual providing standardized reference ranges for SA collection, processing, and result parameters [9]. The most recent version was published in 2009 [10]. Reference values are based on the upper 95% confidence interval of a cohort of fertile men from eight countries on three continents, whose partners had a time to pregnancy of $\leq$ 12 months [9]. While the WHO values are not universally accepted, they are the most commonly used and are generally considered an essential reference for the assessment of human semen.

Technical considerations

The SA provides fundamental information from which clinicians formulate an initial differential diagnosis, so it is imperative that it be performed as accurately as possible. Patients should be counseled on collection techniques and queried for a history of gonadotoxic drugs or medications, including chemotherapy, radiation exposure, cimetidine, sulfasalazine, and nitrofurantoin, as well as tobacco products and anabolic steroids.

Samples should be collected after a period of abstinence ranging from 2 to 7 days [10]. In the first 4 days following ejaculation, semen volume increases by 12% per day [11], and samples collected prematurely may have lower volumes and counts [12]. Conversely, prolonged abstinence can result in an elevated sperm concentration [12] with a decrease in normal forms [13]. Two samples should be analyzed, at least 7 days apart, and the duration of abstinence should be similar between the two samples. If results have over 20% variance, additional samples should be analyzed. Samples should be obtained by masturbation into a sterile container provided by the physician, as many plastics are spermicidal. Lubricants or saliva should be avoided if possible, but if needed should not be applied to the glans, as they may impair sperm motility.

Patients who are unable to obtain their sample through masturbation may alternatively do so using condoms specially designed for semen collection [10]. Ordinary condoms cannot be used because many are inherently spermicidal [10]. Coitus interruptus is inadvisable since the first portion of the ejaculate, which contains the highest concentration of spermatozoa, may be lost using this method. Moreover, there may be cellular and bacteriological contamination of the sample, and the acidic pH of vaginal fluid may adversely affect sperm motility. If the sample is collected off-site, during transport to the laboratory it should be maintained between room temperature (approximately 20 °C) and body temperature (37 °C).

Ideally, sample collection is performed within a dedicated room adjacent to the laboratory, in order to avoid collection- and transportation-related effects. If men experience difficulty achieving erection and ejaculation in the office setting, phosphodiesterase-5 (PDE5) inhibitors or intracavernosal injection of vasoactive agents may be used. Anejaculatory patients with spinal cord or other neurological issues may be able to have an ejaculation with vibratory or electro-ejaculation techniques.

Samples should be evaluated as soon as possible but always within 1 hour of collection. Once the sample has been collected, it is placed into a 37 °C, gently shaking incubator for 30 minutes to allow for liquefaction and mixing. This will optimize homogeneity of the sample. After mixing, 5 μL of seminal fluid is placed on a slide and examined using phase-contrast microscopy. All of these parameters are standardized to ensure that analyses are carried out at a fixed depth (optimally 20 μm), allowing for an assessment of spermatozoa within a single plane without hampering rotational movements. In general, SA characteristics can be classified into two groups: macroscopic and microscopic. Macroscopic characteristics include the gross appearance, volume, pH, and a measurement of liquefaction. Microscopic characteristics include viscosity, agglutination, count and concentration, motility, morphology, viability, and an assessment of the non-sperm cells within the sample.

Macroscopic characteristics

Gross appearance

A normal semen sample has a homogeneous, pearly, gray-opalescent appearance. Samples may appear clear if the sperm concentration is low, or brown if red blood cells are present (hematospermia). A yellow appearance may be due to jaundice, the presence of certain vitamins or drugs, or contamination with urine.

Semen volume

Ejaculated semen is composed of spermatozoa in a milieu composed of seminal vesicle fluid (approximately 65% of the total volume), prostatic secretions (30%), testicular and epididymal fluids (5%), and bulbourethral gland secretions. Volume may be measured by calculating the difference between the weight of the container with and without the sample, or using a graduated cylinder. Semen volume should be greater than 1.5 mL [10]. Large seminal fluid volumes (> 4 mL) are generally not felt to be pathologic and may be found after prolonged sexual abstinence [14]. Low volumes (< 1.5 mL) may be due to improper collection (incomplete sample or a short abstinence period), psychogenic effects, or pathologic causes. Pathologic etiologies include retrograde ejaculation (bladder neck dysfunction or pelvic nerve damage), ductal obstruction, a lack of seminal fluid production from seminal vesicle or prostatic hypoplasia, or hypogonadism [14]. The specific diagnosis can generally be made with a thorough history and physical exam, as well as a few tests such as a post-ejaculate urinalysis, transrectal ultrasound, and serum testosterone level.

pH

The normal pH is of seminal fluid ranges from 7.2 to 8.0 and is established by the acidic secretions of the prostate and alkaline secretions of the seminal vesicles. The seminal vesicles produce the majority of seminal fluid. Acidic seminal fluid may be indicative of vasal or ejaculatory duct obstruction, agenesis (or occlusion) of the seminal vesicles, or incomplete ejaculation in which the seminal vesicles have only been partially emptied. Basic seminal fluid may be indicative of prostatitis resulting in decreased acidic prostate secretions, such as acid phosphatase.

Liquefaction

Normally, semen coagulates upon ejaculation (related to seminal vesicle products) and progressively liquefies within 15 minutes under the effect of the prostatic proteolytic enzyme, fibrinolysin. Semen that does not liquefy within 1 hour is considered abnormal [10]. After liquefaction, an assessment of sperm concentration, count, and other parameters is conducted. Samples which do not liquefy may need additional treatments such as dilution or exposure to bromelin, to make the sample amenable to analysis [12].

Microscopic characteristics

Viscosity

Viscosity is measured after liquefaction is complete, by allowing seminal fluid to drop by gravity from a large-bore pipette and observing the length of the thread formed. A normal sample will leave the needle as small discrete drops, while in cases of abnormal viscosity the drop will form a thread of > 2 cm [12]. Alternatively, a glass rod may be dipped into the semen sample and observed for the thread that forms on withdrawal. Again the thread should not exceed 2 cm [12]. Prolonged liquefaction may indicate poor prostatic enzyme secretion, such as seen in prostatitis, ejaculatory duct obstruction, or congenital absence of the seminal vesicles. Hyperviscous semen is postulated by some to represent a form of minimally expressed cystic fibrosis, and genetic testing may be considered in this population [15].

Hyperviscosity is distinct from agglutination, which is visible microscopically as an adherence and clumping of motile spermatozoa. When seen, agglutination is measured on a scale of 1 (< 10 spermatozoa per agglutinate, many free spermatozoa) to 4 (all spermatozoa agglutinated and interconnected) [15]. A small degree of agglutination is normal [9], but excessive levels are suggestive of anti-sperm antibodies (ASA), infection [15], or malfunction of the accessory sex organs [14]. As such, when either prolonged or excessive agglutination is observed, semen culture (despite its limitations) should be considered.

The full fertility-related implications of viscosity abnormalities remain controversial, although it is well established that excessively viscous specimens may impair sperm motility and availability at the site of fertilization [15]. In-vivo assessment of sperm motility by examination of the cervical fluid after intercourse, the so-called postcoital test, may verify that viscosity abnormalities do not represent impairment to natural sperm motility. Samples with an elevated viscosity can be treated with mucolytic agents such as α-chymotrypsin prior to fertility treatments, although the effects of this on sperm structure are unknown [15].

Count and concentration

The number of sperm in a sample is reported as both the total number and the concentration in millions of

Table 3.3. Nomenclature for sperm density

Polyspermia	Sperm count > 250 million/mL
Normospermia	Sperm count 15–250 million/mL
Mild oligospermia	Sperm count 10–15 million/mL
Moderate oligospermia	Sperm count 5–10 million/mL
Severe oligospermia	Sperm count < 5 million/mL
Azoospermia	No spermatozoa in the ejaculate

Table 3.4. Etiogenesis of azoospermia

Obstructive	Non-obstructive
Congenital bilateral agenesis of the vas deferens ± cystic fibrosis	Klinefelter syndrome
	Sertoli-cell-only syndrome
	Spermatogenic arrest
Bronchiectasia (Young's syndrome)	Mumps orchitis
Ejaculatory duct obstruction	
Rete testis obstruction	
Epididymal obstruction	
Occult vasal injury from previous inguinal or retroperitoneal surgery	

sperm per milliliter. The determination of sperm count may be performed manually using a Neubauer hemocytometer [10], or using specialized counting instruments such as the Makler or Microcell Chambers, or disposable counting chambers [16]. The dilution factor is determined after an initial assessment of the sperm density, with an aim of counting 200 sperm. If the sample appears to have a lower number, it should be centrifuged to prepare an adequate smear. Computer-assisted sperm assessment (CASA), discussed below, can also be used to measure sperm concentration, but is prone to its own set of errors, especially at extremely high or low sperm concentrations, or in the presence of significant agglutination or large amounts of seminal debris [16]. The lower reference limit for sperm concentration is 15 million sperm per mL or 39 million sperm per ejaculate (Table 3.3) [10].

Polyspermia, while having a larger raw number of sperm, may have functional impairments with chromosomal anomalies, decreased adenosine triphosphate (ATP) content, and abnormal acrosomal function [17]. SA reveals a greater prevalence of teratospermia and asthenospermia, which, in one study, has been correlated with a higher risk of miscarriage in women whose partners had a polyspermic semen [17].

Oligospermia may be indicative of partial ductal obstruction, varicocele, cryptorchidism, diabetes, primary testicular failure, or certain medications. Febrile illness may also cause a transient oligospermia or even azoospermia, and if the history is suggestive a repeat SA should be obtained in three months, after a complete spermatogenic cycle of 74 days.

Azoospermia is the complete absence of sperm in the ejaculate, and may be broadly classified into obstructive and non-obstructive (Table 3.4). Obstructive azoospermia is a result of testicular, epididymal, or ejaculatory duct obstruction that prevents the release of spermatozoa. Conditions causing this include congenital bilateral agenesis of the vas deferens (with or without phenotypic cystic fibrosis), Young's

syndrome with inspissated epididymal secretion, or previous inguinal surgery. Non-obstructive azoospermia is seen in conditions of testicular failure, as might be seen with Y-chromosomal microdeletions, Sertoli-cell-only syndrome, Klinefelter syndrome, or spermatogenic arrest. These conditions can be distinguished with hormonal testing (follicle-stimulating hormone and testosterone), karyotyping, and Y-chromosome microdeletion assessment, which will also be vital in future fertility counseling.

In cases of severe oligospermia or azoospermia it is imperative that the sample be centrifuged and the pellet examined for the presence of sperm to confirm the diagnosis. This is of enormous importance with the increasing use of intracytoplasmic sperm injection (ICSI), as the presence of a few spermatozoa may allow for retrieval and in-vitro fertilization (IVF) using the husband/partner's own sperm.

The lower limit of normal is 39 million sperm per ejaculate or 15 million cells per mL [9]. However, there still remains much discussion as to the true "normal" values, as men with lower counts may still achieve natural conception [14]. Other studies have shown that increasing sperm concentrations up to a concentration of 40 million cells/mL result in an increase in the spontaneous pregnancy rates, at which point there is no further improvement [5]. Additionally, the correlation between sperm concentration and the other aspects of semen quality, including motility and morphology [14], cannot be understated, as this may lead to a functional impairment in addition to a limited number of sperm.

Motility

Motility should be assessed at a temperature of 37 °C and within 1 hour of collection, as deviations from either of these can have adverse effects. In recent years, CASA has been investigated to provide an objective assessment of sperm movement characteristics. This is discussed in more detail below.

Motility is notoriously subjective, with a large inter-observer variability. For fertility purposes, the proportion of sperm that demonstrate flagellar movement, as well as forward progression, are both important. Prior versions of the WHO guidelines recommended that progressively motile sperm be categorized as rapid or slow, with "grade A" spermatozoa achieving a speed of > 25 μm/s. However, due to difficulty in accurately defining forward progression, this system has been replaced. The current grading system [10] distinguishes spermatozoa with progressive or non-progressive motility from those that are immotile:

- *Progressive motility* – spermatozoa moving actively, either linearly or in a large circle, regardless of speed
- *Non-progressive motility* – all other patterns of motility with an absence of progression
- *Immotile* – no movement

Sperm are scored both by the total (progressive and non-progressive) and progressive motility, with the lower reference limits being 32% progressive and 40% total motile sperm [10].

Asthenospermia, impaired sperm motility, can be spuriously low due to exposure of sperm to rubber condoms, spermicides, extremes of temperature, prolonged abstinence, or a delay between collection and examination. Truly pathologic asthenospermia, motility < 5–10%, can be associated with ASA, morphological or ultrastructural defects, or necrospermia [14]. In these cases, viability testing may be useful to distinguish between necrospermia and an ultrastructural defect. An underlying structural defect may be identified with electron microscopy, such as absent dynein arms, mitochondrial abnormalities, or abnormal fibrous sheaths around the flagella [14]. Patients found to have an ultrastructural defect may be good candidates for ICSI.

Computer-assisted sperm assessment (CASA)

Traditionally, the assessment of seminal parameters is a subjective measurement. CASA, the use of computer analysis of videomicrography to assess sperm kinetic parameters, was developed in an attempt to more precisely analyze sperm head and flagellar kinematics. The microscopic field is digitized and kinematic values are determined for each spermatozoon, which are then computer analyzed [18]. In specimens with high sperm concentrations (> 40 million/mL), sperm collisions may lead to erroneous results due to computer misinterpretation of overlapping sperm trajectories; thus these samples must be diluted prior to analysis.

The classic parameters of the SA are generated, as well as sperm trajectory characteristics and straight-line velocity, which cannot be determined by standard microscopic evaluation. While these characteristics have been positively correlated with IVF fertilization rates [19], CASA cannot reliably predict spontaneous fertilization rates [20], and requires highly specialized equipment. Therefore, while interesting, this technology is not the standard fashion in which the SA is interpreted, and its role is still being determined [18].

Morphology

Although the intrinsic variability of the human spermatozoon makes "normal" sperm morphology evaluation difficult to determine, attempts have been made based on identification of sperm retrieved from the postcoital endocervical mucus and surface of the zona pellucida. Seminal fluid is "feathered" onto a slide, air-dried, fixed, stained (Papanicolaou, Shorr, Diff-Quik), and then examined using brightfield optics under oil immersion at $1000 \times$ [10].

In an attempt to standardize morphology, both among individuals and among laboratories, several grading systems have been developed. Some of the major classification systems include Williams (1964), Freund (1966), Eliasson (1971), David (1975), Fredricsson (1979), Tygerberg strict criteria (1988), and WHO (1980, 1987, 1992, 1999, 2009) [21–22]. Today the most commonly accepted classification systems are the WHO and Tygerberg strict criteria [23], with the WHO reference values most commonly utilized in US laboratories.

According to these criteria, a normal sperm (Fig. 3.1A) has an oval-shaped head 4.0–5.0 μm long and 2.5–3.5 μm wide, with a smooth, regular surface. The length-to-width ratio is 1.50–1.75. The acrosome, identified as the intensely colored anterior part of the head, should have no vacuoles, and should comprise 40–70% of the total head area. The mid-piece should

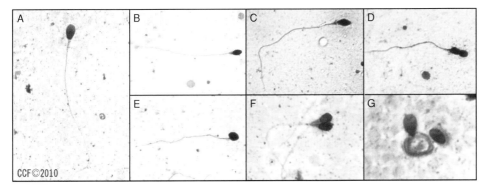

Figure 3.1. (A) Normal sperm; (B) Small head; (C) Tapering head; (D) Pyriform head; (E) Round head; (F) Bicephalic (double head); (G) Coiled tail defect. (Reproduced courtesy of the Cleveland Clinic Foundation.) *See color plate section.*

be slender and regular, about the same length as the head, and aligned with the major axis of the head. The flagella should be 40–50 μm, straight, and without vacuoles [10]. By strict criteria, all sperm deviating from this are considered abnormal.

Abnormalities are classified by their location as well as the presence of cytoplasmic droplets:

- *Head shape defects* – large, small (Fig. 3.1B), tapering (Fig. 3.1C), pyriform (Fig. 3.1D), round (Fig. 3.1E), amorphous, vacuolated (> 2 vacuoles or > 20% of the head area occupied by unstained vacuolar areas, vacuoles in the postacrosomal region), double heads (Fig. 3.1F), or any combination of these
- *Neck and mid-piece defects* – absent, asymmetrically inserted, non-inserted, or bent tail (forming an angle of > 90° to the long axis of the head), distended/irregular/bent mid-piece, abnormally thin mid-piece, or any combination of these
- *Tail defects* – short, multiple, hairpin, broken, irregular width, coiled (Fig. 3.1G), sharply angulated, or any combination of these
- *Excess residual cytoplasm* – more than one-third of the area of a normal sperm head

In cases of teratospermia, defined as < 15% of spermatozoa with normal WHO morphology, it is important to distinguish mixed abnormalities from those in which the majority of sperm show a single uniform defect, as this may indicate a congenital structural anomaly [10]. Round-headed sperm (Fig. 3.1E) may lack an acrosome, rendering them unable to penetrate the zona pellucida. Pin-head sperm may be indicative of a centriole developmental anomaly, resulting

in sperm without heads [10]. Tapered-headed sperm (Fig. 1C) may be seen concurrent with varicocele [16]. Epididymal dysfunction may be suspected when there is coiling of the sperm tail (Fig. 3.1G) or other flagellar abnormalities [16]. A mixed morphology may be indicative of exogenous factors including fever, varicocele, certain drugs, or stress, although it is more frequently idiopathic.

While it is suggested that sperm morphology has predictive value for the fertilizing capacity of sperm [5,24], debate lies in what defines "normal." With time, the cutoff for "normal" has decreased, progressing from 60%, to 30%, to 14%, and currently 4% [9,10,16]. According to the 2009 WHO reference range, the 95% confidence interval for "normal" spermatozoa has a range from 3% to 48%, highlighting our lack of clear criteria to define normal forms.

The full clinical implications of morphology remain controversial, likely due in part to different classification systems, preparation techniques, and the subjective nature of interpretation. In general, semen samples with < 4% normal forms have a poor prognosis for sporadic, IUI [23], and IVF [25] fertilizing ability. When correctable causes of male infertility are not identified, couples with teratospermia may be directed to proceed with ICSI, as this requires only one morphologically and functionally normal spermatozoon to fertilize an oocyte, making morphological imperfections less important [24].

Viability

Motile sperm are readily identified as living, but further testing is required to identify viable but immotile

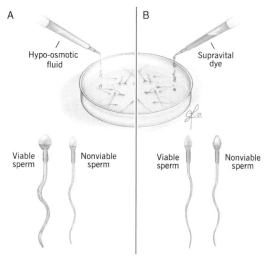
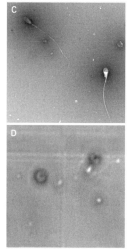

Figure 3.2. (A) Hypo-osmotic sperm swelling test: sperm with an intact cell membrane will swell. (B) Dye exclusion: sperm with an intact cell membrane are able to exclude the dye. (C) Microscopic image of dye exclusion: spermatozoa with dark pink heads are considered dead (membrane-damaged), whereas spermatozoa with white or light pink heads are considered alive (membrane-intact). (D) Endtz test: peroxidase within polymorphonuclear leukocytes is stained, allowing for distinction of seminal leukocytes from immature germ cells. *See color plate section.*

cells. Viability assays are indicated when sperm motility is < 40%, as this may be indicative of either necrospermia or an ultrastructural defect [10].

In general, tests of viability assess the integrity of the sperm cytoplasmic membrane, and include either hypo-osmotic swelling or dye exclusion (Fig. 3.2). The hypo-osmotic sperm swelling test (Fig. 3.2A) involves placing sperm into hypo-osmotic media and assessing their ability to respond osmotically. Water enters the cytoplasm of living cells, causing the spermatozoon's tail to swell [26]. Dye exclusion (Fig. 3.2B,C) involves mixing spermatozoa with a supravital dye such as eosin or trypan blue. Sperm with an intact cell membrane are able to exclude the stain. The lower reference limit for viability is 58% [10].

High viability with low motility is suggestive of an ultrastructural defect, such as primary ciliary dyskinesia or Kartagener syndrome, which may be further evaluated with electron microscopy. Finally, surgically retrieved sperm are often non-motile because they do not pass through the epididymis. In this situation, viability testing may useful to identify sperm suitable for ICSI [27].

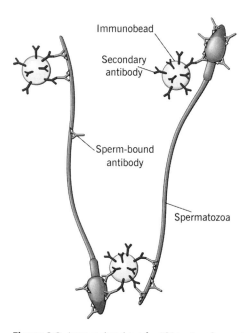

Figure 3.3. Immunobead test for ASA testing. Spermatozoa are mixed with beads that have been coated with IgG class-specific secondary antibodies, and the suspension is observed for agglutination. (Reproduced courtesy of the Cleveland Clinic Foundation.) *See color plate section.*

Anti-sperm antibodies (ASA)

Sperm autoantibodies are present in 4–8% of infertile men and are most commonly IgA or IgG. Their formation is induced by breaching of the blood–testis barrier, either during development, traumatically, surgically, or due to infection. Sperm agglutination on SA, severely impaired sperm motility, an abnormal postcoital test, or abnormalities of cervical mucus interaction or penetration, may prompt ASA testing. The diagnosis of ASA is made by the mixed antiglobulin reaction or, more commonly, the immunobead test (Fig. 3.3). Spermatozoa are mixed with beads that have been coated with IgG class-specific secondary antibodies, and observed for agglutination. Antibodies are considered clinically significant when ≥ 50% of spermatozoa are coated, when spermatozoa are unable to penetrate the preovulatory human cervical mucus, or when they demonstrate impaired fertilizing capacity [10].

The presence of ASA has been shown to negatively affect sperm function at nearly every step of sperm transit through the female reproductive tract and penetration through the oocyte. When IVF is used, patients with ASA have lower pregnancy rates and higher miscarriage rates [28]. Steroids may be given to lower titers prior to IUI, but are unnecessary if ICSI is used [29].

Other cell types

Non-sperm elements which may be present on seminal microscopic examination include immature germ cells, epithelial cells, and leukocytes [30]. When present in high numbers, epithelial cells may be indicative of vaginal contamination if coitus interruptus was the method of collection. Red blood cells are often present in semen. In small quantities they can represent a normal finding, but larger quantities can suggest infection, ductal obstruction, genital tract tumors, or vascular abnormalities.

Leukocytes are normally found throughout the male reproductive tract and are found in almost every human ejaculate [31]. Immature germ cells may be visually confused with leukocytes as both are round, non-flagellated cells. However, their clinical implications are quite different. Whereas pyospermia may suggest a genital tract infection, immature germ cells are most commonly of no clinical significance. Excessive numbers of spermatogenic cells may suggest pathology at the level of the seminiferous epithelium with the premature release of immature forms, or alternatively hypospermatogenesis or varicocele [17]. Elevated numbers of leukocytes may be associated with infection or inflammation of the accessory glands [12], which may have an unfavorable effect on spermatozoal motility as well as genetic integrity [12].

When > 5 round cells per high-powered field are seen, immunocytochemistry with CD45 or the Endtz test (Fig. 3.2D) may be used to distinguish them, based on the presence of peroxidase within leukocytes [32]. Seminal leukocyte levels > 1 million/mL have been correlated with a reduction in normal semen parameters [33] and defective sperm function, as well as compromised sperm structural integrity and acrosomal damage [31]. Seminal leukocytes are powerful generators of reactive oxygen species (ROS), and their full role in fecundity is still being elucidated. Currently we know that antibiotic therapy in men with genital infections leads to a reduction in seminal leukocytes and ROS production, with a subsequent improvement in sperm motility and an improvement in natural conception [34]. Therefore, when leukocytospermia is identified, semen cultures are indicated.

Biochemical analysis

The prostate, seminal vesicles, and epididymis each produce unique seminal components, which may then serve as surrogates for the glands that produce them [17]:

- *Prostate* – citric acid, zinc, calcium, magnesium, Y glutamyl transferase, prostate-specific antigen (PSA), acid phosphatase
- *Seminal vesicles* – fructose, semenogelin, prostaglandin, seminal plasma motility inhibitor
- *Epididymis* – free L-carnitine, glycerophosphocholine, α-glucosidase

Of these, zinc and citric acid are most commonly assayed for the prostate, fructose and semenogelin for the seminal vesicles, and α-glucosidase for the epididymis. Each component has a specific function in male fertility, and all interact with each other. One example of this is the interaction between semenogelin, a coagulum released by the seminal vesicles, and PSA, released from the prostate. PSA rapidly cleaves semenogelin, leading to semen liquefaction and the initiation of sperm motility. An abnormality in either of these compounds would lead to hyperviscous semen, preventing sperm motility and fertilization [35].

Semen analysis in cancer patients

The gonadotoxic effects of cancer treatments on fertility are well established [36]. However, evidence suggests that the disease process itself influences spermatogenesis [37]. Before starting any therapy, oligospermia is seen in up to 57% of patients with leukemia, 28% of those with testicular cancer, 33% of those with gastrointestinal malignancies, and 70% of those with Hodgkin's lymphoma [37]. The type of cancer may also have implications for semen quality [38].

The reason for this baseline impairment in fertility is likely multifactorial and will be covered in more detail in subsequent chapters of this text. In general, malignancy is associated with a hypercatabolic state, which may lead to cachexia and an impaired reproductive capacity [39]. The hormones associated with malignancy may further dysregulate the hormones involved in fertility, including gonadotropin-releasing hormone (GnRH), prolactin, luteinizing hormone (LH), and follicle-stimulating hormone (FSH) [39]. Supporting this, in patients with testicular cancer, the level of spermatogenic impairment is highest in the testicular tissue closest to the tumor [40]. In Hodgkin's lymphoma, a cancer with one of the highest documented levels of spermatogenic impairment, infertility is thought to be due to imbalances in T lymphocytes [41]. However, spermatogenic impairment is also seen in central nervous system tumors, implying that centrally mediated endocrine processes play a role [42].

Predictive parameters for successful fertility

The role of semen parameters as predictive markers of fertility potential has been a matter of debate since 1951, when MacLeod proposed cutoff values for sperm counts to distinguish fertile from subfertile men [12]. However, subsequent studies have shown that many men with counts below these thresholds are able to conceive naturally [43].

In general, sperm concentration, motility, and morphology are usually considered the parameters most closely linked to the probability of conception [4–5]. In a classic article, Bonde et al. found that the probability of conception increased with increasing sperm concentration up to 40×10^5/mL, but that higher values were not associated with a higher likelihood of pregnancy [5]. Subsequent studies have confirmed the link between sperm count and fertility, although the actual cutoff value is unclear. Nallella et al. found that a concentration > 27.5 million/mL was a discriminator of fertility [4], and other authors have identified values ranging from 5 to 20 million/mL [44]. Likewise, several studies have shown a correlation between IVF success and concentration [45,46].

Morphology has been a more controversial predictor of fertility. In general, semen with $> 14\%$ normal forms (by Tygerberg criteria) present a good prognosis for both in-vivo and in-vitro fertilization rates. Values between 4% and 14% also have a good prognosis, albeit less than that found with higher percentages of normal forms. Semen with values $< 4\%$ may have a poorer prognosis for fertilizing ability [17]. Nallella et al. found that the percentage of men with normal morphology was significantly higher in men with proven fertility, as measured by both the WHO and Tygerberg's strict criteria [4]. Other groups have found that morphology is related to likelihood of pregnancy independent of other sperm parameters [5,24], and some suggest that morphology is the best predictor for fertility [2,47]. Normal morphology has been associated with improved IUI [23] and IVF outcomes [21,25], early embryo development, and pregnancy outcomes using IVF [21,25]. However, while the relationship between morphology and fertility has support, it appears that the current reference values may need to be reevaluated, as the data show a significant overlap between values for fertile and infertile men [4,5,24,47].

Sperm motility has been shown to be higher in fertile men [4,48]. Both Nallella et al. and Krause found that motility was not simply correlated, but that it was one of the best predictors of fertility outcomes in vivo [4,49], a finding which has been confirmed for IVF [48]. This correlation is not surprising, given that motility is necessary for penetration through the cervical mucus, transit though the female reproductive tract, and penetration through the zona pellucida.

No single test or sperm parameter has been found to be absolute in its prediction of male fertility, as no single sperm function or feature could truly represent the ability of a spermatozoon to accomplish the complex sequence of events leading to a pregnancy. In reality, a combination of sperm characteristics, including volume, count, and the percentage of normal and motile forms, provides the best diagnostic profile. Each semen characteristic contributes a different aspect to fertility potential, which in conjunction with the others yields maximum potency [50].

Conclusion

The semen analysis can help in the diagnosis of many male fertility-related pathologies, and is often crucial in formulating treatment recommendations. With the increasing use of IVF and ICSI the role of the SA continues to be defined. The SA seems to be not so much a direct test of male fertility as an indicator of fertility potential. Men with semen parameters falling outside of normal ranges may be considered "subfertile," but in reality fertility can only be fully demonstrated by a man's ability to effect a pregnancy in vivo, which depends not only on the number of motile spermatozoa, but also on the functional capability of those spermatozoa to reach, bind, and fertilize an oocyte.

The effect of malignancy on male fertility remains an area of intense research. Men harboring a systemic malignancy have impaired spermatogenesis even prior to oncologic treatment. The treatments are well known to be gonadotoxic. Effective treatments for systemic malignancies have led to an increase in survival, making long-term fertility-related issues more important to patients. A baseline knowledge of the SA can help clinicians appropriately counsel their patients on realistic fertility-related expectations, taking into account the growing acceptance of assisted reproductive technologies.

Acknowledgments

The authors would like to thank Dr. Sajal Gupta for her invaluable technical expertise in obtaining images for this chapter. Its quality has been enhanced significantly by her kindness and skill.

References

1. Colpi GM, Colpi EM, Castiglioni F, Grugnetti C. Semen cryopreservation from oncological patients: the Italian experience. *Eur J Obstet Gynecol Reprod Biol* 2004; 113 (Suppl 1): S12–13.

2. Guzick DS, Overstreet JW, Factor-Litvak P, *et al.* Sperm morphology, motility, and concentration in fertile and infertile men. *N Engl J Med* 2001; 345: 1388–93.

3. Bostofte E, Bagger P, Michael A, Stakemann G. Fertility prognosis for infertile men: results of follow-up study of semen analysis in infertile men from two different populations evaluated by the Cox regression model. *Fertil Steril* 1990; 54: 1100–6.

4. Nallella KP, Sharma RK, Aziz N, Agarwal A. Significance of sperm characteristics in the evaluation of male infertility. *Fertil Steril* 2006; 85: 629–34.

5. Bonde JP, Ernst E, Jensen TK, *et al.* Relation between semen quality and fertility: a population-based study of 430 first-pregnancy planners. *Lancet* 1998; 352: 1172–7.

6. Fisch H, Ikeguchi EF, Goluboff ET. Worldwide variations in sperm counts. *Urology* 1996; 48: 909–11.

7. Robbins WA, Elashoff DA, Xun L, *et al.* Effect of lifestyle exposures on sperm aneuploidy. *Cytogenet Genome Res* 2005; 111: 371–7.

8. Alvarez C, Castilla JA, Martinez L, *et al.* Biological variation of seminal parameters in healthy subjects. *Hum Reprod* 2003; 18: 2082–8.

9. Cooper TG, Noonan E, von Eckardstein S, *et al.* World Health Organization reference values for human semen characteristics. *Hum Reprod Update* 2010; 16: 231–45.

10. World Health Organization. *WHO Laboratory Manual for the Examination and Processing of Human Semen*, 5th edn. Geneva: WHO, 2010.

11. Carlsen E, Petersen JH, Andersson AM, Skakkebaek NE. Effects of ejaculatory frequency and season on variations in semen quality. *Fertil Steril* 2004; 82: 358–66.

12. Comhaire F, Vermeulen L. Human semen analysis. *Hum Reprod Update* 1995; 1: 343–62.

13. Pellestor F, Girardet A, Andreo B. Effect of long abstinence periods on human sperm quality. *Int J Fertil Menopausal Stud* 1994; 39: 278–82.

14. McLachlan RI, Baker HW, Clarke GN, *et al.* Semen analysis: its place in modern reproductive medical practice. *Pathology* 2003; 35: 25–33.

15. Elia J, Delfino M, Imbrogno N, *et al.* Human semen hyperviscosity: prevalence, pathogenesis and therapeutic aspects. *Asian J Androl* 2009; 11: 609–15.

16. Overstreet JW. Clinical approach to male reproductive problems. *Occup Med* 1994; 9: 387–404.

17. Andrade-Rocha FT. Semen analysis in laboratory practice: an overview of routine tests. *J Clin Lab Anal* 2003; 17: 247–58.

18. Mortimer ST. CASA: practical aspects. *J Androl* 2000; 21: 515–24.

19. Macleod IC, Irvine DS. The predictive value of computer-assisted semen analysis in the context of a donor insemination programme. *Hum Reprod* 1995; 10: 580–6.

20. Oehninger S, Franken D, Alexander N, Hodgen GD. Hemizona assay and its impact on the identification and treatment of human sperm dysfunctions. *Andrologia* 1992; 24: 307–21.

21. Kruger TF, Acosta AA, Simmons KF, *et al.* Predictive value of abnormal sperm morphology in in vitro fertilization. *Fertil Steril* 1988; 49: 112–17.

22. Menkveld R, Stander FS, Kotze TJ, Kruger TF, van Zyl JA. The evaluation of morphological characteristics of human spermatozoa according to stricter criteria. *Hum Reprod* 1990; 5: 586–92.

23. Van Waart J, Kruger TF, Lombard CJ, Ombelet W. Predictive value of normal sperm morphology in intrauterine insemination (IUI): a structured literature review. *Hum Reprod Update* 2001; 7: 495–500.

24. Zinaman MJ, Brown CC, Selevan SG, Clegg ED. Semen quality and human fertility: a prospective study with healthy couples. *J Androl* 2000; 21: 145–53.

25. Grow DR, Oehninger S, Seltman HJ, *et al.* Sperm morphology as diagnosed by strict criteria: probing the impact of teratozoospermia on fertilization rate and pregnancy outcome in a large in vitro fertilization population. *Fertil Steril* 1994; 62: 559–67.

26. Liu DY, Baker HW. Tests of human sperm function and fertilization in vitro. *Fertil Steril* 1992; 58: 465–83.

27. Wilcox AJ, Weinberg CR, Baird DD. Timing of sexual intercourse in relation to ovulation. Effects on the probability of conception, survival of the pregnancy, and sex of the baby. *N Engl J Med* 1995; 333: 1517–21.

28. Chiu WW, Chamley LW. Clinical associations and mechanisms of action of antisperm antibodies. *Fertil Steril* 2004; 82: 529–35.

29. Bohring C, Krause W. Immune infertility: towards a better understanding of sperm (auto)-immunity. The value of proteomic analysis. *Hum Reprod* 2003; 18: 915–24.

30. Fedder J. Nonsperm cells in human semen: with special reference to seminal leukocytes and their possible influence on fertility. *Arch Androl* 1996; 36: 41–65.

31. Aziz N, Agarwal A, Lewis-Jones I, Sharma RK, Thomas AJ. Novel associations between specific sperm morphological defects and leukocytospermia. *Fertil Steril* 2004; 82: 621–7.

32. Shekarriz M, Sharma RK, Thomas AJ, Agarwal A. Positive myeloperoxidase staining (Endtz test) as an indicator of excessive reactive oxygen species formation in semen. *J Assist Reprod Genet* 1995; 12: 70–4.

33. Wolff H. The biologic significance of white blood cells in semen. *Fertil Steril* 1995; 63: 1143–57.

34. Keck C, Gerber-Schafer C, Clad A, Wilhelm C, Breckwoldt M. Seminal tract infections: impact on male fertility and treatment options. *Hum Reprod Update* 1998; 4: 891–903.

35. de Lamirande E. Semenogelin, the main protein of the human semen coagulum, regulates sperm function. *Semin Thromb Hemost* 2007; 33: 60–8.

36. Sabanegh ES, Jr., Ragheb AM. Male fertility after cancer. *Urology* 2009; 73: 225–31.

37. Chung K, Irani J, Knee G, *et al.* Sperm cryopreservation for male patients with cancer: an epidemiological analysis at the University of Pennsylvania. *Eur J Obstet Gynecol Reprod Biol* 2004; 113 (Suppl 1): S7–11.

38. Ragni G, Somigliana E, Restelli L, *et al.* Sperm banking and rate of assisted reproduction treatment: insights from a 15-year cryopreservation program for male cancer patients. *Cancer* 2003; 97: 1624–9.

39. Agarwal A, Said TM. Implications of systemic malignancies on human fertility. *Reprod Biomed Online* 2004; 9: 673–9.

40. Ho GT, Gardner H, DeWolf WC, Loughlin KR, Morgentaler A. Influence of testicular carcinoma on ipsilateral spermatogenesis. *J Urol* 1992; 148: 821–5.

41. Barr RD, Clark DA, Booth JD. Dyspermia in men with localized Hodgkin's disease: a potentially reversible, immune-mediated disorder. *Med Hypotheses* 1993; 40: 165–8.

42. Hallak J, Kolettis PN, Sekhon VS, Thomas AJ, Agarwal A. Cryopreservation of sperm from patients with leukemia: is it worth the effort? *Cancer* 1999; 85: 1973–8.

43. David G, Jouannet P, Martin-Boyce A, Spira A, Schwartz D. Sperm counts in fertile and infertile men. *Fertil Steril* 1979; 31: 453–5.

44. Lewis SE. Is sperm evaluation useful in predicting human fertility? *Reproduction* 2007; 134: 31–40.

45. Biljan MM, Taylor CT, Manasse PR, *et al.* Evaluation of different sperm function tests as screening methods for male fertilization potential: the value of the sperm migration test. *Fertil Steril* 1994; 62: 591–8.

46. Robinson JN, Lockwood GM, Dokras A, *et al.* Does isolated teratozoospermia affect performance in in-vitro fertilization and embryo transfer? *Hum Reprod* 1994; 9: 870–4.

47. Chia SE, Tay SK, Lim ST. What constitutes a normal seminal analysis? Semen parameters of 243 fertile men. *Hum Reprod* 1998; 13: 3394–8.

48. Branigan EF, Estes MA, Muller CH. Advanced semen analysis: a simple screening test to predict intrauterine insemination success. *Fertil Steril* 1999; 71: 547–51.

49. Krause W. The significance of computer-assisted semen analysis (CASA) for diagnosis in andrology and fertility prognosis. *Int J Androl* 1995; 18 (Suppl 2): 32–5.

50. Agarwal A, Sharma RK, Nelson DR. New semen quality scores developed by principal component analysis of semen characteristics. *J Androl* 2003; 24: 343–52.

Chapter

4

Physiology of ejaculation

John P. Mulhall

Emission and ejaculation

Generally associated with orgasm, ejaculation is the final phase of the sexual response cycle in the male and represents a reflex involving cerebral and spinal centers as well as peripheral nerves. Ejaculation involves a complex interplay between somatic, sympathetic, and parasympathetic pathways involving predominantly dopaminergic and serotonergic neurons [1]. In antegrade ejaculation, three basic phases are involved: emission, ejection/expulsion, and orgasm.

Emission, the first phase of ejaculation, is a sympathetic spinal cord reflex that involves the deposition of seminal fluid into the prostatic urethra. Ejection or expulsion is due to the combined action of sympathetic and somatic pathways. An antegrade ejaculation requires synchronization between periurethral muscle contractions, bladder neck closure, and relaxation of the external urinary sphincter. Orgasm is the pleasurable sensation, processed centrally, in response to increased pressure in the posterior urethra and contraction of the urethral bulb and accessory sexual organs.

Neuroanatomy

The general anatomy of the structures involved in the ejaculatory process is dealt with elsewhere in this book (Chapter 1).

Peripheral anatomy

The pathways involved in the peripheral control of ejaculation include sensory afferents and motor efferents. The sensory input travels along the dorsal nerve to the perineal nerve and then the hypogastric nerve to the upper sacral and the lower lumbar segments of the spinal cord. The majority of sensory information is gathered via free nerve terminals from the penile skin and glans; however, encapsulated receptors called Krause finger corpuscles have also been identified in the glans [2]. In addition, afferents pass via hypogastric nerve fibers, reaching the paravertebral lumbosacral sympathetic chain via thoracolumbar dorsal roots of the spinal cord [3]. The sensory afferents end in the medial dorsal horn and the dorsal gray commissure of the spinal cord [4].

The autonomic efferent nerves primarily extend from the pelvic plexus, where sympathetic and parasympathetic nerve fibers innervate the male sexual organs. The origins of the preganglionic sympathetic neurons are located in the intermediolateral cell column and in the central autonomic region of the thoracolumbar segments of the spinal cord (T12–L2) [5]. The sympathetic fibers leave the spinal column via the ventral roots and synapse in the paravertebral sympathetic chain. From there fibers proceed via the thoracic sympathetic chain to the inferior enteric, splanchnic, and mesenteric plexi, where descending nerves from these ganglia form the hypogastric plexus just inferior to the aortic bifurcation from which the paired hypogastric nerves arise. The confluence of the hypogastric nerve and the parasympathetic pelvic nerve comprises the pelvic plexus. Nerve fibers from this plexus supply the epididymis, vas deferens, seminal vesicle, prostate, bladder neck, and urethra [6].

The origin of the preganglionic parasympathetic neurons is in the intermediolateral cell column of the lumbosacral segments of the spinal cord in the sacral parasympathetic nucleus (S2–S4). Neurons travel in the pelvic nerve to the pelvic plexus. Efferent somatic nerves emerge from Onuf's nuclei in the anterior horn

Fertility Preservation in Male Cancer Patients, ed. John P. Mulhall, Linda D. Applegarth, Robert D. Oates and Peter N. Schlegel. Published by Cambridge University Press. © Cambridge University Press 2013.

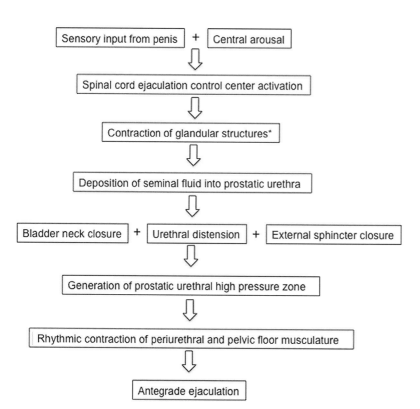

Figure 4.1. The stages of a normal ejaculatory response.

of the sacral segments S2–S4 and travel along the motor branch of the pudendal nerve to innervate the pelvic floor striated muscles, including the bulbospongiosus and ischiocavernosus muscles.

Spinal and central anatomy

Specific neurons in the central gray of laminae 7 and 10 of lumbar segments 3 and 4 (L3–4) are thought to represent the spinal ejaculation control center [7]. These neurons connect with the parvocellular sub-parafascicular thalamic nucleus (SPFp) [8]. These neurons are reported as lumbar spinothalamic (LSt) cells. The LSt cells have connections to somatic motor neurons as well as sympathetic and parasympathetic preganglionic neurons, highlighting their role in the integration of afferent and efferent signals involved in the ejaculatory reflex [7]. The spinal centers are under descending inhibitory and excitatory influences of supraspinal regions involving the medial preoptic area (MPOA), the paraventricular nucleus of the hypothalamus (PVN), the nucleus paragigantocellularis (nPGi), the posterodorsal medial amygdaloid nucleus (MeApd), and the SPFp [9,10].

Physiological control of ejaculation

Thus peripheral and central centers, as well as sympathetic, parasympathetic, and somatic pathways participate in the physiological control of the ejaculatory reflex. A normal ejaculatory response (Fig. 4.1) requires complex coordination of inputs from different levels of the nervous system. In humans, the composition of the ejaculate is released from participating organs in a particular order. The first portion of the ejaculate comes from the bulbourethral glands, followed by some fluid from the prostate including a few spermatozoa. Afterwards, the main fraction of the ejaculate, including the bulk of the spermatozoa, is contributed by the epididymis and vas deferens, combined with the remainder of the prostatic fluid as well as the seminal vesicle contribution. Adequate sensory stimulation of the dorsal penile nerve combined with posterior urethral distention is generally required to trigger an ejaculatory response. This has been proven in humans by the demonstration of electromyographic activity of the bulbospongiosus muscles upon distension of the posterior urethra or sacral root stimulation [11,12].

The emission of the seminal fluid is controlled by the sympathetic nervous system activating propulsive contraction of smooth muscle of the prostate, vas deferens, and seminal vesicles as well as prostatic glandular secretion. Several studies have documented a contractile response of the vasa deferentia, seminal vesicles, prostate, and urethra as a result of sympathetic nervous system activation by stimulation of sympathetic nerve fibers within the hypogastric or splanchnic nerves or by sympathomimetic medications [13].

Besides the adrenergic and cholinergic influences, experimental studies have revealed that vasoactive intestinal polypeptide (VIP) and neuropeptide Y are involved in the contraction and secretion of prostate and seminal vesicles [13]. The important role of the sympathetic pathway in the ejaculatory process in humans is emphasized by the fact that interruption of the innervation of the bladder neck, vas deferens, and the prostate lead to a retrograde ejaculation or, if severe enough, to failure of emission. Protection of sympathetic efferents during surgical procedures in the retroperitoneum or in the pelvis preserves normal ejaculatory function. In patients with spinal cord injury an ejaculation can be achieved clinically though electroejaculation, but it has also been achieved through electric stimulation of the hypogastric plexus activating sympathetic efferents [14].

The somatic nervous system represented by the pudendal nerve is exclusively responsible for the expulsion phase of ejaculation. The synchronous activation of ischiocavernosus, bulbospongiosus, and levator ani muscles, as well as the perineal striated muscles and the anal and urethral external sphincters innervated by the pudendal nerve, causes the powerful thrust of seminal fluid out of the urethra [15]. Patients with sacral spinal cord injuries after trauma (the pudendal nerve arises from sacral segments S2–S4) or patients with neuropathies (e.g., diabetes) typically show a dribbling ejaculation, due to the missing motor innervation of the propulsive pelvic musculature [16].

Summary

Ejaculation is a complex reflex involving sympathetic, parasympathetic, and somatic neural centers and pathways. The precise coordination of events result in bladder neck closure, external sphincter opening, and rhythmic contraction of the periurethral musculature leading to expulsion of semen in an antegrade fashion from the urethral meatus.

References

1. McMahon CG, Abdo C, Incrocci L, *et al.* Disorders of orgasm and ejaculation in men. *J Sex Med* 2004; 1: 58–65.

2. Halata Z, Munger BL. The neuroanatomical basis for the protopathic sensibility of the human glans penis. *Brain Res* 1986; 371: 205–30.

3. Baron R, Janig W. Afferent and sympathetic neurons projecting into lumbar visceral nerves of the male rat. *J Comp Neurol* 1991; 314: 429–36.

4. Ueyama T, Arakawa H, Mizuno N. Central distribution of efferent and afferent components of the pudendal nerve in rat. *Anat Embryol (Berl)* 1987; 177: 37–49.

5. Nadelhaft I. Cholinergic axons in the rat prostate and neurons in the pelvic ganglion. *Brain Res* 2003; 989: 52–7.

6. Sato K., Kihara K. Spinal cord segments controlling the canine vas deferens and differentiation of the primate sympathetic pathways to the vas deferens. *Microsc Res Tech* 1998; 42: 390–7.

7. Truitt WA, Coolen LM. Identification of a potential ejaculation generator in the spinal cord. *Science* 2002; 297: 1566–9.

8. Coolen LM, Veening JG, Wells AB, Shipley MT. Afferent connections of the parvocellular subparafascicular thalamic nucleus in the rat: evidence for functional subdivisions. *J Comp Neurol* 2003; 463: 132–56.

9. Hamson DK, Watson NV. Regional brainstem expression of Fos associated with sexual behavior in male rats. *Brain Res* 2004; 1006: 233–40.

10. Heeb MM, Yahr P. Anatomical and functional connections among cell groups in the gerbil brain that are activated with ejaculation. *J Comp Neurol* 2001; 439: 248–58.

11. Opsomer RJ, Caramia MD, Zarola F, Pesce F, Rossini PM. Neurophysiological evaluation of central-peripheral sensory and motor pudendal fibres. *Electroencephalogr Clin Neurophysiol* 1989; 74: 260–70.

12. Shafik A, El Sibai O. Mechanism of ejection during ejaculation: identification of a urethrocavernosus reflex. *Arch Androl* 2000; 44: 77–83.

13. Giuliano F, Clément P. Neuroanatomy and physiology of ejaculation. *Annu Rev Sex Res* 2005; 16: 190–216.

14. Ohl DA, Sønksen J, Menge AC, McCabe M, Keller LM. Electroejaculation versus vibratory stimulation in spinal cord injured men: sperm quality and patient preference. *J Urol* 1997; 157: 2147–9.

15. Gerstenberg TC, Levin RJ, Wagner G. Erection and ejaculation in man: assessment of the electromyographic activity of the bulbocavernosus and ischiocavernosus muscles. *Br J Urol* 1990; 65: 395–402.

16. Vinik AI, Freeman R, Erbas T. Diabetic autonomic neuropathy. *Semin Neurol* 2003; 23: 365–72.

Chapter

5

History and physical examination

Ndidiamaka Onwubalili and Hossein Sadeghi-Nejad

Clinical diagnosis is an art, and the mastery of an art has no end; you can always be a better diagnostician
Logan Clendening

Introduction

Infertility is a stressful condition for couples who present to the clinician. Coexistence of a diagnosis of infertility after treatment for a malignancy can be devastating. Fortunately, improvement in the understanding of the contributing factors to male infertility and the development of assisted reproductive technologies (ART) have contributed to the management of the infertile couple. The potential for management of infertility in the patient with a history of a malignancy has been broadened as well. The American Society for Reproductive Medicine (ASRM) and the American Urological Association (AUA) have produced guidelines for the evaluation and management of male infertility. Recommendations for fertility preservation in cancer patients have also been developed by ASRM and the American Society of Clinical Oncology (ASCO).

Infertility is defined as the inability to achieve a pregnancy resulting in live birth after one year of unprotected intercourse. Most couples will become pregnant within one year, but about 15% will meet the criteria for infertility [1,2]. In almost 40% of cases, combined male and female factors are responsible for infertility, with approximately 20% of cases due solely to male factors [2]. About 35% of untreated infertile couples will conceive spontaneously over time [3]. During the first two years, conception rates are about 23%, with an additional 10% of couples conceiving over an additional two years [4]. Even in infertile couples, there is a baseline fertility rate of 1–3% per month, and the physician should be cognizant of this during evaluation and interpretation of results. The workup of infertility should be initiated at presentation regardless of whether the one-year time point has been met. The evaluation of the male should be undertaken in concert with that of the female partner to optimize the chances of success.

The goals of evaluation of the infertile male are similar to those in the non-cancer population and include identification of surgically reversible pathologies as well as those irreversible conditions that would benefit from ART. Other aims include unmasking of genetic causes for male infertility, endocrine disorders, malignancies, and those irreversible conditions that cannot be addressed with currently available ART [5,6].

Patients with conditions in this latter category may be appropriate candidates for counseling regarding the use of donor sperm or adoption procedures. Once an abnormality is identified, therapy can be directed towards the underlying condition. In many instances, a cause for an abnormal semen analysis may not be apparent and the empirical use of intrauterine insemination (IUI) or in-vitro fertilization (IVF) with intracytoplasmic sperm injection (ICSI) can offer a chance of conception.

History

A detailed history will not only help uncover underlying fertility issues, but, in combination with the physical examination, will provide a framework for additional imaging and laboratory testing, as well as directions for follow-up care. Young children should be questioned with a parent or primary caregiver. A

Fertility Preservation in Male Cancer Patients, ed. John P. Mulhall, Linda D. Applegarth, Robert D. Oates and Peter N. Schlegel.
Published by Cambridge University Press. © Cambridge University Press 2013.

few screening questions may be directed at the child so as to include him in the discussion. The elicitation of the history in adolescents and young men will require more sensitivity, and privacy should be assured when dealing with patients in this age group. Prefacing any questions with a statement such as "The questions I am about to ask you are routine and will help me to provide you with the best clinical care possible" is very important and serves to strengthen the lines of communication between the provider and the patient. For the cancer patient, a detailed history that includes an account of his cancer and related therapies is the critical starting point in the fertility evaluation. Patients who speak a different language or have impairments that hamper communication should have an appropriate interpreter present to assist in obtaining an accurate history.

A systematic and organized approach will render a more complete picture of the patient's chief complaint and pertinent medical history (Table 5.1). It is important to give the patient time to answer questions appropriately. Multiple interruptions by the clinician can create a difficult and frustrating interaction for even the most organized patient. Given the time constraints experienced by many clinicians in modern-day medicine, new patients who have a complicated medical history due to a chronic illness or malignancy can be challenging for even the most experienced specialists. In these patients, a more focused history and physical exam will be valuable. It is also important to remember that many patients may feel ashamed or embarrassed about symptoms they may have and need reassurance to be able to voice concerns.

Reproductive history

The physician will want to question the couple about the duration of unprotected intercourse. An assessment of the couple's knowledge about appropriate timing and frequency of intercourse in relation to the female ovulatory cycle may also reveal misconceptions about the fertile window in a natural menstrual cycle. Many couples may not realize that the optimal timing for sexual relations is the middle of the menstrual cycle. In a study of 221 women attempting conception naturally, conception occurred only when intercourse was during a six-day window that ended on the day of ovulation [7]. In the same study, daily intercourse demonstrated a cycle fecundability rate of 37%, while sexual intercourse on alternate days had a

Table 5.1. Components of the history of the infertile male

Reproductive history	Duration of infertility Coital frequency Prior pregnancies Previous therapies Partner evaluation
Sexual history	Coital frequency Use of lubricants Erectile dysfunction Premature ejaculation Masturbatory frequency Difficulty attaining orgasm
Childhood conditions	Cryptorchidism and surgical repair Hernia repair Testicular torsion Pubertal delay
Medical history	Systemic illness (hypertension, diabetes mellitus, sickle cell disease, renal disease, hepatic disease) Autoimmune disease History of malignancy Previous/current therapy
Surgical history	Bladder neck surgery Orchiectomy Pelvic surgery Retroperitoneal surgery Hernia repair Vasectomy Pelvic trauma
Infections	Mumps Tuberculosis Sexually transmitted infections Viral/febrile Urinary tract infections
Gonadotoxins	Medications Smoking Marijuana Alcohol
Family history	Malignancy (testicular cancer, lymphoma) Cystic fibrosis Hypogonadism
Review of systems	Headache Anosmia Visual changes Gynecomastia Galactorrhea Respiratory infections

similar rate of 33%. Fecundability dropped dramatically to 15% for couples who had sex once a week [7]. Once ovulation occurs, chances of fertilization are reduced, as the oocyte does not remain in the reproductive tract for very long. Hence, the current recommendation for optimizing natural fertility in couples is for sexual intercourse every two days during the six-day window, ending on the day of presumed ovulation [8].

A thorough assessment for the presence of sexual dysfunction should be undertaken. Sexual dysfunction is a relatively common problem that is influenced by both health-related and psychosocial factors. In an analysis of men representative of the general American sexually active male population aged 18–59 years, the prevalence of sexual dysfunction was approximately 31% [9]. Persistent sexual dysfunction can significantly impair quality of life and can lead to significant interpersonal relationship difficulties and worsen mental health issues. Sexual dysfunction, in both its psychogenic and organic (physiological) forms, can be a significant finding in patients with endocrinopathies or hypogonadism, and in cancer survivors. Sexual dysfunction in the latter category may be secondary to the cancer pathology itself or to the therapies directed at cancer eradication. Sexual dysfunction in male patients may include decreased libido, erectile dysfunction (ED), premature ejaculation, impaired orgasm, or a combination of these factors. Frequency of masturbation should be assessed with directed questioning to determine if sexual dysfunction is also present during masturbation. If normal sexual response occurs with masturbation, the patient may benefit from a psychological evaluation to explore the reasons for impaired performance with his sexual partner.

The use of any lubricants should be ascertained, as some have been shown to have an adverse effect on semen motility in vitro. In one study, over-the-counter lubricants such as K-Y Jelly and Astroglide rendered sperm non-motile and non-viable after in-vitro incubation for 60 minutes, while canola oil had no apparent negative effects [10]. Another study demonstrated a negative effect on semen parameters with olive oil, saliva and K-Y jelly [11], while the lubricant Pre-seed had no apparent detrimental effects on semen motility or chromatin integrity [12]. Couples should be advised to use mineral oil, canola oil, and the hydroxyethylcellulose-based lubricant, Pre-seed, if coital lubrication is needed.

Childhood illnesses and conditions

Any pertinent childhood history should be elicited, including a history of cryptorchidism (undescended testes), inguinal hernia, or testicular torsion. Age at occurrence and surgical management, if any, should also be obtained. Cryptorchidism is a condition where the testes do not descend into the scrotum and the testes can be located anywhere from the inferior pole of the kidney to the external inguinal canal. Prevalence is about 1% [13]. Bilateral cryptorchidism affects fertility more significantly than unilateral cryptorchidism [14,15], with evidence of increased serum FSH, decreased inhibin B, smaller testicular volume, and decreased motility and sperm concentration on semen analysis in patients with bilateral cryptorchidism compared to their counterparts with unilateral cryptorchidism [16]. There is evidence that surgical repair of unilateral cryptorchidism up to eight years of age may not negatively impact fertility potential [16]. However the histological appearance of the testis in patients repaired even after only one year of life is abnormal when compared to those repaired before [17]. One study demonstrated abnormal histology as early as six months of age in patients with cryptorchidism [18]. Based on these data, a recommendation for surgical repair as young as six months of age has been proposed [19]. Cryptorchidism is a major risk factor for the future development of testicular cancer. Approximately 10% of patients with testicular cancer have a history of cryptorchidism [20]. The relative risk for developing testicular cancer after a diagnosis of cryptorchidism was 7.5 in a British cohort study of 1075 boys followed after treatment with orchidopexy or hormones [21].

A history of testicular trauma or torsion should be noted, as either of these can cause testicular atrophy. There is evidence that a history of testicular torsion can impair semen parameters [22]. In addition, patients can develop anti-sperm antibodies regardless of whether they underwent orchidopexy or orchidectomy after testicular torsion [22]. However, the question of whether there is any significant impairment of fertility in patients with a history of unilateral testicular torsion remains controversial [23].

The patient should be questioned about pubertal development, with attention given to any abnormal milestones. An endocrinopathy may be present in patients with delayed pubertal development. A history of mumps orchitis can be a cause of testicular atrophy. With the introduction of the mumps vaccine in 1967, the number of cases of mumps has dropped significantly in the developed world, with a shift in incidence from young children to adolescents and young adults. In 10% of cases, both testes are affected [24,25]. Testicular damage is present in the form of interstitial edema causing increased pressure on the tunica albuginea, atrophy of the germinal epithelium, and hyalinization of the seminiferous tubules with eventual testicular atrophy [26].

Systemic diseases

A history of systemic illness including malignancy, autoimmune disease, sickle cell disease, or neurologic conditions should be elicited. Some of these conditions and their respective treatment modalities may cause sexual dysfunction or impair semen parameters many years later. Patients with diabetes mellitus and neurologic disorders such as multiple sclerosis are at significant risk for impaired urinary and sexual function. Sickle cell disease (SCD) poses a significant risk for erectile dysfunction due to priapism. Lifetime prevalence is approximately 35% in patients with SCD, with a significant number of patients experiencing erectile dysfunction after priapism [27]. SCD patients also have abnormal semen parameters (severe oligospermia or azoospermia) after therapy with hydroxyurea or hematopoietic stem cell transplantation [28], with obvious negative implications for future fertility. Myotonic dystrophy is associated with testicular atrophy [29] and abnormal sperm function [30]. A history of hypertension, especially if uncontrolled, increases the risk for peripheral vascular disease and erectile dysfunction. Patients with active autoimmune diseases such as rheumatoid arthritis, systemic sclerosis, lupus erythematosus, and ankylosing spondylitis are also at risk for hypoactive sexual desire and erectile dysfunction [31]. Patients who have recently experienced an acute febrile illness can have abnormal spermatogenesis for up to two months after the event [32]. An abnormal semen analysis in a patient with a history of recent febrile illness should prompt a repeat analysis over the subsequent 3–6 months for a more accurate assessment [6]. Tuberculosis may cause infertility by causing fibrosis and scarring within the genital tract [33]. Suspicion should arise in patients with a history of tuberculosis exposure or in those from countries with an endemic prevalence.

A history of frequent upper respiratory infections and infertility should alert the clinician to three distinct conditions associated with male infertility. Primary ciliary dyskinesia or immotile cilia syndrome (termed Kartagener syndrome when associated with situs inversus) results in sinusitis, bronchiectasis, and male infertility. Young's syndrome is characterized by azoospermia with chronic sinobronchial disease [34]. The azoospermia in this scenario is caused by epididymal obstruction due to thickening and inspissation of epididymal epithelial secretions. Approximately 97–98% of men with cystic fibrosis (CF) will present with azoospermia and congenital bilateral absence of the vas deferens (CBAVD) [35]. Over 70% of patients with CBAVD will have an identifiable mutation in the cystic fibrosis transmembrane conductance regulator gene (CFTR) [36]. The combination of the 5T allele in one copy of the CFTR gene with a CF mutation in the other is the most common cause of CBAVD [36]. Patients with a history of bilateral epididymitis may also present with obstructive azoospermia due to epididymal occlusion.

In a male infertility patient with headaches, vision changes, and galactorrhea, a high level of suspicion for a pituitary tumor should arise. Patients may also complain of decreased libido and erectile dysfunction. Although prolactinomas are more common in women, they are more likely to be seen as macroprolactinomas in men due to delayed diagnosis [37]. In Kallmann syndrome, patients present with absent or delayed secondary sexual characteristics and anosmia. This syndrome is a form of congenital hypogonadotropic hypogonadism due to gonadotropin-releasing hormone (GnRH) deficiency from the failure of neuroendocrine GnRH cells to migrate to the forebrain from the olfactory epithelium [38]. It has a male preponderance with a prevalence of 1 in 8000, with a much lower prevalence in women [38]. Patients with end-stage renal or hepatic disease may also present with symptoms of hypogonadism due to decreased clearance of prolactin.

Past surgical history

Records of prior surgeries and pathology reports should be requested and reviewed in detail for the safety of the patient and to prevent unnecessary surgical intervention. Prior surgical procedures may be relevant to the patient's current fertility status. Surgery to the bladder neck for voiding dysfunction can cause retrograde ejaculation, in the setting of normal orgasmic sensation. These patients will present with a complaint of low ejaculate volume. Pelvic and retroperitoneal surgery (prostatic surgery, retroperitoneal lymph node dissection) can also cause ejaculatory dysfunction. Sympathomimetic medications such as ephedrine and pseudoephedrine may improve seminal fluid volume in patients with retrograde ejaculation, although most of these patients will still require retrieval of sperm from alkalinized post-ejaculate urine, and processing for IUI or IVF-ICSI.

Complications that can occur after inguinal hernia repair in children include testicular atrophy, injury to the vas deferens, and iatrogenic cryptorchidism [39]. Similarly, any surgery on the scrotum such as removal of a hydrocele can damage the vas deferens and/or the epididymis.

Patients who have had a vasectomy will have obstructive azoospermia. Apart from the patient's cancer history that is relevant to this particular chapter, when vasectomy is identified as the cause of the patient's infertility status, these patients can be offered vasectomy reversal (vasovasostomy or vasoepididymostomy) or testicular sperm aspiration/extraction for use in ART.

Family history

Many conditions that impact the genitourinary system carry familial risk. For example, first-degree relatives of patients with renal cell carcinoma and testicular cancer carry an increased risk of developing the same malignancy [20,40].

Medications

The impact of medications on sexual health can be considerable. Medications used to treat hypertension and psychotropic medications can cause sexual dysfunction. Methotrexate, a commonly used chemotherapeutic agent for the treatment of malignancies and autoimmune disorders, has been associated with gynecomastia and reversible oligospermia [41]. Alkylating agents such as cyclophosphamide, also used to treat autoimmune diseases, can cause more prolonged seminal abnormalities, especially at higher doses, even in those treated prior to puberty [42]. Finasteride, clomiphene, and tricyclic antidepressants can cause gynecomastia. In-utero exposure to diethylstilbestrol (DES) caused a slightly increased risk of cryptorchidism and epididymal cysts in male offspring [43]. Anabolic steroid abuse, common in athletes, causes hypogonadotropic hypogonadism from suppression of the hypothalamic–pituitary–gonadal axis. In these cases, removal of the offending steroidal agent may be sufficient to restore normal hormonal function, although time to normal spermatogenesis is quite variable and additional therapies including gonadotropins are sometimes required [44]. A more inclusive list of spermatotoxic agents is found in Table 5.2.

Table 5.2. Spermatotoxic agents

Alcohol
Alpha-blockers
Anabolic steroids
Calcium channel blockers
Chemotherapeutic agents
Cimetidine
Colchicine
Diethylstilbestrol
Dilantin
Lead
Manganese
Marijuana
Nicotine
Nitrofurantoin
Pesticides
Spironolactone
Sulfasalazine
Valproic acid

Lifestyle exposures and occupational history

The use of cigarettes, alcohol, and other recreational drugs should be assessed, as heavy use can impact sexual function. Patients who smoke cigarettes are at increased risk for renal, bladder, and testicular cancer. Smoking can also cause peripheral vascular disease and worsen erectile dysfunction. The impact of smoking on male fertility has been historically difficult to measure, and data are conflicting [45]. The adverse effects of smoking on semen parameters have been documented [46–48], but translation to a negative impact on fertility in the male has been harder to demonstrate. Regardless, the negative effect of smoking on fertility and ART outcomes in women has been well documented, and men who are attempting to conceive should be actively encouraged to quit, based on the cumulative data [49]. Patients who consume large amounts of alcohol have abnormal reproductive hormone levels and semen parameters [50] and may report difficulty with sexual functioning. Hepatic dysfunction from chronic alcoholism can also cause abnormal liver clearance of estrogens, causing hypogonadism and testicular atrophy. However, moderate alcohol consumption does not appear to impact fertility [51].

Marijuana is associated with impairment of human sperm motility [52] and the acrosome reaction in vitro [53]. Gynecomastia may be secondary to heavy marijuana use, but studies have been conflicting. There has also been an association between cocaine use and low sperm count and motility [54]. Recreational drug abuse reduces inhibitions and leads to an increased risk of contracting sexually transmitted infections. If a positive history of recreational drug use or alcoholism is present, patients should be referred to an appropriate mental health provider. Caffeine use does not appear to have an impact on fertility [55].

Occupational exposures to any pesticides, herbicides, heavy metals, or solvents should also be determined. Accumulating evidence indicates that men who work with glycol ethers are at increased risk for semen analysis abnormalities [56]. There is evidence of impairment of semen parameters in men who use hot tubs or saunas on a regular basis [57]. If the semen analysis is abnormal, behavior modification may improve parameters, but in men with normal semen no modification is recommended [8].

Cancer and cancer therapies

Approximately 62 000 people between the ages of 20 and 39 years were diagnosed with invasive cancer in the United States in 2010 [58]. Many of these patients require potentially gonadotoxic therapy with chemotherapy and/or radiation. In males aged 15–39, tumors with the highest incidence are germ cell gonadal tumors, lymphomas (Hodgkin's and non-Hodgkin's), melanoma, carcinoma of the gastrointestinal tract, and soft tissue sarcomas [59]. In recent decades, survival for these malignancies has improved significantly, with many patients expressing a strong desire to have biological children [60].

Cancer affects fertility in a multipronged fashion by induction of a catabolic state, and through changes in the endocrine and nutritional milieu [61]. There is also a postulated effect of cytokine release on spermatogenesis. Testicular malignancies and Hodgkin's disease (HD) have characteristic endocrinologic derangements that are harmful to spermatogenesis. The effect of sarcomas on fertility remains less clear. Patients who survive one malignancy are at increased risk for a second one. They should be questioned about any stigmata of malignancy such as nodal swelling, lower extremity edema, facial swelling, weakness, or night sweats.

Testicular cancer

This is the most common cancer in men aged 25–40 years, with an estimated 8000 new cases in 2008 [61]. A young man with a retroperitoneal, supraclavicular, or mediastinal mass should be suspected of having an underlying germ cell cancer until proven otherwise

[62]. Risk factors for testicular cancer include contralateral testicular tumor, undescended testis, poor semen analysis, and testicular tumor in a first-degree relative [62]. Testicular tumors disrupt spermatogenesis by destroying surrounding tissue, secretion of beta-human chorionic gonadotropin (β-hCG), elevation of intrascrotal temperature, and changes in local blood flow [61]. Germ cell tumors (GCTs) secrete β-hCG, which increases testicular steroidogenesis with subsequent increases in testosterone and estrogen production. Estrogen is produced in higher amounts, with an increase in the estrogen/androgen ratio. Non-germ cell tumors (NGCTs) cause direct secretion of estrogen from the Leydig cells [63]. Approximately 7–11% of men with testicular cancer have gynecomastia as a presenting symptom [63]. The relative risk for testicular cancer in the contralateral normally descended testis in unilateral cryptorchid men was estimated at 3.6 in a Danish cohort study [64]. On average, survivors of testicular cancer are five times more likely to experience distress about fertility and are six times more likely to experience difficulty in fathering children [65]. However, in patients treated with surgery only or with chemotherapy and surgery, there was no eventual difference in rates of fatherhood compared to controls [65]. In one study, survivors of testicular cancer were three times as likely as their normal counterparts to have hypogonadism with accompanying evidence of impaired Leydig cell function [66]. In another study of survivors of childhood cancers, hypogonadism was six times as likely in subjects compared to controls, with the highest risk factors being brain surgery, chemotherapy, and testicular irradiation [67]. Patients who have been diagnosed with testicular cancer are at increased risk for a contralateral second testicular primary, with a cumulative risk of 2% over 15 years [68]. For patients who have not yet initiated treatment for malignancy, ASCO recommends that semen cryopreservation as an option to preserve fertility is discussed.

Hodgkin's disease (HD)

Survival from HD has improved more than 60% since the 1970s [61]. At the time of diagnosis, 70% of patients with HD will have abnormalities in semen parameters at baseline, prior to chemotherapy [69]. The baseline testicular dysfunction is presumably due to abnormal germ cell genetics, endocrinopathies, systemic cytokine release deleterious to Leydig cells and seminiferous tubules, and adverse local effects from intratesticular lymphatic tissue [61]. In one study of HD patients prior to chemotherapy, presence of B symptoms (night sweats, fever) correlated with worsening semen parameters [70].

Cancer therapies

The three modalities used are surgery, chemotherapy, and radiation. In patients being treated surgically for testicular cancer with retroperitoneal lymph node dissection, retrograde ejaculation is a potential postoperative adverse event. Unilateral nerve-sparing surgery preserves sexual function in a significant number of patients without increasing the risk of local recurrence [71–73]. In a recent retrospective study of 341 patients with testicular cancer who underwent nerve-sparing post-chemotherapy retroperitoneal lymph node dissection (PC-RPLND), 79% of patients reported postoperative antegrade ejaculation, with risk factors for retrograde ejaculation being a right-sided primary testicular tumor and a residual mass ≥ 5 cm [73].

Radiation therapy is a mainstay of treatment for both HD and testicular cancer. Radiation can cause significant sperm DNA damage that can last up to two years after treatment [61]. Gonadotoxicity depends on dosage and delivery method. Even if gonads are shielded, they can still receive a significant amount of scattered radiation. The upper dose limit required to cause permanent azoospermia is not known, but > 1.2 Gy will increase time to resumption of spermatogenesis, and may impede recovery altogether [61]. Total body irradiation is highly associated with infertility, while lesser doses and limited-field radiation are associated with lower rates of gonadal toxicity [74].

Alkylating agents (cyclophosphamide, ifosfamide, nitrosureas, and procarbazine) pose the greatest risk to infertility of the chemotherapeutic agents [74]. ASCO recommends that clinicians inform patients of the detrimental effect of these medications on fertility. Patients may wish to exercise the option to cryopreserve sperm prior to therapy. Agents associated with low or no risk of infertility are methotrexate, fluorouracil, vincristine, bleomycin, and dactinomycin [74].

Physical examination

Prepare the patient for the examination by informing him to remove clothing over areas to be examined. The patient's permission should be obtained before proceeding. Adult patients should be given the option of asking accompanying family members to exit the room for the physical exam. Younger patients may prefer to have family present. Patients should be warned to expect touch during different portions of the exam, which can help to reduce anticipatory anxiety. A warm, well-lit room and suitable chaperones when indicated are recommended for the genitourinary exam.

The patient should be asked to stand without clothing, and inspection of the skin, neck, chest, abdomen, and groin should be performed. Note should be made of any skin changes, gynecomastia, thinness, or obesity. Edema of the genitalia and lower extremities may indicate malignancy. Asymmetry, if present, should be noted for examination. Secondary sexual characteristics should also be noted.

Gloves should be worn for this portion of the physical exam. The male external genitalia should first be inspected. Any skin changes, pigmented nevi, warts, hemorrhagic lesions, or skin piercings should be noted. With the provider seated, the patient should be asked to stand facing the provider, as certain lesions (varicoceles, hernias) may be seen with standing and performance of the Valsalva maneuver. The patient should be examined both in the standing and supine positions. This examination should include the penis, scrotum, and scrotal contents.

Penis

Note the development of the penis and the surrounding pubic hair growth. Penile skin should be inspected for any rashes, warts, or other lesions. If a foreskin is present, retract it and inspect the glans. In an uncircumcised adult male, the foreskin should easily be retracted. The foreskin should be replaced after the glans is examined. If the foreskin cannot be replaced, it can constrict the glans painfully in a condition called paraphimosis. The glans should be free of any nodules or ulcers, which can be indicative of penile cancer. Penile cancer is almost exclusively found in uncircumcised men, and any lesion on the glans in an uncircumcised patient warrants special attention. Inspect the urethral meatus by holding the penis between the thumb and forefinger, paying attention to its position on the glans. Hypospadias refers to a urethral meatus that is located proximally to the tip of the glans on the ventral surface, while a meatus that is on the dorsal surface is termed epispadias. Both of

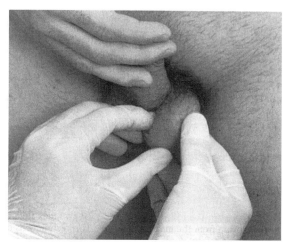

Figure 5.1. Technique for palpation of the testicle. (Reproduced with permission from Swartz MH. Male genitalia and hernias. In *Textbook of Physical Diagnosis: History and Examination*, 6th edn. Philadelphia, PA: Saunders Elsevier, 2010.)

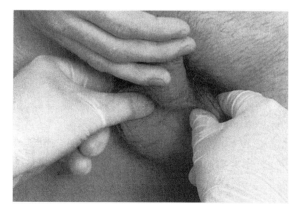

Figure 5.2. Technique for palpation of the spermatic cord. (Reproduced with permission from Swartz MH. Male genitalia and hernias. In *Textbook of Physical Diagnosis: History and Examination*, 6th edn. Philadelphia, PA: Saunders Elsevier, 2010.)

these conditions may interfere with semen deposition in the female genital tract and should be recognized. Note any urethral discharge or tenderness along the ventral penile shaft, which can be a sign of urethritis or mucosal lesions near the urethra. Significant induration or "plaques" involving the tunica albuginea of the penis, most commonly noted along the dorsal or lateral penile shaft, and usually accompanied by shaft deviation in the erect state, is consistent with Peyronie's disease. Ventral plaques along the urethra may also be palpated, and these are attributed to Peyronie's disease or urethral manipulation syndrome, a term used for fibrosis and induration of corpus spongiosum, which is secondary to endoscopic urethral instrumentation (i.e., post-cystourethroscopy).

Scrotum

The scrotum is a loose sac containing the testes and spermatic cord structures. The scrotal wall contains the dartos muscle with investing fascia and the parietal layer of the tunica vaginalis. The scrotum should be lifted and its posterior surface inspected. Note any swelling or asymmetry. A bulge or swelling in the scrotum can be indicative of a hernia or a hydrocele. When a palpable scrotal mass is present, transillumination with a light source in a dark room can help to determine the nature of the mass. A cystic mass such as a hydrocele is easily transilluminated, whereas a solid mass will not transmit light.

The testes are ovoid, smooth, and of firm consistency in the normal state. They should be examined for size, symmetry, descent, and any masses. The normal adult testis is approximately 4.5–5.0 cm in length with a volume of 15–25 mL [75,76]. Examination is performed by grasping the testes between the thumb and fingers and applying gentle pressure (Fig. 5.1). A small and soft testis is indicative of abnormal spermatogenesis or hypogonadism. Any firm or nodular area should be concerning for testicular cancer until proven otherwise.

The epididymis is located posterolateral to the testis and is smooth in contour. An enlarged epididymis should increase suspicion for an epididymal obstruction. An epididymal cyst or spermatocele can be palpated as a solitary, smooth, and rounded outline and is usually benign. A tender epididymis is suggestive of epididymitis and is a common cause of acute scrotal pain [77]. It is more common in sexually active males. Primary tumors of the epididymis are rare, and most findings on exam will be benign.

Each spermatic cord and vas deferens should be palpated by placing the thumb on the anterolateral side of the scrotum, superior to the testicle (Fig. 5.2). The vas deferens should feel like a thick and rubbery string (*al dente* macaroni) that is distinct from the spermatic cord. The two sides should be compared while being palpated simultaneously. A thickened vas deferens may be indicative of chronic infection, but interestingly, the vasa are often normal to palpation in cases of testicular malignancy ("the sign of the vas") [78]. Absence of the vas deferens is usually bilateral, although it can be unilateral as well. Both of these conditions are well-recognized causes of obstructive azoospermia. Obstructive azoospermia can also be seen in unilateral vasal agenesis when there is contralateral atresia of the vas deferens or seminal vesicle [79]. A varicocele is a dilation of the testicular vein and pampiniform plexus. About 15% of adult men have a varicocele, with the rate increasing to 40% in infertile men [77,80]. This can be visually noted as fullness in the scrotum above the testis with inspection. This frequently described "bag of worms" is seen usually on the left side and increases with size on standing (grade 3) or Valsalva (grade 2). A grade 1 varicocele is palpable with Valsalva in the standing position. This fullness should disappear with the supine position, and if it persists a retroperitoneal mass or cord lipoma should be suspected. Subclinical varicoceles are not palpable on exam and are only seen with imaging modalities.

Digital rectal examination

Patients without mobility impairments should be asked to place both elbows on the examination table and feet apart with the backside to the physician. In a patient who may be unable to assume this position, having him lie on the examination table in the left lateral position will suffice.

The buttocks should be spread apart and the skin examined. Any warts, rash, or fissures should be noted. With a generous amount of lubrication applied, the index finger should first rest near the anal sphincter and then be inserted carefully into the anal canal. A slight pause to allow the patient to adjust should then be followed by full insertion of the finger. Sphincter tone is assessed by asking the patient to squeeze around the finger. Examine the posterior and lateral walls of the rectum by sweeping the finger 180 degrees. Any masses, polyps, or extreme tenderness should be noted.

The prostate gland is a walnut-sized organ that should be about 4 cm in length and width. Its surface should be smooth with a rubbery consistency. Palpate the medial sulcus and the lateral lobes. If there is prostatitis, the prostate may be indurated or tender, and may be very hard with prostate cancer. Symmetrical enlargement of the gland with loss of the median sulcus is consistent with bilateral prostatic hyperplasia and should not be present in a young man. Once the exam is concluded, the color of any fecal material

is noted before removing the glove and a fecal occult blood screen is performed if indicated.

Summary

The history and physical examination are critical components in the evaluation of the infertility patient. Sexual dysfunction is commonly encountered in the cancer patient and may not only impair fertility, but can also have a significant adverse effect on the patient's quality of life as well. The optimal fertility preservation strategy will start with a thorough history and physical examination to lay the foundations for arriving at the best management plan and to avoid unnecessary interventions.

References

1. Hull MG, Glazener CM, Kelly NJ, *et al*. Population study of causes, treatment, and outcome of infertility. *Br Med J* 1985; 291: 1693–7.

2. Thonneau P, Marchand S, Tallec A, *et al*. Incidence and main causes of infertility in a resident population (1,850,000) of three French regions (1988–1989). *Hum Reprod* 1991; 6: 811–16.

3. Collins JA, Wrixon W, Janes LB, Wilson EH. Treatment-independent pregnancy among infertile couples. *N Engl J Med*. 1983; 309: 1201–6.

4. Aafjes JH, van der Vijver JC, Schenck PE. The duration of infertility: an important datum for the fertility prognosis of men with semen abnormalities. *Fertil Steril* 1978; 30: 423–5.

5. Sadeghi-Nejad H. Evaluation of the infertile male: part 1. *Postgrad Obstet Gynecol* 2009; 29: 1–7.

6. Sigman M, Jarow J. Male infertility. In Wein AJ, Kavoussi LR, Novick AC, Partin AW, Peters CA. *Campbell–Walsh Urology*, 9th edn. Philadelphia, PA: Saunders, 2007;

7. Wilcox AJ, Weinberg CR, Baird DD. Timing of sexual intercourse in relation to ovulation. Effects on the probability of conception, survival of the pregnancy, and sex of the baby. *N Engl J Med* 1995; 333: 1517–21.

8. Optimizing natural fertility. *Fertil Steril* 2008; 90 (5 Suppl): S1–6.

9. Laumann EO, Paik A, Rosen RC. Sexual dysfunction in the United States: prevalence and predictors. *JAMA* 1999; 281: 537–44.

10. Kutteh WH, Chao CH, Ritter JO, Byrd W. Vaginal lubricants for the infertile couple: effect on sperm activity. *Int J Fertil Menopausal Stud* 1996; 41: 400–4.

11. Anderson L, Lewis SE, McClure N. The effects of coital lubricants on sperm motility in vitro. *Hum Reprod* 1998; 13: 3351–6.

12. Agarwal A, Deepinder F, Cocuzza M, Short RA, Evenson DP. Effect of vaginal lubricants on sperm motility and chromatin integrity: a prospective comparative study. *Fertil Steril* 2008; 89: 375–9.

13. Berkowitz GS, Lapinski RH, Dolgin SE, *et al.* Prevalence and natural history of cryptorchidism. *Pediatrics* 1993; 92: 44–9.

14. Cendron M, Keating MA, Huff DS, *et al.* Cryptorchidism, orchiopexy and infertility: a critical long-term retrospective analysis. *J Urol* 1989; 142: 559–62.

15. Lee PA. Fertility after cryptorchidism: epidemiology and other outcome studies. *Urology* 2005; 66: 427–31.

16. Trsinar B, Muravec UR. Fertility potential after unilateral and bilateral orchidopexy for cryptorchidism. *World J Urol* 2009; 27: 513–9.

17. McAleer IM, Packer MG, Kaplan GW, *et al.* Fertility index analysis in cryptorchidism. *J Urol* 1995; 153: 1255–8.

18. Hadziselimovic F, Herzog B. The importance of both an early orchidopexy and germ cell maturation for fertility. *Lancet* 2001; 358: 1156–7.

19. Hutson JM, Hasthorpe S. Testicular descent and cryptorchidism: the state of the art in 2004. *J Pediatr Surg* 2005; 40: 297–302.

20. Shaw J. Diagnosis and treatment of testicular cancer. *Am Fam Physician* 2008; 77: 469–74.

21. Swerdlow AJ, Higgins CD, Pike MC. Risk of testicular cancer in cohort of boys with cryptorchidism. *BMJ* 1997; 314: 1507–11.

22. Arap MA, Vicentini FC, Cocuzza M, *et al.* Late hormonal levels, semen parameters, and presence of antisperm antibodies in patients treated for testicular torsion. *J Androl* 2007; 28: 528–32.

23. Puri P, Barton D, O'Donnell B. Prepubertal testicular torsion: subsequent fertility. *J Pediatr Surg* 1985; 20: 598–601.

24. Ternavasio-de la Vega HG, Boronat M, Ojeda A, *et al.* Mumps orchitis in the post-vaccine era (1967–2009): a single-center series of 67 patients and review of clinical outcome and trends. *Medicine (Baltimore)* 2010; 89: 96–116.

25. Werner CA. Mumps orchitis and testicular atrophy; occurrence. *Ann Intern Med.* 1950; 32: 1066–74.

26. Hviid A, Rubin S, Muhlemann K. Mumps. *Lancet* 2008; 371: 932–44.

27. Adeyoju AB, Olujohungbe AB, Morris J, *et al.* Priapism in sickle-cell disease; incidence, risk factors and complications – an international multicentre study. *BJU Int* 2002; 90: 898–902.

28. Lukusa AK, Vermylen C, Vanabelle B, *et al.* Bone marrow transplantation or hydroxyurea for sickle cell anemia: long-term effects on semen variables and hormone profiles. *Pediatr Hematol Oncol* 2009; 26: 186–94.

29. Bolanos F, Lopez-Amor E, Vasquez G, Lisker R, Morato T. Hypothalamic-pituitary-gonadal function in two siblings with Prader-Willi syndrome. *Rev Invest Clin* 1974; 26: 53–62.

30. Hortas ML, Castilla JA, Gil MT, *et al.* Decreased sperm function of patients with myotonic muscular dystrophy. *Hum Reprod* 2000; 15: 445–8.

31. Ostensen M. New insights into sexual functioning and fertility in rheumatic diseases. *Best Pract Res Clin Rheumatol* 2004; 18: 219–32.

32. Carlsen E, Andersson AM, Petersen JH, Skakkebaek NE. History of febrile illness and variation in semen quality. *Hum Reprod* 2003; 18: 2089–92.

33. Kumar R. Reproductive tract tuberculosis and male infertility. *Indian J Urol* 2008; 24: 392–5.

34. de Iongh R, Ing A, Rutland J. Mucociliary function, ciliary ultrastructure, and ciliary orientation in Young's syndrome. *Thorax* 1992; 47: 184–7.

35. van der Ven K, Messer L, van der Ven H, Jeyendran RS, Ober C. Cystic fibrosis mutation screening in healthy men with reduced sperm quality. *Hum Reprod* 1996; 11: 513–17.

36. Chillon M, Casals T, Mercier B, *et al.* Mutations in the cystic fibrosis gene in patients with congenital absence of the vas deferens. *N Engl J Med* 1995; 332: 1475–80.

37. Carter JN, Tyson JE, Tolis G, *et al.* Prolactin-screening tumors and hypogonadism in 22 men. *N Engl J Med* 1978; 299: 847–52.

38. Hardelin JP, Dode C. The complex genetics of Kallmann syndrome: KAL1, FGFR1, FGF8, PROKR2, PROK2, *et al. Sex Dev* 2008; 2: 181–93.

39. Brandt ML. Pediatric hernias. *Surg Clin North Am* 2008; 88: 27–43, vii–viii.

40. Karami S, Schwartz K, Purdue MP, *et al.* Family history of cancer and renal cell cancer risk in Caucasians and African Americans. *Br J Cancer* 2010; 102: 1676–80.

41. Pandhi D, Gupta R, Singal A. Gynaecomastia with oligospermia: an unusual complication of low-dose methotrexate for pustular psoriasis. *Clin Exp Dermatol* 2006; 31: 138–40.

42. Kenney LB, Laufer MR, Grant FD, Grier H, Diller L. High risk of infertility and long term gonadal damage in males treated with high dose cyclophosphamide for sarcoma during childhood. *Cancer* 2001; 91: 613–21.

43. Whitehead ED, Leiter E. Genital abnormalities and abnormal semen analyses in male patients exposed to diethylstilbestrol in utero. *J Urol* 1981; 125: 47–50.

44. Gazvani MR, Buckett W, Luckas MJ, *et al.* Conservative management of azoospermia following steroid abuse. *Hum Reprod* 1997; 12: 1706–8.

45. Dikshit RK, Buch JG, Mansuri SM. Effect of tobacco consumption on semen quality of a population of hypofertile males. *Fertil Steril* 1987; 48: 334–6.

46. Gaur DS, Talekar M, Pathak VP. Effect of cigarette smoking on semen quality of infertile men. *Singapore Med J* 2007; 48: 119–23.

47. Vine MF, Tse CK, Hu P, Truong KY. Cigarette smoking and semen quality. *Fertil Steril* 1996; 65: 835–42.

48. Elshal MF, El-Sayed IH, Elsaied MA, El-Masry SA, Kumosani TA. Sperm head defects and disturbances in spermatozoal chromatin and DNA integrities in idiopathic infertile subjects: association with cigarette smoking. *Clin Biochem* 2009; 42: 589–94.

49. Waylen AL, Metwally M, Jones GL, Wilkinson AJ, Ledger WL. Effects of cigarette smoking upon clinical outcomes of assisted reproduction: a meta-analysis. *Hum Reprod Update* 2009; 15: 31–44.

50. Muthusami KR, Chinnaswamy P. Effect of chronic alcoholism on male fertility hormones and semen quality. *Fertil Steril* 2005; 84: 919–24.

51. Olsen J, Bolumar F, Boldsen J, Bisanti L. Does moderate alcohol intake reduce fecundability? A European multicenter study on infertility and subfecundity. European Study Group on Infertility and Subfecundity. *Alcohol Clin Exp Res* 1997; 21: 206–12.

52. Rossato M, Ion Popa F, Ferigo M, Clari G, Foresta C. Human sperm express cannabinoid receptor Cb1, the activation of which inhibits motility, acrosome reaction, and mitochondrial function. *J Clin Endocrinol Metab* 2005; 90: 984–91.

53. Whan LB, West MC, McClure N, Lewis SE. Effects of delta-9-tetrahydrocannabinol, the primary psychoactive cannabinoid in marijuana, on human sperm function in vitro. *Fertil Steril* 2006; 85: 653–60.

54. Bracken MB, Eskenazi B, Sachse K, *et al.* Association of cocaine use with sperm concentration, motility, and morphology. *Fertil Steril* 1990; 53: 315–22.

55. Curtis KM, Savitz DA, Arbuckle TE. Effects of cigarette smoking, caffeine consumption, and alcohol intake on fecundability. *Am J Epidemiol* 1997; 146: 32–41.

56. Cherry N, Moore H, McNamee R, *et al.* Occupation and male infertility: glycol ethers and other exposures. *Occup Environ Med* 2008; 65: 708–14.

57. Saikhun J, Kitiyanant Y, Vanadurongwan V, Pavasuthipaisit K. Effects of sauna on sperm movement characteristics of normal men measured by computer-assisted sperm analysis. *Int J Androl* 1998; 21: 358–63.

58. Bleyer A, Barr R. Cancer in young adults 20 to 39 years of age: overview. *Semin Oncol* 2009; 36: 194–206.

59. SEER cancer statistics review, 1975–2007. National Cancer Institute. Bethesda, MD. http://seer.cancer.gov/csr/1975_2007 (accessed September 2010).

60. Schover LR, Rybicki LA, Martin BA, Bringelsen KA. Having children after cancer. A pilot survey of survivors' attitudes and experiences. *Cancer* 1999; 86: 697–709.

61. Sabanegh ES, Jr., Ragheb AM. Male fertility after cancer. *Urology* 2009; 73: 225–31.

62. Krege S, Beyer J, Souchon R, *et al.* European consensus conference on diagnosis and treatment of germ cell cancer: a report of the second meeting of the European Germ Cell Cancer Consensus group (EGCCCG): part I. *Eur Urol* 2008; 53: 478–96.

63. Hassan HC, Cullen IM, Casey RG, Rogers E. Gynaecomastia: an endocrine manifestation of testicular cancer. *Andrologia* 2008; 40: 152–7.

64. Prener A, Engholm G, Jensen OM. Genital anomalies and risk for testicular cancer in Danish men. *Epidemiology* 1996; 7: 14–19.

65. Kim C, McGlynn KA, McCorkle R, *et al.* Fertility among testicular cancer survivors: a case-control study in the U.S. *J Cancer Surviv* 2010; 4: 266–73.

66. Nord C, Bjoro T, Ellingsen D, *et al.* Gonadal hormones in long-term survivors 10 years after treatment for unilateral testicular cancer. *Eur Urol* 2003; 44: 322–8.

67. Romerius P, Stahl O, Moell C, *et al.* Hypogonadism risk in men treated for childhood cancer. *J Clin Endocrinol Metab.* 2009 Nov; 94(11): 4180–6.

68. Fossa SD, Chen J, Schonfeld SJ, *et al.* Risk of contralateral testicular cancer: a population-based study of 29,515 U.S. men. *J Natl Cancer Inst* 2005; 97: 1056–66.

69. Rueffer U, Breuer K, Josting A, *et al.* Male gonadal dysfunction in patients with Hodgkin's disease prior to treatment. *Ann Oncol* 2001; 12: 1307–11.

70. van der Kaaij MA, Heutte N, van Echten-Arends J, *et al.* Sperm quality before treatment in patients with early stage Hodgkin's lymphoma enrolled in EORTC-GELA Lymphoma Group trials. *Haematologica* 2009; 94: 1691–7.

71. Nonomura N, Nishimura K, Takaha N, *et al.* Nerve-sparing retroperitoneal lymph node dissection for advanced testicular cancer after chemotherapy. *Int J Urol* 2002; 9: 539–44.

72. Miki T, Mizutani Y, Nakamura T, *et al.*
    Post-chemotherapy nerve-sparing retroperitoneal
    lymph node dissection for advanced germ cell tumor.
    Int J Urol 2009; 16: 379–82.

73. Pettus JA, Carver BS, Masterson T, Stasi J, Sheinfeld J.
    Preservation of ejaculation in patients undergoing
    nerve-sparing postchemotherapy retroperitoneal
    lymph node dissection for metastatic testicular cancer.
    Urology 2009; 73: 328–31.

74. Lee SJ, Schover LR, Partridge AH, *et al.* American
    Society of Clinical Oncology recommendations on
    fertility preservation in cancer patients. *J Clin Oncol*
    2006; 24: 2917–31.

75. Prader A. Testicular size: assessment and clinical
    importance. *Triangle* 1966; 7: 240–3.

76. Tishler PV. Diameter of testicles. *N Engl J Med* 1971;
    285: 1489.

77. Wampler SM, Llanes M. Common scrotal and
    testicular problems. *Prim Care* 2010; 37:
    613–26.

78. Bailey H, Lumley JSP. *Hamilton Bailey's Physical Signs:
    Demonstrations of Physical Signs in Clinical Surgery*,
    18th edn. Oxford: Butterworth Heinemann,
    1997.

79. American Urological Association. *The Evaluation of
    the Azoospermic Male: AUA Best Practice Statement*,
    2010.

80. Dubin L, Amelar RD. Varicocelectomy: 986 cases in a
    twelve-year study. *Urology* 1977; 10: 446–9.

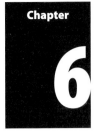

Chapter

6

Abnormalities of semen parameters

Daniel H. Williams IV and Jay I. Sandlow

Introduction

A critical component of the initial evaluation of a man's fertility potential is to obtain at least one and preferably several semen analyses. As described in Chapter 3, the core semen parameters include semen volume, sperm concentration, percentage of motile sperm, and an assessment of sperm morphology. In the strictest sense, an "abnormal" semen parameter refers to one that falls out of the reference range established by the laboratory performing the semen analysis. Most andrology laboratories adhere to the principles and methodology of performing and reporting semen analyses according to the WHO laboratory manual for the examination and processing of human semen [1]. However, other centers may have different reference ranges that are considered to be "normal." When a semen parameter falls below the lower fifth percentile, it is considered to be abnormal.

In this chapter, we review the various etiologies of abnormal semen parameters and highlight the potential impact of cancer and cancer therapy on them. Tests of sperm function, including sperm DNA fragmentation, are reviewed.

It is important to bear in mind that an abnormality of any given semen parameter does not necessarily mean that a man is infertile. Similarly, having semen parameters that are above the fifth percentile does not guarantee that a man is fertile, nor does it obviate the need for the male partner in an infertile couple to undergo a formal infertility evaluation.

Some men with "normal" semen parameters are faced with infertility, as defined by failure to achieve pregnancy within a 12-month period. Conversely, men with "abnormal" semen parameters often achieve paternity. A couple's success or failure in becoming pregnant can be due to multiple factors, both male and female. Additionally, having normal or abnormal semen parameters does not account for other important components of a man's reproductive function, nor is it a measurement or a predictor of a given sperm's ability to fertilize an egg or of the embryo's ability to develop normally.

Herein lies the challenges and frustrations for patients and providers alike when faced with interpreting abnormalities in semen parameters and how these abnormalities may or may not affect a couple's journey through the fertility process.

Low-volume ejaculate

A seminal volume of less than 1.5 mL falls below the fifth percentile [2] and may be considered "abnormal." If the volume of semen is low, then the overall total motile sperm count will be low. For example, even if sperm concentration and motility are within normal parameters, the total motile sperm count may not be adequate for fertilization if there is a low volume of ejaculate.

Causes of low-volume ejaculate (Table 6.1) can include anatomical conditions such as complete ejaculatory duct obstruction, partial ejaculatory duct obstruction, atresia, or absence of seminal vesicles; neurological conditions or medications that lead to ejaculatory dysfunction or retrograde ejaculation, including spinal cord injury, diabetes, multiple sclerosis, alpha-blockers, and selective serotonin uptake inhibitors; and physiological conditions such as hypogonadism. Therefore, these causes can be due to blockage of the outflow tract, absence of the required organs, neurologic dysfunction which prevents transport of the semen through the tract (including

Fertility Preservation in Male Cancer Patients, ed. John P. Mulhall, Linda D. Applegarth, Robert D. Oates and Peter N. Schlegel. Published by Cambridge University Press. © Cambridge University Press 2013.

Table 6.1. Causes of low-volume ejaculate

Ejaculatory duct obstruction (partial or complete)
Congenital bilateral absence of the vas deferens
Atresia/absence of seminal vesicles
Bladder neck incompetence
Transurethral resection/incision of the prostate
Retrograde ejaculation
Anejaculation
Spinal cord injury
Stroke or traumatic brain injury
Low abdominal or pelvic surgery
Retroperitoneal lymph node dissection
Diabetes
Multiple sclerosis
Peripheral neuropathy
Myelodysplasia
Antidepressants
Alpha receptor antagonists
Hypogonadism
Anorgasmia
Idiopathic

Table 6.2. Differential diagnosis of oligospermia

Primary testicular failure
Secondary testicular failure
Pituitary disorder
Varicocele
Numerical chromosome anomaly
Structural chromosomal anomaly
Y-chromosome microdeletion
Sperm chromosome aneuploidy
Environmental exposure to certain pesticides
Epididymal obstruction
Pituitary disorder
Pituitary tumor
Prolactinoma
Hypogonadism
Hypothyroidism
Cryptorchidism
Obesity
Idiopathic

medications), and hormonal dysfunction leading to decreased semen production.

The evaluation of low-volume ejaculate includes taking a focused medical history, reviewing any current medications, checking a post-ejaculatory urinalysis, and performing a transrectal ultrasound. It is also important to ask the patient about difficulties in collecting the entire ejaculate, as men who are not comfortable with masturbation may not catch the entire sample in the collection apparatus.

Prior to the transrectal ultrasound, patients should be instructed to ejaculate within 24 hours of the procedure to reduce the chance that a finding of seminal vesicle enlargement is due to infrequent ejaculation. If the patient has undergone antibiotic and enema prep, seminal vesicle aspiration may be performed, should they be enlarged. The fluid is examined under light microscopy for sperm. While there is no specific finding that is diagnostic of complete or partial ejaculatory duct obstruction, some authors report that > 3 sperm per high-power field is highly suggestive of an obstructive process [3].

Certain cancers and their treatment can put men at risk for having low-volume ejaculate. Following radical prostatectomy for prostate cancer, men will have no ejaculate. Likewise, radiotherapy for prostate cancer may effectively scar the ejaculatory ducts. For testicular cancer, the management of low-stage non-seminomatous germ cell tumors as well as persistent post-chemotherapy retroperitoneal lymphadenopathy can include retroperitoneal lymph node dissection (RPLND). Because the sympathetic nerves, which control ejaculation, are located in the same area as these lymph nodes, surgical node dissection can damage these nerves, leading to ejaculatory dysfunction. Although nerve-sparing templates have been developed to reduce the risk of ejaculatory dysfunction following RPLND, some men are still affected by this postoperative anejaculation, although in experienced hands the rate of this complication is approximately 5% [4].

Oligospermia

A sperm concentration of less than 15 million/mL falls below the fifth percentile for fertile men [2] and may be considered "abnormal." Conversely, the average "fertile" male most likely has a sperm concentration of 40–60 million/mL. Muddying the water even further, some feel that total sperm number per ejaculate is more important than sperm concentration [5]. Therefore, the use of terms such as "normal" can be misleading when referring to sperm production. A man's sperm concentration may be low if there is a problem with sperm production, if there is an obstruction in his reproductive tract, or less commonly if he has both a production and obstruction problem (Table 6.2). Isolated oligospermia is often idiopathic. Varicoceles may cause isolated oligospermia, but can also be accompanied by other abnormalities such as asthenospermia and teratospermia. See Chapter 8 for a more detailed discussion of varicoceles and their management.

In patients with less than 10 million sperm per mL, serum studies including follicle-stimulating hormone (FSH) and testosterone should be obtained. It is the authors' preference also to obtain a serum estradiol

Table 6.3. Differential diagnosis of asthenospermia

Environmental exposures
Exposure to excess heat
Varicoceles
Tobacco smoke
Excess seminal oxidants
Genital tract infections
Pyospermia
Partial ejaculatory duct obstruction
Defective transport through the genital ductal system
Presence of anti-sperm antibodies
Prolonged periods of abstinence
Sperm ultrastructural defects
Primary ciliary dyskinesia
Contaminants within the collection container
Human immunodeficiency virus
Obesity
Idiopathic

Table 6.4. Differential diagnosis of teratospermia

Idiopathic
Varicocele
Excess heat exposure
Ultrastructural defects
Illness
Drugs
Physical stress
Psychological stress

level, particularly if the man is overweight, as increased aromatization of testosterone to estradiol in adipose tissue can suppress FSH levels via a negative feedback to the pituitary gland. If abnormalities in these hormones are identified, a complete endocrine evaluation should be performed. An elevated FSH is suggestive of primary testicular failure, whereas a low or low-normal FSH in the setting of oligospermia suggests secondary (central) hypogonadism and should be further evaluated accordingly.

When sperm concentration is less than 5 million/mL, genetic testing is indicated. Specifically, a karyotype (analysis of chromosome number) and Y-chromosome gene microdeletion assay should be obtained [6].

Asthenospermia

A total sperm motility (progressive plus non-progressive) of less than 40% falls below the fifth percentile for fertile men [2] and may be considered "abnormal." Sperm motility is necessary for sperm to travel through the cervical mucus into the uterus and the fallopian tubes. While non-motile sperm in the ejaculate generally are considered non-viable, sperm viability assays can help determine between necrospermia (dead sperm) and viable sperm (see below).

Common causes of asthenospermia include chronic exposure to heat, toxins, radiation, environmental exposures, smoking, oxidants, genital tract infections associated with elevated seminal white blood cells, partial ejaculatory duct obstruction (EDO), anti-sperm antibodies, and periods of prolonged abstinence (Table 6.3). Whereas prolonged

abstinence and partial EDO cause motility problems from sperm stasis and death, anti-sperm antibodies are thought to attach to the sperm, causing clumping and lack of forward progression.

Sperm clumping (agglutination) may also result in low sperm motility. If sperm clumping is present, testing for anti-sperm antibodies may be considered. If anti-sperm antibodies are found, patients may require treatment with immunosuppressive agents. However, the success of medical therapy in treating anti-sperm antibodies is low, and such patients are often best served by proceeding with assisted reproduction, such as intrauterine insemination (IUI) or in-vitro fertilization with intracytoplasmic sperm injection (IVF-ICSI).

Severely low sperm motility (less than 5–10%) or the complete absence of motility raises the suspicion of ultrastructural defects in the sperm. When viability assays have demonstrated that non-motile sperm are indeed viable, electron microscopy may be performed. The most common sperm ultrastructural defect is primary ciliary dyskinesia, or immotile cilia syndrome. Kartagener syndrome refers to primary ciliary dyskinesia in the setting of situs inversus. Whereas the normal sperm exhibits the familiar 9×2 arrangement of dynein arms, these syndromes are characterized by either a lack of this arrangement or loss of these structures, resulting in poor flagellar movement and little or no motility.

Teratospermia

If the proportion of morphologically normal-appearing sperm is less than 4%, this falls below the fifth percentile for fertile men [2] and may be considered "abnormal." The cause of teratospermia is often idiopathic (Table 6.4). Varicoceles and exposure to excess heat may cause teratospermia [7]. Any debilitating illness, exposure to certain drugs, and physical and psychological stress may produce an increase in the number of abnormal sperm. Severe

Table 6.5. Differential diagnosis of leukocytospermia

Genitourinary tract infection
Orchitis
Epididymitis
Vasitis
Seminal vesiculitis
Prostatitis
Urethritis
Spinal cord injury
Human immunodeficiency virus
Idiopathic

sperm defects, such as globospermia, may be treated with ICSI, but pregnancy rates have been low.

The clinical significance, treatment, and implications of isolated teratospermia remain unclear because having "abnormal" sperm does not mean that a man has abnormal fertility potential [8,9]. Results of strict morphology (Tygerberg criteria) as it affects pregnancy rates with intrauterine insemination are mixed [10,11]. Similarly, some studies have shown a positive predictive value of strict morphology with IVF while others have not [12–14]. Lastly, there is a significant overlap of sperm parameters between fertile and infertile men, and sperm morphology has been shown not to be a useful discriminator between the two groups [15]. As such, a high number of abnormal sperm in a man's semen is most likely reflective of a spermatogenic defect arising from the testis and/or epididimis, but it does not necessarily represent a fertility problem per se, since many of these men are fertile [8].

Leukocytospermia

Leukocytospermia, or pyospermia, refers to the WHO threshold of $\geq$ 1 million white blood cells per mL of semen. Leukocytes in the semen can exert a deleterious effect on sperm and sperm function via a number of mechanisms including increased release of anti-sperm antibodies from plasma cells and cytokine-mediated release of reactive oxygen species and elastase from granulocytes. These pathways ultimately result in increased lipid peroxidation and DNA damage leading to spermatozoa dysfunction.

Genitourinary infection and/or inflammation can result in the presence of white blood cells (WBCs) in the semen. This process can occur anywhere in the reproductive tract including the testes, epididymides, prostate, seminal vesicles, or urethra (Table 6.5). The diagnosis of leukocytospermia requires more than simple quantification of round cells by light microscopy alone, as WBCs and immature germ cells share similar morphology. Quantification of seminal WBCs by immunohistochemical staining using CD45 antigens is considered the "gold standard." This technique provides the most accurate way to detect and quantify leukocytospermia. The peroxidase test may also be used to detect granulocytes, but it has lower sensitivity than immunohistochemistry.

Treatment of leukocytospermia is directed towards the underlying etiology and can include antimicrobials, anti-inflammatory agents, antioxidants, and antihistamines. In the setting of genitourinary infection, the choice of antimicrobial therapy depends on the identified organism and/or the suspected organ system that is affected. Certain antimicrobials penetrate the genitourinary tract better than others. Doxycycline, trimethoprim–sulfamethoxazole, and fluoroquinolones are typically the agents of choice for genitourinary tract infections because of their excellent tissue penetration. However, the efficacy of empirical use of antibiotics for leukocytospermia in the absence of a documented infection remains in question [16–18]. Non-steroidal anti-inflammatory medications can be used to lower seminal WBCs, particularly in the absence of infection [19]. Antioxidant therapy also has been shown to optimize semen parameters in the setting of leukocytospermia [20], as has the use of antihistamines [21]. Semen cultures may be obtained to assess for atypical organisms, and, if positive, directed antimicrobial therapy can be instituted.

Tests of sperm function

As noted above, the predictive value of conventional semen parameters is variable: men with "normal" parameters may have difficulty achieving paternity, while some men with semen parameters that fall below the fifth percentile are fertile. A number of tests of sperm function have been developed to assess a sperm's ability to fertilize an egg and to help predict whether or not the embryo will develop normally. Some of these tests include sperm penetration assay (SPA), hemizona assay, zona pellucida binding, sperm–oocyte fusion, acrosome reactions, viability assays, reactive oxygen species (ROS). Tests of sperm DNA integrity will be discussed in the following section.

Each of these studies examines only a very specific component of a sperm's fertility potential. Thus, none of these tests alone can determine if a man is fertile or infertile. Also, because of the low frequency of abnormal findings and the low predictive values of test results, coupled with the relatively high cost of running these assays, the clinical use of most of these tests has fallen out of favor. Additionally, the success of advanced reproductive technologies (ART), including ICSI, has undermined much of the clinical utility of these tests of sperm function. However, many of these tests are still used in the laboratory setting, for example in sperm toxicology studies.

While sperm motility is necessary for a sperm to reach an egg and fertilize it, a non-motile sperm is not necessarily a dead sperm. While unlikely to fertilize an egg on its own, a non-motile yet viable sperm may be used for ICSI. Tests of sperm viability include special stains assay such as trypan blue or eosin [1] as well as the hypo-osmotic swelling test. Currently, these tests typically are employed when sperm motility is less than 10%.

The acrosome is the structure surrounding the sperm head, and it contains enzymes that help the sperm penetrate the zona pellucida. When a sperm comes into contact with an egg, the zona pellucida will trigger the fusion of the acrosome with the sperm plasma membrane, which results in the release of these enzymes. The acrosome reaction can be induced in a laboratory setting and can help determine if there is a defect in this process. If the stimulated acrosome reaction scores are poor, then couples are often recommended ICSI over conventional IVF [22,23]. This test is generally reserved for men with "normal" semen quality prior to proceeding with ART.

The sperm penetration assay (SPA) is a test that evaluates the ability for a sperm to penetrate an egg. This test utilizes hamster ova that have had their zona pellucida removed by enzymes. Capacitated human sperm are then incubated with the hamster oocytes. Results are considered normal if more than 10–30% of the eggs have been penetrated by sperm [24]. There are many different protocols used for this assay, and failure for human sperm to penetrate hamster ova does not always predict failure with IVF. For these reasons, SPA is not used routinely in fertility evaluations. Some laboratories will use SPA results to direct couples towards ICSI over conventional IVF. However, if semen parameters are poor, couples will be directed towards ICSI anyway and may not benefit from this test.

The hemizona assay evaluates the ability of sperm to bind to the zona pellucida. Zonae pellucidae from non-living, non-fertilizable human eggs are divided in half. Each half is incubated with either the patient's sperm or fertile donor's sperm. A ratio of sperm binding is calculated, called the hemizona index. Historically, patients with poor hemizona indices have had poor outcomes with IUI and conventional IVF [25]. In the era of ICSI, couples who have failed conventional IVF are directed to ICSI. Therefore, results of hemizona assays have less clinical relevance now than prior to ICSI. Additionally, the practical utility of this test is limited by the availability of human oocytes.

Seminal reactive oxygen species (ROS) are necessary in small amounts for a number of critical sperm functions, including capacitation and the acrosome reaction. However, if there is an imbalance between ROS production and degradation or scavenging by antioxidants, then high levels of seminal ROS can be found [26]. This high level of ROS can, in turn, lead to abnormalities of cellular function and even cell death. Semen leukocytes have been shown to generate ROS, and ROS levels are significantly higher in infertile men as compared to controls [27,28]. Determination of semen ROS levels can be clinically useful and can guide therapeutic interventions [29].

Tests of sperm DNA integrity

Successful fusion of male and female gametes depends, in part, on integrity of the sperm DNA. Beyond a certain level of damage, pregnancy and embryo development are impaired. Sperm chromatin structure assay (SCSA) parameters are related to fertilization, blastocyst development, and ongoing pregnancy in IVF and ICSI cycles. Sperm of infertile men typically have higher DNA damage than sperm of fertile men, and elevated levels of DNA damage can predict poor fertility outcomes [30]. Data from smaller studies suggest low pregnancy rates via intercourse and IUI in men with elevated sperm DNA damage [31,32]. Studies of IVF-ICSI in men with elevated levels of sperm DNA damage suggest no significant correlation between fertilization rates and DNA damage [33]. However, sperm DNA damage has been associated with an increased risk of pregnancy loss with IVF-ICSI [34].

The etiology of sperm DNA damage is multifactorial, and can include exposure to environmental hazards and gonadotoxins such as chemotherapy, radiation, heat, and tobacco smoke, as well as host factors including impaired germ cell apoptosis, inflammation, infection, varicocele, testicular hyperthermia, and advanced paternal age.

Impact of cancer and cancer therapies on semen parameters

As illustrated throughout this book, both cancer and cancer therapies can adversely affect almost any aspect of a man's reproductive function, including spermatogenesis, testosterone production, erectile function, and ejaculatory function. While many of these effects are reversible with time and/or various treatments, others are irreversible. Semen cryopreservation prior to the initiation of cancer therapy remains the most effective way for a man to maintain his future fertility after being treated for cancer. However, as illustrated above, there are many potential etiologies of abnormal semen parameters, regardless of a prior history of treated or untreated malignancy. Therefore, it is critical for any man with cancer or a history of cancer who is faced with infertility to undergo a formal male-factor infertility evaluation by a urologist or other specialist in male reproduction, to look for other causes of or contributors to male infertility.

Summary

With the improvement in cancer treatment options and outcomes for men of reproductive age, fertility has become an important issue for these men and their partners. Although some of the treatments, as well as the diseases themselves, can be associated with fertility problems, it is important to be aware of concomitant factors that can affect fertility, as they are often treatable. The healthcare practitioner should be prepared to evaluate and treat these men as they would any other man who presents with infertility. Potentially reversible causes such as varicoceles, endocrinopathies, and obstruction should all be considered and treated when applicable, as well as cessation of gonadotoxins and treatment of infections. Paramount regarding all of these issues is the counseling of cancer patients to cryopreserve semen prior to any treatment. This should become part of the pretreatment protocol, thus providing fertility options for cancer survivors.

References

1. World Health Organization. *WHO Laboratory Manual for the Examination and Processing of Human Semen*, 5th edn. Geneva: WHO, 2010.

2. Cooper TG, Noonan E, von Eckardstein S, *et al.* World Health Organization reference values for human semen characteristics. *Hum Reprod Update* 2010; 16: 231–45.

3. Jarow JP. Seminal vesicle aspiration in the management of patients with ejaculatory duct obstruction. *J Urol* 1994; 152: 899–901.

4. Donohue JP, Foster RS, Rowland RG, *et al.* Nerve-sparing retroperitoneal lymphadenectomy with preservation of ejaculation. *J Urol* 1990; 144: 287–91.

5. Amann RP. Considerations in evaluating human spermatogenesis on the basis of total sperm per ejaculate. *J Androl* 2009; 30: 626–41.

6. American Urological Association. *The Optimal Evaluation of the Infertile Male: AUA Best Practice Statement.* Linthicum, MD: AUA, 2010. www.auanet.org/content/media/optimalevaluation2010.pdf (accessed January 2012).

7. Brun B, Clavert A. [Morphologic acrosomal changes in a man exposed to heat]. *J Gynecol Obstet Biol Reprod (Paris)* 1977; 6: 907–11.

8. Kruger TF, Acosta AA, Simmons KF, *et al.* Predictive value of abnormal sperm morphology in in vitro fertilization. *Fertil Steril* 1988; 49: 112–17.

9. Mortimer D, Menkveld R. Sperm morphology assessment–historical perspectives and current opinions. *J Androl* 2001; 22: 192–205.

10. Spiessens C, Vanderschueren D, Meuleman C, D'Hooghe T. Isolated teratozoospermia and intrauterine insemination. *Fertil Steril* 2003; 80: 1185–9.

11. Matorras R, Corcostegui B, Perez C, *et al.* Sperm morphology analysis (strict criteria) in male infertility is not a prognostic factor in intrauterine insemination with husband's sperm. *Fertil Steril* 1995; 63: 608–11.

12. Ombelet W, Fourie FL, Vandeput H, *et al.* Teratozoospermia and in-vitro fertilization: a randomized prospective study. *Hum Reprod* 1994; 9: 1479–84.

13. Coetzee K, Kruge TF, Lombard CJ. Predictive value of normal sperm morphology: a structured literature review. *Hum Reprod Update* 1998; 4: 73–82.

14. Morgentaler A, Fung MY, Harris DH, Powers RD, Alper MM. Sperm morphology and in vitro fertilization outcome: a direct comparison of World Health Organization and strict criteria methodologies. *Fertil Steril* 1995; 64: 1177–82.

15. Guzick DS, Overstreet JW, Factor-Litvak P, *et al.* Sperm morphology, motility, and concentration in fertile and infertile men. *N Engl J Med* 2001; 345: 1388–93.

16. Erel CT, Senturk LM, Demir F, Irez T, Ertungealp E. Antibiotic therapy in men with leukocytospermia. *Int J Fertil Womens Med* 1997; 42: 206–10.

17. Omu AE, al-Othman S, Mohamad AS, al-Kaluwby NM, Fernandes S. Antibiotic therapy for seminal infection. Effect on antioxidant activity and T-helper cytokines. *J Reprod Med* 1998; 43: 857–64.

18. Yanushpolsky EH, Politch JA, Hill JA, Anderson DJ. Antibiotic therapy and leukocytospermia: a prospective, randomized, controlled study. *Fertil Steril* 1995; 63: 142–7.

19. Lackner JE, Herwig R, Schmidbauer J, *et al.* Correlation of leukocytospermia with clinical infection and the positive effect of antiinflammatory treatment on semen quality. *Fertil Steril* 2006; 86: 601–5.

20. Vicari E, La Vignera S, Calogero AE. Antioxidant treatment with carnitines is effective in infertile patients with prostatovesiculoepididymitis and elevated seminal leukocyte concentrations after treatment with nonsteroidal anti-inflammatory compounds. *Fertil Steril* 2002; 78: 1203–8.

21. Oliva A, Multigner L. Ketotifen improves sperm motility and sperm morphology in male patients with leukocytospermia and unexplained infertility. *Fertil Steril* 2006; 85: 240–3.

22. Bastiaan HS, Windt ML, Menkveld R, *et al.* Relationship between zona pellucida-induced acrosome reaction, sperm morphology, sperm–zona pellucida binding, and in vitro fertilization. *Fertil Steril* 2003; 79: 49–55.

23. Katsuki T, Hara T, Ueda K, Tanaka J, Ohama K. Prediction of outcomes of assisted reproduction treatment using the calcium ionophore-induced acrosome reaction. *Hum Reprod* 2005; 20: 469–75.

24. Yanagimachi R, Yanagimachi H, Rogers BJ. The use of zona-free animal ova as a test-system for the assessment of the fertilizing capacity of human spermatozoa. *Biol Reprod* 1976; 15: 471–6.

25. Burkman LJ, Coddington CC, Franken DR, *et al.* The hemizona assay (HZA): development of a diagnostic test for the binding of human spermatozoa to the human hemizona pellucida to predict fertilization potential. *Fertil Steril* 1988; 49: 688–97.

26. Aitken J, Fisher H. Reactive oxygen species generation and human spermatozoa: the balance of benefit and risk. *Bioessays* 1994; 16: 259–67.

27. Athayde KS, Cocuzza M, Agarwal A, *et al.* Development of normal reference values for seminal reactive oxygen species and their correlation with leukocytes and semen parameters in a fertile population. *J Androl* 2007; 28: 613–20.

28. Iwasaki A, Gagnon C. Formation of reactive oxygen species in spermatozoa of infertile patients. *Fertil Steril* 1992; 57: 409–16.

29. Agarwal A, Sharma RK, Nallella KP, *et al.* Reactive oxygen species as an independent marker of male factor infertility. *Fertil Steril* 2006; 86: 878–85.

30. Zini A, Bielecki R, Phang D, Zenzes MT. Correlations between two markers of sperm DNA integrity, DNA denaturation and DNA fragmentation, in fertile and infertile men. *Fertil Steril* 2001; 75: 674–7.

31. Bungum M, Humaidan P, Axmon A, *et al.* Sperm DNA integrity assessment in prediction of assisted reproduction technology outcome. *Hum Reprod* 2007; 22: 174–9.

32. Duran EH, Morshedi M, Taylor S, Oehninger S. Sperm DNA quality predicts intrauterine insemination outcome: a prospective cohort study. *Hum Reprod* 2002; 17: 3122–8.

33. Benchaib M, Lornage J, Mazoyer C, *et al.* Sperm deoxyribonucleic acid fragmentation as a prognostic indicator of assisted reproductive technology outcome. *Fertil Steril* 2007; 87: 93–100.

34. Zini A, Boman JM, Belzile E, Ciampi A. Sperm DNA damage is associated with an increased risk of pregnancy loss after IVF and ICSI: systematic review and meta-analysis. *Hum Reprod* 2008; 23: 2663–8.

Chapter

Azoospermia

Cara B. Cimmino and Robert D. Oates

Introduction

The initial diagnosis of azoospermia is made when no spermatozoa are detected upon microscopic evaluation of two separate semen samples. The prevalence of azoospermia is 1% among all men, and ranges between 8% and 15% among infertile men [1]. This condition should be distinguished from *aspermia*, in which there is complete absence of seminal fluid emission during ejaculation.

Classification of azoospermia into diagnostic categories

The initial evaluation of azoospermia is directed at finding the cause for this abnormality in order to most effectively select a treatment option. Etiologies for azoospermia are conveniently divided into three main categories: pre-testicular, testicular, and post-testicular (Fig. 7.1). Included in the pre-testicular category are hypothalamic and pituitary abnormalities that negatively effect spermatogenesis and androgenesis, leading to "secondary" testicular failure. Testicular causes of spermatogenic compromise ("primary" testicular failure) include known autosomal and sex-chromosomal genetic aberrations, and a presumed host of uncharacterized genetic anomalies involved in the complex process of spermatogenesis. External forces such as chemotherapy and radiotherapy may also impair spermatogenesis. Post-testicular azoospermia stems from problems related to delivery of sperm to the urethral meatus and female reproductive tract, as sperm production is normal, and it includes issues such as ejaculatory dysfunction and obstruction of the male reproductive ductal system. Often, many patients with pre- and post-testicular causes may be amenable

to corrective strategies, while a smaller percentage of those with primary testicular failure will be.

More broadly, then, these patients can be divided into those with obstructive azoospermia (post-testicular, OA) and those with non-obstructive azoospermia (pre-testicular and testicular, NOA).

Initial evaluation of the azoospermic male

Patients who present for workup of azoospermia should be evaluated to determine the cause of their condition in order to plan appropriate therapeutic options [2]. The initial assessment should include a complete history, physical examination, and often measurement of testosterone and follicle-stimulating hormone (FSH). Other potentially useful hormonal studies include those for luteinizing hormone (LH), prolactin, and estradiol, depending on the accumulated findings of the history and physical exam.

History begins with questions pertaining to prior fertility of the patient and his partner, frequency and timing of intercourse, and duration of infertility. Investigation of childhood disorders and illnesses such as cryptorchidism, viral orchitis, or testicular torsion is also important. Additionally, it is critical to elicit a history of epididymitis, urethritis, sexually transmitted diseases, and recent febrile illness. Any history of genital trauma and pelvic or inguinal surgery should be assessed, especially as it relates to prior testis, bladder, or prostate cancer. A complete list of medications, a history of radiation and chemotherapy, which may have already occurred in the azoospermic male, and exposure to heat, gonadotoxins, alcohol, and tobacco should be obtained as well. It is critically important to ask specifically if the patient is taking any type

Fertility Preservation in Male Cancer Patients, ed. John P. Mulhall, Linda D. Applegarth, Robert D. Oates and Peter N. Schlegel. Published by Cambridge University Press. © Cambridge University Press 2013.

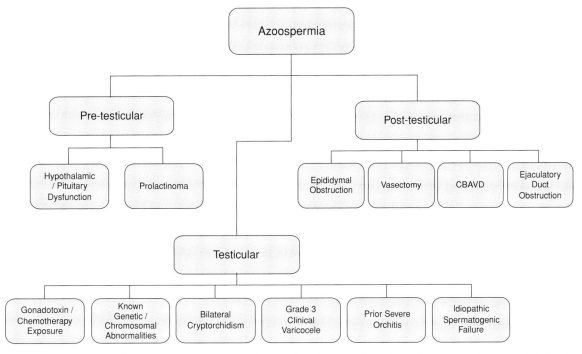

Figure 7.1. Classification of azoospermia. Azoospermia can be more broadly grouped into obstructive azoospermia (post-testicular) and non-obstructive azoospermia (pre-testicular and testicular). CBAVD, congenital bilateral absence of the vas deferens.

of illicit anabolic steroid or prescribed testosterone pharmaceutical, as exogenous androgenic compounds are suppressive to spermatogenesis and are being used commonly in the male population (reviewed in Chapter 30) [3,4]. Finally patients should be asked about family history of infertility, birth defects of any kind, cystic fibrosis, or disorders of sexual differentiation.

Physical exam should note testis size, volume, and consistency, as well as presence or absence of the vasa deferentia. Normal adult testicular size ranges between 18 and 20 mL, and small testes indicate probable impairment of spermatogenesis [5]. The consistency of the epididymides, scrotal or inguinal surgical scars, and a clinically palpable varicocele should be documented. The presence of gynecomastia, the pattern of hair distribution, and the nature of the secondary sex characteristics are important to describe.

It is also vital that the patient has had two separate semen analyses performed in which the sample provided has been centrifuged and the pellet examined microscopically for any spermatozoa that may be present. Up to 21% of men initially diagnosed with NOA upon initial semen analysis were found to have tiny numbers of motile sperm present in a centrifuged

pellet of their ejaculate [6]. These patients would be considered severely oligospermic, rather than truly azoospermic, and these small numbers of ejaculate spermatozoa may be able to be cryopreserved to save future fertility and biological paternity. Measurement of serum FSH can be helpful if it is unclear from the history and/or physical examination whether sperm production is normal (implying OA) or deficient to a severe degree (implying NOA) [7]. The value of FSH that is found in a male with optimal and adequate spermatogenesis is always at the lower end of the "reference range" supplied with each assay. With spermatogenic failure, there is a compensatory rise in pituitary secretion of FSH with a consequent elevation in the serum value above the lower part of the reference range. The exact value does not need to be "above the upper limits of normal" to indirectly (inversely) indicate a problem with spermatogenesis. In unclear circumstances (no suggestive history or physical examination findings), the measurement of FSH can be of great help in delineating the azoospermia as likely obstructive or non-obstructive.

Once the diagnosis of azoospermia has been confirmed, it is necessary to characterize the cause as obstructive or non-obstructive. Obstruction is definite if the patient has bilateral absence of the vas (as occurs in congenital bilateral absence of the vas deferens and clinical cystic fibrosis) [8]. Blockage to normal spermatozoal flow will necessarily occur if the patient had a prior radical prostatectomy or radical cystoprostatectomy, as the distal ductal system (seminal vesicles, vasal ampullae, ejaculatory ducts, and prostate) are removed, as may occur in cases of prostate carcinoma, transitional cell carcinoma of the bladder, or rhabdomyosarcoma of either organ. Previous hernia repair or epididymitis may lead to occlusion of the proximal ductal system (vas and epididymis), and the vas or epididymis may feel full and firm to careful and directed palpation because of the downstream blockage to flow.

Those patients found to have NOA should undergo genetic testing to rule out possible karyotypic abnormalities or Y-chromosome microdeletions if the history does not offer an obvious etiology such as prior chemotherapy. The prevalence of karytotype anomalies in azoospermic men is approximately 10–15% (the majority being 47,XXY Klinefelter syndrome) [9,10]. Similarly, Y-chromosome microdeletions are seen in 10–15% of men with azoospermia (the majority being microdeletion of the AZFc region which imparts no predisposition to gonadal or somatic malignancy) [11]. Karyotypic findings such as 46,XX testicular disorder of sex development occurs in approximately 1 in 20 000 males and, while a rare cause of NOA, there will be no sperm production potential whatsoever since nearly the entire Y chromosome is missing. Similarly, when NOA men have a microdeletion of the AZFa or AZFb region of the Y chromosome (detected on Y-chromosomal microdeletion assay), they will have no sperm production potential, as genes necessary for spermatogenesis reside in the stretches of Y-chromosomal DNA that have been deleted, and hence they are not present in the genome. While specific findings such as these are not related to tumor development of any type, they are unfortunately prognostic for the patient and not only explain why he is azoospermic but also inform him that further fertility preservation schemes and options (e.g., testis tissue extraction) do not need to be pursued [9].

Occasionally, the nature of the tumor and the genetic basis underlying the azoospermia are indeed linked. For example, breast cancer, Leydig cell tumors, leukemia, lymphomas, mediastinal and intracranial germ cell tumors may all occur at higher frequency in men with Klinefelter syndrome [12–14]. Therefore,

in these circumstances, the baseline spermatogenic potential of the patient is already severely compromised (only an extremely rare Klinefelter patient will have any sperm in the ejaculate; approximately 50% will have individual spermatozoa found within the parenchyma of the testes that can be used in conjunction with in-vitro technologies to effect pregnancy) [15]. Chemotherapy or radiotherapy will only compromise this further, perhaps to the point that no sperm exist in the testes. Patients with disorders of sex development (DSD), such as androgen insensitivity, may have spermatogenic failure as a consequence of their genetic and phenotypic anomalies as well as be at risk for certain malignancies such as gonadoblastoma [16]. Finally, men with testicular dysgenesis syndrome (TSD) may have a combination of cryptorchidism, germ cell malignancy, and spermatogenic dysfunction. Therefore, it is not unusual to see severe oligospermia or NOA in a male with a prior history of cryptorchidism or testis cancer [17,18]. In males presenting with a gonadal germ cell malignancy, up to 20% will be azoospermic (and many oligospermic) at time of discovery and/or orchiectomy as a byproduct of the "global dysgenesis" that affects some testes, the hormonal aberrations induced by markedly elevated levels of beta-human chorionic gonadotropin (β-hCG), or by overwhelming metastatic disease [19–21].

Malignancy itself can have detrimental effects on gonadal function leading to azoospermia. Cancer patients may be found to have lower levels of reproductive hormones and serum testosterone secondary to the stress of disease, metabolic changes, or downregulation by release of endocrine substances from the tumors themselves, such as β-hCG released by some testicular germ cell tumors [22]. Cancer may also lead to suboptimal spermatogenesis secondary to malnutrition, with deficiencies in minerals, vitamins, and trace elements. In non-testis malignancy, there may be no direct linkage to the testis and the process of spermatogenesis but sperm quantity and quality may be reduced. As reported by van der Kaaij et al., sperm density was below 20 million/mL in 59% of young men with low-stage Hodgkin's lymphoma prior to any chemotherapy at the time of attempted cryopreservation [23]. However, azoospermia was present in only 3% of those men, about three times higher than would be expected in the general population but still a fairly low percentage. Meguro et al. reported on the results of pre-treatment semen cryopreservation in 38 men with a variety of hematologic malignancies, including acute promyelocytic leukemia, acute lymphoblastic leukemia, and non-Hodgkin's lymphoma [24]. All but two had normal sperm concentration and motility (one showed low motility and the other oligospermia) and no male had azoospermia. Even the vast majority of adolescent boys (aged 12–18 years) will have cryopreservable sperm in their ejaculate (collected through masturbation, penile vibratory stimulation, or rectal probe electroejaculation), roughly 12% being azoospermic at the time of collection [25]. Therefore, except for those with testicular carcinoma, in whom initial azoospermia is more likely, it is unusual to have azoospermia at presentation with most other types of malignancy, and so other reasons (which may even be completely unrelated to the cancer) need to be searched for, including obstructive processes and known genetic causes of NOA, as described above.

Indications for treatment of men with azoospermia

As mentioned above, azoospermia may be caused by obstruction of the extratesticular ductal system (obstructive azoospermia, OA) or abnormalities with spermatogenesis (non-obstructive azoospermia, NOA). Patients typically demonstrate different clinical findings depending on the cause for their disorder.

Men presenting with OA typically have normal-sized testes, fullness of the epididymides, and a normal FSH. Those with NOA typically possess smaller than normal testes, and elevated FSH.

Treatment of non-obstructive azoospermia

NOA indicates an inherent problem with spermatogenesis, rather than a problem with delivery of spermatozoa to the female reproductive tract, as is the case with OA. Although these patients have deficient spermatogenesis, recent studies have suggested that approximately 60% of these men will have some evidence of sperm production within the testes when microsurgical dissection and exploration of the testis (testicular sperm extraction, TESE) is carried out [26]. On histologic evaluation of these patients, several abnormal patterns will be seen, including seminiferous tubules lined only by Sertoli cells, hypospermatogenesis, or maturation arrest. However, some interspersed small areas of ongoing sperm production can be found using a microsurgical approach (microsurgical TESE:

see Chapter 28). The testis tissue that contains whole spermatozoa can then be cryopreserved for later use by the patient (perhaps even years later) in conjunction with intracytoplasmic sperm injection (ICSI) to effect pregnancy. Therefore, if the history, physical examination, laboratory data, and genetic studies all point to a diagnosis of NOA with the possibility of extremely low levels of ongoing sperm production, the patient should be referred for TESE prior to ablative surgery (radiotherapy or spermatotoxic chemotherapy: see Chapters 12 and 13).

Treatment of obstructive azoospermia

If bilateral ejaculatory duct obstruction is discovered (low semen volume, low semen pH, dilated ejaculatory ducts, or a midline prostatic cyst on transrectal ultrasound imaging of the distal male reproductive ductal system), transurethral resection of the ejaculatory ducts (TURED) can be performed in the operating room prior to surgical tumor treatment, radiation, or chemotherapy [27]. Studies demonstrate that success rates of this procedure are associated with location of obstruction, with midline cysts being most amenable to surgical treatment. If time permits, a semen analysis can be obtained just a few weeks after TURED, and this may show enough motile sperm to making semen cryopreservation worthwhile. If treatment of the malignancy needs to be carried out sooner than TURED can be accomplished, at least testis tissue can be harvested and cryopreserved, as spermatogenesis is usually normal in these males.

Congenital bilateral absence of the vas deferens (CBAVD) can be diagnosed, as discussed above, by physical exam alone. Further imaging is generally not required. Because of the embryologic relationship between the vas deferens and seminal vesicles, the majority of men with CBAVD demonstrate hypoplasia or absence of the seminal vesicles, leading to the characteristic low-volume, acidic, azoospermic semen analysis (the seminal vesicles contribute approximately 70% of the fluid to the ejaculate and all of the alkalinity) [28]. These men (and their partners if they are presently trying to conceive) need to have cystic fibrosis (CF) mutation analysis. The CF genes encode the cystic fibrosis transmembrane conductance regulator (CFTR), a protein that helps maintain proper ion concentrations and fluidity/viscosity in certain epithelial lined tubes such as in the pulmonary and pancreatic ductal systems. At least two-thirds of men with CBAVD have detectable mutations of the CFTR gene, and conversely almost all men with clinical cystic fibrosis have CBAVD [29]. Most men with CBAVD demonstrate normal spermatogenesis, allowing them to be candidates for surgical epididymal sperm aspiration or testicular sperm extraction for use with IVF-ICSI as either fresh or frozen/thawed specimens [30,31]. However, before the couple proceeds with any therapies, genetic testing should be offered to the female partner to rule out the possibility that she is a carrier of a CFTR mutation. As for bilateral ejaculatory duct obstruction, sperm retrieval and cryopreservation should be accomplished prior to definitive oncologic treatment.

This concept also applies to all of the other etiologies of OA that may exist when a malignancy is first discovered, such as prior vasectomy, post-inflammatory epididymitis, and ejaculatory duct occlusion secondary to prostatic malignancy. Finally, prior intravesical BCG therapy for superficial transitional cell carcinoma may precipitate granulomatous prostatitis or orchitis. This may be a consideration in the right circumstances [32].

Conclusion

While few male oncology patients will present with confirmed azoospermia prior to definitive therapy, it is imperative to define the etiology of the azoospermia for those that do. In cases of OA, treatment of the underlying cause can be carried out to restore normal sperm flow to the ejaculate, if time permits, that also allows for semen cryopreservation. If the timeline of chemotherapy, for example, does not permit this, either microsurgical epididymal sperm aspiration or testis tissue extraction should be offered, with cryopreservation of the sperm to ensure an opportunity for biological fatherhood in the future. If NOA is present and there are no absolutely limiting genetic abnormalities, e.g., an AZFa or AZFb microdeletion of the Y chromosome, the patient should be offered TESE prior to the initiation of surgical, chemical, or radiation therapy.

References

1. Practice Committee of the American Society for Reproductive Medicine in collaboration with Society for Male Reproduction and Urology. Evaluation of the azoospermic male. *Fertil Steril* 2008; 90(5 Suppl): S74–7.

2. Sigman S, Lipshultz L, Howards S. Office evaluation of the subfertile male. In Lipshultz L, Howards S, Niederberger C, eds. *Infertility in the Male*, 4th edn. New York, NY: Cambridge University Press; 2009; pp. 153–76.

3. Dohle GR, Smit M, Weber RF. Androgens and male fertility. *World J Urol* 2003; 21: 341–5.

4. Lombardo F, Sgro P, Salacone P, *et al.* Androgens and fertility. *J Endocrinol Invest* 2005; 28(3 Suppl): 51–5.

5. Chipkevitch E, Nishimura RT, Tu DG, Galea-Rojas M. Clinical measurement of testicular volume in adolescents: comparison of the reliability of 5 methods. *J Urol* 1996; 156: 2050–3.

6. Jaffe TM, Kim ED, Hoekstra TH, Lipshultz LI. Sperm pellet analysis: a technique to detect the presence of sperm in men considered to have azoospermia by routine semen analysis. *J Urol* 1998; 159: 1548–50.

7. Sokol R. Endocrine evaluation. In Lipshultz L, Howards S, Niederberger C, eds. *Infertility in the Male*, 4th edn. New York, NY: Cambridge University Press, 2009; pp. 199–214.

8. Samli H, Samli MM, Yilmaz E, Imirzalioglu N. Clinical, andrological and genetic characteristics of patients with congenital bilateral absence of vas deferens (CBAVD). *Arch Androl* 2006; 52: 471–7.

9. Oates R, Lamb D. Genetic aspects of infertility. In Lipshultz L, Howards S, Niederberger C, eds. *Infertility in the Male*, 4th edn. New York, NY: Cambridge University Press, 2009; pp. 251–76.

10. Oates RD. Clinical evaluation of the infertile male with respect to genetic etiologies. *Syst Biol Reprod Med* 2010; 57: 72–7.

11. Stahl PJ, Masson P, Mielnik A, *et al.* A decade of experience emphasizes that testing for Y microdeletions is essential in American men with azoospermia and severe oligozoospermia. *Fertil Steril* 2010; 94: 1753–6.

12. Aguirre D, Nieto K, Lazos M, *et al.* Extragonadal germ cell tumors are often associated with Klinefelter syndrome. *Hum Pathol* 2006; 37: 477–80.

13. Machatschek JN, Schrauder A, Helm F, Schrappe M, Claviez A. Acute lymphoblastic leukemia and Klinefelter syndrome in children: two cases and review of the literature. *Pediatr Hematol Oncol* 2004; 21: 621–6.

14. Queipo G, Aguirre D, Nieto K, *et al.* Intracranial germ cell tumors: association with Klinefelter syndrome and sex chromosome aneuploidies. *Cytogenet Genome Res* 2008; 121: 211–14.

15. Forti G, Corona G, Vignozzi L, Krausz C, Maggi M. Klinefelter's syndrome: a clinical and therapeutical update. *Sex Dev* 2010; 4: 249–58.

16. Pleskacova J, Hersmus R, Oosterhuis JW, *et al.* Tumor risk in disorders of sex development. *Sex Dev* 2010; 4: 259–69.

17. Jorgensen N, Meyts ER, Main KM, Skakkebaek NE. Testicular dysgenesis syndrome comprises some but not all cases of hypospadias and impaired spermatogenesis. *Int J Androl* 2010; 33: 298–303.

18. Toppari J, Virtanen HE, Main KM, Skakkebaek NE. Cryptorchidism and hypospadias as a sign of testicular dysgenesis syndrome (TDS): environmental connection. *Birth Defects Res A Clin Mol Teratol.* 2010; 88: 910–9.

19. Fossa SD, Klepp O, Molne K, Aakvaag A. Testicular function after unilateral orchiectomy for cancer and before further treatment. *Int J Androl* 1982; 5: 179–84.

20. Liguori G, Trombetta C, Bucci S, *et al.* Semen quality before and after orchiectomy in men with testicular cancer. *Arch Ital Urol Androl* 2008; 80(3): 99–102.

21. Petersen PM, Skakkebaek NE, Vistisen K, Rorth M, Giwercman A. Semen quality and reproductive hormones before orchiectomy in men with testicular cancer. *J Clin Oncol* 1999; 17: 941–7.

22. Dohle GR. Male infertility in cancer patients: review of the literature. *Int J Urol* 2010; 17(4): 327–31.

23. van der Kaaij MA, Heutte N, van Echten-Arends J, *et al.* Sperm quality before treatment in patients with early stage Hodgkin's lymphoma enrolled in EORTC-GELA Lymphoma Group trials. *Haematologica* 2009; 94: 1691–7.

24. Meguro A, Muroi K, Miyoshi T, *et al.* Sperm cryopreservation in patients with hematologic malignancies. *Int J Hematol* 2008; 88: 351–4.

25. Hagenas I, Jorgensen N, Rechnitzer C, *et al.* Clinical and biochemical correlates of successful semen collection for cryopreservation from 12–18-year-old patients: a single-center study of 86 adolescents. *Hum Reprod* 2010; 25: 2031–8.

26. Schlegel PN. Nonobstructive azoospermia: a revolutionary surgical approach and results. *Semin Rreprod Med* 2009; 27: 165–70.

27. Smith JF, Walsh TJ, Turek PJ. Ejaculatory duct obstruction. *Urol Clin North Am* 2008; 35: 221–7, viii.

28. Oates RD. The genetic basis of male reproductive failure. *Urol Clin North Am* 2008; 35: 257–70, ix.

29. Bareil C, Guittard C, Altieri JP, *et al.* Comprehensive and rapid genotyping of mutations and haplotypes in congenital bilateral absence of the vas deferens and other cystic fibrosis transmembrane conductance regulator-related disorders. *J Mol Diagn* 2007; 9: 582–8.

30. Van Peperstraten A, Proctor ML, Johnson NP, Philipson G. Techniques for surgical retrieval of sperm prior to intra-cytoplasmic sperm injection (ICSI) for azoospermia. *Cochrane Database Syst Rev* 2008; (2): CD002807.

31. Wald M, Ross LS, Prins GS, *et al.* Analysis of outcomes of cryopreserved surgically retrieved sperm for IVF/ICSI. *J Androl* 2006; 27: 60–5.

32. Harving SS, Asmussen L, Roosen JU, Hermann G. Granulomatous epididymo-orchitis, a rare complication of intravesical bacillus Calmette-Guerin therapy for urothelial cancer. *Scand J Urol Nephrol* 2009; 43: 331–3.

Chapter

8

Varicocele

Peter J. Stahl and Marc Goldstein

Introduction

Varicocele is an abnormal dilation of the pampini-form plexus within the spermatic cord, which is the main route of venous drainage from the testis. Varicoceles are identifiable in approximately 15% of men in the general population and in 35–40% of subfertile men [1,2]. The higher prevalence of varicoceles in the subfertile male population suggests that varicoceles cause or contribute to testicular dysfunction. This notion is supported by studies that have demonstrated that varicocele is associated with a progressive and duration-dependent decline in testicular function [3–5]. Varicocele repair ameliorates further damage to testicular function [4,6] and results in improved spermatogenesis in a large percentage of men. Furthermore, varicocelectomy may enhance Leydig cell function and lead to stabilization or improvement of serum androgen levels in hypogonadal men [7–9]. For these reasons, surgical correction of varicocele is by far the most commonly performed procedure for the treatment of male subfertility [10].

Although the role of varicocele treatment for the specific indication of male fertility preservation has not yet been the subject of dedicated studies, it is of paramount importance that health practitioners treating men who face a threat to their fertility be familiar with the diagnosis and management of this highly prevalent clinical condition. In this chapter we briefly review the pathophysiology and clinical features of varicocele, key components of the clinical evaluation of men with suspected varicocele, and the indications for varicocele treatment. We also discuss special considerations pertaining to varicocele in men with cancer, and suggest an algorithmic approach to varicocele management in this unique population of patients.

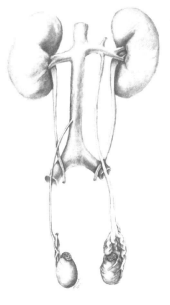

Figure 8.1. Spermatic vein anatomy.

Pathophysiology of varicocele

The embryological descent of the testicles from the pararenal retroperitoneum into the scrotum results in long internal spermatic veins that must withstand significant hydrostatic pressure. Any degree of venous valvular incompetence may result in high intravenous pressures, retrograde venous flow, and development of the venous dilation and tortuosity that characterize varicoceles. This sequence of pathophysiologic changes is more likely on the left, where the internal spermatic vein is longer, drains perpendicularly into the left renal vein, and may be externally compressed by the superior mesenteric artery. In contrast, the right internal spermatic vein typically drains directly into the inferior vena cava via an oblique insertion. The differences in venous anatomy (Fig. 8.1) likely account

Fertility Preservation in Male Cancer Patients, ed. John P. Mulhall, Linda D. Applegarth, Robert D. Oates and Peter N. Schlegel. Published by Cambridge University Press. © Cambridge University Press 2013.

for the significantly higher prevalence of left-sided varicoceles.

Multiple hypotheses have been suggested to explain the association between varicocele and testicular dysfunction. The most widely accepted theory is that varicocele disturbs countercurrent heat exchange within the pampiniform plexus and results in scrotal hyperthermia [11]. Elevated testicular temperatures have been observed in several studies of varicocele [12,13], and varicocele repair has been demonstrated to reverse testicular hyperthermia [14]. The mechanism by which scrotal hyperthermia impairs testicular function is incompletely understood but may relate to alterations in serum gonadotropin levels [15], thermal-induced germ cell apoptosis [16], or up-regulation of testicular mRNA transcripts such as heat shock proteins [17]. Varicocele may also induce testicular dysfunction through reflux of renal or adrenal metabolites into the internal spermatic vein, though the gonadotoxicity of these metabolites is not established [18]. Additionally, increased hydrostatic pressure within the internal spermatic vein may impair testicular function [19].

Clinical features of varicocele

Whatever the underlying mechanisms may be, varicocele is associated with measurable impairments in testicular function within the subfertile male population. Varicocele has been associated with testicular atrophy, low semen quality, and most recently with androgen deficiency. Less commonly, varicocele is associated with chronic scrotal pain. Additionally, patients with varicoceles often present with a chief complaint of scrotal mass and may be concerned about testicular cancer.

The impact of varicocele on male fertility is perhaps most evident by its association with testicular atrophy [5,20,21]. Two thousand years ago the Greek physician Celsus noted that "The veins are swollen and twisted over the testicle, which becomes smaller than its fellow, in as much as its nutrition has become defective" [22]. Celsus' observation has been corroborated by numerous contemporary studies. Zini et al. used scrotal ultrasound and demonstrated that left testicular volume is less than right testicular volume in subfertile men with a left varicocele [23]. These authors also showed that the degree of discrepancy between left and right testicular volume in men with unilateral left varicocele is correlated with varicocele grade, although other groups have performed similar studies that failed to show a relationship between testicular atrophy and varicocele grade [24].

The relationship between varicocele and seminal fluid abnormalities is well established among subfertile men, though not all subfertile men with varicoceles have abnormal semen parameters. Varicocele exerts a negative modulatory effect on semen quality and may result in decreased sperm concentration, decreased sperm motility, increased percentage of abnormal morphologic forms, and increased presence of immature germ cells in the ejaculate [25]. In the largest published analysis of semen quality with respect to varicocele presence, the World Health Organization studied 9034 male partners of subfertile couples and observed varicoceles in 25.4% of men with abnormal semen parameters, compared with 11.7% of men with normal semen analyses [26]. These data strongly support the notion that varicocele is a significant risk factor for abnormal semen quality.

However, the relationship between varicocele and semen quality is less clear within the general population. Several studies have demonstrated an association and several have failed to do so. Johnson et al. found semen abnormalities in 70% of unselected military recruits with a palpable varicocele [27]. In a more recent similarly designed study, however, Zargooshi found normal semen parameters in the majority of young military recruits with palpable varicoceles [28]. Such conflicting observations are common in the varicocele literature, and therefore a causal relationship between varicocele and male infertility has not been definitively established.

Beyond its deleterious effects on spermatogenesis, varicocele may also exert a negative modulatory impact on testicular androgen production. Animal models have demonstrated decreased secretion of androgens by Leydig cells when a varicocele is present [29], and in humans varicocele has been associated with Leydig cell vacuolization and atrophy [30]. At our institution, we analyzed early-morning testosterone levels in 325 men with varicoceles and in 510 vasectomy reversal patients without varicoceles who served as controls. We found that men with varicocele had significantly lower testosterone levels than controls (416 ± 156 vs. 469 ± 192 ng/dL, $p < 0.001$) [31], supporting the notion that varicocele may be a clinically important cause of androgen deficiency.

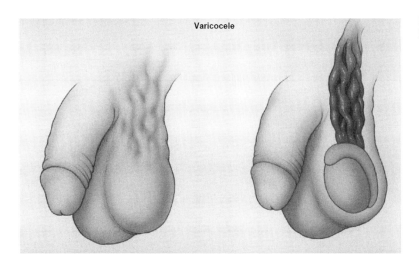

Figure 8.2. Illustration demonstrating large left varicocele.

Evaluation of men with suspected varicoceles

The clinical evaluation of male fertility should always include evaluation for the presence of varicoceles and their possible clinical sequelae. A proper reproductive and sexual history should be obtained. Patients should be asked about their prior fertility history, and about symptoms of androgen deficiency such as low energy level, depressed mood, and low libido. If a patient is aware of his varicocele, particular attention should be given to the presence or absence of scrotal discomfort and to the onset and progression of the varicocele. Rapidly progressive varicoceles should raise suspicion for vena caval or retroperitoneal pathology and should prompt further investigation.

Physical examination provides the cornerstone of diagnosis. The scrotum should be warmed with a heating pad prior to examination to achieve relaxation of the cremasteric muscle fibers, which facilitates accurate assessment of the spermatic cord, epididymis, and testicles. Scrotal examination should first be performed with the patient supine. The spermatic cord is visually inspected and palpated to assess for dilation of the pampiniform plexus, which is facilitated by manual exclusion of the vas deferens from the remainder of the cord. The testis is examined for the presence of masses. Testicular consistency (soft or hard) should be noted and testicular size should be measured with an orchidometer and recorded.

At this point the patient should stand and the examination should be repeated, both prior to and during abdominal straining. Any dilation of the

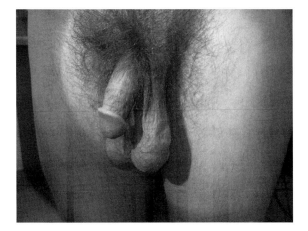

Figure 8.3. Grade 3 varicocele.

pampiniform plexus that is visible or palpable with or without abdominal straining is diagnostic of varicocele. Varicocele severity is graded based upon physical diagnosis. Grade 1 varicoceles are palpable impulses felt during active abdominal straining. Grade 2 varicoceles are palpable with the patient standing even without Valsava maneuver, but are not visible. Grade 3 varicoceles are easily visible through the scrotal skin during standing (Figs. 8.2 and 8.3)

Scrotal ultrasonography is a useful adjunct to diagnosis when adequate physical examination of the scrotum is not possible, and should be reserved for such cases. Examples of common clinical situations when ultrasonography may be necessary include presence of other scrotal pathology such as a hydrocele, history of prior scrotal or inguinal surgery, inability to obtain adequate relaxation of the cremasteric muscles, ectopic testicular location in the high scrotum or inguinal canal, and morbid obesity. Unfortunately sonographic criteria for varicocele diagnosis have not been standardized. We consider the presence of veins greater than 2.5 mm in diameter in which retrograde flow is demonstrated during Valsava maneuver to be consistent with varicocele.

The final component of the clinical assessment of patients with varicoceles is a laboratory investigation. This should include a semen analysis to assess semen quality, and an early-morning serum testosterone level to assess for androgen deficiency. The need for further laboratory testing is directed by results of the semen analysis and the testosterone level. The degree to which the seminal fluid is abnormal and the degree, if any, to which testosterone prouduction is impaired will determine the need for varicocele treatment.

Indications for varicocele treatment

While the management of varicocele is dealt with elsewhere (Chapter 34), some discussion of indications for treatment is warranted. Varicocele treatment for subfertility should be limited to men with palpable varicoceles, impaired semen quality, and documented infertility who have a female partner with normal fertility or correctable infertility [10]. Varicocele repair should not be offered as a fertility treatment to men with normal semen parameters or in men with non-palpable varicoceles detected by ultrasonography, as the evidence has failed to demonstrate a benefit of treatment in such men.

Scrotal pain is another common indication for varicocele treatment. Treatment of varicoceles for pain relief must be approached cautiously, as pain will not resolve in all patients after treatment. In these cases, particular attention should be paid to the characteristics and timing of scrotal pain. Pain associated with varicoceles is typically described as dull or aching, typically worsens during prolonged activity in the standing position, and is typically relieved by lying down. Varicocelectomy has been shown to provide complete or partial pain relief in up to 94% of properly selected patients [32].

Varicocele treatment is also recommended for adolescents in whom the varicocele is associated with abnormal semen parameters or ipsilateral testicular atrophy. The latter indication is far more common, as

few physicians routinely obtain semen analyses in adolescent boys with varicoceles. Though the definition of testicular atrophy is not standardized, most clinicians feel that a volume discrepancy of 2 mL or 20% between the affected and contralateral testis is diagnostic. In these cases varicocele repair may halt or even reverse testicular atrophy.

Lastly, evidence is emerging that varicocele treatment should also be considered in men with varicoceles and androgen deficiency. In such cases, varicocele repair may improve Leydig cell function and increase serum testosterone levels, thereby avoiding the need for lifelong androgen replacement in some men. Other relative indications for varicocele treatment include patient anxiety about subsequent infertility resulting from an untreated varicocele, and cosmetic bother.

Special considerations in men with cancer

Several important considerations pertain to the evaluation and treatment of varicoceles in men with cancer, which are highlighted in the algorithmic approach to varicocele in cancer patients that we have provided (Fig. 8.4).

First, the diagnosis of varicocele in a cancer patient should trigger concern that the varicocele has resulted from pathologic processes related to malignancy, which may be critically important to identify and treat. Cancer predisposes to thrombotic events that could cause obstruction of the vena cava, and most cancer patients are at risk for the development of retroperitoneal masses or adenopathy that could obstruct venous drainage from the testis and cause varicocele. Malignant varicoceles may be distinguished from incidental varicoceles that are unrelated to cancer on the basis of history and physical examination. Varicoceles that are rapidly progressive, that are only present on the right side, or that do not collapse in the supine position should prompt investigative imaging.

The indications for varicocele treatment in cancer patients are similar to indications for treatment in the general population. Usually treatment is non-urgent and may be deferred until a later date that is convenient for the patient and does not interfere with cancer treatment. However, prompt varicocele treatment may be beneficial and should be considered in several unique clinical scenarios. One such scenario is the presence of a large varicocele in a solitary testis, which

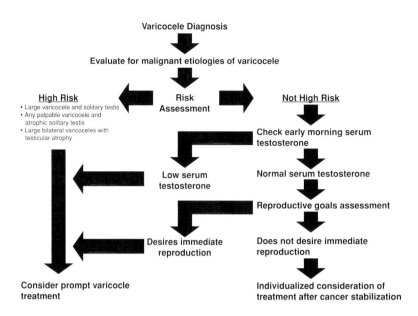

Figure 8.4. Clinical care algorithm for varicocele in men with cancer.

may be the case after radical orchiectomy for testicular germ cell tumor, or in patients with a history of testicular torsion or trauma. These patients typically have limited testicular reserve due to the presence of a solitary testis, which has often been subjected to the gonadotoxicity of chemotherapy. Progressive damage to germ cells and Leydig cells may occur in the presence of a large varicocele, which may lead to irreversible testicular damage in these patients. A similar argument in favor of aggressive varicocele treatment may be applied to men with cancer who have large bilateral varicoceles. The presence of testicular atrophy in either of these scenarios may indicate impending testicular failure, and suggests that prompt varicocele treatment may be warranted.

Most cancer patients with varicoceles have two testicles and are at lower risk for progressive testicular dysfunction. In these men, decisions about whether or not and when to treat the varicocele depend upon the reproductive goals of the patient and the feasibility of varicocele treatment in the context of the patient's cancer treatment. Patients who are actively trying to reproduce in whom treatment does not interfere with cancer therapy should be evaluated and treated similarly to men without cancer. When indicated, varicocelectomy should be performed without delay. In men with varicocele and cancer who are not actively trying to reproduce, decisions about varicocele treatment should not be rushed and should be tailored to the needs and desires of the individual patient.

Special consideration for varicocele treatment should also be given to men with cancer who have large varicoceles and low serum testosterone levels. Testosterone deficiency causes low energy level, depressed mood, depressed libido, muscle wasting, and loss of bone mineral density. These symptoms of hypogonadism may significantly decrease quality of life in cancer patients, who are doubly at risk for these symptoms because of their underlying malignancies. Varicocele treatment may lead to significant improvements in serum testosterone [31] without the need for medical therapy, which may lead to significant quality of life improvement.

Finally, cancer and cancer therapy are significant risk factors for non-obstructive azoospermia, in which sperm are completely absent from the ejaculate [33]. In men with non-obstructive azoospermia who have palpable varicoceles, sperm return to the ejaculate in a significant proportion of men after microsurgical varicocelectomy, allowing in-vitro fertilization with intracytoplasmic sperm injection (IVF-ICSI) with ejaculated sperm and obviating the need for testicular sperm extraction (TESE), which is especially important in a patient with a solitary testis. Rarely, varicocelectomy may enable reproduction via intrauterine insemination (IUI) or even natural conception in some cases [34].

Summary

It is highly likely that health practitioners who care for men who face a clinical threat to their fertility will encounter varicocele, which is the most commonly identified abnormality in subfertile men and also a relatively common finding in the general population. Familiarity with the management of varicocele is therefore critically important. In this chapter we have provided an overview of the pathophysiology, clinical features, and evaluation of varicocele, as well as the indications for varicocele treatment. We have also provided a suggested algorithmic approach to varicocele management which we hope will be useful for health practitioners who care for men with cancer but are not specialized in male infertility.

References

1. Clarke BG. Incidence of varicocele in normal men and among men of different ages. *JAMA*. 1966; 198: 1121–2.

2. Fretz PC, Sandlow JI. Varicocele: current concepts in pathophysiology, diagnosis, and treatment. *Urol Clin North Am* 2002; 29: 921–37.

3. Nagler HM, Li XZ, Lizza EF, Deitch A, White RD. Varicocele: temporal considerations. *J Urol* 1985; 134: 411–13.

4. Gorelick JI, Goldstein M. Loss of fertility in men with varicocele. *Fertil Steril* 1993; 59: 613–16.

5. Witt MA, Lipshultz LI. Varicocele: a progressive or static lesion? *Urology* 1993; 42: 541–3.

6. Kass EJ, Belman AB. Reversal of testicular growth failure by varicocele ligation. *J Urol* 1987; 137: 475–6.

7. Su LM, Goldstein M, Schlegel PN. The effect of varicocelectomy on serum testosterone levels in infertile men with varicoceles. *J Urol* 1995; 154: 1752–5.

8. Cayan S, Kadioglu A, Orhan I, *et al.* The effect of microsurgical varicocelectomy on serum follicle stimulating hormone, testosterone and free testosterone levels in infertile men with varicocele. *BJU Int* 1999; 84: 1046–9.

9. Tanrikut C, Goldstein M. Varicocele repair for treatment of androgen deficiency. *Curr Opin Urol* 2010; 20: 500–2.

10. Sharlip ID, Jarow JP, Belker AM, *et al.* Best practice policies for male infertility. *Fertil Steril* 2002; 77: 873–82.

11. Zorgniotti AW. Testis temperature, infertility, and the varicocele paradox. *Urology* 1980; 16: 7–10.

12. Tessler AN, Krahn HP. Varicocele and testicular temperature. *Fertil Steril* 1966; 17: 201–3.

13. Lewis RW, Harrison RM. Contact scrotal thermography: application to problems of infertility. *J Urol* 1979; 122: 40–2.

14. Wright EJ, Young GP, Goldstein M. Reduction in testicular temperature after varicocelectomy in infertile men. *Urology* 1997; 50: 257–9.

15. Mieusset R, Bujan L, Plantavid M, Grandjean H. Increased levels of serum follicle-stimulating hormone and luteinizing hormone associated with intrinsic testicular hyperthermia in oligospermic infertile men. *J Clin Endocrinol Metab* 1989; 68: 419–25.

16. Lue YH, Lasley BL, Laughlin LS, *et al.* Mild testicular hyperthermia induces profound transitional spermatogenic suppression through increased germ cell apoptosis in adult cynomolgus monkeys (*Macaca fascicularis*). *J Androl* 2002; 23: 799–805.

17. Ferlin A, Speltra E, Patassini C, *et al.* Heat shock protein and heat shock factor expression in sperm: relation to oligozoospermia and varicocele. *J Urol* 2010; 183: 1248–52.

18. Comhaire F, Vermeulen A. Varicocele sterility: cortisol and catecholamines. *Fertil Steril* 1974; 25: 88–95.

19. Shafik A, Bedeir GA. Venous tension patterns in cord veins. I. In normal and varicocele individuals. *J Urol* 1980; 123: 383–5.

20. Lipshultz LI, Corriere JN, Jr. Progressive testicular atrophy in the varicocele patient. *J Urol* 1977; 117: 175–6.

21. Pinto KJ, Kroovand RL, Jarow JP. Varicocele related testicular atrophy and its predictive effect upon fertility. *J Urol* 1994; 152: 788–90.

22. Saypol DC, Howards SS, Turner TT, Miller ED. Influence of surgically induced varicocele on testicular blood flow, temperature, and histology in adult rats and dogs. *J Clin Invest* 1981; 68: 39–45.

23. Zini A, Buckspan M, Berardinucci D, Jarvi K. The influence of clinical and subclinical varicocele on testicular volume. *Fertil Steril* 1997; 68: 671–4.

24. Alukal JP, Zurakowski D, Atala A, *et al.* Testicular hypotrophy does not correlate with grade of adolescent varicocele. *J Urol* 2005; 174: 2367–70.

25. MacLeod J. Seminal cytology in the presence of varicocele. *Fertil Steril* 1965; 16: 735–57.

26. World Health Organization. The influence of varicocele on parameters of fertility in a large group of men presenting to infertility clinics. *Fertil Steril* 1992; 57: 1289–93.

27. Johnson DE, Pohl DR, Rivera-Correa H. Varicocele: an innocuous condition? *South Med J* 1970; 63: 34–6.

28. Zargooshi J. Sperm count and sperm motility in incidental high-grade varicocele. *Fertil Steril* 2007; 88: 1470–3.

29. Rajfer J, Turner TT, Rivera F, Howards SS, Sikka SC. Inhibition of testicular testosterone biosynthesis following experimental varicocele in rats. *Biol Reprod* 1987; 36: 933–7.

30. Sirvent JJ, Bernat R, Navarro MA, *et al.* Leydig cell in idiopathic varicocele. *Eur Urol* 1990; 17: 257–61.

31. Tanrikut C, Goldstein M, Rosoff JS, *et al.* Varicocele as a risk factor for androgen deficiency and effect of repair. *BJU Int* 2011; 108: 1480–4.

32. Park HJ, Lee SS, Park NC. Predictors of pain resolution after varicocelectomy for painful varicocele. *Asian J Androl* 2010; 13: 754–8.

33. Stahl PJ, Stember DS, Hsiao W, Schlegel PN. Indications and strategies for fertility preservation in men. *Clin Obstet Gynecol* 2010; 53: 815–27.

34. Pasqualotto FF, Sobreiro BP, Hallak J, Pasqualotto EB, Lucon AM. Induction of spermatogenesis in azoospermic men after varicocelectomy repair: an update. *Fertil Steril* 2006; 85: 635–9.

Chapter

Disorders of ejaculation

9

Doron S. Stember and John P. Mulhall

Introduction

Ejaculatory dysfunction is a common male sexual disorder and can cause severe distress in men of all ages. Although orgasm in men usually accompanies ejaculation, it represents a distinct cognitive and emotional cortical process. In a survey of nearly 13 000 men aged 50–80 years, 46% reported reduced amount of ejaculation and 5% reported a complete absence of ejaculate within the previous month. Patients' level of bother from ejaculatory problems was independent of age and ranged from 52% to 80%, with worse bother for patients with worse voiding dysfunction [1]. An intact ejaculatory process is particularly important, for the purposes of intromission, to men interested in fertility.

In clinical practice, four main ejaculatory disorders are commonly encountered: anejaculation (AE), retrograde ejaculation (RE), premature ejaculation (PE), and retarded or delayed ejaculation (DE). Although PE and DE are well-recognized disorders of sexual function that cause serious bother, they are not typically associated with impaired fertility. For the purpose of discussion of ejaculatory dysfunction as it relates to fertility preservation, this chapter will focus on AE and RE. We will also review normal reproductive anatomy and physiology and present diagnostic and management strategies.

Reproductive anatomy

A working knowledge of the relevant anatomy is critical to understanding the processes underlying ejaculatory dysfunction. The organs related to ejaculation include the testis, epididymis, vas deferens, seminal vesicles, prostate, bladder neck, and periurethral

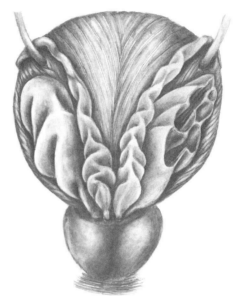

Figure 9.1. Posterior bladder anatomy, demonstrating vasal ampullae (medial) and seminal vesicles (lateral).

skeletal muscle, along with intact thoracolumbar spinal nerves (Figs. 9.1 and 9.2).

Spermatozoa are produced in the seminiferous tubules that comprise the majority of the volume of the paired testes. The tubules drain towards the mediastinum, which is located at the superior and posterior aspect of the testes. The mediastinum coalesces into 5–10 efferent ductules. The ductules leave the testis to enter the head of the epididymis, which is positioned immediately superior and posterior to the testis. The multiple tubules coalesce into a single epididymal duct. Spermatozoa are transported from the caput (head) to the cauda (tail) of the epididymis. As they migrate, interactions between the secretory

Fertility Preservation in Male Cancer Patients, ed. John P. Mulhall, Linda D. Applegarth, Robert D. Oates and Peter N. Schlegel. Published by Cambridge University Press. © Cambridge University Press 2013.

products of sperm surface and epididymal epithelial cells allow the spermatozoa to acquire the capacities for forward motility and fertility.

The epididymal tubule is continuous with the vas (ductus) deferens, a 30–35 cm tubular conduit for sperm that is surrounded by three distinct muscular layers that facilitate seminal emission. In addition to propelling spermatozoa forward, the vas also acts as a reservoir for sperm. The vas begins in the cauda epididymis, ascends in the spermatic cord, travels through the inguinal canal, and enters the pelvis. The vasal ampullae join the seminal vesicles, which are located posterior to the bladder, to form the ejaculatory ducts. The ejaculatory ducts travel for a short course through the prostate and empty into the posterior urethra just lateral to the verumontanum. During ejaculation, sperm rapidly transit the vas deferens towards the vasal ampullae.

The seminal vesicles are paired structures that are located between the bladder and rectum. They secrete fructose-rich, alkaline fluid that mixes with spermatozoa as the seminal vesicle ducts empty into the ejaculatory ducts. Prostatic secretions also mix with seminal fluid as it enters the prostatic urethra and serve to liquefy semen, thus facilitating contact between the spermatozoa and ovum.

Ejaculatory physiology

Ejaculation is a complex process that involves closely coordinated neurological and muscular events. The central and peripheral nervous systems both play critical roles in ejaculation. Spinal ejaculatory centers are controlled by supraspinal regions (cognitive arousal) and peripheral sensory afferents from the genitals (reflex stimulation) [2]. Thoracolumbar and lumbosacral nuclei produce efferent stimulation of the anatomical structures involved in ejaculation (Fig. 9.2). Two distinct phases can be identified, which occur in sequence during the ejaculatory response: emission and expulsion.

Progressive sexual stimulation leads to ejaculatory inevitability. Emission is initiated by the thoracolumbar sympathetic nerves, which arise from sympathetic nerves that exit the spinal cord at levels T10–L2. The nerves cause contraction of smooth muscle in the vas deferens, seminal vesicles, and prostate. Sperm flows from the testicular end of the vas towards the abdominal end and merges with

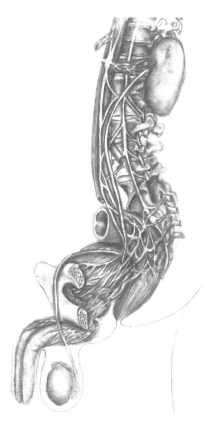

Figure 9.2. Illustration of the sympathetic nerve fibers involved in ejaculation emanating from the spinal cord.

seminal vesicle fluid at the level of the ejaculatory ducts. Smooth muscle contraction similarly expels seminal vesicle fluid into the ejaculatory ducts. The mixed components from the vas and seminal vesicles constitute the seminal fluid, which is then deposited into the prostatic urethra. During seminal emission, the bladder neck (BN) contracts forcefully to prevent the fluid from flowing retrograde into the bladder.

The next phase, expulsion, occurs just after emission. The seminal fluid bolus distends the posterior urethra, stimulating a reflex arc. The pudendal nerve, which originates from spinal cord levels S2–S4, mediates involuntary contractions of the striated periurethral (bulbospongiosus and ischiocavernosus) and pelvic floor muscles. These rhythmic contractions forcibly eject the seminal fluid in an antegrade fashion (assuming that the BN is adequately closed) from the posterior urethra towards, and through, the urethral meatus [3].

Failure of the initial step, emission, causes the condition of anejaculation (AE). Failure of antegrade expulsion due to inadequate BN closure defines retrograde ejaculation (RE).

Anejaculation

AE is defined as the complete absence of seminal emission into posterior urethra. The diagnosis should be suspected in patients with the total absence of an antegrade ejaculate, in patients with spinal cord injury (SCI), and in men with autonomic neuropathy associated with severe diabetes mellitus (DM). Psychogenic anejaculation may need to be considered if the patient complains of sudden inability to ejaculate, especially if no other causes can be identified.

The most common causes of AE are SCI and retroperitoneal lymph node dissection (RPLND) surgery, respectively. These two etiologies alone account for almost 90% of AE [4], although the incidence of anejaculation secondary to RPLND has dramatically decreased over the past 20 years as operative technique has evolved to ensure routine nerve sparing, even after chemotherapy. SCI patients with upper motor neuron lesions above spinal cord level T9 frequently have some degree of impaired erectile function, although complete absence of the ejaculatory reflex represents the most significant issue with regard to fertility [5]. The combination of erectile and ejaculatory dysfunction ensures that only about 5% of men with SCI will be able to procreate without medical intervention [6].

RPLND is a diagnostic and therapeutic surgical procedure performed in men with testicular cancer. The goal of the operation is to resect nodal tissue around the great vessels that are potential or known sites of testicular cancer metastasis. Anejaculation can result from trauma to the sympathetic chains or postganglionic branches of the lumbar sympathetic nerves. Prior to 1984, the rate of ejaculatory dysfunction following RPLND was 36% [7]. A nerve-sparing dissection modification of RPLND, developed in the 1980s, has greatly reduced this problem [8]. RPLND with prospective identification and sparing of the sympathetic chains, postganglionic sympathetic nerve fibers, and hypogastric plexus is associated with excellent preservation of antegrade ejaculation with excellent oncologic outcomes. Antegrade ejaculatory function remains threatened, however, when nerve-sparing

techniques are not carefully performed or when sparing nerves is not feasible for oncologic safety or in men who have previously undergone chemotherapy. The Indiana University group studied 176 men 3–9 years after primary RPLND, and found that 97% preserved antegrade emission. Of the 135 men who had undergone a nerve-sparing procedure, 99% could ejaculate, as could 89% who underwent non-nerve-sparing surgery [9].

Post-chemotherapy RPLND (PC-RPLND) is technically more difficult to perform than primary RPLND due to fibrosis and scarring of the retroperitoneum. In a series of 341 patients who underwent PC-RPLND by a single surgeon, nerve sparing was deemed oncologically safe and feasible in 136 (40%). Of these 136 men, 107 (79%) reported postoperative antegrade ejaculation without sympathomimetic agents. On multivariable analysis, predictors of antegrade ejaculation included a residual mass size > 5 cm (OR 0.1, 95% CI 0.0–0.7, $p = 0.020$) and right-sided testicular primary tumor (OR 0.4, 95% CI 0.1–1.0, $p = 0.044$), both of which were negatively associated with ejaculation recovery [10]. In another large analysis of patients undergoing PC-RPLND, 62/81 (77%) of men had postoperative antegrade ejaculation, closely mirroring the results of the aforementioned study [11].

Diabetes mellitus (DM) is a well-known cause of autonomic neuropathy that can affect both erectile and ejaculatory function. Neuropathy associated with DM is commonly associated with RE due to incomplete BN closure. In more severe cases, absence of vasal and seminal vesicle peristalsis causes failure of seminal emission. The overall prevalence in subjects with DM is difficult to determine, since it is likely that many older men who develop DM have previously fathered children, are no longer interested in fertility, and are therefore unrecognized. In a review of 54 men (mean age 36 years) with DM, a 6% incidence of RE was observed [12]. The prevalence of DM among men evaluated for subfertility is low. In a review of 466 consecutive patients presenting to a male infertility clinic, only 3 (0.7%) had insulin-dependent DM [13]. More recently, Sexton and Jarow reviewed 466 consecutive men (mean age 32 years) who presented to an infertility clinic and found that only 5 (1.1%) had insulin-dependent DM [14].

In addition to the medical and surgical causes of anejaculation, multiple drugs that interfere with ejaculation have been identified. Psychotropic drugs, in particular, have been associated with ejaculatory dysfunction. It is extremely challenging to accurately ascertain the incidence of ejaculatory dysfunction in men using psychotropic drugs because of multiple factors including variability of physician assessment, frequently poor patient communication of adverse effects, and impaired sexual function due to the underlying psychiatric condition itself. Psychotropics that are considered to have a high capacity to cause AE or RE include thioridazine, isocarboxazid, and phenelzine. Fluphenazine, trifluoperazine, and tranylcypromine have moderate capacity to result in ejaculatory dysfunction. Chlorpromazine and pimozide have minor ability to cause these adverse effects [15]. In a prospective, multicenter, open-label study conducted by the Spanish Working Group for the Study of Psychotropic-Related Sexual Dysfunction, 412 men and 610 women were interviewed using a questionnaire that included questions about erectile function, libido, ejaculation, and overall sexual satisfaction [16]. The rate of male sexual dysfunction with use of antidepressants, when all types were considered, was 62%. Unfortunately, the authors did not distinguish between anorgasmia and anejaculation with orgasm and, worse, did not report separate figures in that category for men versus women.

Alpha-1-adrenoreceptors are present in the smooth muscle of the prostate, urethra, and bladder neck. Alpha-1-adrenoreceptor antagonists, given for symptomatic relief of lower urinary tract symptoms (LUTS) caused by benign prostatic hypertrophy (BPH), are commonly associated with abnormal ejaculation. The incidence of ejaculatory dysfunction with these medications has been reported to be between 4% and 11% [17]. The mechanism is related to relaxation of the bladder neck, vas deferens, or seminal vesicles. Modification of the typically prescribed daily regimen has been proposed as a method for decreasing the side-effect profile. A prospective study was performed to evaluate the impact of intermittent tamsulosin on abnormal ejaculation. The study included 405 men with LUTS who were initially treated with 0.4 mg tamsulosin daily for three months, of whom 30 patients (7.3%) had treatment-related abnormal ejaculation (RE in 4.4%, decreased volume in 1.7%, absent ejaculate in 1.2%). In the second phase of the study, these 30 patients received tamsulosin 0.4 mg

every other day. Ejaculatory function recovered during the intermittent treatment period in 19 cases (63.3%), including 12 men with RE and 7 with decreased or absent ejaculate. Intermittent therapy was shown to be equally efficacious for LUTS as the daily regimen [18].

Retrograde ejaculation

RE is the most common cause of ejaculatory dysfunction. This is a condition in which ejaculate is deposited into the posterior urethra but makes its way into the bladder, and it is the cause of infertility in 0.3–2% of men with fertility problems [19,20]. Emitted semen, once deposited into the urethra, will take the path of least resistance. In the normal state, the BN closes with high pressure and ejaculation is antegrade. With impaired or absent BN closure, however, the semen is propelled in a retrograde fashion into the bladder.

RE is typically categorized into anatomic, neurogenic, and pharmacologic etiologies [4]. Anatomic etiologies can be further classified as acquired (transurethral resection of prostate [TURP], retropubic prostatectomy, bladder neck surgery, and trauma such as pelvic fracture) or congenital (posterior urethral valves, utricular cysts, and exstrophy). Mechanical anatomic obstruction, such as urethral stricture, can also cause RE. Neurogenic causes of RE include spinal cord lesions, surgical injury (lumbar sympathectomy, retroperitoneal lymphadenectomy, aortoiliac surgery, and abdomino-perineal resection), and neuropathies such as diabetes mellitus and multiple sclerosis. The major drug categories associated with RE are alpha-adrenergic blockers and antipsychotics.

The diagnosis of RE can often be made, or at least suggested, by taking a careful patient history, including medications and surgical procedures. RE is part of the differential diagnosis in men who present with absent or low-volume ejaculate. The patient may report that his post-orgasmic urine has a cloudy appearance due to the presence of semen. Postcoital urinalysis revealing sperm, seminal fluid, or fructose confirms the diagnosis [4,21].

Since closure of the BN is under sympathetic control, any underlying pathology that interferes with sympathetic nerve function, such as DM or retroperitoneal surgery, can result in RE. Medications that inhibit closure of the BN can temporarily cause RE. Mechanical disruption of the BN, as commonly occurs during transurethral surgical treatment of prostate enlargement, can also cause RE. In a recent prospective evaluation of 72 men with symptomatic BPH who underwent transurethral photoselective vaporization of the prostate (PVP), there was a new-onset incidence of RE in 30% of patients [22]. In a prospective, randomized trial of 121 men with BPH, 41% of men undergoing TURP experienced RE, compared with 0% of patients who underwent transurethral needle ablation of the prostate (TUNA). Follow-up time was five years from TURP or TUNA procedure, and evaluation was performed annually [23]. Although TUNA appears to have a lower incidence of ejaculatory dysfunction than either TURP or PVP, it is generally considered less effective than those procedures in terms of treating BPH.

Alpha-blockers are commonly used to treat BPH. There are currently five alpha-blockers approved for use by the US Food and Drug Administration (FDA). Although the FDA maintains that the alpha-blockers are equally effective in treatment of BPH symptoms, they have varying impact on ejaculatory function [24]. For example, Hellstrom and Sikka showed that tamsulosin 0.8 mg/day significantly reduced ejaculate volume in 90% of healthy volunteers. In similar patients treated with alfusozin, significantly reduced ejaculate volume was seen in 21% of men. Of patients taking placebo, 13% had significantly reduced volumes. Of patients on tamsulosin, 35% had anejaculation, compared with no cases of anejaculation in patients taking either alfusozin or placebo [25].

Medical treatment for ejaculatory dysfunction

Pharmacotherapy

The treatment of ejaculatory dysfunction depends to a large extent on the cause. Anatomic causes, such as TURP, are generally not reversible. Neurologic causes of AE or RE are often irreversible, particularly with SCI. In patients with partial neurologic injuries (e.g., secondary to DM), however, medications may induce antegrade ejaculation. Pharmacological success is generally better achieved in men with partial neural impairment (RE) compared to men with

complete neural injury (AE). The goal of medical treatment is to increase sympathetic tone, or decrease parasympathetic activity, of the BN so that semen is propelled antegrade. Medication is taken in close proximity to the time of ejaculation. Several alpha-adrenergic agonists have been used, including midodrine, pseudoephedrine, and ephedrine sulfate.

In a systematic review of 40 studies of men with anejaculation, Kamischke and Nieschlag determined an overall success rate of 12% in inducing antegrade ejaculation with various alpha-agonists [4]. The authors also reviewed 38 studies of medical treatment of RE. In all, 264 patients were treated with alpha-agonists, anticholinergic, and antihistamine agents. A total of 560 patients with AE and 205 with RE were reported among the 76 total studies reviewed. The overall calculated success rate of medical treatment for men with AE (as defined by the absence of antegrade ejaculation) was 12%, with only two spontaneous pregnancies after alpha-agonist drug therapy. In contrast, medical therapy yielded a 50% success rate in inducing antegrade ejaculation for men with RE. Among men with a documented desire for pregnancy it was achieved in 34% of cases. The authors note that only uncontrolled clinical trials comparing efficacy of the different drugs and regimens were available for review.

The tricyclic antidepressant imipramine has also been used successfully. Imipramine has alpha-adrenergic activity and causes an increase in the pressure profile of the posterior urethra [26]. Ochsenkuhn et al. evaluated 11 patients with iatrogenic RE (secondary to RPLND for testis cancer in 10 and aortic and thromboendarterectomy in 1) [27]. All patients received an ovarian cycle-dependent dose regime consisting of daily oral imipramine at 25 mg for four days, followed by 50 mg daily for the next three days. On day 8 of treatment, patients ejaculated and ejaculate parameters were measured. In all 11 patients, antegrade ejaculate was induced with imipramine (between 0.5 and 3.2 mL, sperm concentration between 5.4 and 276 million spermatozoa/mL) and two spontaneous pregnancies were reported within six months of start. Furthermore, every patient reported that antegrade ejaculation persisted for 1–2 days after the final dose of imipramine. Although five patients experienced minor side effects such as dizziness and sweating, no major side effects were seen. Despite the impressive results of this study, however, the published success rates for restoring antegrade ejaculation vary from 0% to 100% [28].

Midodrine is an alpha-adrenergic agonist that modifies arterial resistance and is primarily used for treatment of orthostatic hypotension. Animal and human studies have suggested that midodrine also stimulates sympathetically innervated structures, including the vasa deferentia, prostate, and seminal vesicles, in a manner that promotes the rhythmic muscle contraction required during ejaculation. The efficacy of midodrine for treatment of ejaculatory dysfunction was demonstrated in a large study from France. The authors reviewed their experience with 449 SCI patients referred for anejaculation. Ejaculation was achieved in 65% of these men using penile vibratory stimulation (PVS). The remaining 158 men who failed to ejaculate were treated with midodrine within 30–120 minutes prior to repeat PVS. The procedure was repeated weekly with dose increases of 7.5 mg up to a maximum dose of 30 mg. Ejaculation was achieved in 65% of men at a mean midodrine dose of 18.7 mg [29].

Pseudoephedrine is a sympathomimetic that increases the tone of the BN. Pseudoephedrine may be used to effect antegrade ejaculation, and may be used prior to attempts at conception, semen analysis with post-ejaculatory urinalysis, or assisted reproduction for men with AE or RE. In a retrospective review of 26 men with advanced testicular cancer presenting with infertility after post-chemotherapy RPLND, Hsiao *et al.* studied the implementation of a clinical pathway using pseudoephedrine. Four men had RE, and 50% were converted to antegrade ejaculation with pseudoephedrine. Twenty-two patients had AE, and no patients converted to antegrade ejaculation with medication [30].

There are some data to suggest that combination therapy is superior to single drug treatment. In a study of 33 diabetic men with RE (23 complete and 10 partial), antegrade ejaculation was successfully achieved in 39% of men taking imipramine, 48% of men taking pseudoephedrine, and 62% of patients using combined imipramine and pseudoephedrine. Among the men with partial RE at initial presentation, there was a significant increase in both semen volume and sperm count using either drug or combination therapy [31].

Assisted ejaculation procedures

In men who cannot be pharmacologically converted to antegrade ejaculation, more invasive methods are required to harvest sperm. Sperm retrieval procedures are also appropriate for men with SCI or in whom pharmacologic management is contraindicated. The two approaches are penile vibratory stimulation (PVS) and electroejaculation (EEJ). These procedures will be briefly described here. A through review of PVS and EEJ is given in Chapter 27.

Penile vibratory stimulation

In men with SCI, penile vibratory stimulation (PVS) is an effective procedure that involves placing a vibrator in the perifrenular region of the glans penis for 2–3 minutes, or until antegrade ejaculation occurs. For PVS to induce ejaculation, the thoracolumbar spinal cord, that is the ejaculatory reflex arc, must be functioning. Specifically, the sensory system from the penis, the spinal cord at the levels of sensory input (S2–S4) and efferent exit (T10–L2), and peripheral sympathetic outflow must be intact. Therefore, the best candidates for PVS are SCI patients with lesions above the T10 spinal cord level [32].

Sønksen and Ohl evaluated the ejaculatory response to PVS in men with SCI to determine the optimal parameters [32]. They found that vibrator amplitude level of 2.5 mm and frequency of 100 Hz produced ejaculation (antegrade ± retrograde) in 96% of patients, compared with an ejaculatory rate of only 32% when the amplitude was 1 mm with a frequency of 100 Hz. These results led to the development of a medical grade vibrator for PVS (FertiCare Personal, Multicept A/S, Copenhagen, Denmark) that remains the only FDA-approved device for ejaculation of men with SCI.

Success rates with PVS are significantly higher in patients with an intact ejaculatory reflex. In men with SCI at level T10 or higher, PVS resulted in ejaculation in 88% of cases, compared with a 15% success rate in patients with an injury at T11 or below [33]. Even if PVS is unsuccessful as a first treatment, SCI patients have an excellent chance of ejaculation when EEJ is used as a second option. In a review of 28 SCI men and their partners, an overall ejaculation rate of 100% was achieved (79% via PVS and the remaining 21% via EEJ). Median total sperm count was 65 million (range 0.1–480) with a median motility of 13%

(range 1–60%). Using assisted reproductive techniques, including vaginal self-insemination, intrauterine insemination, in-vitro fertilization, and intracytoplasmic injection, nearly a third of the couples (9/28) achieved pregnancy [34].

PVS is generally well tolerated and may be performed in the office. Great caution must be applied in SCI patients with lesions above T6, however, since PVS may potentially induce autonomic dysreflexia (AD) in these men [35]. AD is a syndrome of large-magnitude reflex sympathetic discharge that travels up the spinal cord but cannot pass the spinal lesion. Dangerously high systemic blood pressure can lead to seizure, stroke, or death. For at-risk SCI patients, pre-treatment with 20 mg sublingual or oral nifedipine and constant monitoring of vital signs during the procedure is essential. Further, spinal or general anesthesia is highly effective at ablating AD and should be strongly considered as opposed to no anesthesia [36]. Minor skin abrasions may also occur at the site of PVS application, but this usually requires no treatment and is unlikely to occur when a medical grade vibrator is used.

Bladder sperm harvesting

Anejaculation is defined as the persistent absence of antegrade seminal fluid at ejaculation. In order to distinguish failure of emission from RE, retrograde semen analysis is performed (Table 9.1). Patients are instructed to void to completion at the semen analysis laboratory. The purpose of voiding immediately prior to ejaculation is to avoid large volumes of urine upon voiding making the search for sperm difficult. The patient is then instructed to masturbate to orgasm and collect any ejaculated fluid into a sterile collection cup. He then waits 10–15 minutes before voiding into a second sterile collection container. For patients unable to void, urethral catheterization may be required. The post-orgasmic voided sample is evaluated for the presence of seminal fluid and is immediately centrifuged. The spun pellet is evaluated for the presence of sperm. If any seminal fluid or sperm are seen in the urine specimen, the patient meets the definition for RE. Sperm harvested from an alkalinized urine sample can be used for assisted reproductive technologies. Absence of seminal fluid or sperm in the post-orgasmic urine sample defines failure of emission.

Table 9.1. Instructions for the performance of a retrograde semen analysis

(1) Patient should abstain from ejaculation for 2–4 days prior to collection.
(2) Urine should not be diluted by excessive fluid intake during 12 hours prior to collection. If sperm is being retrieved for banking, urine acidity, which is toxic to sperm, may be counteracted by utilizing sodium bicarbonate 500 mg, 12 and 2 hours prior to collection (or alternatively potassium citrate).
(3) At the time of collection, patient should void in bathroom prior to masturbation. Alternatively, patient may be catheterized to evacuate urine.
(4) After voiding, patient should be given two sterile collection cups, labeled #1 and #2, and placed in private room for stimulation and ejaculation. Saliva and lubricants should be avoided.
(5) Patient should hold cup #1 to tip of penis and collect semen.
(6) Patient should return to waiting room for 15 minutes and refrain from drinking liquid during this time.
(7) Patient should return to bathroom and urinate into cup #2. Alternatively, patient may be recatheterized to ensure complete collection of specimen.
(8) Send both collection cups to laboratory for semen analysis and inform technician to survey urine for semen and not just sperm.

Conclusion

Ejaculatory dysfunction is common and is associated with significant patient anxiety and bother. It also represents a distinct cause of male-factor infertility. Anejaculation (AE) may be psychogenic in nature but is more often secondary to systemic medical conditions such as DM, medications such as alpha-1 blockers, or previous surgery such as TURP or RPLND. Retrograde ejaculation (RE) may be partial or complete and is characterized by the presence of semen in the bladder following orgasm. RE can be classified according to anatomic, neurogenic, or pharmacologic etiologies, and, while similar in many respects to AE, can be distinguished by a post-orgasmic urinalysis.

Medical therapy is based on mechanisms of action that increase sympathetic tone of the bladder neck so that semen is propelled antegrade. Medication should be taken within close proximity prior to the time of ejaculation and is generally more effective for RE than AE. For patients who do not respond to pharmacologic therapy, more invasive methods are required to harvest sperm. PVS and EEJ are effective methods for harvesting sperm but carry a risk of AD in men with spinal cord lesions above T6.

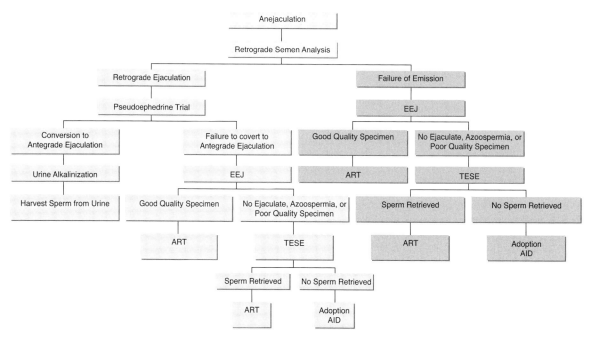

Figure 9.3. Clinical care algorithm for anejaculation.

An organized and rational approach to the patient who presents with failure of antegrade ejaculation is required to optimize therapeutic success. A suggested clinical care pathway is presented in Fig. 9.3.

References

1. Rosen R, Altwein J, Boyle P, *et al.* Lower urinary tract symptoms and male sexual dysfunction: the multinational survey of the aging male (MSAM-7). *Eur Urol* 2003; 44: 637–49.

2. Betocchi C, Verze P, Palumbo F, *et al.* Ejaculatory disorders: pathophysiology and management. *Nat Clin Pract Urol* 2008; 5: 93–103.

3. Hershlag A, Schiff SF, DeCherney AH. Retrograde ejaculation. *Hum Reprod* 1991; 6: 255–8.

4. Kamischke A, Nieschlag E. Update on medical treatment of ejaculatory disorders. *Int J Androl* 2002; 25: 333–44.

5. Biering-Sørensen F, Sønksen J. Sexual function in spinal cord lesioned men. *Spinal Cord* 2001; 39: 455–70.

6. Ohl DA, Quallich SA, Sonksen J, Brackett NL, Lynne CM. Anejaculation: an electrifying approach. *Semin Reprod Med* 2009; 27: 179–85.

7. Jones DR, Norman AR, Horwich A, *et al.* Ejaculatory dysfunction after retroperitoneal lymphadenectomy. *Eur Urology* 1993, 23: 169–71.

8. Jewett MA, Kong YS, Goldberg SD, *et al.* Retroperitoneal lymphadenectomy for testis tumor with nerve sparing for ejaculation. *J Urol* 1998; 139: 1220–4.

9. Beck SD, Bey AL, Bihrle R, *et al.* Ejaculatory status and fertility rates after primary retroperitoneal lymph node dissection. *J Urol* 2010; 184: 2078–80.

10. Pettus JA, Carver BS, Masterson T, *et al.* Preservation of ejaculation in patients undergoing nerve-sparing postchemotherapy retroperitoneal lymph node dissection for metastatic testicular cancer. *Urology* 2009; 73: 328–31.

11. Coogan CL, Hejase MJ, Wahle GR, *et al.* Nerve sparing post-chemotherapy retroperitoneal lymph node dissection for advanced testicular cancer. *J Urol* 1996; 156: 1656–8.

12. Dinulovic D, Radonjic G. Diabetes mellitus/male infertility. *Arch Androl* 1990; 25: 277–93.

13. Greenberg SH, Lipshultz LI, Wein AJ. Experience with 425 subfertile male patients. *J Urol* 1978; 119: 507–10.

14. Sexton WJ, Jarow JP. Effect of diabetes mellitus upon male reproductive function. *Urology* 1997; 49: 508–13.

15. Shiloh R, Strijer R, Weizman A, Nutt D (eds). Drugs affecting sexual function. In *Atlas of Psychiatric Pharmacotherapy*, 2nd edn. Abingdon: Taylor Francis, 2006; pp. 105–13.

16. Montejo AL, Llorca G, Izquierdo JA, *et al.* Incidence of sexual dysfunction associated with antidepressant agents: a prospective multicenter study of 1022 outpatients. Spanish Working Group for the Study of Psychotropic-Related Sexual Dysfunction. *J Clin Psychiatry* 2001; 62 (Suppl 3): 10–21.

17. Hofner K, Claes H, De Reijke TM, *et al.* Tamsulosin 0.4 mg once daily: effect on sexual function in patients with lower urinary tract symptoms suggestive of benign prostatic obstruction. *Eur Urol* 1999; 36: 335.

18. Goktas S, Kibar Y, Kilic S, *et al.* Recovery of abnormal ejaculation by intermittent tamsulosin treatment. *J Urol* 2006; 175: 650–3.

19. Vernon M, Wilson E, Muse K, *et al.* Successful pregnancies from men with retrograde ejaculation with the use of washed sperm and gamete intrafallopian tube transfer (GIFT). *Fertil Steril* 1988; 50; 822–4.

20. Yavetz H, Yogev L, Hauser R, *et al.* Retrograde ejaculation. *Hum Reprod* 1994; 9: 381–6.

21. Colpi G, Weidner W, Jungwirth A, *et al.* EAU guidelines on ejaculatory dysfunction. *Eur Urol* 2004; 46: 555–8.

22. Spaliviero M, Strom KH, Gu X, *et al.* Does Greenlight HPS (TM) laser photoselective vaporization prostatectomy affect sexual function? *J Endourol* 2010: 24: 2051–7.

23. Hill B, Belville W, Bruskewitz R, *et al.* Transurethral needle ablation versus transurethral resection of the prostate for the treatment of symptomatic benign prostatic hyperplasia: 5-year results of a prospective, randomized, multicenter clinical trial. *J Urol* 2004; 171: 2336–40.

24. Kaplan SA. Side effects of alpha-blocker use: retrograde ejaculation. *Rev Urol* 2009; 11(Suppl 1): S14–8.

25. Hellstrom WJ, Sikka SC. Effects of acute treatment with tamsulosin versus alfuzosin on ejaculatory function in normal volunteers. *J Urol* 2006; 176: 1529–33.

26. Goldwasser B, Jonas MP, Lunefeld B, *et al.* Imipramine for the treatment of sterility in patients following retroperitoneal lymph node dissection. *Andrologia* 1983; 15: 588–591.

27. Ochsenkuhn R, Kamischke A, Nieschlag E. Imipramine for successful treatment of retrograde ejaculation caused by retroperitoneal surgery. *Int J Androl* 1999; 22: 173–7.

28. Kamischke A, Nieschlag E. Treatment of retrograde ejaculation and anejaculation. *Hum Reprod Update* 1999; 5: 448–74.

29. Soler JM, Previnaire JG, Plante P, *et al.* Midodrine improves ejaculation in spinal cord injured men. *J Urol* 2007; 178: 2082–6.

30. Hsiao W, Deveci W, Mulhall JP. Outcomes of post-chemotherapy retroperitoneal lymph node dissection-associated anejaculation management. *BJU Int* (in press). (doi:10.1111/j.1464-410X.2011. 10852.x).

31. Arafa M, El Tabie O. Medical treatment of retrograde ejaculation in diabetic patients: a hope for spontaneous pregnancy. *J Sex Med* 2008; 5: 194–8.

32. Sønksen J, Ohl DA. Penile vibratory stimulation and electroejaculation in the treatment of ejaculatory dysfunction. *Int J Androl* 2002; 25: 324–32.

33. Kafetsoulis A, Brackett NL, Ibrahim E, *et al.* Current trends in the treatment of infertility in men with spinal cord injury. *Fert Steril* 2006; 86: 781–9.

34. Sønksen J, Sommer P, Biering-Sørensen F, *et al.* Pregnancy after assisted ejaculation procedures in men with spinal cord injury. *Arch Phys Med Rehabil.* 1997; 78: 1059–61.

35. Comarr AE. Sexuality and fertility among spinal cord and/or cauda equina injuries. *J Am Paraplegia Soc* 1985; 8: 67–75.

36. Brackett NL, Lynne CM, Ibrahim E, *et al.* Treatment of infertility in men with spinal cord injury. *Nat Rev Urol* 2010; 7: 162–72.

Chapter 10

Androgen deficiency in the male

Gregory C. Mitchell and Wayne J. G. Hellstrom

Introduction

When used to describe the male patient, hypogonadism most commonly refers to a decrease in circulating testosterone levels. In the clinic, however, this definition must be augmented to account for the diverse array of patient presentations that fall under the definition of hypogonadism. For example, it is possible for a man with a low-normal range level of testosterone to present with all of the classic symptoms of hypogonadism, such as depression, fatigue, and erectile dysfunction. Similarly, another man with completely normal sexual function and energy levels may be found to have low circulating testosterone levels only discovered incidentally. It is important to note that testosterone exhibits numerous end-organ effects, and different patients conceivably possess different thresholds at which those effects occur. For this reason, laboratory measurements of serum androgens need to be correlated with signs and symptoms of hypogonadism in order to arrive at the standard clinical diagnosis of hypogonadism. To that end, validated questionnaires have been developed to help provide some objective assessment of symptoms associated with hypogonadism (Androgen Deficiency in the Aging Male questionnaire, International Index of Erectile Function) [1,2]. The effective management of hypogonadism requires not only a diagnosis and treatment, but also understanding of the underlying causes of the deficit, and a familiarity with the numerous systemic effects of androgens. This chapter will provide an orientation to these concepts.

Physiology of the hypothalamic–pituitary–gonadal axis

The male reproductive axis involves the secretion of multiple signaling proteins from various levels that alter downstream hormonal release (Fig. 10.1). Neurons located in the preoptic area of the hypothalamus release gonadotropin-releasing hormone (GnRH) into the portal circulation surrounding the pituitary gland. GnRH is released from the hypothalamus in a pulsatile fashion and can also vary based on the season and time of day. Secretion tends to be highest in the spring. Also, levels tend to be highest in the morning and can vary throughout the day with a peak in secretion every 90–120 minutes. GnRH release directly stimulates production of luteinizing hormone (LH) and follicle-stimulating hormone (FSH) in the anterior pituitary. Changes in the pulse frequency of GnRH secretion can alter gonadotropin secretion from the pituitary. For instance, an increase in GnRH secretion interval (longer interval) results in an increase in the response amplitude for LH secretion. Alternatively, a decrease in GnRH secretion interval (shorter interval) results in a profound decrease in LH release, thus serving as the basis for androgen ablation with GnRH analogs.

The pituitary gland is divided into two segments, the anterior and posterior pituitary. The posterior pituitary gland is directly innervated by hypothalamic neurons that function to control the release of arginine-vasopressin (AVP, or antidiuretic hormone) and oxytocin. The anterior pituitary is a collection of cells involved in the tightly regulated release of

Fertility Preservation in Male Cancer Patients, ed. John P. Mulhall, Linda D. Applegarth, Robert D. Oates and Peter N. Schlegel. Published by Cambridge University Press. © Cambridge University Press 2013.

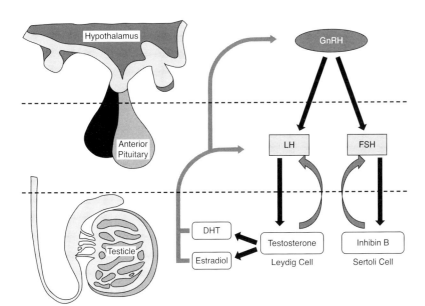

Figure 10.1. The male hypothalamic–pituitary–gonadal (HPG) axis. The antegrade actions of hormonal signals at the levels of the hypothalamus, pituitary, and testicle are shown in black arrows, while feedback actions are shown in gray arrows. DHT, dihydrotestosterone; FSH, follicle-stimulating hormone; GnRH, gonadotropin-releasing hormone; LH, luteinizing hormone.

stimulating hormones, including prolactin, thyroid-stimulating hormone (TSH), adrenocorticotropic hormone (ACTH), growth hormone (GH), LH, and FSH. This review of physiology will concentrate on the sex-steroid hormone axis involving LH and FSH. However, alterations in the secretion of any of the pituitary hormones can have dramatic effects on the release of others.

Release of LH and FSH relies on a tightly regulated system of stimulatory and inhibitory signals. Pulsatile GnRH release from the hypothalamus causes periodic release of gonadotropins from the pituitary gland. Both LH and FSH exert their endocrine effects in the male testis. LH stimulates Leydig cells in the testes to produce testosterone. FSH exerts its effects on Sertoli cells lining the seminiferous tubules to promote and maintain spermatogenesis.

Feedback mechanisms are primarily responsible for the tightly regulated control of gonadotropin release and hormone production. Testosterone acts mainly at the level of the hypothalamus and the pituitary by binding to androgen receptors to inhibit GnRH release and subsequent LH release. Metabolites of testosterone also act to regulate gonadotropin release. Testosterone is converted to estradiol in the periphery by the enzyme aromatase. Estradiol binds to estrogen receptors at the level of the pituitary to inhibit gonadotropin release. Even dihydrotestosterone (DHT) regulates gonadotropin release. Men with genetic 5-alpha-reductase deficiency have been

shown to have higher circulating levels of LH. In addition to steroids and their metabolites regulating gonadotropin release, other molecules are also involved in the regulatory process. Inhibin B is secreted by Sertoli cells and acts at the level of the pituitary to block transcription and release of FSH. In fact, evidence suggests that Inhibin B is the predominant negative regulator of FSH release. Additionally, activins are secreted by Sertoli cells and locally by the pituitary gland to stimulate production of FSH. It is intuitive that alterations in any of these feedback loops can have dramatic effects on gonadotropin release and circulating hormone levels.

Causes of hypogonadism

Patients may exhibit low levels of circulating androgens for several different reasons. Etiologies of hypogonadism, subdivided by gonadotropin secretion status, are categorized in Table 10.1. Primary hypogonadism, also known as testicular failure, refers to a defect in androgen production by the testicle. This condition is also referred to as "hypergonadotropic hypogonadism," as the serum levels of the gonadotropins LH and FSH, which are critical for androgen production and sperm production by the testicle, are typically elevated in this situation.

Testicular failure can be further subdivided as primary or secondary (shown graphically in Fig. 10.2). In primary testicular failure, congenital defects

Table 10.1. Causes of male hypogonadism. Hypergonadotropic hypogonadism refers to any cause of testicular failure and resultant decreased testosterone synthesis in the presence of normal hypothalamic and pituitary function. Hypogonadotropic hypogonadism can result from any interruption in normal pituitary or hypothalamic cellular function, thereby decreasing release of gonadotropins. Pathologic process is displayed on the left, with corresponding examples on right.

Hypergonadotropic hypogonadism: testicular failure (primary hypogonadism)	
Congenital	Klinefelter syndrome, male XX syndrome, anorchia, testicular dysgenesis syndrome
Trauma	Testicular torsion, traumatic anorchia
Inflammatory/infectious diseases	Tuberculosis, mumps orchitis
Drug use	Glucocorticoids, opioids, ketoconazole
Chemotherapy	
Radiation	
Tumor	
Aging	

Hypogonadotropic hypogonadism: decreased gonadotropin release (secondary hypogonadism)	
Congenital	Kallmann syndrome
Tumor	Pituitary adenoma (prolactinoma), craniopharyngioma, Hand–Schuller–Christian syndrome, metastatic lesions, glioma
Inflammatory/infectious diseases	Tuberculosis, sarcoidosis
Hemorrhage/ischemia	Simmond's disease
Medications	LHRH-agonists
Surgery	
Radiation therapy	
Aging	

lead to low levels of androgen production, typified by Klinefelter syndrome in the male. These patients may demonstrate a 47,XXY karyotype or a mosaic pattern 46,XY/47,XXY karyotype. Interestingly, some patients may have normal testosterone levels but have low bioavailable testosterone as a result of elevated estrogen and sex-hormone binding globulin (SHBG) levels (a summary of the diverse conditions that are associated with changes in SHBG levels is shown in Table 10.2). However, LH is usually elevated and FSH is markedly elevated in these individuals. For the readership of this book, the most likely cause of testicular failure is patient exposure to chemotherapy or testicular

radiation resulting in Leydig cell damage. Other causes of testicular failure include any incident that reduces the testicle's capacity to produce androgens, ranging from infection and trauma to drug use. Severe cases of mumps orchitis can irreversibly impair testicular function, including Leydig cell production of testosterone. Testicular torsion or trauma resulting in anorchia are common adolescent etiologies of secondary testicular failure.

Secondary hypogonadism, or "hypogonadotropic hypogonadism," generally refers to conditions that develop as a result of decreased release of LH and/or FSH. The causative defect may be in the hypothalamus or the pituitary. The classic example of hypogonadotropic hypogonadism is Kallmann syndrome. This congenital hypogonadal syndrome is characterized clinically by findings resulting from decreased or absent GnRH secretion, including anosmia, and various midline defects (cleft lip/palate, color blindness, seizures). This syndrome is thought to result from impaired migration of GnRH-releasing neurons to the hypothalamus during the embryonic period, and these patients typically present with delayed puberty. Idiopathic hypogonadotropic hypogonadism presents as a similar clinical scenario to Kallmann syndrome. Any damage to the hypothalamus or pituitary can lead to low circulating gonadotropin levels. At a cancer center, pituitary surgery or brain radiation can lead to pituitary dysfunction. Other insults such as infection, tumor, and infarction of the hypothalamus or pituitary gland can lead to low levels of gonadotropins and result in hypogonadism. As an example, pituitary prolactinomas elevate prolactin secretion, leading to decreased gonadotropin secretion and subsequent hypogonadism.

Another prevalent and often unappreciated secondary cause of hypogonadism is aging. In 2002, Harman *et al.* used data from the Baltimore Longitudinal Study on Aging to note that the prevalence of low serum testosterone levels in men aged 70–79 ranged from 28% (based on serum total testosterone) to 68% (based on free testosterone index) [3]. The fact that SHBG levels tend to rise with age, resulting in an even lower level of bioavailable testosterone, can help to explain the greater prevalence of hypogonadism as defined by free testosterone index [3]. Some men may exhibit an increase in LH secretion resulting from the low serum testosterone levels, while others may have low or inappropriately normal LH levels. These findings indicate not only

Table 10.2. Factors associated with fluctuation in sex-hormone binding globulin (SHBG) levels

Increases in SHBG level	Decreases in SHBG level
Mutations in the SHBG gene (ASN327, possibly D327N)	Elevated insulin, IGF-1
Dietary (isoflavones, reduced caloric intake leading to significant weight loss)	Elevated androgen levels
Elevated growth hormone	Elevated transcortin (corticosteroid binding globulin, CBG) levels
Elevated estrogen	Obesity
Hyperthyroidism (elevated thyroxine)	Coronary artery disease
Aging	
Frailty in elderly men	
Klinefelter syndrome	

a primary testicular defect but also secondary alterations in the hypothalamic–pituitary axis. Several monikers have been assigned to this phenomenon, including "androgen deficiency in the aging male," "late-onset hypogonadism," "testosterone deficiency syndrome," and "andropause." Symptoms of this condition resemble those of "normal" aging and include changing body composition, decreased libido, erectile dysfunction, and decreased cognitive function.

Chemotherapy and radiation have been scrutinized for their effects on gonadal function. Chemotherapy is well known to cause azoospermia. Although many cases of post-chemotherapy azoospermia are temporary, and reproductive function can show recovery over time, certain chemotherapeutic agents, such as alkylating agents, result in much lower rates of subsequent fertility. For example, males with Hodgkin's lymphoma suffer a very high incidence of infertility (in some studies, up to 100%) when treated with certain protocols that make use of alkylating agents, such as MOPP (nitrogen mustard, vincristine, procarbazine, prednisone) [4]. Newer chemotherapeutic protocols attempt to preserve reproductive function in male patients. Although past research has reported on the possible return of reproductive function following chemotherapy, the detrimental effects of such agents on overall gonadal function have only recently been investigated in detail. The majority of studies have shown that, even in men who retain reproductive function, hypogonadism persists after treatment. Eberhard *et al.* studied over 140 men with testicular cancer who received either chemotherapy or radiation as adjuvant treatment [5]. They found that hypogonadism, here defined as low serum testosterone, was prevalent and that those men with decreased circulating testosterone prior to adjuvant therapy with chemotherapy or radiation were at a higher risk for persistent hypogonadism up to three years after their adjuvant treatment. Further, Greenfield *et al.* studied 176 cancer survivors where 97% had undergone chemotherapy and 40% had received radiation [6]. The authors measured total testosterone levels and calculated free testosterone levels, which they then compared to levels from 213 control patients. Cancer survivors had significantly lower levels of testosterone, along with greater fat mass, higher serum insulin and glucose levels, and

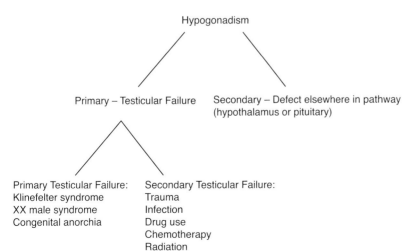

Figure 10.2. Schematic of causes of primary and secondary hypogonadism.

decreased sexual function when compared to control subjects.

Historically, evidence suggested that Leydig cells were generally radio-resistant and androgen production was not significantly impaired by radiation therapy. However, more recent studies have challenged this assumption. Schmiegelow et al. studied 30 male patients with childhood cranial tumors [7]. These patients were treated with radiation and/or chemotherapy, and mean follow-up for the study was 18 years. Despite the small sample size, the results demonstrated that both patients receiving radiation only and those receiving radiation plus chemotherapy had chronically low levels of testosterone following their treatment. Cranial radiation also depressed levels of LH, suggesting direct damage to the hypothalamic–pituitary axis. Additionally, inhibin B levels were significantly lower in patients receiving radiation and chemotherapy, which implicates a component of primary gonadal failure being present.

One of the most thoroughly studied hormonal therapies known to induce hypogonadism is manipulation of the hypothalamic–pituitary–gonadal (HPG) axis for the treatment of metastatic prostate cancer. Charles Huggins received the Nobel Prize for Medicine for demonstrating that metastatic prostate cancer responded to hormonal ablation, and the primary modality by which advanced prostate cancer was treated became surgical castration. Although significant clinical improvements in cancer-related symptoms were noted soon after castration, prominent side effects of androgen ablation became evident, such as decreased libido, erectile dysfunction, and hot flashes.

Understanding the physiology of the HPG axis led to the development and use of several agents that effectively accomplish the goal of reducing circulating androgen levels without surgical castration. Estrogens such as diethylstilbestrol (DES) were administered in order to block release of LH at the level of the pituitary gland. Identification and purification of GnRH led to the production of GnRH agonists, which exert their effect by making the normally pulsatile release of LH constant. Although GnRH agonists cause an initial surge in testosterone levels after administration, they eventually lead to down-regulation of LH release and medical castration. Therapeutic blockade of the androgen receptor using both steroidal and non-steroidal antiandrogens has been employed clinically. Cyproterone acetate, a steroidal antiandrogen, exhibits both antiandrogen effects (by blocking the androgen receptor) and estrogen-like effects (by blocking release of LH at the level of the pituitary gland). As a result, it causes typical hypogonadal symptoms in addition to direct androgen blockade. By comparison, non-steroidal antiandrogens (flutamide, nilutamide, bicalutamide) exert their effect only by competitive inhibition of the androgen receptor. These molecules lead to a rise in circulating LH and testosterone levels, theoretically ameliorating some of the clinical symptoms of hypogonadism, while still reducing androgenic stimulation of prostate cancer cells. One notable side effect of these medications is that elevated levels of circulating testosterone lead to an increased peripheral conversion to estradiol, causing gynecomastia and breast tenderness in some men [8].

Effects of hypogonadism

The effects of circulating testosterone on the body are many and varied (Table 10.3).

Metabolic effects

Recent evidence has detailed extensive metabolic effects caused by low androgen levels, which include insulin resistance, type 2 diabetes, lipid alterations, and higher rates of obesity [9,10]. Additionally, men with preexisting diabetes who were treated with androgen deprivation therapy had increased levels of glycosylated hemoglobin (HbA1C) [11], and required higher doses of self-administered insulin to maintain glycemic control [12]. An analysis of a population of 849 hypogonadal men showed a high prevalence of coincident cardiometabolic risk factors that were correlated to total testosterone levels, including obesity, systolic blood pressure, body mass index (BMI), and fasting glucose [13].

There is some evidence to suggest that testosterone replacement therapy has the potential to reverse some of the metabolic effects associated with hypogonadism. When diabetic men were treated with supplemental testosterone, they demonstrated a significant improvement in insulin sensitivity and glycemic control [14,15]. Page et al. studied hypogonadal men given testosterone replacement therapy, and found marked improvements in body composition and lipid profiles, increases in lean body mass, decreases in total body fat, decreases in low-density lipoprotein (LDL), and reduced triglyceride levels [16]. Interestingly,

Table 10.3. Effects of testosterone on various body systems

Organ/function	Effect
Metabolic	Improved insulin sensitivity Decreased triglyceride levels Decreased low-density lipoprotein (LDL) levels
Cardiovascular	Possible improvement in endothelial function (increased vasodilation) Possible decreased risk of atherosclerosis Decreased pro-inflammatory cytokines (IL-1, TNF-α)
Bone	Closure of epiphyses Reduced bone resorption Increased bone mineral density Accelerated linear bone growth
Body composition	Increased muscle mass Decreased fat mass via attenuation of lipoprotein lipase activity
Cognition/mood	Possible improvement in depressive symptoms in select populations Possible improvement in memory and visuospatial learning Improvement in libido Possible decreased risk of Alzheimer's disease
Sexual function	Improvement in libido Short-term improvement in erectile function
Male sexual organs	Spermatogenesis Prostate growth and function Penile growth
Skin	Hair growth Sebum production Balding
Kidney	Stimulation of erythropoietin production

there was no improvement in high-density lipoprotein levels.

Multiple mechanisms that explain these associations have been postulated. It is possible that insulin resistance and the development of obesity lead to an increase in peripheral conversion of testosterone to estradiol and resultant hypogonadal symptoms. This could then exacerbate the initial problem by increasing body fat mass and altering lipid profiles, further worsening glucose and lipid homeostasis. Alternatively, initially low androgen levels could lead to increased body fat mass and insulin resistance. Even though there is no direct evidence to establish a causal relationship between hypogonadism and the previously noted metabolic derangements, the entities are clearly meaningfully connected, and therefore merit further investigation.

Cardiovascular effects

As the body of evidence regarding the link between hypogonadism and cardiovascular risk factors such as the metabolic syndrome continues to emerge, it is necessary to examine the cardiovascular implications of androgen deficiency. Several studies have suggested a link between hypogonadism and cardiovascular disease [17–19]. Hak *et al.* demonstrated a direct correlation between low testosterone levels and elevated risk of atherosclerosis which was independent of a variety of factors, including age, BMI, smoking status, total cholesterol, or diabetes [20]. Another study found that a six-month course of androgen deprivation therapy for androgen-responsive prostate cancer led to an earlier onset of fatal myocardial infarction [21]. An observational study reviewing data collected from over 70 000 men undergoing androgen deprivation therapy for prostate cancer identified elevated risk of diabetes, coronary artery disease, myocardial infarction, and sudden cardiac death in men treated with GnRH agonists [22]. Additionally, men undergoing orchiectomy were shown to be at an increased risk for developing diabetes, but not coronary artery disease or myocardial infarction.

Several preclinical and clinical studies have suggested the mechanisms of action of androgens on the cardiovascular system involve endothelial function. Microscopic evaluation of endothelial tissue from castrated rats demonstrated significant damage to the endothelial lining, which, in a later experiment, was partially reversed with androgen supplementation [23]. In a related finding, pro-inflammatory cytokines such as tumor necrosis factor-alpha (TNF-α) and interleukin-1 (IL-1), believed to increase the risk of atherosclerotic disease when present in excess, were decreased in hypogonadal men following treatment with testosterone supplementation [24].

The question of whether early identification and treatment of hypogonadism can halt, or perhaps reverse, any endothelial damage has yet to be answered. The relationships between obesity, lipid profiles, insulin resistance, and endothelial dysfunction do indeed suggest that lowered serum testosterone can lead to increased cardiovascular risk.

Bone

It has been well documented in men with advanced prostate cancer that low circulating androgen levels as a result of deprivation therapy significantly decrease bone mineral density (BMD) and increase fracture risk, particularly in weight-bearing areas such as the hip and spine [25]. A recent study demonstrated a fracture risk of 19.4% in men undergoing androgen deprivation therapy for prostate cancer, compared to 12.6% in the control group [26]. Clinical and molecular evidence suggests that both testosterone and estrogens play an important role in bone health, and that bioavailable testosterone is a better correlate for BMD than is total serum testosterone [27]. Several population-based studies have shown that BMD in elderly men was directly related to serum estrogen levels, and that mildly decreased serum testosterone as a physiologic effect of aging had little correlation with changes in BMD [28]. Estrogen appears to exert its effects on BMD by stimulating osteoblastic activity that augments bone deposition, whereas testosterone appears to inhibit osteoclastic activity [29]. Further, estrogens, by activating osteoblasts and enhancing production of osteoprotegerin, inhibit osteoclastic bone resorption. As estrogen production in men requires aromatization of testosterone to estradiol and androstenedione to estrone, low testosterone levels not only lead to an increase in osteoclast-induced bone resorption via a disruption of its direct effects, but also secondarily lead to reduced bone deposition resulting from low circulating levels of estrogens.

Body composition

As men age and androgen levels diminish, muscle mass decreases and a subsequent increase in adipose tissue leads to a change in body shape and composition [30]. Testosterone exerts effects on muscle mass by initiating an increase in muscle protein synthesis [31], thereby causing muscle fiber hypertrophy. The cross-sectional volume of muscle fibers has been shown to increase in a dose-dependent manner in healthy men administered supplemental testosterone in the form of injections [32].

Studies of men with hypogonadism and patients undergoing androgen deprivation therapy for prostate cancer have shown increases in weight and overall body fat mass along with decreases in lean body mass accompanying reduced androgen levels [33–35]. Androgens are likely to exert significant effects on the regional body distribution of adipose tissue. Analyses performed on a cohort of Rancho Bernardo men aged 30–79 followed over 12 years showed that serum total testosterone levels were inversely correlated with

central adiposity [36]. Additionally, testosterone replacement therapy in hypogonadal men decreases the total amount of adiposity and alters its distribution, while increasing lean body mass [37]. Testosterone's catabolic effect on adipose tissue is believed to result from the inhibition of lipoprotein lipase, which leads to lipolysis [38].

Cognition and mood

Several studies have explored the link between serum testosterone and cognitive function. One study found a relationship between low serum testosterone levels and significant declines in visuospatial performance and memory [39]. Animal studies have demonstrated that areas of the brain involved in spatial learning such as the hippocampus are targets of androgens, and that androgenic stimulation leads to an up-regulation of local nicotinic receptors. Testosterone has also been shown to up-regulate the expression of nerve growth factors, and to induce an increase in acetylcholine release in these areas [40].

Recent prospective studies have identified an association between low circulating androgen levels in aging men and an increased risk of Alzheimer's dementia [41,42]. In-vitro studies also suggest that low levels of testosterone may lead to more intracranial beta-amyloid deposition and decreased neuronal survival in response to a toxic insult [43,44]. Unfortunately, there is presently no direct evidence that low androgen levels lead to Alzheimer's disease.

The effect of hypogonadism on mood is also difficult to establish. Studies examining the efficacy of testosterone replacement therapy on the resolution of depressive symptoms have revealed conflicting results, which may be attributable to relatively small subject numbers and heterogeneous patient populations [45,46]. However, a recent placebo-controlled clinical trial showed that supplemental testosterone injections led to significant improvements in depressive symptoms in a cohort of men with late-onset dysthymia [47]. At present, testosterone is not indicated as a broadly effective antidepressant therapy, but its use may be justified in carefully selected patient populations, such as hypogonadal men, antidepressant-resistant men, and HIV-infected men [48].

Sexual function

Androgens such as testosterone are recognized to play a significant role in sexual function. That being said, erectile function may not directly depend on the presence of androgens. The literature offers studies with differing conclusions regarding the effect of androgen supplementation and erectile function. These studies are plagued by heterogeneous populations and discordant inclusion criteria [49,50]. Testosterone supplementation appears to provide a lasting improvement in libido, but resultant improvement in erectile function, when assayed using validated questionnaires, is short-lived [51]. Hypogonadal men with erectile dysfunction (ED) who were treated with a combination of testosterone supplementation and phosphodiesterase-5 (PDE5) inhibitors were observed to have improvement in erectile function for a limited time, based on validated questionnaire results [52].

Preclinical and clinical studies do provide a connection between erectile function and androgen levels. As there is a clear association between endothelial dysfunction and hypogonadism, and there is evidence of a link between ED and endothelial dysfunction, some authorities suggest that men presenting with significant ED should undergo a full cardiac evaluation, as ED may be a harbinger of comorbid and yet-undiscovered coronary artery disease [53]. The effects of testosterone supplementation on endothelial dysfunction have been quantified by observing an improvement in brachial artery flow-mediated dilation following administration [54]. In-vitro studies have offered possible mechanisms of action of androgens on endothelial function. Androgens, including testosterone and dehydroepiandrosterone (DHEA), may activate endothelial nitric oxide synthase (eNOS) in the endothelial lining of the vascular wall [55], thereby leading to smooth muscle relaxation and increased blood flow. In contrast, testosterone-dependent vasodilation has been successfully demonstrated in denuded endothelium, suggesting that vasodilation is not dependent on an endothelial mechanism [56]. Further in-vitro evidence suggests that testosterone-mediated vasodilation may result from inhibition of calcium entry into endothelial smooth muscle cells [57].

Diagnosis of hypogonadism

As previously noted, the diagnosis of hypogonadism can be challenging for the clinician. Routine reliance on laboratory testing can sometimes lead to a missed diagnosis of hypogonadism in the event of an atypical testosterone level/symptom complex. Importantly,

the presence of significant clinical symptoms often impacts the diagnostic algorithm. An objective evaluation of subjective symptoms, especially in aging males, can be difficult as well. Validated questionnaires assessing symptoms related to androgen deficiency have been developed, may aid with the diagnosis, and are often employed as screening tools. While prospective evaluations of these questionnaires have demonstrated less than perfect assessment of symptoms, these questionnaires, which include the Androgen Deficiency in the Aging Male questionnaire [2], the Aging Male Survey [58], and the International Index of Erectile Function [1], remain useful screening tools. The results of these questionnaires can be used in conjunction with clinical symptoms and laboratory measurements of androgen levels to make the clinical diagnosis of hypogonadism.

There are inherent difficulties in using serum total testosterone measurements to make the diagnosis of hypogonadism. Testosterone circulates in the blood either free or bound to various proteins. The majority (∼60%) of circulating testosterone is tightly bound to SHBG and considered inactive. Approximately one-third of circulating testosterone is loosely bound to albumin, which leaves only 1–2% of testosterone as free and directly available to enter cells and elicit downstream activity. The fraction of testosterone bound to albumin is easily released, and when added to the free testosterone, it is referred to as "bioavailable testosterone." Measurements of total testosterone, which do not distinguish between bound and bioavailable testosterone, can therefore vary greatly, since circulating levels of SHBG are able to fluctuate in association with several conditions (Table 10.2). Accordingly, total testosterone levels may not accurately reflect the level of bioavailable testosterone.

Laboratory measurement of serum testosterone levels can be accomplished in a variety of ways. Most laboratories use either chemiluminescence assays or radioimmunoassay to measure total testosterone. Testosterone can also be measured by high-performance liquid chromatography mass spectrometry or gas chromatography mass spectrometry. There can be wide variability in testosterone measurements using any of these techniques, and standard reference values for testosterone levels can vary among different laboratories and different assay manufacturers, thus making accurate diagnosis of hypogonadism difficult [59]. Although measurement of free testosterone would be the most accurate method of determining true bioavailable testosterone levels, this measurement is difficult and costly to obtain. Ultrafiltration and equilibrium dialysis methods are historically the most accurate means by which one can determine accurate free testosterone values, and are therefore considered the gold standard, but these procedures are only available in select centers. Isotope dilution mass spectrometry has also been advocated, but results vary significantly [60]. Free testosterone and bioavailable testosterone levels can be estimated using accurate measurements of total testosterone and SHBG using the following equation [61]:

$$[T] = [T_{Free}] + [T_{Albumin\text{-}bound}] + [T_{SHBG\text{-}bound}]$$

A calculator tool using this method to calculate bioavialable testosterone is available online at **www.issam.ch/freetesto.htm**. Measurement of bioavailable testosterone can be accurately accomplished using ammonium sulfate precipitation techniques, which precipitate the SHBG-bound fraction of testosterone and then measure remaining testosterone in the supernatant. As with free testosterone assays, this test may not be readily available. Newer methods to measure testosterone levels are being developed, such as salivary testosterone, but these methods still require further investigation and standardization [62].

As a result of the myriad factors that can alter symptoms and measurements of serum testosterone, there is presently no standard reference laboratory value for the diagnosis of hypogonadism. Clinical assessment of symptoms, when judiciously combined with laboratory measurements, guide the clinician toward a diagnosis. While reference values for total testosterone vary significantly, most authors would agree that a morning serum total testosterone measurement of 200–300 ng/dL would be classified as low. However, given the variability in testing for total and bioavailable testosterone, a patient with low-normal testosterone levels and clinical symptoms of hypogonadism may be a candidate for a trial of testosterone replacement [63,64].

Treatment

Treatment of male hypogonadism varies significantly, depending on the underlying cause. As a general rule, treatment involves replacement of either pituitary gonadotropins to stimulate endogenous androgen production or simply administration of replacement androgens, usually testosterone.

The most appropriate treatment for men with hypogonadotropic hypogonadism depends on the individual's desire for future fertility. Testosterone replacement therapy is the easiest and most cost-effective form of treatment, but exogenous testosterone administration results in suppression of the endogenous HPG axis, resulting in infertility and potentially testicular atrophy. If future fertility is desired, treatment can be administered by supplementation with human chorionic gonadotropin (hCG – an analog of LH), human menopausal gonadotropin (hMG – mimics both LH and FSH), or the oral agent clomiphene citrate. Both supplementation of GnRH in a pulsatile fashion and supplementation of LH and FSH can result in adequate sperm production in hypogonadotropic hypogonadal men. The pulsatile delivery of GnRH can be accomplished via the use of an infusion pump, but this requires the patient to have an intact and functional pituitary gland, as LH and FSH are released by the pituitary following GnRH stimulation. Therefore, patients with previous pituitary surgery, trauma, or possibly radiation must be evaluated before they are declared to be candidates for hCG therapy. Gonadotropin supplementation may be administered by injection 2–3 times weekly (1000–2500 IU of hCG). This therapy is sufficient to initiate sperm production, but usually FSH supplementation permits quantitative spermatogenesis. FSH can be supplemented either by administering recombinant FSH 2–3 times weekly (75 IU) or by administering hMG, which contains both FSH and LH [65]. Assuming that the patient has functional testicular tissue, testosterone levels are usually normalized with supplementation of gonadotropins. Clomiphene citrate (CC) is a selective estrogen receptor modulator (SERM) that effectively blocks the retrograde inhibitory signal of estrogen on the hypothalamus (Fig. 10.1), resulting in an increase in released LH and FSH. A study has shown that prolonged CC therapy (3–9 months) at titrated dosages ranging from 25 to 75 mg per day in patients with non-obstructive azoospermia led to ejaculated sperm of sufficient quantity to perform intracytoplasmic sperm injection (ICSI) in approximately 70% of treated patients, as well as improved likelihood of sperm recovery during surgical sperm extraction [66]. Additionally, the administration of CC in dosages ranging from 25 to 100 mg every other day has been shown to be effective in raising serum

Table 10.4. A comparison of currently available treatment modalities for hypogonadism

Agent	Common regimen	Cost	Advantages	Disadvantages
1% Testosterone gel	Apply 5–10g of T gel containing 50–100 mg T once or twice daily	$320 per month at 50 mg T qd	Flexibility of dosing, ease of application, good skin tolerability	Potential for transfer to others by skin to skin contact, potential for skin rash in some users
Transdermal testosterone patch	1–2 patches per day, each delivering 5–10 mg T per 24 h	$280 per month at 1 × 5 mg patch qd	Ease of application, once-daily application	Frequent skin irritation in patch application areas
Testosterone enanthate or cypionate	150–200 mg injected IM every 2 weeks, or 75–100 mg per week	$34–50 per month at 1 × 200 mg injection every 2 weeks	Flexibility of dosing; relatively inexpensive if self-administered	Injection required; pharmacokinetics of depot injection lead to peaks and valleys in T concentration early and late in administration, respectively
Testosterone pellets	Subcutaneous implantation of 3–6 pellets; concentration of T varies with formulation	Pricing varies by provider, placement performed, and billed by surgeon	Long duration of therapeutic effect with little time investment	Surgical incision required for placement of pellets; potential for spontaneous extrusion of pellets
Buccal, bioadhesive testosterone tablets	30 mg controlled-release bioadhesive tablets used twice daily	$311 per month at 1 × 30 mg buccal tablet bid	Ease of use	Alteration of taste; adverse reactions in gum tissue in some users
Oral methyltestosterone	10–50 mg orally 1–2 × daily	$748 per month at 1 × 10 mg tablet bid	Convenience of oral administration	High person-to-person variability in serum T levels achieved; high DHT: T ratio
Testosterone in adhesive-matrix patch	2 × 60 cm² patches deliver ~4.8 mg of T per day	Not available in US market	Lasts for 2 days	Skin irritation seen in some users
Long-acting injectable T undecanoate in oil	1000 mg injected IM, then 1000 mg IM in 6 weeks, with 1000 mg every 10–14 weeks thereafter	Not available in US market	Long duration of therapeutic effect	IM injection of large volume (4 mL); immediate post-injection cough reported in some users
Clomiphene citrate	25–100 mg orally every other day	$83 per month at 50 mg qod	Relatively inexpensive, oral dosing	Not functional in men with hypogonadism due to testicular failure

Adapted from information presented in Bhasin S, Basaria S. Diagnosis and treatment of hypogonadism in men. *Best Pract Res Clin Endocrinol Metab* 2011; 25: 251–70 [72]. Estimated retail pricing information gathered from www.drugstore.com.

testosterone levels to values comparable to those achieved with testosterone gel replacement therapy, but at a significantly reduced cost [67].

If future fertility is not a concern for the hypogonadal patient, then supplementation with testosterone alone is provided. Testosterone can be administered several different ways, including intramuscular injections of testosterone preparations (testosterone enanthate, testosterone cypionate, testosterone undecanoate), or applying testosterone gels (Androgel [Abbot Laboratories, Abbot Park, IL], Testim [Auxilium, Mavern, PA]), patches (Androderm [Watson Pharmaceuticals, Parsippany, NJ], Testoderm [Alza Corporation, Mountain View, CA]), and buccal

testosterone tablets. Long-acting subcutaneous pellets of testosterone are popular longer-term solutions to testosterone supplementation (Testopel, Slate Pharmaceuticals, Durham, NC). Novel topical testosterone preparations have been developed for application to the underarm (Axiron [Lilly, Indianapolis, IN]) or inner thigh (Fortesta [Endo Pharmaceuticals, Newark, DE]). Additionally, long-acting depot testosterone injections (Nebido, Bayer, Berlin, Germany) are available in most countries in the world, although not yet in the USA, providing another treatment option.

Each method of supplementation confers different risks and benefits (Table 10.4). Injectable forms are typically the most cost-effective, but can cause significant fluctuations in testosterone levels. Transdermal forms of testosterone replacement are able to offer steadier, physiologic levels of testosterone, but these are more costly and carry the risk of person-to-person transfer of androgen. As a general rule, blood counts need to be periodically monitored in those receiving testosterone replacement, especially with injectable forms of testosterone. With any form of testosterone replacement therapy, routine digital rectal exam (DRE) and prostate-specific antigen (PSA) monitoring needs to be performed, given the potential for hormonal responsiveness of an undetected prostate carcinoma. Patients presenting with abnormal DRE and/or elevated PSA must undergo further evaluation prior to continuing with or initiating testosterone replacement therapy. Treatment of hypogonadal men with a history of prostate cancer is controversial, but recent evidence suggests that the practice is safe with regular follow-up [68–70]. As it appears that testosterone replacement has no significant impact on lower urinary tract symptoms in the short term, the evaluation of urinary symptoms in males on testosterone replacement therapy is considered optional [71].

Conclusion

Androgen deficiency can be primary, secondary, or a combination of both, and result from a plethora of factors, ranging from congenital, idiopathic, medication-induced, infectious, inflammatory, iatrogenic, malignancy, or as a consequence of aging. Making an absolute diagnosis of hypogonadism can be challenging for the clinician, but the combination of subjective clinical symptoms suggestive of hypogonadism (sometimes with the aid of a validated questionnaire) in conjunction with laboratory measures offers an appropriate standard of care starting point. Treatment depends on the underlying cause but generally involves replacement. In men, either gonadotropin administration is used to stimulate endogenous androgen production, or testosterone supplementation is used in one of many currently available forms. The goal of therapy in the male with hypogonadism is centered on restoring physiologic androgen levels while alleviating the clinical symptoms of androgen deficiency. All patients receiving hormone replacement therapy need appropriate clinical observation and follow-up. Androgen replacement

therapy should be tailored to an individual patient's needs, preferences, and risk factors.

References

1. Rosen RC, Riley A, Wagner G, *et al*. The international index of erectile function (IIEF): a multidimensional scale for assessment of erectile dysfunction. *Urology* 1997; 49: 822–30.

2. Morley JE, Charlton E, Patrick P, *et al*. Validation of a screening questionnaire for androgen deficiency in aging males. *Metabolism* 2000; 49: 1239–42.

3. Harman SM, Metter EJ, Tobin JD, Pearson J, Blackman MR. Longitudinal effects of aging on serum total and free testosterone levels in healthy men. Baltimore Longitudinal Study of Aging. *J Clin Endocrinol Metab* 2001; 86: 724–31.

4. Kiserud CE, Fossa A, Bjoro T, *et al*. Gonadal function in male patients after treatment for malignant lymphomas, with emphasis on chemotherapy. *Br J Cancer* 2009; 100: 455–63.

5. Eberhard J, Stahl O, Cwikiel M, *et al*. Risk factors for post-treatment hypogonadism in testicular cancer patients. *Eur J Endocrinol* 2008; 158: 561–70.

6. Greenfield DM, Walters SJ, Coleman RE, *et al*. Prevalence and consequences of androgen deficiency in young male cancer survivors in a controlled cross-sectional study. *J Clin Endocrinol Metab* 2007; 92: 3476–82.

7. Schmiegelow M, Lassen S, Poulsen HS, *et al*. Gonadal status in male survivors following childhood brain tumors. *J Clin Endocrinol Metab* 2001; 86: 2446–52.

8. Sharifi N, Gulley JL, Dahut WL. An update on androgen deprivation therapy for prostate cancer. *Endocr Relat Cancer* 2010; 17: R305–15.

9. Ding EL, Song Y, Malik VS, Liu S. Sex differences of endogenous sex hormones and risk of type 2 diabetes: a systematic review and meta-analysis. *JAMA* 2006; 295: 1288–99.

10. Grossmann M, Thomas MC, Panagiotopoulos S, *et al*. Low testosterone levels are common and associated with insulin resistance in men with diabetes. *J Clin Endocrinol Metab* 2008; 93: 1834–40.

11. Derweesh IH, Diblasio CJ, Kincade MC, *et al*. Risk of new-onset diabetes mellitus and worsening glycaemic variables for established diabetes in men undergoing androgen-deprivation therapy for prostate cancer. *BJU Int* 2007; 100: 1060–5.

12. Haidar A, Yassin A, Saad F, Shabsigh R. Effects of androgen deprivation on glycaemic control and on cardiovascular biochemical risk factors in men with

advanced prostate cancer with diabetes. *Aging Male* 2007; 10: 189–96.

13. Miner MM, Khera M, Bhattacharya RK, Blick G, Kushner H. Baseline data from the TRiUS registry: symptoms and comorbidities of testosterone deficiency. *Postgrad Med* 2011; 123: 17–27.

14. Boyanov MA, Boneva Z, Christov VG. Testosterone supplementation in men with type 2 diabetes, visceral obesity and partial androgen deficiency. *Aging Male* 2003; 6: 1–7.

15. Kapoor D, Goodwin E, Channer KS, Jones TH. Testosterone replacement therapy improves insulin resistance, glycaemic control, visceral adiposity and hypercholesterolaemia in hypogonadal men with type 2 diabetes. *Eur J Endocrinol* 2006; 154: 899–906.

16. Page ST, Amory JK, Bowman FD, *et al.* Exogenous testosterone (T) alone or with finasteride increases physical performance, grip strength, and lean body mass in older men with low serum T. *J Clin Endocrinol Metab* 2005; 90: 1502–10.

17. Makinen J, Jarvisalo MJ, Pollanen P, *et al.* Increased carotid atherosclerosis in andropausal middle-aged men. *J Am Coll Cardiol* 2005; 45: 1603–8.

18. Basaria S. Androgen deprivation therapy, insulin resistance, and cardiovascular mortality: an inconvenient truth. *J Androl* 2008 Sep-Oct; 29: 534–9.

19. Makinen JI, Perheentupa A, Irjala K, *et al.* Endogenous testosterone and serum lipids in middle-aged men. *Atherosclerosis* 2008; 197: 688–93.

20. Hak AE, Witteman JC, de Jong FH, *et al.* Low levels of endogenous androgens increase the risk of atherosclerosis in elderly men: the Rotterdam study. *J Clin Endocrinol Metab* 2002; 87: 3632–9.

21. D'Amico AV, Denham JW, Crook J, *et al.* Influence of androgen suppression therapy for prostate cancer on the frequency and timing of fatal myocardial infarctions. *J Clin Oncol* 2007; 25: 2420–5.

22. Keating NL, O'Malley AJ, Smith MR. Diabetes and cardiovascular disease during androgen deprivation therapy for prostate cancer. *J Clin Oncol* 2006; 24: 4448–56.

23. Lu YL, Kuang L, Zhu H, *et al.* Changes in aortic endothelium ultrastructure in male rats following castration, replacement with testosterone and administration of 5alpha-reductase inhibitor. *Asian J Androl* 2007; 9: 843–7.

24. Malkin CJ, Pugh PJ, Jones RD, *et al.* The effect of testosterone replacement on endogenous inflammatory cytokines and lipid profiles in hypogonadal men. *J Clin Endocrinol Metab* 2004; 89: 3313–18.

25. Melton LJ, 3rd, Alothman KI, Khosla S, *et al.* Fracture risk following bilateral orchiectomy. *J Urol* 2003; 169: 1747–50.

26. Shahinian VB, Kuo YF, Freeman JL, Goodwin JS. Risk of fracture after androgen deprivation for prostate cancer. *N Engl J Med* 2005; 352: 154–64.

27. van den Beld AW, de Jong FH, Grobbee DE, Pols HA, Lamberts SW. Measures of bioavailable serum testosterone and estradiol and their relationships with muscle strength, bone density, and body composition in elderly men. *J Clin Endocrinol Metab* 2000; 85: 3276–82.

28. Amin S, Zhang Y, Sawin CT, *et al.* Association of hypogonadism and estradiol levels with bone mineral density in elderly men from the Framingham study. *Ann Intern Med* 2000; 133: 951–63.

29. Michael H, Harkonen PL, Vaananen HK, Hentunen TA. Estrogen and testosterone use different cellular pathways to inhibit osteoclastogenesis and bone resorption. *J Bone Miner Res* 2005; 20: 2224–32.

30. Vermeulen A. Androgen secretion after age 50 in both sexes. *Horm Res* 1983; 18: 37–42.

31. Griggs RC, Kingston W, Jozefowicz RF, *et al.* Effect of testosterone on muscle mass and muscle protein synthesis. *J Appl Physiol* 1989; 66: 498–503.

32. Sinha-Hikim I, Artaza J, Woodhouse L, *et al.* Testosterone-induced increase in muscle size in healthy young men is associated with muscle fiber hypertrophy. *Am J Physiol Endocrinol Metab* 2002; 283: E154–64.

33. Chen Z, Maricic M, Nguyen P, *et al.* Low bone density and high percentage of body fat among men who were treated with androgen deprivation therapy for prostate carcinoma. *Cancer* 2002; 95: 2136–44.

34. Smith MR, Finkelstein JS, McGovern FJ, *et al.* Changes in body composition during androgen deprivation therapy for prostate cancer. *J Clin Endocrinol Metab* 2002; 87: 599–603.

35. Bhasin S. Regulation of body composition by androgens. *J Endocrinol Invest* 2003; 26: 814–22.

36. Khaw KT, Barrett-Connor E. Lower endogenous androgens predict central adiposity in men. *Ann Epidemiol* 1992; 2: 675–82.

37. Wang C, Swerdloff RS, Iranmanesh A, *et al.* Transdermal testosterone gel improves sexual function, mood, muscle strength, and body composition parameters in hypogonadal men. *J Clin Endocrinol Metab* 2000; 85: 2839–53.

38. Rebuffe-Scrive M, Marin P, Bjorntorp P. Effect of testosterone on abdominal adipose tissue in men. *Int J Obes* 1991; 15: 791–5.

39. Moffat SD, Zonderman AB, Metter EJ, *et al.* Longitudinal assessment of serum free testosterone concentration predicts memory performance and cognitive status in elderly men. *J Clin Endocrinol Metab* 2002; 87: 5001–7.

40. Janowsky JS. The role of androgens in cognition and brain aging in men. *Neuroscience* 2006; 138: 1015–20.

41. Moffat SD, Zonderman AB, Metter EJ, *et al.* Free testosterone and risk for Alzheimer disease in older men. *Neurology* 2004; 62: 188–93.

42. Rosario ER, Chang L, Stanczyk FZ, Pike CJ. Age-related testosterone depletion and the development of Alzheimer disease. *JAMA* 2004; 292: 1431–2.

43. Ramsden M, Nyborg AC, Murphy MP, *et al.* Androgens modulate beta-amyloid levels in male rat brain. *J Neurochem* 2003; 87: 1052–5.

44. Ramsden M, Shin TM, Pike CJ. Androgens modulate neuronal vulnerability to kainate lesion. *Neuroscience* 2003; 122: 573–8.

45. Seidman SN, Spatz E, Rizzo C, Roose SP. Testosterone replacement therapy for hypogonadal men with major depressive disorder: a randomized, placebo-controlled clinical trial. *J Clin Psychiatry* 2001; 62: 406–12.

46. Pope HG, Cohane GH, Kanayama G, Siegel AJ, Hudson JI. Testosterone gel supplementation for men with refractory depression: a randomized, placebo-controlled trial. *Am J Psychiatry* 2003; 160: 105–11.

47. Seidman SN, Orr G, Raviv G, *et al.* Effects of testosterone replacement in middle-aged men with dysthymia: a randomized, placebo-controlled clinical trial. *J Clin Psychopharmacol* 2009; 29: 216–21.

48. Amiaz R, Seidman SN. Testosterone and depression in men. *Curr Opin Endocrinol Diabetes Obes* 2008; 15: 278–83.

49. Jain P, Rademaker AW, McVary KT. Testosterone supplementation for erectile dysfunction: results of a meta-analysis. *J Urol* 2000; 164: 371–5.

50. Isidori AM, Giannetta E, Gianfrilli D, *et al.* Effects of testosterone on sexual function in men: results of a meta-analysis. *Clin Endocrinol (Oxf)* 2005; 63: 381–94.

51. Mulhall JP, Valenzuela R, Aviv N, Parker M. Effect of testosterone supplementation on sexual function in hypogonadal men with erectile dysfunction. *Urology* 2004; 63: 348–52.

52. Shabsigh R, Kaufman JM, Steidle C, Padma-Nathan H. Randomized study of testosterone gel as adjunctive therapy to sildenafil in hypogonadal men with erectile dysfunction who do not respond to sildenafil alone. *J Urol* 2004; 172: 658–63.

53. Costa C, Virag R. The endothelial–erectile dysfunction connection: an essential update. *J Sex Med* 2009; 6: 2390–404.

54. Kang SM, Jang Y, Kim JY, *et al.* Effect of oral administration of testosterone on brachial arterial vasoreactivity in men with coronary artery disease. *Am J Cardiol* 2002; 89: 862–4.

55. Liu D, Dillon JS. Dehydroepiandrosterone activates endothelial cell nitric-oxide synthase by a specific plasma membrane receptor coupled to Galpha(i2,3). *J Biol Chem* 2002; 277: 21379–88.

56. Murphy JG, Khalil RA. Decreased [Ca(2+)](i) during inhibition of coronary smooth muscle contraction by 17beta-estradiol, progesterone, and testosterone. *J Pharmacol Exp Ther* 1999; 291: 44–52.

57. Crews JK, Khalil RA. Gender-specific inhibition of Ca2+ entry mechanisms of arterial vasoconstriction by sex hormones. *Clin Exp Pharmacol Physiol* 1999; 26: 707–15.

58. Moore C, Huebler D, Zimmermann T, Heinemann LA, Saad F, Thai DM. The Aging Males' Symptoms scale (AMS) as outcome measure for treatment of androgen deficiency. *Eur Urol* 2004; 46: 80–7.

59. Lazarou S, Reyes-Vallejo L, Morgentaler A. Wide variability in laboratory reference values for serum testosterone. *J Sex Med* 2006; 3: 1085–9.

60. Van Uytfanghe K, Stockl D, Kaufman JM, *et al.* Validation of 5 routine assays for serum free testosterone with a candidate reference measurement procedure based on ultrafiltration and isotope dilution-gas chromatography-mass spectrometry. *Clin Biochem* 2005; 38: 253–61.

61. Vermeulen A, Verdonck L, Kaufman JM. A critical evaluation of simple methods for the estimation of free testosterone in serum. *J Clin Endocrinol Metab* 1999; 84: 3666–72.

62. Wood P. Salivary steroid assays: research or routine? *Ann Clin Biochem* 2009; 46: 183–96.

63. Sattler FR, Castaneda-Sceppa C, Binder EF, *et al.* Testosterone and growth hormone improve body composition and muscle performance in older men. *J Clin Endocrinol Metab* 2009; 94: 1991–2001.

64. Wang C, Nieschlag E, Swerdloff R, *et al.* Investigation, treatment, and monitoring of late-onset hypogonadism in males: ISA, ISSAM, EAU, EAA, and ASA recommendations. *J Androl* 2009; 30: 1–9.

65. Schiff JD, Ramirez ML, Bar-Chama N. Medical and surgical management male infertility. *Endocrinol Metab Clin North Am* 2007; 36: 313–31.

66. Hussein A, Ozgok Y, Ross L, Niederberger C. Clomiphene administration for cases of nonobstructive azoospermia: a multicenter study. *J Androl* 2005; 26: 787–91; discussion 92–3.

67. Taylor F, Levine L. Clomiphene citrate and testosterone gel replacement therapy for male hypogonadism: efficacy and treatment cost. *J Sex Med* 2010; 7: 269–76.

68. Kaufman JM, Graydon RJ. Androgen replacement after curative radical prostatectomy for prostate cancer in hypogonadal men. *J Urol* 2004; 172: 920–2.

69. Khera M, Lipshultz LI. The role of testosterone replacement therapy following radical prostatectomy. *Urol Clin North Am* 2007; 34: 549–53, vi.

70. Morgentaler A. Testosterone replacement therapy and prostate cancer. *Urol Clin North Am* 2007; 34: 555–63, vii.

71. Morales A. Androgen replacement therapy and prostate safety. *Eur Urol* 2002; 41: 113–20.

72. Bhasin S, Basaria S. Diagnosis and treatment of hypogonadism in men. *Best Pract Res Clin Endocrinol Metab* 2011; 25: 251–70.

Infertility and male sexual dysfunction

Raanan Tal

Introduction

The term male sexual dysfunction (MSD) includes erectile dysfunction (ED), ejaculatory disorders, male hypogonadism, and alterations in orgasm. MSD may coexist with male infertility, may be the cause, or may even be the result of male infertility. Both MSD and infertility are associated with significant emotional burden for men, their partners, and their relationship as a couple. The purpose of this chapter is to present the epidemiology and pathophysiology of MSD in the male partner of the infertile couple, to discuss the association of MSD and infertility, and to describe the possible impact of MSD-related therapeutic interventions on male infertility.

Epidemiology of combined morbidity: MSD and infertility

The first large-scale population-based epidemiologic study reporting on the prevalence of ED was the Massachusetts Male Aging Study (MMAS) [1]. The MMAS was a cross-sectional population-based survey of community-dwelling American men, conducted from 1987 to 1989. This study, which comprised 1290 men surveyed in Boston, MA, estimated ED of various severities in 52% of men aged 40–70 years, with a strong age dependency. Unfortunately, the MMAS, as well as multiple other ED epidemiologic studies that followed, failed to report on other aspects of MSD and did not focus on males of reproductive age.

A landmark study in MSD epidemiology is the National Health and Social Life Survey (NHSLS), a probability sample study of sexual behavior in a demographically representative 1992 cohort of US adults, men and women, aged 18–59 [2]. According to the NHSLS, sexual dysfunction in men of reproductive age (18–39) included "lacked interest in sex" (13–14%), "inability to achieve orgasm" (7%), "climax too early" (30–32%), "sex not pleasurable" (8–10%), "anxiety about performance" (17–19%), and "trouble maintaining or achieving an erection" (7–9%). Interestingly, the most common sexual dysfunction among young men in the NHSLS study was "climax too early", i.e., premature ejaculation. These data represent sexual dysfunction in the general male population of young to middle age, and not specifically in male partners of infertile couples.

A recent Iranian study specifically addressed the prevalence of sexual function among 100 infertile couples, men and women [3]. MSD in men aged 22–52 years (mean age 32) was assessed by the International Index of Erectile Function (IIEF), and the mean reported scores by domain were 23.2/30 for erectile function (mild ED), 8.4/10 for orgasmic function, 6.1/10 for sexual desire, 10.7/15 for intercourse satisfaction, and 7/10 for overall satisfaction. Only 2% of men reported severe ED, while moderate and mild ED were reported by 5% and 22%, respectively, higher than the 6% reported incidence of ED among the general population of Iranian men aged 20–39 [3,4]. The authors suggested that stress associated with infertility is a potential contributor to the development of ED in male partners of infertile couples. At this time, it is unclear if these interesting findings, derived from a survey of a limited-size population with specific social, cultural, and religious characteristics, are readily generalized to western societies.

O'Brien et al. addressed the incidence of ED in males presenting for evaluation of infertility in a controlled study using the Sexual Health Inventory for Men (SHIM) questionnaire [5]. They compared the

Fertility Preservation in Male Cancer Patients, ed. John P. Mulhall, Linda D. Applegarth, Robert D. Oates and Peter N. Schlegel. Published by Cambridge University Press. © Cambridge University Press 2013.

incidence of ED in 302 infertile males to a control group of males seeking vasectomy and found that 28% of infertile males had a SHIM score less than 22 (mild ED) and 8% less than 17 (moderate ED), while only 11% of fertile subjects had a SHIM score of less than 22 and none had a score of less than 17. However, this study failed to specify either the definition or the duration of infertility, potential contributing factors to the stress associated with infertility and the resultant psychogenic ED.

The impact of male infertility on sexual desire and sexual satisfaction was addressed in a study by Ramezanzadeh *et al.* [6]. Using a proprietary, non-validated patient interview in which responses were ranked on a five-point scale, approximately half of male partners of infertile couples reported a reduction in sexual desire and in sexual satisfaction after the diagnosis of infertility, inversely related to the duration of infertility. Baseline sexual desire and satisfaction in this study were obtained by patient recall and therefore are subject to potential bias.

Shindel *et al.* studied the prevalence of premature ejaculation, but not of other sexual dysfunctions, among male partners of couples presenting for infertility evaluation [7]. Their study design was unique in that not only men were asked about premature ejaculation but also their partners. Respondents completed a demographic survey, the Short Form-36 (SF-36), and the Center for Epidemiological Studies Depression (CES-D) scale. Both partners also completed a gender-specific survey instrument to detect premature ejaculation and distress related to the condition. Male partners completed the IIEF and the Self-Esteem and Relationship Quality (SEAR) scale. Female partners completed the Female Sexual Function Index (FSFI) and a modified version of the SEAR. The study results showed that 50% of men reported that they ejaculated more rapidly than they wished. When men reported premature ejaculation, their partners agreed with the diagnosis in 47% of cases. Female partners of men who did not report premature ejaculation reported premature ejaculation in 11% of cases. Partner frustration related to premature ejaculation was reported by 30% of men. Partners agreed that they were frustrated in 43% of these cases. Among the 70% of men who did not report partner frustration from premature ejaculation, 93% of the partners agreed that they were not frustrated. There was a statistically significant negative association between male and female report of premature ejaculation and SEAR scores but no other

statistically significant associations between premature ejaculation responses and demographic variables, IIEF, FSFI, CES-D, and SF-36 scores. The reported premature ejaculation prevalence in this study is significantly higher than the reported prevalence of 30–32% in a comparable American population [2]. Despite the paucity of epidemiologic studies on MSD and infertility, it appears that MSD is prevalent in infertile couples, significantly more than it is in the general population.

Etiology of combined morbidity: MSD and infertility

Although MSD and infertility are closely linked, the medical literature on the etiology of combined morbidity, infertility, and MSD is scarce. However, MSD and infertility do share common risk factors and common etiologies, and moreover there are medical conditions in which MSD and infertility are likely to coexist.

Psychogenic MSD and male infertility

There is some evidence to support the concept that infertile couples experience significant stress, for both male and female partners [8]. Infertility is not a discrete stressful event, but an evolving long-lasting process, involving hope and despair with every treatment cycle. The stress associated with infertility stems from the fact that infertility evaluation and treatment is an uncontrollable and unpredictable situation, with possibly negative consequences and a real threat of childlessness. Although there are no specific data to directly link stress of male partners in an infertile couple with sexual dysfunction, stress in general is highly correlated with ED [9]. The primary erectolytic neurotransmitter is epinephrine, a chemical that abounds in the setting of stress. Epinephrine limits arterial inflow and causes excessive venous outflow, resulting in poor and short-lived erection.

A cohort observational study from India looked at ED and anxiety, specifically in a subgroup of men who failed to ejaculate with masturbation or with sexual intercourse to produce sperm for semen analysis, 11% of the total infertile male population in this study [10]. This study reported a significant deterioration in IIEF scores and the concomitant development of severe anxiety over the course of infertility evaluation. Stress and anxiety may not only affect erectile function, but may also be involved in the pathogenesis of acquired premature ejaculation, associated with increased secretion of adrenergic neurotransmitters. Stress itself, and in conjunction with the resultant ED and premature ejaculation, may adversely affect sexual desire of infertile couples. Elia *at al.* studied sexual function in 171 infertile couples and compared erectile function, orgasmic function, sexual desire, and satisfaction with intercourse when sexual intercourse is performed for reproductive purposes and when it is performed for pleasure [11]. They found that the prevalence of sexual dysfunction was 23.7% when intercourse was performed for reproductive purposes and only 8.9% when it was performed for pleasure. These findings further emphasize the psychological impact of infertility, infertility interventions, and the demand to perform on sexual function. Sexual encounters may be conceived as a tool to achieve pregnancy, rather than as an emotional and intimate interaction. For men, the rigid, structured "sex on demand" approach to sex may also be accompanied by depression, guilt, ambivalence about parenthood and relationship, loss of self-esteem, negative impact on body image, and inability to perform as expected when ED and premature ejaculation ensues, all contributing significantly to psychologically based lack of sexual interest [8]. The psychosocial implications of infertility and its causative association with MSD mandate addressing these issues, and point to the evaluation of MSD as a part of a comprehensive approach to the management of infertility.

Hormonal disorders associated with MSD and male infertility

MSD in infertile men may not only be psychological and stress-related, but may also be the result of hormonal abnormalities. The most common hormonal disorder associated with MSD is hypogonadism (decreased testosterone levels). Symptoms of low testosterone may include decreased libido, infertility, alteration in body hair distribution and in fat distribution, decreased muscle mass and bone mineral density, mood changes, and fatigability. Ninety-five percent of a man's testosterone is secreted by Leydig cells in the testis, in response to luteinizing hormone (LH) stimulation, and the remaining 5% is secreted by the adrenal gland. Not only follicle-stimulating hormone (FSH), but also testosterone (intratesticular in particular) is required for normal spermatogenesis. Hypogonadism is classified as primary, due to testicular failure, or secondary, due to hypothalamic–pituitary–gonadal

(HPG) axis abnormalities. The incidence of hypogonadism among infertile males is considerably higher than that of age-matched fertile males.

Sussman *et al.* reported their results surveying men attending an infertility clinic and found that the incidence of hypogonadism (defined as morning serum testosterone level < 300 ng/dL) was 45% in men with non-obstructive azoospermia, 43% with oligospermia, 35% with normal semen analysis, and 17% with obstructive azoospermia [12]. The incidence of MSD among men with low testosterone is unknown, but low testosterone level is clearly associated with low desire and lower overall sexual activity [13]. A meta-analysis of 17 randomized placebo-controlled studies conducted by Isidori *et al.* showed that testosterone treatment in men with testosterone levels below 12 nmol/L (343 ng/dL) improved the number of nocturnal erections, sexual thoughts and motivation, number of successful intercourses, scores of erectile function, and overall sexual activity, although a cutoff value to predict treatment effect could not be defined [14].

The role of testosterone in the erectile response is yet to be completely defined. Animal studies have clearly demonstrated that androgen deprivation induces specific intrapenile changes such as smooth muscle cell degeneration and apoptosis with associated fibrosis of the corpus cavernosum; reduction in the expression of neuronal nitric oxide synthase (nNOS); decrease of arterial inflow and increase in venous outflow in the corpus cavernosum; enhanced response to mediators of vasoconstriction and smooth muscle contraction such as alpha-adrenergic stimuli; decrease in nitric oxide (NO)-mediated smooth muscle relaxation during sexual stimuli, which is likely due to a direct effect of androgens on phosphodiesterase-5 (PDE5) activity [15]. Clinical human data show that hypogonadal men are capable of achieving erections in response to visual erotic stimuli. However, nocturnal erections are of shorter duration and amplitude in hypogonadal men, corresponding to the diurnal variation in testosterone level. The testosterone level that is required for adequate erectile tissue health is unknown; indeed, some castrated men are capable of obtaining erections. It has been suggested that spontaneous but not stimulation-induced erections depend on testosterone. The mechanism of testosterone involvement in the regulation of the erectile response is yet to be elucidated, but it has been shown to have a role in the NO pathway and is required for cavernosal smooth muscle integrity [13].

Orgasmic dysfunction, low libido, and ejaculatory dysfunction have also been reported as sexual dysfunctions of hypogonadal men. Schmidt *et al.* reported on a unique study in which they evaluated sexual function in healthy men at baseline, after induction of hypogonadism with leuprolide acetate (a GnRH analog), and after hypogonadism reversal with testosterone administration [16]. Using a validated questionnaire, they found significant decrease in global and domain-specific sexual function scores, including: (1) sexual cognition and fantasy (e.g., erotic thoughts and dreams), (2) sexual arousal (e.g., level of arousal during sexual behaviors), (3) sexual behavior and experience (e.g., masturbation, foreplay, and intercourse), (4) quality of orgasm, and (5) sexual drive and relationship (e.g., level of satisfaction with sexual relationships). This decrease in sexual function score was corrected by testosterone administration. The limitations of this study are the limited size of the study group (only 20 subjects) and the use of a pharmacologic agent that results in profound and sudden, nonphysiologic hypogonadism (mean testosterone level of 34 ng/dL). Testosterone may also be involved in ejaculatory function. An association between ejaculatory dysfunction and testosterone levels was suggested by Corona *et al.*, who studied a selected population of men presenting for evaluation of sexual dysfunction and reported a lower prevalence of hypogonadism among men with premature ejaculation (12%) and a higher prevalence of hypogonadism among men with delayed ejaculation (26%), compared to the prevalence of hypogonadism in men without premature or delayed ejaculation (17%) [17]. These results should be viewed with caution, awaiting the elucidation of the mechanism of testosterone involvement in the ejaculatory process and the role of testosterone replacement in the treatment of ejaculatory dysfunction.

Not only testosterone, but also its metabolites are involved in sexual function. In males, testosterone is converted by aromatase to estrogen, a hormone that adversely affects spermatogenesis [12]. Estradiol has also been suggested to adversely affect sexual function. Adaikan and Srilatha have shown that animals treated with exogenous estradiol have prolongation of ejaculation latency, impaired erectile response, and cavernosal tissue damage [18]. Clinical evidence supporting the role of estradiol in the etiology of ED is scarce, but elevated estradiol levels have been reported in patients with venous leak of unknown etiology, and furthermore it has been reported that sustained improvement in sexual function with chronic phosphodiesterase-5 inhibitor (PDE5i) treatment is associated with increase in testosterone-to-estradiol ratio [19,20].

The sex hormones testosterone and estradiol are not the only hormones involved in regulation of sperm production and sexual function. Prolactin, secreted by the anterior pituitary, has an important role in reproduction. In seasonally breeding animals, prolactin is the signal to start reproductive activity. Physiologic levels of prolactin are required to support testosterone biosynthesis and to modulate the response of Leydig cells to testosterone. Prolactin increases the number of LH receptors on Leydig cells, thereby enhancing their sensitivity to LH, while it also increases the binding of androgens to target reproductive tissues [21]. On the other hand, in a state of hyperprolactinemia, prolactin has an inhibitory effect on the pulsatile secretion of gonadotropin-releasing hormone (GnRH), suppresses the pulsatile secretion of LH, and to lesser extent of FSH, and, not surprisingly, men with hyperprolactinemia commonly have lower testosterone levels [21]. Colao *et al.* studied the clinical features of subjects with hyperprolactinemia and found a low testosterone prevalence of 50% among men with microadenomas and a prevalence of 82% among men with macroadenomas [22]. It is important to emphasize that hyperprolactinemia induces hypogonadism mostly by an indirect mechanism. Only giant prolactinomas directly compress pituitary gonadotropic cells, reducing their number, leading to markedly reduced LH, FSH, and, consequently, markedly reduced testosterone levels [21]. The hypogonadism that occurs in hyperprolactinemia induces impairment of spermatogenesis and impaired sperm motility, and produces morphologic testicular changes similar to those observed in prepubertal testes [21]. Hyperprolactinemia may cause infertility and sexual dysfunction: in fact, the most common presenting symptoms of hyperprolactinemia are depressed libido and ED [13]. Hyperprolactinemia is present in 16% of patients with erectile dysfunction and in 11% of men with oligospermia [21]. Among men with sexual dysfunction, the most common endocrinopathies are low testosterone and hyperprolactinemia [23]. Hyperprolactinemia may be caused by medications, physiologic stress, psychological stress, or pituitary tumors, or it may be idiopathic.

Thyroid dysfunction may also cause both MSD and male infertility. One study suggested that hyperthyroidism is associated with reduced sperm quality. The mechanism involved is not fully understood: hyperthyroidism interferes with steroid hormone synthesis and causes elevation of sex-hormone binding globulin (SHBG) and total testosterone, but free testosterone is usually not elevated [12]. In hypothyroidism, although LH response to GnRH stimulation is blunted, semen quality seems to be unaffected and infertility is uncommon. The association between the described hormonal disorders not only with infertility but also with MSD warrants an evaluation of sexual function of an infertile male who is found to have an endocrinopathy. It is not unreasonable to conceive that the treatment of the underlying hormonal disorder may improve both fertility and sexual function.

Cancer, MSD, and male infertility

Cancer and cancer-related interventions may have a profound effect on male sexual health and male fertility. Sexual dysfunction and decline in self-reported sexual activity may be apparent from the early stages of a diagnostic evaluation, even before cancer treatments take their toll, and may persist long after cure has been achieved [24]. Cancer-related sexual dysfunction includes ED, reduced libido, ejaculatory dysfunction, and orgasm alterations. The etiology of sexual dysfunction in men with cancer may be psychological, secondary to anatomic structural damage, hormonal, drug-induced, or related to physical symptoms [24]. Psychogenic MSD is a consequence of changes in physical appearance, impaired body image and loss of perceived sexual attractiveness, or resulting from unrealistic fear that sexual activity will be harmful or will harm the sexual partner, or difficulties in expressing sexual thoughts and desire when cancer is confronted. Anatomic structural changes leading to MSD include direct damage to organs or systems involved in sexual function (radical pelvic surgery for prostate, bladder, or colorectal cancer, orchiectomy for testicular cancer), blood supply interruption, and nerve damage. Hormonal MSD, hypogonadism secondary to transient or permanent Leydig cell dysfunction, has been described in patients with hematologic malignancies after intensive chemotherapy or total-body irradiation. Hypogonadism in cancer patients has also been reported with chronic opioid use for pain control or as a part of endocrine insufficiency in cancer and other systemic illnesses, worsening with disease progression [24].

MSD pharmacotherapy and infertility

Phosphodiesterase-5 inhibitors and infertility

Sildenafil citrate (Viagra), the first PDE5i, was introduced in 1998, and currently PDE5is are the first-line treatment for ED of various etiologies. Not long after the introduction of sildenafil, in 1999, Tur-Kaspa *et al.* published a case report on the successful use of sildenafil 50 mg in three men who had difficulties providing sperm for intrauterine insemination (IUI) or in-vitro fertilization (IVF) [25]. Additional patients in their case series were able to provide sperm after reassurance that sildenafil could be given if needed to help overcome anxiety-induced ED, without actually taking the drug. Although their clinical description corresponds more closely to ejaculation failure rather than to ED, they suggested that sildenafil may be considered as a treatment for male partners of couples treated with assisted reproductive technologies (ART) who develop ED when asked to provide sperm on demand, to avoid stress, frustration, delays in fertilization, or missing a cycle. Jannini *et al.* studied 25 men who had to provide a sperm sample for IUI and 12 men who had a postcoital test (PCT), with no preexisting ED [26]. They found ED of various severities in 72% of the IUI group and 67% of the PCT group, when they were required to ejaculate for the procedure. All subjects were treated with sildenafil 50 mg. In addition to improved ability to obtain and maintain erections, greater confidence, and, interestingly, higher sexual desire in both groups (in contradistinction to all pivotal phase III trials for the three currently available PDE5 inhibitors), they found also an increase in sperm concentration and in total sperm count in the IUI group, and an increase in total number of spermatozoa in the cervical mucus and in the number of spermatozoa with linear progressive motility in the PCT group. They hypothesized that treatment with sildenafil reduced the stress associated with fertility procedures, facilitating a more complete ejaculation and improved sperm quality.

Despite over 25 million men treated and over a billion pills of sildenafil citrate prescribed, our understanding of the mechanisms linking PDE5i and fertility is incomplete, and the literature is mostly limited to the effect of PDE5i on semen parameters and reproductive hormone levels (Tables 11.1, 11.2). In the erectile response, NO is synthesized in nerve endings as well as the endothelium by nNOS and eNOS,

Table 11.1. Effect of PDE5i on sperm quality and fertilization: laboratory evidence

Author	Year	Study type	PDE5i	Main outcomes
Foresta et al. [28]	2010	In vitro	Tadalafil Vardenafil	PDE5i isoforms A1, A2 are expressed in spermatozoal neck and acrosome regions Increased progressive motility, velocity, and intracellular calcium No effect on sperm capacitation, acrosome reaction, apoptosis, and penetration
Glenn et al. [29]	2009	Animals (mice)	Sildenafil	Reduced fertilization rate, impaired early embryo development
Glenn et al. [30]	2007	In vitro	Sildenafil	Increase in sperm motility, premature acrosome reaction
Mostafa [31]	2007	In vitro	Sildenafil	Concentration-related stimulation of sperm motility
Mostafa [32]	2007	In vitro	Tadalafil	Concentration-related stimulation of sperm motility, decreased motility at high dose
Andrade et al. [33]	2000	In vitro	Sildenafil	No effect on motility at low dose, reduced motility at high dose
Lefievre et al. [34]	2000	In vitro	Sildenafil	Dose-dependent increase in sperm motility and capacitation No triggering of acrosome reaction
Cuadra et al. [35]	2000	In vitro	Sildenafil	Dose-dependent increase in sperm motility, premature acrosome reaction
Burger et al. [36]	2000	In vitro	Sildenafil	No effect on motility, viability, membrane integrity, penetration characteristics

respectively, activating guanylate cyclase to form cyclic guanosine monophosphate (cGMP). cGMP functions as a second messenger activating cGMP-dependent protein kinases to lower sarcoplasmic calcium levels, leading to corporal smooth muscle relaxation. PDE5is inhibit the breakdown of cGMP by PDE5 and augment the smooth muscle relaxation response. Both eNOS and nNOS are present in human spermatozoa and synthesize spermatozoal NO. The NO effect on sperm motility and viability is dose-dependent: at low doses NO improves sperm motility, whereas high doses of NO adversely affect sperm motility, probably promoting the generation of free radicals (such as peroxynitrite) causing oxidative damage to spermatozoal membranes [27]. Activation of guanylate cyclase by NO has a beneficial effect on sperm motility, capacitation, and acrosomal reactivity and promotes sperm interaction with the oocyte. Several studies have documented the presence of various PDE isoforms in human spermatozoa, including PDE1A, PDE1B, PDE3A, PDE3B, PDE4A, PDE4B, and PDE8, and these support the role of PDE in the regulation of spermatozoal cytosolic nucleotides [27].

Selective serotonin reuptake inhibitors and infertility

Selective serotonin reuptake inhibitors (SSRIs) are widely used in general and psychiatric medicine and also in sexual medicine: they are the most commonly prescribed treatment for premature ejaculation by urologists, either as an on-demand treatment or as daily-use agents [45]. SSRIs may also be used to alleviate performance-anxiety-induced ED, and it has been suggested that their use in combination with PDE5is may be of benefit in males with ejaculatory failure during ART treatments [46].

Elevated prolactin can impair fertility at the hypothalamic level through elevating dopamine, which suppresses GnRH release, or at the pituitary level by suppression of LH and FSH release [47]. High levels of prolactin also inhibit LH binding to Leydig cells in the testes, leading to significant yet reversible suppression of spermatogenesis [48]. Despite this apparent association of serotoninergic antidepressants, prolactin, and impaired spermatogenesis, elevated prolactin levels are not consistently found in men with infertility attributed to SSRI use. Kumar et al. showed that SSRIs, including fluoxetine, citalopram, fluvoxamine, paroxetine, and sertraline, possess a direct spermicidal activity, with fluoxetine being most spermicidal [49]. In their in-vitro study, serotonin itself was not spermicidal; therefore they suggested that SSRI spermicidal properties are mediated by inhibition of oxidative phosphorylation and adenosine triphosphate (ATP) synthesis in the sperm mitochondria or by interaction with sulfhydryl groups in the sperm cell membrane and not by increasing

Table 11.2. Effect of PDE5i on sperm quality and reproductive hormones: clinical evidence

Author	Year	Design	n	PDE5i	Duration	Treatment	Main outcomes
Jannini et al. [26]	2004	Open-label, repeated measurements – before and after treatment	37	Sildenafil	1 hour	Single dose: sildenafil 50 mg	No change: volume, pH, non-linear progressive motility, morphology Increased: count, concentration, linear progressive motility
Dimitriadis et al. [37]	2010	Prospective, randomized, controlled	75	Vardenafil Sildenafil	12 weeks	Daily vardenafil, vs. sildenafil, vs. carnitine, vs. no treatment	Increased insulin-like-3 peptide concentration (Leydig cell function) Increased sperm concentration, motility, and improved morphology
Hellstrom et al. [38]	2008	Prospective, randomized, double-blind, placebo-controlled, multicenter	253	Tadalafil	9 months	Daily placebo, vs. tadalafil 20 mg	Equivocal decrease in sperm concentration. No change: total count, motility, morphology Mild increase in total testosterone No change in free testosterone, FSH, LH
Jarvi et al. [39]	2008	Prospective, randomized, double-blind, placebo-controlled, parallel group, multicenter	200	Sildenafil Vardenafil	6 months	Daily placebo, vs. sildenafil 100 mg, vs. vardenafil 20 mg	No change in semen parameters No change in FSH, LH
Pomara et al. [40]	2007	Prospective, randomized, double-blind, crossover	18	Sildenafil Tadalafil	1–2 hours	Single dose: sildenafil 50 mg vs. tadalafil 20 mg	Sildenafil: increased motility (37 vs. 28.5%) Tadalafil: decreased motility (21.5 vs. 28.5%)
du Plessis et al. [41]	2004	Prospective, double-blind, placebo-controlled, crossover	20	Sildenafil	1 hour	Single dose: sildenafil 50 mg vs. placebo	No change: count, concentration, morphology, % motile, % progressive motile, % static Increased: smoothed path velocity, straight line velocity, % rapid cells
Hellstrom et al. [42]	2003	Prospective, randomized, placebo-controlled	421	Tadalafil	6 months	Daily placebo, vs. tadalafil 10 mg, vs. tadalafil 20 mg	No change: total count, concentration, morphology, motility
Purvis et al. [43]	2002	Prospective, randomized, double-blind, placebo-controlled, crossover	17	Sildenafil	1.5, 4 hours	Single dose: sildenafil 100 mg	No change: volume, count, density, morphology, motility, vitality, viscosity
Aversa et al. [44]	2000	Prospective, randomized, double-blind, placebo-controlled, crossover	20	Sildenafil	1 hour	Single dose: sildenafil 100 mg	No change: count, motility, morphology

serotonin levels. A controlled study by Safarinejad proposed that structural DNA damage is the underlying mechanism for SSRI-induced impaired sperm quality [50]. In males taking an SSRI, this study showed a decline in semen parameters related to the duration of treatment, independent of the specific SSRI used (citalopram, escitalopram, fluoxetine, paroxetine, or sertraline), and a significant increase in DNA damage as measured by sperm chromatin structure assay, which was negatively correlated with sperm motility.

Testosterone replacement therapy and infertility

Testosterone replacement therapy (TRT), used in the treatment of hypogonadism, suppresses spermatogenesis by inhibiting the HPG axis through a negative feedback mechanism, causing a decrease in GnRH, LH, and FSH. Exogenously administered testosterone is also aromatized to estrogens in fat tissue, further suppressing spermatogenesis [48]. In fact, testosterone in combination with progestins may be the future of male contraceptives [51]. For hypogonadal men who desire fertility, normalization of testosterone levels should be achieved without suppression of gonadotropins. Clomiphene citrate (an orally administered centrally acting antiestrogen), hCG (an LH analog), or aromatase inhibitors are all viable options. Clomiphene citrate has been shown to increase testosterone level, improve testosterone-to-estrogen ratio, improve FSH and LH levels, induce sperm in the ejaculate of patients with idiopathic non-obstructive azoospermia, allowing in-vitro fertilization with intracytoplasmic sperm injection (IVF-ICSI) to be performed, and facilitate testicular surgical sperm extraction [52–54]. Clomiphene treatment is most likely to benefit patients with low-normal LH levels, but it is worthwhile mentioning that this use of clomiphene citrate for treatment of hypogonadism is an off-label use, not FDA-approved, and therefore patients should be informed accordingly. Clomiphene doses used vary greatly, from 25 mg every other day titrated according to testosterone levels to 100 mg daily. Another medical treatment option in the patient with low testosterone and low testosterone-to-estrogen ratio is the use of aromatase inhibitors, to decrease the conversion of testosterone to estrogen in adipose tissue. Raman and Schlegel have shown that subfertile men with a low testosterone-to-estradiol ratio had an increase in testosterone-to-estrogen ratio and improvement in semen parameters [55].

Conclusion

MSD in infertile men may include ED, reduced libido, ejaculatory dysfunction, and orgasm alterations. Infertility, and MSD are closely related: male partners of infertile couples are more likely to experience MSD, MSD can cause difficulties to "perform on demand" and compromise infertility treatment outcomes, certain medical conditions are common risk factors for both infertility and MSD, and finally, certain therapies for MSD may impact on male fertility potential. Therefore, it is prudent to actively address sexual health issues in every couple presenting with infertility and throughout the course of infertility evaluation and treatments – to obtain a sexual history from the couple, to actively seek common risk factors for MSD and infertility, to accurately diagnose MSD, and to treat MSD with fertility-friendly interventions. The best option to preserve reproductive potential in men with cancer is semen cryopreservation before treatment. Fertility issues should therefore be discussed early, before treatment begins.

References

1. Feldman HA, Goldstein I, Hatzichristou DG, Krane RJ, McKinlay JB. Impotence and its medical and psychosocial correlates: results of the Massachusetts Male Aging Study. *J Urol* 1994; 151: 54–61.

2. Laumann EO, Paik A, Rosen RC. Sexual dysfunction in the United States: prevalence and predictors. *JAMA* 1999; 281: 537–44.

3. Khademi A, Alleyassin A, Amini M, Ghaemi M. Evaluation of sexual dysfunction prevalence in infertile couples. *J Sex Med* 2008; 5: 1402–10.

4. Safarinejad MR. Prevalence and risk factors for erectile dysfunction in a population-based study in Iran. *Int J Impot Res* 2003; 15: 246–52.

5. O'Brien JH, Lazarou S, Deane L, Jarvi K, Zini A. Erectile dysfunction and andropause symptoms in infertile men. *J Urol* 2005; 174: 1932–4.

6. Ramezanzadeh F, Aghssa MM, Jafarabadi M, Zayeri F. Alterations of sexual desire and satisfaction in male partners of infertile couples. *Fertil Steril* 2006; 85: 139–43.

7. Shindel AW, Nelson CJ, Naughton CK, Mulhall JP. Premature ejaculation in infertile couples: prevalence and correlates. *J Sex Med* 2008; 5: 485–91.

8. Burns LH. Psychiatric aspects of infertility and infertility treatments. *Psychiatr Clin North Am* 2007; 30: 689–716.

9. Rosen RC. Psychogenic erectile dysfunction: classification and management. *Urol Clin North Am* 2001; 28: 269–78.

10. Saleh RA, Ranga GM, Raina R, Nelson DR, Agarwal A. Sexual dysfunction in men undergoing infertility evaluation: a cohort observational study. *Fertil Steril* 2003; 79: 909–12.

11. Elia J, Delfino M, Imbrogno N, Mazzilli F. The impact of a diagnosis of couple subfertility on male sexual function. *J Endocrinol Invest* 2010; 33: 74–6.

12. Sussman EM, Chudnovsky A, Niederberger CS. Hormonal evaluation of the infertile male: has it evolved? *Urol Clin North Am* 2008; 35: 147–55, vii.

13. Bhasin S, Enzlin P, Coviello A, Basson R. Sexual dysfunction in men and women with endocrine disorders. *Lancet* 2007; 369: 597–611.

14. Isidori AM, Giannetta E, Gianfrilli D, *et al.* Effects of testosterone on sexual function in men: results of a meta-analysis. *Clin Endocrinol* 2005; 63: 381–94.

15. Aversa A, Isidori AM, Greco EA, *et al.* Hormonal supplementation and erectile dysfunction. *Eur Urol* 2004; 45: 535–8.

16. Schmidt PJ, Steinberg EM, Negro PP, *et al.* Pharmacologically induced hypogonadism and sexual function in healthy young women and men. *Neuropsychopharmacology* 2009; 34: 565–76.

17. Corona G, Jannini EA, Mannucci E, *et al.* Different testosterone levels are associated with ejaculatory dysfunction. *J Sex Med* 2008; 5: 1991–8.

18. Adaikan PG, Srilatha B. Oestrogen-mediated hormonal imbalance precipitates erectile dysfunction. *Int J Impot Res* 2003; 15: 38–43.

19. Greco EA, Pili M, Bruzziches R, *et al.* Testosterone: estradiol ratio changes associated with long-term tadalafil administration: a pilot study. *J Sex Med* 2006; 3: 716–22.

20. Mancini A, Milardi D, Bianchi A, Summaria V, De Marinis L. Increased estradiol levels in venous occlusive disorder: a possible functional mechanism of venous leakage. *Int J Impot Res* 2005; 17: 239–42.

21. De Rosa M, Zarrilli S, Di Sarno A, *et al.* Hyperprolactinemia in men: clinical and biochemical features and response to treatment. *Endocrine* 2003; 20: 75–82.

22. Colao A, Sarno AD, Cappabianca P, *et al.* Gender differences in the prevalence, clinical features and response to cabergoline in hyperprolactinemia. *Eur J Endocrinol* 2003; 148: 325–31.

23. El-Sakka AI, Hassoba HM, Sayed HM, Tayeb KA. Pattern of endocrinal changes in patients with sexual dysfunction. *J Sex Med* 2005; 2: 551–8.

24. Tal R, Mulhall JP. Sexual health issues in men with cancer. *Oncology (Williston Park)* 2006; 20: 294–300.

25. Tur-Kaspa I, Segal S, Moffa F, Massobrio M, Meltzer S. Viagra for temporary erectile dysfunction during treatments with assisted reproductive technologies. *Hum Reprod* 1999; 14: 1783–4.

26. Jannini EA, Lombardo F, Salacone P, Gandini L, Lenzi A. Treatment of sexual dysfunctions secondary to male infertility with sildenafil citrate. *Fertil Steril* 2004; 81: 705–7.

27. Dimitriadis F, Giannakis D, Pardalidis N, *et al.* Effects of phosphodiesterase-5 inhibitors on sperm parameters and fertilizing capacity. *Asian J Androl* 2008; 10: 115–33.

28. Foresta C, Pati MA, Perilli L, *et al.* Expression of phosphodiesterase type 5A in human spermatozoa and influence of its inhibition on motility and functional sperm parameters. *J Endocrinol Invest* 2010 [epub ahead of print].

29. Glenn DR, McClure N, Cosby SL, Stevenson M, Lewis SE. Sildenafil citrate (Viagra) impairs fertilization and early embryo development in mice. *Fertil Steril* 2009; 91: 893–9.

30. Glenn DR, McVicar CM, McClure N, Lewis SE. Sildenafil citrate improves sperm motility but causes a premature acrosome reaction in vitro. *Fertil Steril* 2007; 87: 1064–70.

31. Mostafa T. In vitro sildenafil citrate use as a sperm motility stimulant. *Fertil Steril* 2007; 88: 994–6.

32. Mostafa T. Tadalafil as an in vitro sperm motility stimulant. *Andrologia* 2007; 39: 12–15.

33. Andrade JR, Traboulsi A, Hussain A, Dubin NH. In vitro effects of sildenafil and phentolamine, drugs used for erectile dysfunction, on human sperm motility. *Am J Obstet Gynecol* 2000; 182: 1093–5.

34. Lefievre L, De Lamirande E, Gagnon C. The cyclic GMP-specific phosphodiesterase inhibitor, sildenafil, stimulates human sperm motility and capacitation but not acrosome reaction. *J Androl* 2000; 21: 929–37.

35. Cuadra DL, Chan PJ, Patton WC, Stewart SC, King A. Type 5 phosphodiesterase regulation of human sperm motility. *Am J Obstet Gynecol* 2000; 182: 1013–15.

36. Burger M, Sikka SC, Bivalacqua TJ, Lamb DJ, Hellstrom WJ. The effect of sildenafil on human sperm motion and function from normal and infertile men. *Int J Impot Res* 2000; 12: 229–34.

37. Dimitriadis F, Tsambalas S, Tsounapi P, *et al.* Effects of phosphodiesterase-5 inhibitors on Leydig cell

secretory function in oligoasthenospermic infertile men: a randomized trial. *BJU Int* 2010; 106: 1181–5.

38. Hellstrom WJ, Gittelman M, Jarow J, *et al.* An evaluation of semen characteristics in men 45 years of age or older after daily dosing with tadalafil 20mg: results of a multicenter, randomized, double-blind, placebo-controlled, 9-month study. *Eur Urol* 2008; 53: 1058–65.

39. Jarvi K, Dula E, Drehobl M, *et al.* Daily vardenafil for 6 months has no detrimental effects on semen characteristics or reproductive hormones in men with normal baseline levels. *J Urol* 2008; 179: 1060–5.

40. Pomara G, Morelli G, Canale D, *et al.* Alterations in sperm motility after acute oral administration of sildenafil or tadalafil in young, infertile men. *Fertil Steril* 2007; 88: 860–5.

41. du Plessis SS, de Jongh PS, Franken DR. Effect of acute in vivo sildenafil citrate and in vitro 8-bromo-cGMP treatments on semen parameters and sperm function. *Fertil Steril* 2004; 81: 1026–33.

42. Hellstrom WJ, Overstreet JW, Yu A, *et al.* Tadalafil has no detrimental effect on human spermatogenesis or reproductive hormones. *J Urol* 2003; 170: 887–91.

43. Purvis K, Muirhead GJ, Harness JA. The effects of sildenafil on human sperm function in healthy volunteers. *Br J Clin Pharmacol* 2002; 53 (Suppl 1): 53S–60S.

44. Aversa A, Mazzilli F, Rossi T, *et al.* Effects of sildenafil (Viagra) administration on seminal parameters and post-ejaculatory refractory time in normal males. *Hum Reprod* 2000; 15: 131–4.

45. Shindel A, Nelson C, Brandes S. Urologist practice patterns in the management of premature ejaculation: a nationwide survey. *J Sex Med* 2008; 5: 199–205.

46. Lu S, Zhao Y, Hu J, *et al.* Combined use of phosphodiesterase-5 inhibitors and selective serotonin reuptake inhibitors for temporary ejaculation failure in couple undergoing assisted reproductive technologies. *Fertil Steril* 2009; 91: 1806–8.

47. Hendrick V, Gitlin M, Altshuler L, Korenman S. Antidepressant medications, mood and male fertility. *Psychoneuroendocrinology* 2000; 25: 37–51.

48. Nudell DM, Monoski MM, Lipshultz LI. Common medications and drugs: how they affect male fertility. *Urol Clin North Am* 2002; 29: 965–73.

49. Kumar VS, Sharma VL, Tiwari P, *et al.* The spermicidal and antitrichomonas activities of SSRI antidepressants. *Bioorg Med Chem Lett* 2006; 16: 2509–12.

50. Safarinejad MR. Sperm DNA damage and semen quality impairment after treatment with selective serotonin reuptake inhibitors detected using semen analysis and sperm chromatin structure assay. *J Urol* 2008; 180: 2124–8.

51. Amory JK. Progress and prospects in male hormonal contraception. *Curr Opin Endocrinol Diabetes Obes* 2008; 15: 255–60.

52. Whitten SJ, Nangia AK, Kolettis PN. Select patients with hypogonadotropic hypogonadism may respond to treatment with clomiphene citrate. *Fertil Steril* 2006; 86: 1664–8.

53. Shabsigh A, Kang Y, Shabsigh R, *et al.* Clomiphene citrate effects on testosterone/estrogen ratio in male hypogonadism. *J Sex Med* 2005; 2: 716–21.

54. Hussein A, Ozgok Y, Ross L, Niederberger C. Clomiphene administration for cases of nonobstructive azoospermia: a multicenter study. *J Androl* 2005; 26: 787–91.

55. Raman JD, Schlegel PN. Aromatase inhibitors for male infertility. *J Urol* 2002; 167: 624–9.

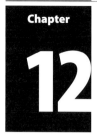

Chapter

12

Radiation effects on spermatogenesis

Fabio Firmbach Pasqualotto and Ashok Agarwal

Introduction

Human fertility is dependent on the maturation of germ cells through meiosis and their association with supporting cells. These processes are sensitive to radiotherapy. Infertility is functionally defined as the inability to conceive after one year of intercourse without contraception [1]. Rates of permanent infertility and compromised fertility after cancer treatment vary and depend on many factors [2]. The effects of radiation therapy depend on the size/location of the radiation field, dose, dose intensity, disease, and the age and pre-treatment fertility status of the patient [2]. Male infertility may result from the disease itself (best documented in patients with testicular cancer and Hodgkin's disease), anatomic problems (e.g., retrograde ejaculation or anejaculation), primary or secondary hormonal insufficiency, or, more frequently, from damage or depletion of the germinal stem cells [3]. The measurable effects of radiation therapy include a decrease in the number of spermatozoa, decreased motility, abnormal morphology, and reduced DNA integrity. Radiation therapy increases the DNA fragmentation index, whereas this value decreases after chemotherapy [4–6]. The biologic implications of such changes in sperm DNA after cancer therapy have, to date, not been fully elucidated.

Cancer and radiation therapy

Spermatogenesis is a long, complex, and finely tuned process; during this process, the developing germ cells are sensitive to endogenous and exogenous stress. Cancer therapies such as radiation and chemotherapy can cause temporary or permanent impairment of fertility in male cancer patients who are of reproductive age.

A total of 1 596 670 new cancer cases and 571 950 deaths from cancer are projected to occur in the United States in 2011. Overall cancer incidence rates were stable in men in the most recent time period after decreasing by 1.9% per year from 2001 to 2005; in women, incidence rates have been declining by 0.6% annually since 1998 [5]. Testicular germ cell carcinoma is the most common malignant disease among young men, and the incidence is increasing. In view of the excellent prognosis, with a cure rate surpassing 95%, the clinical challenge of today lies in minimizing the long-term effects of the treatment. The prognosis of patients with testicular cancer has considerably improved in recent years: whereas in 1970 the mean survival of such patients was only 10%, since 1990 it has risen to 90%. This can be attributed to notable diagnostic and surgical advances and new radiotherapy and chemotherapy protocols, to which testicular tumors are especially sensitive.

From an infertility point of view, patients with testicular germ cell carcinoma represent a particular challenge. Not only is the reproductive function affected by the treatment given (i.e., chemotherapy and/or radiation therapy), but the tumor is also known to be associated with male sub/infertility and undescended testicles, all of which are considered to be part of the testicular dysgenesis syndrome [4].

The cytotoxic effect of radiation therapy on the spermatogenetic cells has led to great interest in studying post-therapy sperm parameter alterations in testicular cancer subjects. Numerous articles report studies of antineoplastic therapy on sperm quality, but these can be limited by the low number of patients examined and methodological errors which reduce their validity. Radiotherapy is used to treat malignancies such as Hodgkin's lymphoma, lymphosarcoma,

Fertility Preservation in Male Cancer Patients, ed. John P. Mulhall, Linda D. Applegarth, Robert D. Oates and Peter N. Schlegel.
Published by Cambridge University Press. © Cambridge University Press 2013.

and testicular cancers, many of which strike patients of young or childbearing age. Radiation doses range from 3000 to 7000 cGy – doses that are thousands of times higher than those used in diagnostic radiology. The effects of such high doses can be mutagenic, embryotoxic, embryolethal, and teratogenic. When possible, the gonads are shielded to reduce exposure to the radiation.

Spermatogenesis is initiated from the most primitive type of spermatogonium, the type A-single (As) or stem cell spermatogonium, which has two possible fates: self-renewal or committed differentiation. The As spermatogonia give rise to A-pair (Apr) and then A-aligned (Aal) spermatogonia, which are then able to differentiate into A1, A2, A3, A4, intermediate (In), and B spermatogonia. When a type B spermatogonium enters the last mitotic division, it generates two primary spermatocytes, which initiate meiosis by replicating the DNA before they pass through a number of stages that end with the two nuclear divisions distinguished as meiosis I and II. After the meiotic divisions each primary spermatocyte results in the formation of four haploid round spermatids. The spermatids proceed through a long differentiation process (designated spermiogenesis) resulting in the release of spermatozoa [2–9].

Radiation induces germinal depletion in a dose-dependent manner, with immature cells being the most radiosensitive. It has been hypothesized that spermatogonia – which are the most radiosensitive cells because of their intense mitotic activity – and spermatids are affected by ionizing radiation. Spermatids are unprotected because they lose their DNA damage repair mechanisms during post-meiotic differentiation and chromatin condensation. Any radiation damage that occurs may not be apparent initially, as many spermatocytes generally survive the first round of radioactive impact and go on to mature and produce spermatozoa [2]. Ultimately, radiotherapy damages the DNA, impeding the cell from replicating itself and causing its death. This therapy is especially effective in cancer cells, which replicate more quickly, but also affects normal cells, especially those with a high replication rate such as spermatogonia. Radiation induces material ionization both directly, through excitation of the atoms making up the DNA molecule, and indirectly, through its interaction with non-DNA molecules, which induce the ionization of the genetic material by emitting secondary electrons [2,6].

The germinal epithelium is damaged by doses as low as 1 Gy, while Leydig cells are damaged by doses of 20–30 Gy [1]. Doses as low as 0.1–1.2 Gy may damage dividing spermatogonia and may result in oligospermia. In prepubertal males, doses to the testes in excess of 20 Gy may result in delayed puberty. These doses result from irradiation to the pelvis for conditions including bladder, rectal, and anal tumors as well as for germ cell tumors of the testes. Total-body irradiation also causes permanent impairment of spermatogenesis but has variable effects on Leydig cell function.

The observed activation of reserve stem cells after a gonadotoxic insult demonstrates that a single insult is less damaging to the seminiferous epithelium than multiple insults of lower intensity. In men following single measured doses of 6 Gy and above, and low-dose fractionated irradiation of 1.5 Gy and above, irreversible damage of spermatogenesis can be expected [2–10]. Testicular irradiation with doses of 20 Gy is associated with Leydig cell dysfunction in prepubertal boys [7]. Apart from the dose and fractionation, other factors such as source, field of treatment, type of radiation, age, and individual susceptibility influence the gonadotoxicity of irradiation.

Virtually the entire population of spermatogonia will die if exposed to sufficiently high x-ray doses, and especially a fractionated irradiation. Considering the mean dose (2600 rad) as the discriminating value, at 12 months, the reduction in total sperm count is statistically significant in subjects having undergone a total dose > 2600 cGy in comparison with those subjected to a dose ≤ 2600 cGy. This difference is not statistically significant at 24 months after therapy. This confirms that the total dose of radiation administered is a discriminating and predictive factor of the time necessary to recover spermatogenesis [2].

Recovery may however be increased at very high doses with a fractionated irradiation. After exposure to irradiation, spermatocytes and spermatids continue normal development and ultimately leave the testis as spermatozoa. If stem cells (As spermatogonia) survive the irradiation, they may in some cases quickly initiate the recovery of spermatogenesis and repopulate the seminiferous epithelium. The remaining As spermatogonia will either first replenish their own numbers before they enter spermatogenic differentiation, so that in time spermatogenesis spreads along the length of the tubule, or they can remain "arrested" in the testis as isolated spermatogonia in atrophic tubules. In some cases a delay before spermatogenesis reinitiates

Table 12.1. Effects of radiation therapy on spermatogenesis

Testicular dose (cGy)	Effect on spermatogenesis
<10	No effect
10–30	Temporary oligospermia
30–50	Temporary azoospermia at 4–12 months after radiation; 100% recovery by 48 months
50–100	100% temporary azoospermia for 3–17 months after radiotherapy; recovery begins at 8–26 months
100–200	100% azoospermia from 2 months to at least 9 months; recovery begins at 11–20 months
200–300	100% azoospermia beginning at 1–2 months; may lead to permanent azoospermia; if recovery takes place, it may take years
1200	Permanent azoospermia
2400	Permanent azoospermia

has been observed. Currently there is little evidence for damage to the somatic elements of the testis after moderate doses of radiation or chemotherapy. However, as the germ cells are dependent on Sertoli cells for survival, it is difficult to assess whether it is germ cells or somatic cells that are damaged by radiation.

Boys with acute leukemia requiring marrow-ablative chemoradiotherapy and hematopoietic stem cell transplantation (HSCT) are at extremely high risk for infertility, with 85% of adult patients found to be azoospermic after total-body irradiation and cyclophosphamide administration [8].

Ionizing radiation has adverse effects on gonadal function in men of all ages, with the degree and persistence of the damage being dependent on the dose (Table 12.1) [9]. In many cases, men are azoospermic after treatment, and those who do regain spermatogenesis some time after treatment exhibit low sperm counts, decreased motility, and an increased rate of chromosomal abnormalities [10]. Compared with the testicles, the ovaries are more resistant, mainly because of the biology of the germ cells present in the ovary. These do not divide until completion of the first meiotic division at ovulation, in contrast to the constant cell division that occurs during sperm production in the testes.

Studies in animals

Studies involving animals have shown that radiation has direct mutagenic effects on germ cells in relation to the dose. High doses lead to dominant lethal effects, point mutations, and chromosomal abnormalities [11]. Testicular irradiation in mice, rats, monkeys, and men uniformly decreases the number of differentiating spermatogonia and later depletes the more advanced spermatogenic cells [12].

The mutagenic effects of radiation therapy are well known from animal studies. Total-body irradiation, which is used in myeloablative stem cell transplantation, is highly associated with infertility, while lesser doses or limited radiation fields have less gonadal toxicity [6]. In rhesus monkeys and humans after single doses of 4 and 6 Gy it takes five years or more for spermatogenesis to return to pre-irradiation germinal cell numbers and sperm concentrations [13–18]. Others have used doses of 1–4 Gy for the depletion of the seminiferous epithelium, or for studies on gonadal protection in rhesus monkeys [16–18].

Most of the studies performed in rats and one study in two baboons have shown that blocking gonadotropin secretion can lead to hormonal protection even if the treatment is applied after irradiation [19–24]. In monkeys, after gonadotropin withdrawal, high amounts of testicular androgens remain, which should not severely affect spermatogenic regulation in primates [25–28].

In one study, 20 adult male monkeys were randomized to receive either recombinant human follicle-stimulating hormone (FSH), gonadotropin-releasing hormone (GnRH) antagonist, or saline injections for 36 days [29]. Testicular volume and inhibin B decreased significantly in all irradiated groups compared with baseline and with the non-irradiated control group, followed by a gradual recovery of these parameters, which was, especially at the earlier time points, significantly better in the FSH-treated group than in both other irradiated groups. Irradiation caused a drastic decrease of sperm parameters in all groups, followed by a partial recovery of sperm parameters, which was significantly slower in the early phases of recovery in the GnRH antagonist group compared with the vehicle group. Testicular histology showed a significant depletion on study day 261 in all irradiated animals. In contrast to rodent studies, therefore, GnRH antagonist treatment did not provide gonadal protection in this primate model. FSH treatment resulted in slightly better recovery of spermatogenesis, which appears to be of no or only little clinical relevance.

A study in rat testes demonstrated that radiation-induced block in spermatogonial differentiation may in fact be caused by damage to the somatic environment, i.e., the Sertoli cells, and not to the germ cells [30]. Indeed, transplantation of Sertoli cells into irradiated testes has been shown to stimulate recovery of endogenous host spermatogenesis. Stimulation might, however, be indirect, as the endocrine androgen–estrogen balance seems crucial in stimulating spermatogonial recovery [30,31].

A recent study has shown that irradiation of mice testis created a gap in spermatogenesis, which was initiated by loss of A1 to B spermatogonia [12]. The gap lasted for approximately 10 days and successively extinguished germ cells at different developmental stages. Spermatogonial stem cells were, however, able to repopulate the seminiferous epithelia, which was reconstituted 42 days after irradiation. Also, gene expression can be a useful tool to describe reconstitution of testicular tissue after irradiation or chemotherapy, which otherwise relies on detailed histological descriptions that require carefully trained pathologists.

Studies in humans

In humans, most men are azoospermic for at least a year following radiation therapy, and studies of semen samples taken three years following treatment have found an increased frequency of sperm chromosomal abnormalities (both numerical and structural) in 20.9% of the patients compared with a control rate of 8.5%. These studies have also found a greater frequency of hypohaploidy relative to hyperhaploidy, suggesting that radiation therapy causes chromosomal loss rather than non-dysfunction [32]. There is also a suggestion that high doses of paternal irradiation preconception may increase induction of lymphomyeloid malignancies in the offspring if they are exposed after birth to a recognized inducer of leukemia [33].

In humans, a number of studies have shown that the frequency of autosomal and sex chromosome aneuploidy in sperm samples increases after radiation therapy, but the data suggest that these changes are transient. Results of studies of patients with testicular germ cell carcinoma indicate that sperm DNA might be damaged post-orchiectomy, even before radiation therapy [4]. The risk of damage to sperm DNA due to cancer or its treatment is a source of potential concern. Children who are fathered by cancer survivors do not seem to be at an increased risk for genetic abberations, although this conclusion is largely based on data from small case series. In addition, the vast majority of large studies represent a follow-up of survivors of pediatric cancer [2–4]. It can be assumed that the sensitivity of DNA damage of a prepubertal germ cell is less pronounced than in the proliferating postpubertal cells of spermatogenesis. Finally, these surveys were based on conceptions that had occurred naturally.

Paternal exposure to ionizing radiation can produce dramatic effects on reproduction resulting in a decrease in fertility, which may be associated with a drop in sperm production and an increase in dominant lethal mutations in offspring [34]. Evidence from animal studies suggests that a high risk of transmissible defects exists that results from increases in the frequency of germline mutations [35,36], predisposing future generations to risks such as cancer [36].

Even though radiation therapy may damage DNA, the extent, duration, and biologic significance of such an effect on sperm chromatin integrity is not known [33]. A dose-dependent increase in DNA damage in testis cells 14 days after radiation therapy has been reported [37]. The overall results show that DNA damage induced in pre-meiotic germ cells is detectable in primary spermatocytes and is still present in mature spermatozoa. Other animal studies have shown that pregnancies resulting from mating with an irradiated male are associated with impaired fetal development, pregnancy loss, abnormal somatic development, and tumor induction in the fetus [38].

Genetic instability was detected in children whose fathers previously had been exposed to radiation therapy [39], but no increase in malformation rates or in tumor induction was observed [40].

The DNA fragmentation index (DFI) was found to be significantly increased in men who received radiation therapy [33]. The potential risk of using sperm samples with post-irradiation DNA damage for advanced techniques of assisted reproduction is emphasized by the results of studies using the human sperm–hamster oocyte technique. In such models, the fertilization ability remained despite radiation-induced sperm DNA damage. Therefore, the risk of transmitting defective DNA to the offspring is apparent [41,42].

Regarding semen parameters, there is a statistically significant decrease in ejaculate volume, sperm concentration per mL, total sperm count, and forward motility and a statistically significant increase in abnormal forms up to 12 months following cancer therapy. In one study, there were no differences at the beginning and 24 months post-therapy for any semen parameter except volume, indicating that sperm quality had returned to pre-radiotherapy values [4]. However, even after 24 months, sperm volume remained lower than before treatment. In contrast with the chemotherapy group, alteration in sperm parameters were most relevant six months after the end of radiotherapy.

Gonadal shielding

Semen quality has been reported in men who received external-beam irradiation for testicular cancer without gonadal shielding, and it has been found that while 51% of patients had low sperm counts before therapy, all of them had low sperm counts two years after treatment, and 82% of them had persistently low counts at a mean of eight years after therapy [3]. With pelvic irradiation of 5000 cGy, a shield should provide a 99% block. It has also been demonstrated that gonadal shielding before radiation is effective in protecting testicular function following bone marrow transplantation in childhood and adolescence [43].

Conclusions

Quality of life is an important issue for childhood and adult cancer patients. Radiation treatment for testicular or other cancers may damage the testis, leaving permanent problems with sperm production. Reduced fertility or sterility after radiation therapy depends on the dose received by the testis. Therefore, physicians should discuss the side effects of radiation therapy on fertility potential with their patients before beginning the treatment.

References

1. Galarneau GJ, Nagler HM. Cost-effective infertility therapies in the '90s: to treat or to cure? *Contemp Urol* 1999; 11: 32–45.

2. Gandini L, Sgro P, Lombardo F, *et al.* Effect of chemo- or radiotherapy on sperm parameters of testicular cancer patients. *Hum Reprod* 2006; 21: 2882–9.

3. Lass A, Akabosu F, Brinsden P. Sperm banking and assisted reproduction treatment for couples following cancer treatment of the male partner. *Hum Reprod Update* 2001; 7: 370–7.

4. Stahl O, Eberhard J, Jepson K, *et al.* The impact of testicular carcinoma and its treatment on sperm DNA integrity. *Cancer* 2004; 100: 1137–44.

5. Siegel R, Ward E, Brawley O, Jemal A. Cancer Statistics, 2011. The impact of eliminating socioeconomic and racial disparities on premature cancer deaths. *CA Cancer J Clin* 2011; 61: 212–36.

6. Lee SJ, Schover LR, Partridge AH, *et al.* American Society of Clinical Oncology recommendations on fertility preservation in cancer patients. *J Clin Oncol* 2006; 24: 2917–31.

7. Shalet SM, Tsatsoulis A, Whitehead E, Read G. Vulnerability of the human Leydig cell to radiation damage is dependent upon age. *J Endocrinol* 1989; 120: 161–5.

8. Anserini P, Chiodi S, Spinelli S, *et al.* Semen analysis following allogeneic bone marrow transplantation. Additional data for evidence-based counselling. *Bone Marrow Transplant* 2002; 30: 447–541.

9. Arnon J, Meirow D, Lewis-Roness H, Ornoy A. Genetic and teratogenic effects of cancer treatments on gametes and embryos. *Hum Reprod Update* 2001; 7: 394–403.

10. Martin RH, Hildebrand K, Yamamoto J. An increased frequency of human sperm chromosomal abnormalities after radiotherapy. *Mutat Res* 1986; 174: 219–25.

11. Brent RL. Utilization of developmental basic science principles in the evaluation of reproductive risks form pre and postconception environmental radiation exposures. *Teratology* 1999; 59: 182–204.

12. Shah FJ, Tanaka M, Nielsen JE, *et al.* Gene expression profiles of mouse spermatogenesis during recovery from irradiation. *Reprod Biol Endocrinol* 2009; 7: 130.

13. Rowley MJ, Leach DR, Warner GA, Heller CG. Effect of graded doses of ionizing radiation on the human testis. *Radiat Res* 1974; 59: 665–78.

14. van Alphen MM, van de Kant HJ, de Rooij DG. Depletion of the spermatogonia from the seminiferous epithelium of the rhesus monkey after X irradiation. *Radiation Research* 1988; 113: 473–86.

15. van Alphen MM, van de Kant HJ, de Rooij DG. Repopulation of the seminiferous epithelium of the rhesus monkey after X irradiation. *Radiation Research* 1988; 113: 487–500.

16. van Alphen MM, van de Kant HJ, de Rooij DG. Follicle stimulating hormone stimulates spermatogenesis in the adult monkey. *Endocrinology* 1988; 123: 1449–55.

17. van Alphen MM, van de Kant HJ, Davids JA, *et al.* Dose-response studies on the spermatogonial stem cells of the rhesus monkey (*Macaca mulatta*) after X irradiation. *Radiation Research* 1989; 119: 443–51.

18. van Alphen MM, van de Kant HJ, de Rooij DG. Protection from radiation-induced damage of spermatogenesis in the rhesus monkey (*Macaca mulatta*) by follicle-stimulating hormone. *Cancer Research* 1989; 49: 533–6.

19. Clifton DK, Bremner WJ. The effect of testicular X-irradiation on spermatogenesis in man. A comparison with the mouse. *J Andrology* 1983; 4: 387–92.

20. Huhtaniemi I, Nikula H, Parvinen M, Rannikko S. Pituitary–testicular function of prostatic cancer patients during treatment with a gonadotropin-releasing hormone agonist analog. II. Endocrinology and histology of the testis. *J Androl* 1987; 8: 363–73.

21. Meistrich ML. Hormonal stimulation of the recovery of spermatogenesis following chemo or radiotherapy. *Acta Pathol Microbiol Immunol* 1998; 106: 37–46.

22. Meistrich ML, Wilson G, Huhtaniemi I. Hormonal treatment after cytotoxic therapy stimulates recovery of spermatogenesis. *Cancer Res* 1999; 59: 3557–60.

23. Meistrich ML, Wilson G, Kangasniemi M, Huhtaniemi I. Mechanism of protection of rat spermatogenesis by hormonal pretreatment: stimulation of spermatogonial differentiation after irradiation. *J Androl* 2000; 21: 464–9.

24. Shuttlesworth GA, de Rooij DG, Huhtaniemi I, *et al.* Enhancement of A spermatogonial proliferation and differentiation in irradiated rats by gonadotropin-releasing hormone antagonist administration. *Endocrinology* 2000; 141: 37–49.

25. Morse HC, Horike N, Rowley MJ, Heller CG. Testosterone concentrations in testes of normal men: effects of testosterone propionate administration. *J Clin Endocrinol Metabol* 1973; 37: 882–6.

26. Weinbauer GF, Nieschlag E. The role of testosterone in spermatogenesis. In Nieschlag E, Behre HM, eds. *Testosterone: Action, Deficiency, Substitution*, 2nd edn. Heidelberg: Springer, 1998; pp. 143–68.

27. Weinbauer GF, Gromoll J, Simoni S, Nieschlag E. Physiology of testicular function. In Nieschlag E, Behre HM, eds. *Andrology: Male Reproductive Health and Dysfunction*, 2nd edn. Heidelberg: Springer, 2000; pp. 23–61.

28. McLachlan RI, O'Donnell L, Stanton PG, *et al.* Effects of testosterone plus medroxyprogesterone acetate on semen quality, reproductive hormones, and germ cell populations in normal young men. *J Clin Endocrinol Metabol* 2002; 87: 546–56.

29. Kamischke A, Kuhlmann M, Weinbauer GF, *et al.* Gonadal protection from radiation by GnRH antagonist or recombinant human FSH: a controlled trial in a male nonhuman primate (*Macaca fascicularis*). *J Endocrinol* 2003; 179; 183–94.

30. Nielsen J, Hansen M, Jørgensen M, *et al.* Germ cell differentiation-dependent and stage-specific expression of LANCL1 in rodent testis. *Eur J Histochem* 2003; 47: 215–22.

31. Almstrup K, Nielsen J, Hansen M, *et al.* Analysis of cell-type-specific gene expression during mouse spermatogenesis. *Biol Reprod* 2003; 70: 1751–61.

32. Fattibene P, Mazzei F, Nuccetelli C, Risica S. Prenatal exposure to ionizing radiation: sources, effects and regulatory aspects. *Acta Paediatr* 1999; 88: 693–702.

33. Lord BI. Transgenerational susceptibility to leukaemia induction resulting from preconception paternal irradiation. *Int J Radiat Biol* 1999; 75: 801–10.

34. Meistrich ML. Critical components of testicular function and sensitivity to disruption. *Biol Reprod* 1986; 34: 17–28.

35. Brinkworth MH. Paternal transmission of genetic damage: findings in animals and humans. *Int J Androl* 2000; 23: 123–35.

36. Russell WL, Bangham JW, Russell LB. Differential response of mouse male germ-cell stages to radiation-induced specific-locus and dominant mutations. *Genetics* 1998; 148: 1567–78.

37. Stahl O, Eberhard J, Jepson K, *et al.* Risk of birth abnormalities in the offspring of men with a history of cancer: the impact of testicular carcinoma and its treatment on sperm DNA integrity. *Cancer* 2004; 100: 1137–44.

38. Cordelli E, Fresegna AM, Leter G, *et al.* Evaluation of DNA damage in different stages of mouse spermatogenesis after testicular X irradiation. *Radiat Res* 2003; 160: 443–51.

39. Dubrova YE, Nesterov VN, Krouchinsky NG, *et al.* Human mini-satellite mutation rate after the Chernobyl accident. *Nature* 1996; 380: 683–6.

40. Byrne J, Rasmussen SA, Steinhorn SC, *et al.* Genetic disease in offspring of long-term survivors of childhood and adolescent cancer. *Am J Hum Genet* 1998; 62: 45–52.

41. Kamiguchi Y, Tateno H. Radiation- and chemical-induced structural chromosome aberrations in human spermatozoa. *Mutat Res* 2002; 504: 183–91.

42. Stahl O, Boyd HA, Giwercman A, *et al.* Risk of birth abnormalities in the offspring of men with a history of cancer: a cohort study using Danish and Swedish national registries. *J Natl Cancer Inst* 2011; 103: 398–406.

43. Ishiguro H, Yasuda Y, Tomita Y, *et al.* Gonadal shielding to irradiation is effective in protecting testicular growth and function in long-term survivors of bone marrow transplantation during childhood or adolescence. *Bone Marrow Transplant* 2007; 39: 483–90.

Chapter

13

Chemotherapy effects on spermatogenesis

Akanksha Mehta and Mark Sigman

Introduction

Every year in the United States, cancer is diagnosed in over 9000 males between 15 and 35 years of age, and in over 4000 children under the age of 15 [1]. Testicular cancer, lymphoma, and leukemia are the most common malignancies diagnosed in these young men, but a variety of other solid-organ malignancies have also been described. Advances in diagnostic techniques and treatment modalities have markedly improved the chances of cure or long-term remission in these patients, with overall cure rates now approaching 90% [1].

Along with surgery and radiation, chemotherapy is a mainstay of cancer therapy. The improved survival of cancer patients has naturally been accompanied by concerns for the short- and long-term toxicity associated with chemotherapeutic agents, including reproductive dysfunction. According to a recent survey, 51% of men with cancer desired children in the future, including 77% of men who were childless when their cancer was diagnosed [2]. In many cancer patients, sperm quality is already impaired before they receive any form of treatment. Further deterioration in endocrine and semen parameters due to the damaging effects of chemotherapy may be temporary or permanent. While our understanding of the gonadotoxic effects of specific chemotherapy regimens is improving, it is impossible to distinguish those patients who will continue to have impaired spermatogenesis following therapy from those who will have sufficient recovery of gonadal function to re-establish normal spermatogenesis.

Advances in assisted reproductive technologies (ART) have undoubtedly improved the fertility potential of cancer patients of reproductive age. However, semen quality can be imperfect despite the recovery of gonadal function following chemotherapy, and there remains some controversy as to the safety of ART when using sperm from post-chemotherapy patients.

This chapter reviews the biologic basis and clinical aspects of chemotherapy and its effects on spermatogenesis and fertility in male cancer patients. Ethical considerations concerning the use of cryopreservation, assisted reproduction, and stem cell transplantation in this patient population are also discussed.

Overview of spermatogenesis

Spermatogenesis is an elaborate and closely regulated cell-differentiation process, which requires approximately 74 days in humans, beginning with the spermatogonial stem cell and terminating with a fully differentiated and highly specialized male gamete called the spermatozoon.

The testis consists of seminiferous epithelium arranged in tubules, and testosterone-producing Leydig cells in the interstitial region between the tubules. The seminiferous tubules, in turn, contain stem and differentiating spermatogonia, as well as Sertoli cells, which support and regulate spermatogenesis. Histologic examination of the normal human seminiferous tubule shows two classes of spermatogonial stem cells lining the base of the seminiferous epithelium: type A and type B cells. The type A spermatogonia are subdivided into pale type (Ap) and dark type (Ad) cells (Fig. 13.1). Ap spermatogonia are mitotically active, and give rise to Ap as well as type B spermatogonia. The type B spermatogonia undergo mitotic division to produce primary spermatocytes, which then undergo two meiotic divisions to form the haploid spermatids (Fig. 13.2). Spermatids undergo further maturation

Fertility Preservation in Male Cancer Patients, ed. John P. Mulhall, Linda D. Applegarth, Robert D. Oates and Peter N. Schlegel. Published by Cambridge University Press. © Cambridge University Press 2013.

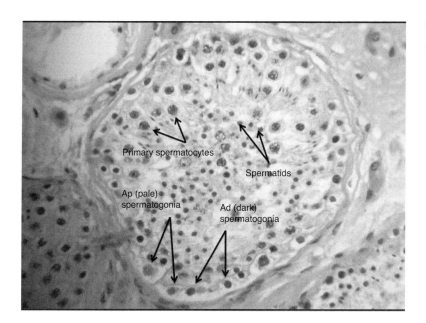

Figure 13.1. Cross-sectional view of a normal seminiferous tubule. *See color plate section.*

Primary spermatocytes

Spermatids

Ap (pale) spermatogonia

Ad (dark) spermatogonia

in order to develop into spermatozoa, via a process termed spermiogenesis. Ap spermatogonia are, therefore, responsible for replenishing their own populations, as well as the entire spermatogenic process. In contrast, Ad spermatogonia rarely divide, and are believed to represent dormant germ cells. When the number of Ap spermatogonia is diminished, Ad spermatogonia become active, transform into Ap spermatogonia, and then start to proliferate [3].

Because of their mitotic activity, spermatogonial stem cells are particularly susceptible to cytotoxic therapies that target rapidly dividing cell populations. Sertoli cells, Leydig cells, and spermatids, which are comparatively quiescent, and spermatocytes, which carry out meiotic divisions, are all less vulnerable to the damaging effects of chemotherapy than spermatogonia.

The hormonal regulation of spermatogenesis is via the hypothalamic–pituitary–gonadal (HPG) axis, which is based on hormonal feedback mechanisms. Pulsatile release of gonadotropin-releasing hormone (GnRH) from the hypothalamus regulates the pulsatile release of luteinizing hormone (LH) and follicle-stimulating hormone (FSH) from the anterior pituitary. LH acts on Leydig cells to regulate testosterone (T) secretion, while FSH acts on Sertoli cells to initiate and sustain spermatogenesis. Elevated serum levels of FSH and LH, and low serum levels of testosterone, have been associated with impaired spermatogenesis.

The role of testosterone in the regulation of spermatogenesis is complex. Although testosterone is essential to both the initiation and perpetuation of spermatogenesis, elevated intratesticular concentrations of testosterone have been shown to have a paradoxical and detrimental effect on spermatogonial differentiation in animal studies. De Rooij and Russell maintain that testosterone levels are actually very low during normal early pubertal development, when spermatogonial divisions are very active [3]. Fine regulation of intratesticular testosterone concentration during spermatogenesis is essential for normal sperm production and differentiation. Exposure to chemotherapy has been associated with the development of a block in spermatogonial differentiation, and some authors have shown that suppression of testosterone production promotes spermatogonial development in rodents exposed to chemotherapeutic agents [4]. A similar phenomenon is thought to occur in humans, and forms the basis of attempts at hormonal manipulation to restore fertility in cancer patients.

Normal Sertoli cell function is also essential for spermatogenesis. Because each Sertoli cell supports a defined number of germ cells, any reduction in the Sertoli cell population directly impairs spermatogenesis. Elevated serum levels of FSH have traditionally been used as a marker of abnormal Sertoli cell function. Recently, inhibin B, secreted by Sertoli cells, has been proposed as a marker for Sertoli cell function,

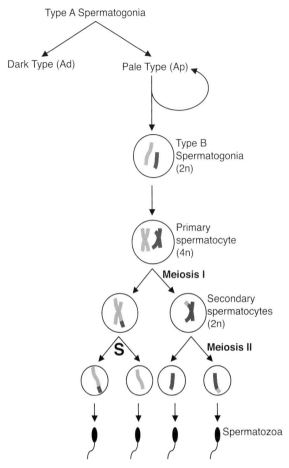

Figure 13.2. Overview of spermatogenesis. *See color plate section.*

particularly in men treated with chemotherapy. Bordallo *et al.* compared inhibin B/FSH ratios in 21 males after chemotherapy for Hodgkin's lymphoma with 20 healthy, matched controls [5]. There was no significant difference in LH, T, inhibin B concentrations, or T/LH ratio between the groups, but serum inhibin B was correlated with serum FSH levels and inhibin B/FSH ratio was positively correlated with sperm count. The authors concluded that serum inhibin B levels may be an important marker of Sertoli cell function in men treated with chemotherapy, and should be interpreted in the context of serum FSH.

Effect of cancer on spermatogenesis

Malignant disease, in and of itself, can have a detrimental impact on spermatogenesis well before the initiation of any cytotoxic therapy. In a recent study on

semen quality in 205 adolescent males with various solid and hematologic malignancies, semen parameters such as sperm count, motility, and semen volume were all found to be significantly lower in cancer patients than in age-matched controls [6]. The adverse effect of cancer on sperm production is mediated by various hormonal alterations and metabolic conditions [7]. Increased physiologic stress, tumor-released endocrine substances, and tumor invasion of endocrine organs can all lead to down-regulation of reproductive hormones. Malnutrition and constitutional symptoms, such as fever, can have a direct negative influence on spermatogenesis. The development of anti-sperm antibodies as a result of disruption of the blood–testis barrier, leading to poor semen analysis results, has also been described [8]. Lastly, tumor-released cytokines such as interleukins and tumor necrosis factor (TNF) can also exert a paracrine effect on spermatozoal development, leading to low sperm motility [9].

Men with testicular tumors have been shown to have significantly lower sperm quality than men with hematologic malignancies or other solid tumors [10]. Based on sperm concentrations alone, a striking 50–75% of patients with unilateral testicular carcinoma are subfertile at the time of diagnosis, with sperm concentrations below 10 million/mL [11]. In part, this observation may be explained by the association between cryptorchidism and testicular cancer, the possibility of existing Leydig cell dysfunction in testicular cancer, or the possible presence of concomitant carcinoma in situ in testicular cancer patients, all of which can independently impact spermatogenesis [12,13].

While semen parameters are comparable in men with hematological malignancies as a whole versus other solid tumors, subset analysis shows that patients with Hodgkin's lymphoma do have significantly poorer sperm quality than patients with non-Hodgkin's lymphoma [10]. Advanced Hodgkin's lymphoma is a metabolically active disease, often presenting with systemic symptoms and elevated markers of inflammation, and may thus have a more significant impact on spermatogenesis than other hematological malignancies [14].

The institution of chemotherapy, therefore, often adds insult to a preexisting impairment in spermatogenesis. As such, it is not surprising that the effects of chemotherapy on sperm production and semen quality can be prolonged, or even irreversible. However, there is no concrete evidence to support the hypothesis that pre-treatment spermatogenic function predicts post-treatment spermatogenic function. On the contrary, patients who are azoospermic prior to the initiation of cancer therapy can go on to have normal sperm parameters after treatment. This observation has led some authors to suggest that the mechanism of infertility before treatment is reversible and distinct from the mechanism of infertility following treatment for cancer [15]. Minimizing gonadotoxicity in the selection of chemotherapeutic regimens should be considered for all patients, irrespective of any preexisting impairment of spermatogenic function.

Gonadotoxicity of chemotherapy versus radiation

The most common cancers in men of reproductive age are leukemia, lymphoma, and testicular germ cell tumors. The role of chemotherapy, and the choice of chemotherapeutic regimen used, is cancer-specific. Patients with testicular cancer undergo radical orchiectomy, followed by retroperitoneal lymph node dissection (RPLND), chemotherapy, or radiation, depending on tumor histology and stage. For patients with leukemia and lymphoma, chemotherapy is the primary mode of treatment, with or without concomitant radiation therapy. Over the past two decades, bone marrow transplantation has become an important treatment modality for hematological malignancies, and a combination of high-dose chemotherapy and total-body irradiation is frequently used in preparative regimens before transplantation.

Radiation therapy has been shown to have more deleterious effect on fertility than chemotherapy [16]. In a large, retrospective study of 451 patients with testicular germ cell tumors treated with either orchiectomy and chemotherapy or orchiectomy and radiation, conception rates were much lower for patients treated with radiotherapy compared to those treated with chemotherapy [16]. Even when multimodal therapy is used, the irradiation component of therapy appears to have a more significant and lasting impact on the spermatogenesis cycle than chemotherapy. Anserini et al. examined semen parameters in bone marrow transplant patients conditioned with one alkylating agent, two alkylating agents, or an alkylating agent and total-body irradiation [17]. Recovery of some degree of spermatogenesis was significantly better in patients receiving single- or dual-agent

chemotherapy (90% and 50%, respectively), compared to those receiving single-agent chemotherapy and irradiation (17%).

Mechanism of action of chemotherapeutic agents

Chemotherapeutic agents can be divided into classes based on their mechanisms of action (Table 13.1). Some of these agents are cell-cycle-specific. Alkylating agents such as cyclophosphamide impair cell function by alkylating specific functional groups and thereby chemically modifying cell DNA. Cisplatin and carboplatin, which act by DNA cross-linking, are considered "alkylating-like" agents in their mechanism of action. The antimetabolites such as methotrexate and gemcitabine interfere with DNA and RNA synthesis by preventing purines and pyrimidines from becoming incorporated into DNA and RNA strands during the S phase of the cell cycle. Alkaloids inhibit microtubule function and therefore interrupt cell division in the M phase of the cell cycle, while topoisomerase inhibitors such as etoposide interfere with the transcription and replication of DNA by upsetting proper DNA coiling (Fig. 13.3).

Most men undergoing chemotherapy become azoospermic within 50–60 days after the first course of treatment. Chemotherapeutic agents primarily affect the rapidly proliferating type B spermatogonia. The comparatively quiescent type A spermatogonia have the potential to restore the spermatogonial population. If partial or complete destruction of type A spermatogonia occurs as a result of chemotherapy, then sustained or irreversible loss of spermatogenesis can ensue. It was initially thought that prepubertal boys undergoing chemotherapy might be protected from its cytotoxic effects, as the less mature testicles would be less susceptible to these agents. Follow-up studies of these patients, however, show no difference in cytotoxic effects such as impaired semen parameters and elevated serum hormone levels compared to postpubertal boys, providing cogent evidence that the prepubertal testis is not afforded protection from cytotoxic insult [18,19].

Certain classes of chemotherapeutic agents are more gonadotoxic than others. If treatment avoids agents that eradicate stem spermatogonia or block their differentiation, then normospermia can be restored within three months after therapy [20]. With the use of more gonadotoxic agents, surviving stem

Table 13.1 Classification of chemotherapy agents

Group	Agent	Risk of permanent impairment of spermatogenesis	Cell-cycle-specific
Alkylating agents			
Nitrogen mustards	Mechlorethamine	High	No
Nitrosureas	Chlorambucil	High	No
Others	Cyclyphosphamide	High	No
	Melphalan	High	
	Ifosfamide	High	
	Carmustine	Medium	
	Lomustine	Medium	
	Busulfan	High	
Antimetabolites			
Folate antagonists	Methotrexate	Low	Yes
Pyrimidine analogs	Cytarabine	Medium	Yes
Purine analogs	Fluorouracil	Low	Yes
	Gemcitabine	Low	
	Mercaptopurine	Low	
	Thioguanine	Low	
Cytotoxic antibiotics			
Anthracyclines	Doxorubicin	Medium	Yes
Others	Bleomycin	Low	Yes
	Dactinomycin	Low	
Plant alkaloids			
Vinca alkaloids	Vincristine	Low	Yes
Topoisomerase inhibitors	Vinblastine	Low	Yes
	Etoposide	Low	
Others			
Platinum compounds	Cisplatin	Medium	No
Miscellaneous	Carboplatin	Medium	No
	Procarbazine	High	
	Dacarbazine	Low	

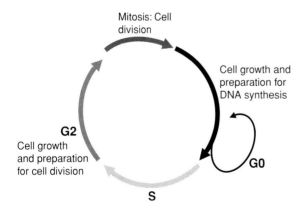

Figure 13.3. Overview of the cell cycle. *See color plate section.*

cells can remain in the testis but may fail to differentiate into spermatozoa for several years after the cytotoxic insult [1].

The risk of permanent azoospermia after chemotherapy is drug-specific and dose-dependent.

Pont and Albrecht concluded in their review that cumulative doses of > 400 mg/m^2 of cisplatin given to testicular cancer patients led to irreversible impairment of gonadal function [21]. Similarly, gonadal dysfunction is well documented in over 80% of patients who receive > 300 mg/m^2 of cyclophosphamide, and in over 50% of patients who receive a cumulative dose of > 4 g/m^2 of procarbazine [22,23]. The cumulative dose of chemotherapeutic agents received by patients is, in turn, dependent on the type of malignancy as well as cancer stage. The dosing of cisplatin for testicular cancer is 100 mg/m^2/cycle. Most patients receive 2–4 cycles of chemotherapy, or a dose of 200–400 mg/m^2. Cyclophosphamide and procarbazine are used in the BEACOPP regimen for Hodgkin's lymphoma. Depending upon cancer stage, the dose of cyclophosphamide can range from 650 to 1250 mg/m^2/cycle, for a total of 4–8 treatment cycles. In the United States, the ABVD regimen is more commonly used for Hodgkin's lymphoma, and it is associated with lower risk of infertility. More detailed information on the infertility risk associated with various chemotherapeutic agents can be found on the website for Fertile Hope (www.fertilehope.org), a national initiative dedicated to providing reproductive information to cancer patients whose medical treatments present the risk of infertility.

Maymon *et al.* have argued that chemotherapy-induced Sertoli cell damage may be a contributory factor to treatment-induced azoospermia [24]. Histologic examination of specially stained testicular biopsy specimens by the authors identified de-differentiation of Sertoli cells following chemotherapy for testicular cancer. As Sertoli cells are responsible for maintaining the blood–testis barrier, as well as supporting spermatogonial development, damage to even a fraction of Sertoli cells in a given tubule can have a disproportionately larger impact on spermatogenesis.

The loss of germ cells, with the added possibility of damage to Sertoli cells, has secondary effects on the HPG axis. Inhibin secretion by Sertoli cells declines, and consequently serum FSH levels rise. Testicular blood flow is reduced, leading to less testosterone being distributed into the circulation [20]. LH levels rise in an attempt to maintain constant serum testosterone levels.

Toxicity of chemotherapeutic regimens

Cytotoxic agents are seldom administered alone; most patients receive combination chemotherapy, and the gonadotoxicity associated with each individual agent becomes cumulative. For example, vincristine, vinblastine, and dacarbazine have been shown to be minimally gonadotoxic on their own, but can contribute to azoospermia when used with other gonadotoxic agents [15]. Careful selection of the various components of any regimen is therefore important for preserving fertility. Table 13.2 lists the commonly used chemotherapeutic regimens for solid and hematologic malignancies in young men.

Testes are highly sensitive to alkylating agents, and chemotherapy regimens that include alkylating agents are more gonadotoxic than those that do not contain alkylating agents. The use of mechlorethamine, vincristine, procarbazine, and prednisone (MOPP), or a comparable regimen for the treatment of lymphoma resulted in prolonged azoospermia in 90–100% of patients. In contrast, non-alkylating regimens such as doxorubicin, bleomycin, vinblastine, and dacarbazine

Table 13.2. Common chemotherapeutic regimens used in the treatment of solid and hematological malignancies in young men (from Guidelines of the National Comprehensive Cancer Network 2010–2011: www.nccn.org/professionals/physician_gls/f_guidelines.asp)

Malignancy	Chemotherapy agents
Testicular cancer	BEP (bleomycin, etoposide, cisplatin) VIP (ifosfamide, etoposide, cisplatin)
Osteosarcoma	MAP (methotrexate, doxorubicin, cisplatin) ± ifosfamide Ifosfamide and etoposide Ifosfamide, epirubicin, cisplatin
Hodgkin's lymphoma	ABVD (doxorubicin, bleomycin, vinblastine, dacarbazine) Sanford V (doxorubicin, vinblastine, mechlorethamine, etoposide, vincristine, bleomycin, prednisone) BEACOPP (bleomycin, etoposide, doxorubicin, cyclophosphamide, vincristine, procarbazine, prednisone)
Non-Hodgkin's lymphoma	CHOP (doxorubicin, bleomycin, vinblastine, dacarbazine) CVP (cyclophosphamide, vincristine, prednisone) EPOCH (cyclophosphamide, doxorubicin, etoposide, vincristine, prednisone) Fludarabine, cyclophosphamide, dexamethasone

(ABVD) cause transient azoospermia in about one-third of patients, but the majority will realize full recovery of spermatogenesis [15].

Meistrich *et al.* evaluated the recovery of spermatogenesis in 58 men receiving mitoxantrone, vincristine, vinblastine, and prednisone (NOVP) for Hodgkin's lymphoma [25]. After a transient decrease in sperm counts, excellent recovery was noted within 3–4 months after therapy, with 63% of patients achieving normospermic levels. Further calculations showed that type B spermatogonia were the most sensitive to the chemotherapy regimen, with only 1% of the population surviving each course. Late spermatids and meiotic cells were only moderately sensitive to chemotherapy, with 4–30% surviving each course. Stem spermatogonia were relatively resistant to chemotherapy, with over 90% surviving each course [25]. Decreased toxicity of this regimen to stem cell populations was likely responsible for more timely recovery of spermatogenesis in this population of patients. The ideal regimen for any patient, of course, must balance efficacy against cancer with minimizing side effects.

Both FSH and inhibin B have been evaluated as serum markers for spermatogenesis following chemotherapy. A large study by the European Organisation for Research and Treatment of Cancer (EORTC) compared FSH levels as a measure of fertility in men treated with alkylating versus non-alkylating chemotherapy agents, and found that FSH was elevated in 60% of patients treated with alkylating chemotherapy, compared to 8% of patients treated with non-alkylating chemotherapy [26]. Those who received alkylating agents had poorer recovery of spermatogenesis, manifested by a slower and less likely return to normal FSH levels.

Van Beek *et al.* followed 56 men with a history of Hodgkin's lymphoma over a period of 15 years after completion of chemotherapy [27]. Serum concentrations of FSH, LH, and testosterone were correlated with sperm concentration and sperm DNA integrity. The number of courses of MOPP chemotherapy was significantly correlated with FSH and inhibin B levels, but only inhibin B showed an independent correlation with sperm concentration. The authors concluded that inhibin B may be a valuable long-term serum marker of gonadal function after chemotherapy.

While much of the chemotherapy literature consists of studies in lymphoma patients, chemotherapeutic regimens for testicular cancer have also been associated with significant gonadotoxicity. Most patients receiving cisplatin-based chemotherapy for testis cancer become azoospermic, but approximately 50% resume spermatogenesis within two years and 80% after five years [21]. Recovery is more likely in those with normal pre-treatment sperm densities than in those with pre-treatment oligospermia. Various authors have demonstrated a drastic decrease in the number and motility of spermatozoa produced, as well as an increase in the proportion of morphologically abnormal sperm and DNA-damaged sperm in samples from men receiving bleomycin, etoposide and cisplatin (BEP) for testicular cancer [28,29]. A high-dose chemotherapy regimen for testicular cancer has also been reported, consisting of carboplatin, etoposide, and ifosfamide. In a study of ten patients subject to this regimen, spermatogenesis recovered in five, and two patients went on to father children [30]. Further investigation is needed to compare the long-term toxicity of this regimen with the more commonly used BEP regimen.

DNA damage

Controversy exists as to the degree and reversibility of DNA damage secondary to chemotherapy exposure. Our knowledge of the susceptibility of male gametes in various stages of spermatogenesis to chemotherapy-induced damage is limited. However, the DNA repair capability of late spermatids appears to be reduced compared to early spermatids and other spermatogenic cell types, and therefore damage induced during late stages of spermatogenesis may be more likely to be transmitted than repaired [31]. DNA and chromosomal aberrations that can be transmitted by sperm include aneuploidy, structural aberrations, epigenetic modifications, nucleotide repeats, and gene mutations. Unfortunately, most studies addressing this topic are very limited in size. Exactly how many chemotherapeutic agents are capable of inducing DNA damage, and whether specific agents are associated with specific types of aberrations, is unknown.

It is apparent that commonly used chemotherapy regimens can disrupt spermatozoal DNA and result in deleterious effects on embryo development in animal models [19]. In testicular cancer patients treated with bleomycin, etoposide, and cisplatin chemotherapy, Spermon *et al.* similarly found an abnormally high percentage of DNA-damaged sperm [28]. But in a separate cohort of childhood cancer survivors, Thomson *et al.* found no significant difference in sperm DNA integrity between non-azoospermic patients and healthy, age-matched controls [19]. Despite reduced sperm concentrations, sperm produced by patients in this study carried as healthy DNA as sperm produced by controls.

The induced DNA damage may be temporary. In a study of eight patients with Hodgkin's lymphoma treated with novanthrone, oncovin, vinblastine, and prednisone, the use of fluorescence in-situ hybridization (FISH) revealed a fivefold increase in disomies, diploidies, and complex aneuploidies involving chromosomes X, Y and 8. The aneuploidy effects were found to be transient, and declined to pre-treatment levels within approximately 100 days after the cessation of chemotherapy [32]. More recently, Thomas *et al.* have reiterated the absence of long-term effects of chemotherapy on sperm aneuploidy rates, based on a cohort of 38 patients [33]. In contrast, Tempest *et al.* reported increased sperm aneuploidy frequencies following chemotherapy for 18–24 months [34]. In addition to aneuploidy, sperm generated after chemotherapy have been shown to maintain a significant degree of chromatin damage as well. O'Flaherty *et al.* compared semen parameters and the presence of DNA strand breaks in patients with testicular cancer and Hodgkin's lymphoma to community volunteers, before and after chemotherapy at 6, 12, 18, and 24 months [35]. Sperm DNA damage was higher in the cancer patients prior to chemotherapy, increased further at 6 months, and remained elevated 24 months after treatment completion.

In light of the combined evidence from animal and human studies, most authors recommend a post-chemotherapeutic delay of at least six months, but preferably up to 18–24 months from the cessation of treatment to attempt of pregnancy by either natural conception or assisted reproduction. Given the duration of one cycle of spermatogenesis in humans, a six-month delay should allow for newly produced sperm to be present in semen. However, the quality of this sperm remains a matter of debate, as does the degree to which specific chemotherapeutic regimens may differentially influence the recovery of normal spermatogenesis. The only available guidelines on this matter have been put forth by the European Society for Medical Oncology (ESMO), which recommends deferring childbearing for at least 12 months in all male and female patients after cancer therapy [36]. This is a grade C recommendation, based on level IV evidence, which further illustrates the lack of reliable data and clinical consensus on the safe return to unprotected sexual activity following chemotherapy.

Summary

Improved survival rates for young men with cancer are accompanied by an increasing awareness of the gonadotoxicity associated with chemotherapy and the concern for preservation of fertility potential. The degree of impairment of spermatogenesis associated with a particular chemotherapy regimen may be difficult to predict accurately, as malignancy itself can lead to impaired gonadal function, and many patients receive multimodal therapy with added potential for gonadal dysfunction. Recovery of spermatogenic function after completion of chemotherapy is possible, and may even occur over a period of years, depending on the extent of cytotoxic insult. Avoidance of high doses of alkylating agents is likely to be beneficial in early restoration of spermatogenesis. Sperm cryopreservation should be discussed with all patients prior to

the initiation of chemotherapy. Assisted reproductive technologies have improved the chances for men with post-chemotherapy azoospermia to father children, but most experts recommend a wait period of approximately 18 months after completion of therapy before attempting conception. While exposure to chemotherapy has been associated with sperm DNA damage and mutations, several studies show these to be temporary. There is presently no evidence to suggest that the offspring of post-chemotherapy patients are at increased risk of congenital anomalies or malignancies.

References

1. Schrader M, Müller M, Straub B, Miller K. The impact of chemotherapy on male fertility: a survey of the biologic basis and clinical aspects. *Reprod Toxicol* 2001; 15: 611–17.

2. Schover LR, Brey K, Lichtin A, Lipshultz LI, Jeha S. Knowledge and experience regarding cancer, infertility, and sperm banking in younger male survivors. *J Clin Oncol* 2002; 20: 1880–9.

3. De Rooij D, Russell LD. All you wanted to know about spermatogonia but were afraid to ask. *J Androl* 2000: 21; 776–98.

4. Meistrich ML, Wilson G, Huhtaniemi I. Hormonal treatment after cytotoxic therapy stimulates recovery of spermatogenesis. *Cancer Res* 1999; 59: 3557–60.

5. Bordallo MA, Guimaraes MM, Pessoa CH, *et al.* Decreased serum inhibin B/FSH ratio as a marker of Sertoli cell function in male survivors after chemotherapy in childhood and adolescence. *J Pediatr Endocr Metab* 2004; 17: 879–87.

6. Bahadur G, Ling KL, Hart R, *et al.* Semen quality and cryopreservation in adolescent cancer patients. *Hum Reprod* 2002; 17: 3157–61.

7. Dohle GR. Male infertility in cancer patients: review of the literature. *Int J Urol* 2010; 17: 327–31.

8. Foster RS, Rubin LR, McNulty A, Bihrle R, Donohue JP. Detection of antisperm-antibodies in patients with primary testicular cancer. *Int J Androl* 1991; 14: 179–85.

9. Ho GT, Gardner H, DeWolf WC, Loughlin KR, Morgentaler A. Influence of testicular carcinoma on ipsilateral spermatogenesis. *J Urol* 1992; 148: 821–5.

10. Lass A, Akagbosu F, Abusheikha N, *et al.* A programme of semen cryopreservation for patients with malignant disease in a tertiary infertility centre: lessons from 8 years' experience. *Hum Reprod* 1998; 13: 3256–61.

11. Petersen PM, Skakkebaek NE, Giwercman A. Gonadal function in men with testicular cancer: biological and

clinical aspects. *Acta Path Micro IM C* 1998; 106: 24–36.

12. Petersen PM, Giwercman A, Hansen SW, *et al.* Impaired testicular function in patients with carcinoma in situ of the testis. *J Clin Oncol* 1999; 17: 173–9.

13. Jacobsen KD, Fosså SD, Bjøro TP, *et al.* Gonadal function and fertility in patients with bilateral testicular germ cell malignancy. *Eur Urol* 2002; 42: 229–38.

14. Sieniawski M, Reineke T, Josting A, *et al.* Assessment of male fertility in patients with Hodgkin's lymphoma treated in the German Hodgkin Study Group (GHSG) clinical trials. *Annals Oncology* 2008; 19: 1795–801.

15. van der Kaaij MA, van Echten-Arends J, Simons AH, Kluin-Nelemans HC. Fertility preservation after chemotherapy for Hodgkin lymphoma. *Hematol Oncol* 2010; 28: 168–79.

16. Huyghe E, Matsuda T, Daudin M, *et al.* Fertility after testicular cancer treatments: results of a large multicenter study. *Cancer* 2004; 100: 732–7.

17. Anserini P, Chiodi S, Spinelli S, *et al.* Semen analysis following allogeneic bone marrow transplantation. *Bone Marrow Transplant* 2002; 30: 447–51.

18. Puscheck E, Philip PA, Jeyendran RS. Male fertility preservation and cancer treatment. *Cancer Treat Rev* 2004; 30: 173–80.

19. Thomson AB, Campbell AJ, Irvine DC, *et al.* Semen quality and spermatozoal DNA integrity in survivors of childhood cancer: a case-control study. *Lancet* 2002; 360: 361–7.

20. Shetty G, Meistrich ML. Hormonal approaches to preservation and restoration of male fertility after cancer treatment. *J Natl Cancer Inst Monogr* 2005; 34: 36–9.

21. Pont J, Albrecht W. Fertility after chemotherapy for testicular germ cell cancer. *Fertil Steril* 1997; 68: 1–5.

22. Howell SJ, Shalet SM. Spermatogenesis after cancer treatment: damage and recovery. *J Natl Cancer Inst Monogr* 2005; 34: 12–17.

23. Schrader M, Heicappell R, Müller M, Straub B, Miller K. Impact of chemotherapy on male fertility. *Onkologie* 2001; 24: 326–30.

24. Maymon BB, Yogev L, Marks A, *et al.* Sertoli cell inactivation by cytotoxic damage to the human testis after cancer chemotherapy. *Fertil Steril* 2004; 81: 1391–4.

25. Meistrich ML, Wilson G, Mathur K, *et al.* Rapid recovery of spermatogenesis after mitoxantrone, vincristine, vinblastine, and prednisone chemotherapy for Hodgkin's disease. *J Clin Oncol* 1997; 15: 3488–95.

26. van der Kaaij MA, Heutte N, Le Stang N, *et al.* Gonadal function in males after chemotherapy for early-stage Hodgkin's lymphoma treated in four subsequent trials by the European Organisation for Research and Treatment of Cancer: EORTC Lymphoma Group and the Groupe d'Etude des Lymphomes de l'Adulte. *J Clin Oncol* 2007; 25: 2825–32.

27. van Beek RD, Smit M, van den Heuvel-Eibrink MM, *et al.* Inhibin B is superior to FSH as a serum marker for spermatogenesis in men treated for Hodgkin's lymphoma with chemotherapy during childhood. *Hum Reprod* 2007; 22: 3215–22.

28. Spermon JR, Ramos L, Wetzels AM, *et al.* Sperm integrity pre- and post-chemotherapy in men with testicular germ cell cancer. *Hum Reprod* 2006; 21: 1781–6.

29. Stephenson WT, Poirier SM, Rubin L, Einhorn LH. Evaluation of reproductive capacity in germ cell tumor patients following treatment with cisplatin, etoposide, and bleomycin. *J Clin Oncol* 1995; 13: 2278–80.

30. Ishikawa T, Kamidono S, Fujisawa M. Fertility after high-dose chemotherapy for testicular cancer. *Urology* 2004; 63: 137–40.

31. Wyrobek AJ, Schmid TE, Marchetti F. Relative susceptibilities of male germ cells to genetic defects induced by cancer chemotherapies. *J Natl Cancer Inst Monogr* 2005; 34: 31–5.

32. Robbins WA, Meistrich ML, Moore D, *et al.* Chemotherapy induces transient sex chromosomal and autosomal aneuploidy in human sperm. *Nat Genet* 1997; 16: 74–8.

33. Thomas C, Cans C, Pelletier R, *et al.* No long-term increase in sperm aneuploidy rates after anticancer therapy: sperm fluorescence in situ hybridization analysis in 26 patients treated for testicular cancer or lymphoma. *Clin Cancer Res* 2004; 10: 6535–43.

34. Tempest HG, Ko E, Chan P, *et al.* Sperm aneuploidy frequencies analyzed before and after chemotherapy in testicular cancer and Hodgkin's lymphoma patients. *Hum Reprod* 2008; 23: 251–8.

35. O'Flaherty C, Hales BF, Chan P, Robaire B. Impact of chemotherapeutics on advanced testicular cancer or Hodgkin's lymphoma on sperm deoxyribonucleic acid. *Fertil Steril* 2010; 94: 1374–9.

36. Pentheroudakis G, Orecchia R, Hoekstra HJ, Pavlidis N; ESMO Guidelines Working Group. Cancer, fertility and pregnancy: ESMO Clinical Practice Guidelines for diagnosis, treatment, and follow-up. *Ann Oncol* 2010; 21 (Suppl 5): v266–73.

Chapter 14

Effects of therapy for solid tumors

Gretchen A. Gignac and Leonard H. Wexler

Introduction

Much is known about the effects of cancer therapy in adult males in regards to germ cell tumors and Hodgkin's lymphoma, as these are the models of a curable neoplasm afflicting men in the childbearing years. However, many solid malignancies can become evident in young men who still have the potential to father a child. The age range for childbearing as a whole in modernized countries has moved to later in life. According to the United Nations report on world fertility patterns, among the 45 developed countries with more than 100 000 inhabitants in 2008, 12 countries had a mean age at childbearing surpassing 30 years [1]. With cancer therapeutics leading to patients living longer and living better in the face of active disease, addressing fertility concerns needs to remain a consideration when caring for patients with both curable and incurable neoplasia.

Thankfully, the treatments available for patients with solid tumors are rapidly expanding. However, most chemotherapeutic agents are not studied in such a way that effects on fertility are always clear. This can be disconcerting both to patients and to the physicians caring for them, given the uncertainty regarding the concerns for increased risk of future infertility, cancer in the offspring, birth defects, and abnormal growth and development patterns. Despite this uncertainty it is evident, based on published guidelines from the American Society of Clinical Oncology, that a dialog regarding these issues needs to become a part of standard oncologic practice [2].

There are some class effects on fertility that are well known, such as those of the alkylating agents, but the newer agents that are now available may have no data to aid in counseling a patient. And the effects that are seen with single-agent therapy may not be representative of combination therapy. The disruption of the germinal epithelium and spermatogenesis is by far the largest contributor to male infertility, more so than declines in androgen production [3]. The rapidly dividing spermatogonia are the most sensitive to the toxic effects of chemotherapy [4,5]. Additionally, the degree of gonadotoxicity can be transient or permanent, and it is dependent on the type of drug or radiation treatment, how it is delivered, the dose (how much, how long), as well as patient-related indices such as baseline fertility [2]. For example, germ cell tumors themselves can have an effect on spermatogenesis in that up to 50% of these patients have decreased spermatogenesis prior to treatment [6]. Sperm count is the lowest in the six months after the completion of therapy, but impaired spermatogenesis may be temporary and may improve even two years after therapy completion [7].

Post-chemotherapy, the data do not support significant increases in congenital malformations or genetic diseases in children born naturally; however, most children conceived following treatment are born more than two years after the completion of therapy [8–10]. There are no firm consensus recommendations on the duration of contraceptive use for men after treatment for cancer, but certain classes of chemotherapy agents are mutagenic and teratogenic, and contraception is essential during treatment. Some studies have shown that an increase in sperm aneuploidy persists for up to 18 months after the start of chemotherapy, and recommendations for continuing contraception post-chemotherapy range between one and two years [11,12].

Understanding that fertility preservation is complex and unique to each individual patient's case, we will endeavor to outline the data available regarding

Fertility Preservation in Male Cancer Patients, ed. John P. Mulhall, Linda D. Applegarth, Robert D. Oates and Peter N. Schlegel. Published by Cambridge University Press. © Cambridge University Press 2013.

classes of systemic therapies in use in practice with respect to the treatment of solid tumors. Class effects will be reviewed, and representative chemotherapeutic agents most often used in solid tumor oncology discussed. A more detailed discussion of the risks associated with treating the most common types of childhood solid tumors will follow. Treatment effects related to leukemia, lymphoma, transplant, radiation, and surgery are addressed elsewhere in this book.

Alkylating agents

This class of chemotherapeutics causes direct DNA damage, whose effects are not phase-specific. Alkylating therapies are most frequently used in hematologic malignancies, but some are used for solid tumors, especially ifosfamide in germ cell tumors, temozolomide in melanoma, dacarbazine in melanoma and sarcoma, streptozocin in metastatic pancreatic islet cell tumors, and carmustine and lomustine in brain tumors.

As a general rule, most alkylating agents have a high rate of gonadal toxicity with prolonged azoospermia. There is little doubt that cyclophosphamide, busulfan, chlorambucil, and melphalan can profoundly affect fertility in both the short and long term. This is best seen in extensive research on the treatment of hematologic malignancies such as lymphoma [13]. Chlorambucil and cyclophosphamide can produce prolonged azoospermia even when used as single agents [14,15]. Procarbazine also functions in an alkylator-like fashion. It is highly gonadotoxic, and while most data are from its use in lymphomas [16], it is rarely used in solid tumors, generally only as salvage therapy in brain tumors.

The effects of some members of this drug class, such as ifosfamide, may be less detrimental to fertility than others. Although ifosfamide is an alkylator, and is known to be gonadotoxic, it was found that its effects on spermatogenesis are dose-dependent and potentially reversible in the rabbit [17]. In adult men with poor-risk non-seminomatous germ cell tumors who were treated with M-TIP × 4 cycles (methotrexate, ifosfamide 1.2 g/m^2 days 2–6 of each cycle, paclitaxel, cisplatin), of the 21 patients who remained disease-free 17 (80%) recovered spermatogenesis at a median follow-up of 2.3 years (33% were oligospermic and 48% normospermic). Leydig cell function was not affected [18]. Additionally, dose-dependent gonadal dysfunction has been reported at doses of ifosfamide greater than 60 g/m^2 when studied in pediatric and adult sarcoma patients [19]. A similar dose-dependent finding of increased risk of azoospermia and oligospermia was found in patients treated with a multi-agent chemotherapy regimen that included neoadjuvant and adjuvant ifosfamide, as well as cisplatin, doxorubicin, and high-dose methotrexate, although the contribution of these latter agents to the gonadotoxic effect of these regimens is less clear [20].

Platinum analogs

The platinum compounds such as cisplatin, carboplatin, and oxaliplatin are alkylator-like in function in that they are directly DNA-toxic via DNA cross-linking effects. However, unlike the alkylating agents, they are cell-cycle-specific. The platinum compound best studied in adult men is cisplatin, as it is the cornerstone of curative therapy for germ cell tumors. Carboplatin is used in the treatment of multiple solid tumors and oxaliplatin is currently FDA-approved for use in colorectal cancer, which can also occur in young men.

Chemotherapy regimens for male germ cell tumors have undergone many derivations over the years, but it has remained cisplatin-based since this drug was found to have such a profound impact on overall survival. Studies in early testicular cancer patients found that not only was spermatogenesis impaired before treatment, but cisplatin-based combination chemotherapy (cisplatin, vinblastine, bleomycin, +/− doxorubicin) had substantial effects on gonadal function (including azoospermia) as well as recovery after 2–3 years in most [21]. Gonadal damage from cisplatin is dose-dependent. Both Leydig cell dysfunction and decreased spermatogenesis can be persistent in those patients treated with cumulative doses of cisplatin > 400 mg/m^2. In fact, in men with germ cell tumors who receive more than four cycles of platinum-based chemotherapy there is a 50% chance of irreversible infertility [22–25].

Patients treated with carboplatin have a higher likelihood to recover fertility when compared to patients treated with cisplatin [25]. There are no data available on clinical outcomes regarding fertility in males treated with oxaliplatin, but the package insert states that it is mutagenic and clastogenic. Males are advised not to father a child during treatment and for up to six months thereafter. Irreversible infertility is possible [26].

Antimetabolites

The antimetabolites function by interfering with DNA synthesis and transcription. These drugs are cell-cycle-specific, acting mainly in the S phase. Examples of drugs in this class include purine and pyrimidine analogs and antifolates. Those most commonly used in the treatment of adult males with solid tumors are the pyrimidine analogs 5-fluorouracil, capecitabine, and gemcitabine, and the antifolates methotrexate and pemetrexed. In conventional doses 5-fluorouracil, capecitabine, and methotrexate may cause temporary reductions in sperm concentration, but recovery of normal spermatogenesis is expected [27–29]. However, being newer compounds, there are few clinical data available from which to draw conclusions regarding gemcitabine's and pemetrexed's effects on male fertility. One clinical study evaluating taxane-based combinations and fertility showed that the combination of taxanes and gemcitabine may be gonadotoxic, as extrapolated using endpoints of inhibin B and follicle-stimulating hormone (FSH) in short-term follow-up [30].

Cytotoxic antibiotics

Anthracyclines bind with nucleic acids, interfere with enzymes involved with DNA replication, and prevent RNA synthesis. They are active in all phases of the cell cycle. Members of this drug class often used in the treatment of men with solid tumors include doxorubicin, bleomycin, and mitoxantrone. As a rule, anthracyclines do not seem to have a significant effect on male gonadal function. Most of these agents are given in combination with other agents (e.g., ABVD [doxorubicin, bleomycin, vinblastine, dacarbazine] in Hodgkin's lymphoma and BEP [bleomycin, etoposide, cisplatin] in testicular cancer) [13]. Other antineoplastic antibiotics include actinomycin-D, which does not appear to result in decreased fertility, and mitomycin, which has little fertility data in humans [31].

Mitotic inhibitors

Mitotic inhibitors are naturally derived compounds that inhibit mitosis by interrupting microtubule polymerization. By definition they are M-phase-specific, but they can exert damage in all phases. This drug class includes the taxanes, the vinca alkaloids, and the epothilones. Vinca alkaloids, when they are given alone or not in combination with other gonadotoxic drugs such as the alkylators or platinum analogs, are expected to cause only transient effects on sperm counts [32]. The taxanes, as mentioned above, may be gonadotoxic, but most of the published literature studied the taxanes in combination with other gonadotoxic agents.

Topoisomerase inhibitors

Topoisomerase inhibitors interfere with the enzymes necessary for DNA strand breakage during replication and transcription. Examples of topoisomerase I inhibitors are topotecan and irinotecan. Examples of topoisomerase II inhibitors are etoposide, mitoxantrone, and doxorubicin. Effects on male gonadal function and fertility in humans are unknown for the topoisomerase I inhibitors. The topoisomerase II inhibitors have been studied most commonly in combination with other agents in germ cell tumors and lymphomas, and if not combined with alkylators or platinum compounds usually do not result in long-term infertility [4].

Immunomodulators and hormonal agents

Corticosteroids deserve mention, as they are not only the mainstay in some chemotherapy regimens for solid tumors but are frequently an adjunct used as an antiemetic or appetite stimulant, in the prevention of hypersensitivity reactions, or to decrease edema. It is unlikely that corticosteroids impair male fertility. Interferon-alpha remains a treatment option for melanoma, Kaposi's sarcoma, and advanced kidney cancer. There is no evidence that it impacts sperm production [2]. High-dose interleukin-2 (IL2) is occasionally used in melanoma and kidney cancer. It has effects on both adrenal and testicular androgen production in men [27]. Sex hormones and hormone-like drugs such as estrogens, gonadotropin-releasing hormone (GnRH) agonists and antagonists, antiandrogens and mitotane are used in the treatment of hormone-responsive malignancies such as prostate cancer and adrenal cortical carcinoma. These drugs inhibit androgen production or action at the level of the testis and/or adrenals and thereby inhibit libido, erectile function, and fertility. It is controversial whether medical castration may be protective against the cytotoxic effects of cancer treatments. Most hormonal effects are reversible, but this is not always the case [33].

Monoclonal antibodies, tyrosine kinase inhibitors, and other new agents

As the rapid pace of drug development in oncology continues, it remains crucial to continue prospective research on the effects on fertility in men. At this time there are very few data on newer agents such as monoclonal antibodies, tyrosine kinase inhibitors, radiopharmaceuticals, and vaccine therapies. For the most part these treatments have not been studied, and there is not enough clinical experience to draw conclusions regarding effects on gonadal function. Experience with the rapamycin inhibitors, such as sirolimus and everolimus, is available given their use in transplant patients. These drugs seem to impact testicular function via inhibition of a stem cell factor/c-kit-dependent process in the spermatogonia and appear to impair spermatogenesis [34].

Overview of childhood solid tumors

Approximately 15 000 children and adolescents 20 years of age and younger are diagnosed with cancer annually in the United States. The number of cases in children 14 years of age and younger is approximately 2.5 times greater than in older adolescents. Some tumors that are more common in younger children (e.g., neuroblastoma, Wilms' tumor, hepatoblastoma) are very rare in older adolescents. Overall, non-lymphoid solid tumors comprise slightly less than half of all cases of childhood cancer. In order of decreasing frequency, these include (annual incidence): CNS tumors (approximately 3800 cases); neuroblastoma (800 cases); Wilms' tumor (500 cases); soft tissue sarcomas (800 cases, approximately equally divided between cases of rhabdomyosarcoma [350] and the broader "non-rhabdomyosarcoma soft tissue sarcomas" [450]); bone sarcomas (650 cases, primarily osteosarcoma [400 cases] and Ewing sarcoma [250 cases]); germ cell tumors (200 cases); and hepatic tumors (80 cases). Because of the clinical diversity of these tumors, some patients will be treated with local therapy only (e.g., surgery), some will require multimodality local therapy (e.g., surgery and/or radiation), and most will be treated with a combination of chemotherapy and surgery or radiation for "local control." Because the majority of non-metastatic solid tumors of childhood are curable, the impact of therapy on the potential for normal future fertility is typically among the major issues addressed at the time of initial diagnosis.

At the time of initial presentation, the urgency to establish a diagnosis and initiate therapy promptly can be overwhelming. For patients and families already faced with the trauma of an existential crisis, the added trauma of uncertainty about future fertility can be immense. For most parents of young children, and especially for peri- and postpubertal teens and young adults, a careful assessment of the risks of treatment-associated adverse effects on fertility and the options for fertility preservation is very much desired, and should be considered as integral a part of patient education as are discussions of other chemotherapy- or radiation-associated side effects [32,35].

The effects of treatment for childhood cancer on fertility was analyzed recently in a cohort of 20 720 untreated patients 20 years of age or younger at diagnosis who survived at least five years following a diagnosis of cancer between 1970 and 1986 [36,37]. For the 5149 female survivors who were not surgically sterile, the relative risk of ever becoming pregnant was 0.81 compared to female siblings. Factors associated with impaired fertility included radiation exposure to the hypothalamic/pituitary region of ≥ 30 Gy or ovarian/uterine radiation exposure to doses of > 5 Gy; the impact of chemotherapy on the subsequent risk of pregnancy was greatest in those with a summed "alkylating agent dose" (AAD) score of three or four or those who were treated with lomustine or cyclophosphamide. Women treated with pelvic irradiation and/or increasing alkylating agent doses are at increased risk of ovarian failure, premature menopause, and small-for-gestational-age offspring [38,39]. Similarly, gonadal irradiation to a dose of > 7.5 Gy and higher cumulative AAD were risk factors for never siring a pregnancy in 6224 male survivors. In general, males appear more sensitive to the gonadotoxicity of alkylating agents, though subtle but clinically meaningful differences may exist among the risks of treatment-associated infertility with structurally similar agents [19,40]. With increased awareness of the scope of the problem, and the resultant ability to identify patients at greater and lesser risk of developing impaired fertility, fertility preservation options can be targeted in a more rational and informed fashion.

Strategies for fertility preservation in pre- and postpubertal children and adolescents are discussed elsewhere in this book in greater detail. Knowledge of the basic paradigms for treating the most common types of childhood solid tumors is critical to allow the responsible physician to inform the patient and his or her family of the risk that treatment will compromise future fertility, and to discuss in a meaningful way the option of pursuing fertility-preserving technologies.

Central nervous system tumors

Approximately three-quarters of children and adolescents with central nervous system (CNS) tumors will survive five years. The mainstays of treatment are surgical resection and some combination of focal or extended-field CNS radiation and/or chemotherapy. Approximately half of all CNS tumors are treated with surgery alone or surgery plus focal radiation therapy. The remainder of patients, particularly those who have embryonal histologies, are typically treated with chemotherapy following surgical resection and radiation therapy. Alkylating agents, including cyclophosphamide and the nitrosoureas carmustine (CCNU) and lomustine (BNCU), and platinum agents (both cisplatin and carboplatin) are commonly employed to treat CNS tumors and are particularly gonadotoxic. Consequently, depending on whether treatment consists of surgery alone or with involved-field radiation, or whole-brain radiation and/or chemotherapy, the risk of infertility can range from low to very high. Survivors of childhood CNS tumors are at elevated risk for late mortality, second malignant neoplasms, and chronic medical conditions including neurocognitive impairment and endocrinopathies [41]. Post-radiation hypothalamic–pituitary axis dysfunction and secondary gonadal dysfunction can lead to delayed puberty, central precocious puberty, or hypogonadotropic hypogonadism [42]. Although hormonal supplementation can address the secondary gonadal effects of primary hypothalamic–pituitary dysfunction, given the generally younger age of children with CNS tumors, until recently relatively few patients were candidates for fertility preservation techniques prior to initiation of chemotherapy.

Neuroblastoma

Neuroblastoma is the most common extracranial solid tumor of childhood. More than 90% of cases are diagnosed in prepubertal children. Most cases arise in the adrenal gland and present with large, unresectable tumors, typically with bulky regional lymphadenopathy and multiple bone and/or bone marrow metastases. Treatment with intensive doses of alkylator-containing chemotherapy (typically cyclophosphamide and cisplatin) is standard; previously, patients achieving complete or near-complete remissions underwent consolidation with high-dose chemotherapy and autologous stem cell rescue. Retroperitoneal and/or pelvic radiation to doses of 21 Gy are typically given to control microscopic residual disease. Until recently, the majority of children with advanced-stage neuroblastoma died of their disease; however, with modern intensive chemotherapy and the development of targeted biologically based differentiation and immunotherapy, at least half of newly diagnosed patients will survive [43]. The risk of infertility or subfertility is moderate to high in both boys and girls. As survival has improved, newer treatment approaches have tried to limit the cumulative exposure to alkylating agents. Survivors of neuroblastoma are significantly more likely than their healthy siblings to have chronic health conditions: in one of the largest studies of survivors, 13 of 204 evaluable women developed ovarian failure, with radiotherapy to the ovaries identified as the greatest risk factor [44]. Given the generally young age and advanced stage of disease of the typical child with neuroblastoma, fertility preservation options have generally not been realistic for most children.

Wilms' tumor

Wilms' tumor is the second most common extracranial solid tumor of childhood. Most children are prepubertal at the time of diagnosis. The overwhelming majority of children with Wilms' tumor, even those with distant metastases, are cured. Treatment for many children consists of two or three generally non-gonadotoxic chemotherapy agents (vincristine, dactinomycin, doxorubicin) given for 5–8 months. Alkylator-containing therapy (typically cyclophosphamide) is generally reserved for those with unfavorable histologies or metastatic or recurrent disease, though even here the cumulative dose of the alkylating agent may be below the threshold to produce infertility. With careful treatment planning, flank or whole-abdomen radiation to doses of 10.5–10.8 Gy for control of microscopic residual disease at the primary site or in the event of tumor spillage or regional nodal involvement may not invariably lead to fertility problems.

Soft tissue sarcomas

Rhabdomyosarcoma (RMS)

The median age at diagnosis of rhabdomyosarcoma (RMS) is six years; a second peak occurs during adolescence. Approximately 40% of tumors arise in structures of the head and neck, and another 25% arise in the bladder/prostate or male and female reproductive organs (paratestis, vulva/vagina, and cervix/uterus). Between 75% and 80% of patients present without distant metastases, and 65–85% of these patients are cured with modern therapy. Chemotherapy administration is routine and lasts for 5–12 months. Cumulative exposure to alkylating agents differs according to "risk stratification" based on pre-treatment patient characteristics and tumor histology, with patients being divided into groups of "very low," "low," "intermediate," and "high" risk; the majority of patients fall into the intermediate- and high-risk categories. The risk of treatment-related infertility is moderate to high for boys and moderate for girls with intermediate- and high-risk tumors, and low to moderate for children with very-low- and low-risk tumors. Current-generation Children's Oncology Group (COG) protocols administer cumulative cyclophosphamide dosages from as little as 4.8 g/m^2 to children with low-risk tumors, a dose associated with relatively little risk of infertility, to as high as 8.4–16.8 g/m^2 to children with intermediate- and high-risk tumors, doses associated with a risk of oligospermia or azoospermia that may approach 50% at the higher end of this dose range.

Different treatment strategies with potentially significant differences in the risk of infertility have developed in the United States and Canada (as reflected in the COG treatment protocols) and most European cooperative groups with regard to the choice of alkylating agent for inclusion as the "backbone" of treatment. In the trials sponsored by the COG, all patients receive cyclophosphamide, though the cumulative dose varies as outlined above. Conversely, in Europe, the potentially less gonadotoxic analog ifosfamide has largely replaced cyclophosphamide as the alkylating agent of choice. Similar trans-Atlantic philosophical differences exist with regard to the use of radiation therapy for control of unresected or microscopic residual

disease, with the uniform administration of doses of between 36 and 50.4 Gy in COG studies.

In addition to the potentially gonadotoxic effects of systemic chemotherapy, given the common anatomic sites of origin of these tumors, patients with rhabdomyosarcoma may be at risk of radiation-related hypothalamic–pituitary dysfunction, or radiation damage to pelvic structures [45]. Whenever possible, testicular or ovarian transposition should be considered for children with bladder/prostate or reproductive organ tumors that will likely need sterilizing doses of radiation as part of local therapy. Fertility-preserving surgical techniques have been developed for girls with tumors arising in the reproductive organs, though hysterectomy remains the surgical procedure "of choice" at most centers where such highly specialized techniques are not routinely available [46].

Non-rhabdomyosarcoma soft tissue sarcomas (NRSTS)

Non-rhabdomyosarcoma soft tissue sarcomas (NRSTS) comprise a number of histologic entities. Children with these tumors are, on average, older than those with RMS, and NRSTS are more common in adolescence than are RMS. Approximately half of patients with NRSTS are treated with surgery or surgery plus radiation. Depending on the adequacy of initial surgical resection, cure rates range from 50% to 80% for patients without distant metastases. Adjuvant chemotherapy is generally reserved for patients with resected large, invasive, high-grade tumors, and is given to all patients with unresected or metastatic tumors. The choice of chemotherapy agents for patients with NRSTS generally does include one or more alkylating agents, most commonly ifosfamide, typically in combination with doxorubicin. The risk of infertility in patients with NRSTS is low to moderate. When indicated, high doses (45–63 Gy) of radiation are employed to control microscopic or gross residual disease, though in comparison to adult NRSTS relatively few of these tumors arise in the pelvis or retroperitoneum in children and adolescents. Because of the generally older age of newly diagnosed patients with NRSTS, fertility preservation options are more broadly applicable in this group of patients compared to most other childhood solid tumors.

Bone sarcomas

Osteosarcoma

Most patients with osteosarcoma are diagnosed during the second decade of life, typically during or following the adolescent growth spurt. Most tumors arise in the distal femur, proximal tibia, or proximal humerus, and 80% have no radiographically detectable metastases at the time of diagnosis. Modern multimodality therapy consisting of pre- and postoperative multi-agent chemotherapy (typically with cisplatin plus doxorubicin, and high-dose methotrexate) sandwiched around surgical resection, and prosthetic or allograft reconstruction of the primary tumor is curative in nearly two-thirds of patients without radiographically detectable metastases. Historically, most patients did not receive an alkylating agent with significant risk of irreversible gonadal damage, though patients with recurrent tumors and some newly diagnosed patients may be treated with ifosfamide. The risk of treatment-related infertility is low to moderate in boys and low in girls [47], but that risk may be increased based on the still-pending results of an ongoing international clinical trial exploring the potential benefit of adding ifosfamide and etoposide postoperatively to "standard" three-drug chemotherapy for patients whose response to preoperative chemotherapy is suboptimal. Despite the relatively lower risk of treatment-related infertility, sperm banking for boys is routinely offered; referral of adolescent girls and young adult women for oocyte or ovarian (or embryo) cryopreservation has historically been less uniform, in part because of the relatively low risk of treatment-related ovarian failure or premature menopause, combined with the perceived need to delay the initiation of systemic therapy for "too long" a period of time.

Ewing sarcoma

Approximately two-thirds of patients with Ewing sarcoma are diagnosed during the second decade of life. Tumors arise in the bones of the axial and appendicular skeleton with equal frequency. Approximately 75% of patients present without radiographically detectable metastases, and approximately two-thirds are cured with modern therapy. Treatment generally consists of 6–12 months of intensive, multi-agent alkylator-containing chemotherapy and either surgical resection or definitive irradiation of the primary tumor (occasionally both surgery and radiation are employed). The

risk of severe, life-threatening, or disabling chronic health conditions and infertility is elevated in survivors of Ewing sarcoma [48].

As for RMS, there is a divide between North American and European oncologists in the choice of alkylating agents: the former continue to administer both cyclophosphamide and ifosfamide, with an attendant greater risk of treatment-related infertility given the administration of cumulative cyclophosphamide and ifosfamide dosages of 8.4–16.8 g/m^2 and 42–63 g/m^2, respectively, doses associated with a risk of infertility approaching 50% or more at the higher end of the dose range, while the latter have switched almost exclusively to ifosfamide (and generally give a lower cumulative alkylator agent total dose).

Girls with pelvic tumors that are not amenable to surgical resection, or that are surgically resected but treated with postoperative radiation to doses of 45–55.8 Gy, are at elevated risk of ovarian failure and/or uterine fibrosis. Ovarian transposition should be considered for all girls thought likely to need pelvic irradiation where ovarian exposure of > 1000 cGy is likely. Although uterine fibrosis may prevent successful gestation, the use of a gestational surrogate can be offered to young women with preserved ovarian function. Given the high cumulative alkylator exposure, the risk of treatment-related infertility is high for boys and low to moderate for girls (except those with pelvic tumors treated with radiation) [49,50]. Pregnancy is possible in young women who have previously undergone an internal hemipelvectomy; consequently, although there is no clear association between surgery and more favorable outcome in girls with pelvic tumors, surgery may offer a greater chance of preserved fertility.

Most postpubertal boys with Ewing sarcoma are offered semen cryopreservation prior to starting chemotherapy; the use of fertility-preserving techniques for girls has been less consistent, though newer protocols for rapid ovarian stimulation that minimize the delay in starting systemic chemotherapy should lessen the reluctance of treating physicians to refer their female patients, particularly those at high risk based on a potential role for pelvic irradiation.

Summary

Advances in multimodality therapy for children and adolescents with cancer have led to cures for the majority of patients. Treatment of children, adolescents, and young adults with solid tumors is typically intensive, involves the administration of one or more alkylating agents with potentially gonadotoxic effects, and may also involve the administration of moderate to high doses of therapeutic radiation to the hypothalamic–pituitary region or the pelvis. Honest and open discussion about the potential effects of treatment on fertility should begin as early as feasible in the process of staging a child or adolescent with newly diagnosed cancer, particularly for those patients who are likely to receive treatment associated with an elevated risk of infertility. However potentially "awkward" such conversations may be, parents and children, and even more so adolescent and young adult patients, are eager to learn about options for fertility preservation. Nonetheless, knowledge deficits about the risks of infertility are substantial [51]. Until recently, fertility preservation options were not generally available to prepubertal children, and only semen cryopreservation was routinely recommended to postpubertal boys. Newer techniques for rapid ovarian stimulation for oocyte and/or embryo cryopreservation or ovarian tissue cryopreservation [52,53], as well as newer techniques for cryopreservation of prepubertal testicular or ovarian tissue, should result in fertility preservation options being made available to larger numbers of patients. The economic impact of these techniques with regard to reimbursement by third-party payers remains to be seen [54].

References

1. World Fertility Patterns 2009. United Nations Department of Economic and Social Affairs Population Division, 2010. www.un.org/esa/population/publications/worldfertility2009/worldfertility2009.htm (accessed January 2012).

2. Lee SJ, Schover LR, Partridge AH, *et al.* American Society of Clinical Oncology recommendations on fertility preservation in cancer patients. *J Clin Oncol* 2006; 24: 2917–31.

3. Chapman RM, Sutcliffe SB, Rees LH, Edwards CR, Malpas JS. Cyclical combination chemotherapy and gonadal function. Retrospective study in males. *Lancet* 1979; 1: 285–9.

4. Meistrich ML. Male gonadal toxicity. *Pediatr Blood Cancer* 2009; 53: 261–6.

5. Jeruss JS, Woodruff TK. Preservation of fertility in patients with cancer. *N Engl J Med* 2009; 360: 902–11.

6. Petersen PM, Skakkebaek NE, Vistisen K, Rorth M, Giwercman A. Semen quality and reproductive hormones before orchiectomy in men with testicular cancer. *J Clin Oncol* 1999; 17: 941–7.

7. Hart R. Preservation of fertility in adults and children diagnosed with cancer. *BMJ* 2008; 337: a2045.

8. Meistrich ML, Byrne J. Genetic disease in offspring of long-term survivors of childhood and adolescent cancer treated with potentially mutagenic therapies. *Am J Hum Genet* 2002; 70: 1069–71.

9. Blatt J. Pregnancy outcome in long-term survivors of childhood cancer. *Med Pediatr Oncol* 1999; 33: 29–33.

10. Dodds L, Marrett LD, Tomkins DJ, Green B, Sherman G. Case-control study of congenital anomalies in children of cancer patients. *BMJ* 1993; 307: 164–8.

11. Brydoy M, Fossa SD, Dahl O, Bjoro T. Gonadal dysfunction and fertility problems in cancer survivors. *Acta Oncol* 2007; 46: 480–9.

12. Shin D, Lo KC, Lipshultz LI. Treatment options for the infertile male with cancer. *J Natl Cancer Inst Monogr* 2005; 34: 48–50.

13. van der Kaaij MA, van Echten-Arends J, Simons AH, Kluin-Nelemans HC. Fertility preservation after chemotherapy for Hodgkin lymphoma. *Hematol Oncol* 2010; 28: 168–79.

14. Calamera JC, Morgenfeld MC, Mancini RE, Vilar O. Biochemical changes of the human semen produced by chlorambucil, testosterone propionate and human chorionic gonadotropin administration. *Andrologia* 1979; 11: 43–50.

15. Buchanan JD, Fairley KF, Barrie JU. Return of spermatogenesis after stopping cyclophosphamide therapy. *Lancet* 1975; 2: 156–7.

16. Bokemeyer C, Schmoll HJ, van Rhee J, *et al.* Long-term gonadal toxicity after therapy for Hodgkin's and non-Hodgkin's lymphoma. *Ann Hematol* 1994; 68: 105–10.

17. Ypsilantis P, Papaioannou N, Psalla D, *et al.* Effects of subchronic ifosfamide-mesna treatment on testes and semen characteristics in the rabbit. *Reprod Toxicol* 2003; 17: 699–708.

18. Pectasides D, Pectasides E, Papaxoinis G, *et al.* Testicular function in poor-risk nonseminomatous germ cell tumors treated with methotrexate, paclitaxel, ifosfamide, and cisplatin combination chemotherapy. *J Androl* 2009; 30: 280–6.

19. Williams D, Crofton PM, Levitt G. Does ifosfamide affect gonadal function? *Pediatr Blood Cancer* 2008; 50: 347–51.

20. Longhi A, Macchiagodena M, Vitali G, Bacci G. Fertility in male patients treated with neoadjuvant chemotherapy for osteosarcoma. *J Pediatr Hematol Oncol* 2003; 25: 292–6.

21. Drasga RE, Einhorn LH, Williams SD, Patel DN, Stevens EE. Fertility after chemotherapy for testicular cancer. *J Clin Oncol* 1983; 1: 179–83.

22. Petersen PM, Hansen SW, Giwercman A, Rorth M, Skakkebaek NE. Dose-dependent impairment of testicular function in patients treated with cisplatin-based chemotherapy for germ cell cancer. *Ann Oncol* 1994; 5: 355–8.

23. Brydoy M, Fossa SD, Klepp O, *et al.* Paternity following treatment for testicular cancer. *J Natl Cancer Inst* 2005; 97: 1580–8.

24. Gerl A, Muhlbayer D, Hansmann G, Mraz W, Hiddemann W. The impact of chemotherapy on Leydig cell function in long term survivors of germ cell tumors. *Cancer* 2001; 91: 1297–303.

25. Lampe H, Horwich A, Norman A, Nicholls J, Dearnaley DP. Fertility after chemotherapy for testicular germ cell cancers. *J Clin Oncol* 1997; 15: 239–45.

26. Oxaliplatin package insert, version 5.0. Sanofi-Aventis Canada, Inc., 2010.

27. Yeung SC, Chiu AC, Vassilopoulou-Sellin R, Gagel RF. The endocrine effects of nonhormonal antineoplastic therapy. *Endocr Rev* 1998; 19: 144–72.

28. Lee SJ. Preservation of fertility in patients with cancer. *N Engl J Med* 2009; 360: 2680.

29. Shamberger RC, Rosenberg SA, Seipp CA, Sherins RJ. Effects of high-dose methotrexate and vincristine on ovarian and testicular functions in patients undergoing postoperative adjuvant treatment of osteosarcoma. *Cancer Treat Rep* 1981; 65: 739–46.

30. Chatzidarellis E, Makrilia N, Giza L, *et al.* Effects of taxane-based chemotherapy on inhibin B and gonadotropins as biomarkers of spermatogenesis. *Fertil Steril* 2010; 94: 558–63.

31. Aubier F, Flamant F, Brauner R, *et al.* Male gonadal function after chemotherapy for solid tumors in childhood. *J Clin Oncol* 1989; 7: 304–9.

32. Levine J, Canada A, Stern CJ. Fertility preservation in adolescents and young adults with cancer. *J Clin Oncol* 2010; 28: 4831–41.

33. Conn PM, Crowley WF. Gonadotropin-releasing hormone and its analogues. *N Engl J Med* 1991; 324: 93–103.

34. Huyghe E, Zairi A, Nohra J, *et al.* Gonadal impact of target of rapamycin inhibitors (sirolimus and everolimus) in male patients: an overview. *Transpl Int* 2007; 20: 305–11.

35. Fallat ME, Hutter J; Committee on Bioethics, Section on Hematology/Oncology, and Section on Surgery. Preservation of fertility in pediatric and adolescent patients with cancer. *Pediatrics* 2008; 121: e1461–9.

36. Green DM, Kawashima T, Stovall M, *et al.* Fertility of female survivors of childhood cancer: a report from the Childhood Cancer Survivor Study. *J Clin Oncol* 2009; 27: 2677–85.

37. Green DM, Kawashima T, Stovall M, *et al.* Fertility of male survivors of childhood cancer: a report from the Childhood Cancer Survivor Study. *J Clin Oncol* 2010; 28: 332–9.

38. Green DM, Sklar CA, Boice JD, *et al.* Ovarian failure and reproductive outcomes after childhood cancer treatment: results from the Childhood Cancer Survivor Study. *J Clin Oncol* 2009; 27: 2374–81.

39. Johnston RJ, Wallace WHB. Normal ovarian function and assessment of ovarian reserve in the survivor of childhood cancer. *Pediatr Blood Cancer* 2009; 5: 296–302.

40. Ridola V, Fawaz O, Aubier F, *et al.* Testicular function of survivors of childhood cancer: a comparative study between ifosfamide and cyclophosphamide-based regimens. *Eur J Cancer* 2009; 45: 814–18.

41. Armstrong GT, Liu Q, Yasui Y, *et al.* Long-term outcomes among adult survivors of childhood central nervous system malignancies in the Childhood Cancer Survivor Study. *J Natl Cancer Inst* 2009; 101: 946–58.

42. Chemaitilly W, Sklar CA. Endocrine complications in long-term survivors of childhood cancers. *Endocr Relat Cancer* 2010; 17: R141–59.

43. Yu AL, Gilman AL, Ozkaynak F, *et al.* Anti-GD2 antibody with GM-CSF, Interleukin-2, and isotretinoin for neuroblastoma. *N Engl J Med* 2010; 363: 1324–34.

44. Laverdiere C, Liu Q, Yasui Y, *et al.* Long-term outcomes in survivors of neuroblastoma: a report from the Childhood Cancer Survivor Study. *J Natl Cancer Inst* 2009; 101: 1131–40.

45. Mansky P, Arai A, Stratton P, *et al.* Treatment late effects in long-term survivors of pediatric sarcoma. *Pediatr Blood Cancer* 2007; 48: 192–9.

46. Kayton ML, Wexler LH, Lewin SN, *et al.* Pediatric radical abdominal trachelectomy for anaplastic embryonal rhabdomyosarcoma of the uterine cervix: an alternative to radical hysterectomy. *J Pediatr Surg* 2009; 44: 862–7.

47. Greenberg DB, Goorin A, Gebhardt MC, *et al.* Quality of life in osteosarcoma survivors. *Oncology* 1994; 8: 19–25.

48. Ginsberg JP, Goodman P, Leisenring W, *et al.* Long-term survivors of childhood Ewing sarcoma: report from the Childhood Cancer Survivor Study. *J Natl Cancer Inst* 2010; 102: 1–12.

49. Horowitz M, Wexler L. Fertility in females after high cumulative dose alkylating agent therapy for pediatric sarcomas. American Society of Pediatric

127

Hematology/Oncology, Ninth Annual Meeting, Chicago, IL, 1996.

50. Sudour H, Chastagner P, Claude L, *et al.* Fertility and pregnancy outcome after abdominal irradiation that included or excluded the pelvis in childhood tumor survivors. *Int J Radiation Oncol Biol Phys* 2010; 76: 867–73.

51. van den Berg H, Langeveld NE. Parental knowledge of fertility in male childhood cancer survivors. *Psychooncology* 2008; 17: 287–91.

52. Oktay K, Oktem O. Fertility preservation medicine: a new field in the care of young cancer survivors. *Pediatr Blood Cancer* 2009; 53: 267–73.

53. Weintraub M, Gross E, Kadari A, *et al.* Should ovarian cryopreservation be offered to girls with cancer. *Pediatr Blood Cancer* 2007; 48(1): 4–9.

54. Campo-Engelstein L. Consistency in insurance coverage for iatrogenic conditions resulting from cancer treatment including fertility preservation. *J Clin Oncol* 2010; 28: 1284–6.

Chapter

15

Lymphoma and leukemia

Eytan Stein and Ariella Noy

Introduction

Leukemia and lymphoma typically strike the middle-aged and elderly, many of whom already have a family or have decided to forgo having children. But a subset of hematologic malignancies tends to disproportionately affect the young – those that either by choice or circumstance do not yet have children. In this chapter, we will delve into how treatments for lymphomas and leukemias, including high-dose therapy with hematopoietic stem cell transplantation, affect fertility, primarily in young men who may still want to start a family once their disease is cured.

The effects of cytotoxic chemotherapy on male fertility stem primarily from disruption of spermatogenesis rather than from direct effects on androgen production or Leydig cells. The risk of acquired azoospermia and gonadal dysfunction has been attributed to specific cytotoxic agents, with alkylators including cisplatin being the most frequently implicated. The severity of gonadal dysfunction tends to be proportional to the cumulative dose of these agents. As recently reviewed, higher doses of busulfan, chlorambucil, cyclophosphamide, procarbazine, melphalan, and cisplatin predictably produce severe gonadal dysfunction [1]. Microtubule inhibitors and anthracyclines alone do not tend to produce prolonged azoospermia, but can have additive effects with other agents such as alkylators. Topoisomerase inhibitors, antimetabolites, and biological agents tend not to permanently affect gonadal function.

Hodgkin's lymphoma

Hodgkin's lymphoma is the best-studied malignancy affecting young men who do not yet have children.

With a bimodal distribution, males between the ages of 15 and 35 are frequently diagnosed at a time when they are thinking of starting a family. Combination chemotherapy treatment of Hodgkin's lymphoma started in earnest in the 1950s, with a regimen composed of mechlorethamine (a.k.a. nitrogen mustard), vincristine, procarbazine, and prednisone. Although this was highly effective, side effects included both male and female infertility, primarily as a result of the mechlorethamine and procarbazine components. At the time, loss of fertility was a small price to pay for life-saving therapy. With time, side effects such as secondary leukemia and sterility adversely affected the longevity of these cured Hodgkin's lymphoma patients. As detailed below, current Hodgkin's chemotherapeutic regimens are less gonadotoxic than older regimens, allowing young men cured of their disease to father children.

Intriguingly, male Hodgkin's lymphoma patients may have gonadal dysfunction predating chemotherapy. A 1981 study of MVPP (mechlorethamine, vinblastine, procarbazine, prednisone) reported that 16 out of 43 men were "functionally subfertile" with a combination of impotence and inadequate sperm counts before treatment [2]. A 2002 study of 158 patients by the German Hodgkin Study Group (GHSG) revealed that 70% of men had semen parameter abnormalities prior to the onset of treatment (Table 15.1) [3]. Multivariate analysis identified elevated sedimentation rate and advanced stage as prognostic factors for severe fertility damage. The etiology of gonadal dysfunction in male patients with Hodgkin's lymphoma prior to therapy is currently unknown. Theories range from the secretion of cytokines by Hodgkin's lymphoma Reed–Sternberg cells, which may impair spermatogenesis, to an overall

Fertility Preservation in Male Cancer Patients, ed. John P. Mulhall, Linda D. Applegarth, Robert D. Oates and Peter N. Schlegel. Published by Cambridge University Press. © Cambridge University Press 2013.

Table 15.1. Pre-treatment and post-treatment semen analyses in patients with Hodgkin's lymphoma treated by the German Hodgkin Study Group

Treatment regimen	No. of patients	Pre-treatment sperm assessment	Post-treatment sperm assessment
Various: ABVD COPP/ABVD BEACOPP Escalated BEACOPP	Pre-treatment: 202 Post-treatment: 112	Normospermia: 20% Azoospermia: 11% Other dysspermia: 69%	Normospermia: 6% Azoospermia: 64% Other dysspermia: 30%
BEACOPP BEACOPP (escalated)	Pre-treatment: 26 Post-treatment: 26	Normospermia: 23% Azoospermia: 8% Other dysspermia: 69%	Normospermia: 0% Azoospermia: 88% Other dysspermia: 12%

increase in inflammatory activity, as evidenced by erythrocyte sedimentation rates, leading to gonadal dysfunction.

Methodologically, studies studying fertility in male patients after cytotoxic chemotherapy have used surrogate endpoints. While the best endpoint in assessing fertility is percentage conceptions in those attempting to father a child, this has been difficult to study in practice. Because of this difficulty, surrogate endpoints such as levels of follicle-stimulating hormone (FSH), sperm count, sperm motility, and sperm morphology have been used.

Current treatments for Hodgkin's lymphoma around the world tend to be divided into one of three regimens: ABVD (doxorubicin, bleomycin, vinblastine, and dacarbazine), which is used primarily as first-line treatment in the United States; Stanford V (doxorubicin, vinblastine, mechlorethamine, etoposide, vincristine, bleomycin, and prednisone), an alternative regimen in the United States; and BEACOPP (bleomycin, etoposide, doxorubicin, cyclophosphamide, vincristine, procarbazine, and prednisone), a regimen primarily used in Europe.

Sieniawski *et al.* looked at all male patients enrolled in GHSG trials HD4–HD12 for Hodgkin's lymphoma from 1988 to 2003 [3]. Treatment regimens included COPP (cyclophosphamide, vincristine, procarbazine, prednisone)/ABVD, BEACOPP, and COPP/ABV/IMEP. Some studies included involved-field radiation. In pre-treatment analysis ($n = 202$), 20% of patients had normospermia, 11% azoospermia, and 69% other dysspermia. In post-treatment analysis ($n = 112$), 64% of patients had azoospermia, 30% other dysspermia, and 6% normospermia ($p < 0.001$). Of note, BEACOPP, the favored regimen in Germany for higher-risk patients and used

internationally in selected high-risk patients, had a 93% risk of post-treatment azoospermia for the baseline dosing and 87% for the escalated version. A statistically significant difference in post-treatment FSH levels existed between patients with azoospermia and those with preserved spermatogenesis ($p = 0.001$). The median onset to time for recovery of spermatogenesis was 27 months. Among the patients with recovery, return of sperm to the ejaculate was observed in 18% of patients during the first year after treatment, 23% during the second year, 25% during the third year, and 35% after the third year. Regimens containing alkylating agents tended to cause greater decreases in fertility than non-alkylating regimens [4].

The European Organisation for Research and Treatment of Cancer (EORTC) retrospectively analyzed fertility of male Hodgkin's lymphoma patients enrolled in four consecutive randomized controlled trials performed between 1982 and 2004 [5]. In these trials, patients received a variety of chemotherapeutic regimens including MOPP (mechlorethamine, vincristine, procarbazine, prednisone), ABVD, EBVP (epirubicin, bleomycin, vinblastine, prednisone), MOPP/doxorubicin, ABV, or BEACOPP. As with other reports of male fertility, pre-treatment and post-treatment sperm parameters were not routinely obtained in a controlled fashion. As a way to get around this, the researchers in this EORTC study used FSH levels as a surrogate for Sertoli cell function, spermatogenesis, and male fertility. Even with the use of this surrogate endpoint, only 545 of the 2362 male patients in the study had at least one FSH value drawn after treatment, either within nine months of treatment completion or more than one year after completion. In the final analysis a significantly greater proportion of men treated with alkylating chemotherapy had elevated FSH levels. Sixty percent of patients treated with alkylating chemotherapy had elevated FSH levels, compared to only 8% of patients treated with non-alkylator chemotherapy. In addition to alkylating agents, clinical stage, age, and the presence of B symptoms correlated with an elevated FSH post-treatment. As expected, FSH levels tended to return to normal levels as patients got further from the toxic effects of chemotherapy [5].

Male patients with Hodgkin's lymphoma are now routinely offered pre-treatment sperm banking as a way of maintaining fertility post-chemotherapy.

Non-Hodgkin's lymphomas

Non-Hodgkin's lymphomas (NHLs) tend to affect men in middle age and older. Since many men at this age have already had a family and are not as concerned about fathering children, less research has focused on this population. Generally speaking, men treated with CHOP (cylcophosphamide, doxorubicin, vincristine, prednisone)-based chemotherapy for NHLs tend to have fewer issues with fertility than those treated for Hodgkin's lymphoma. In a study of 71 adult patients treated for NHL from 1979 to 1991 with CHOP-based chemotherapy, none of the patients was azoospermic prior to treatment, while during treatment all of the patients developed abnormal semen parameters, using the standards of the World Health Organization [6]. However, seven years post-treatment two-thirds of the patients were normospermic. As with treatment for Hodgkin's lymphoma, the favorable outlook for fertility in men with NHL has been attributed to the use of less gonadotoxic chemotherapy. Bokemeyer *et al.* demonstrated this nicely in a study of 24 patients with NHL and 66 patients with Hodgkin's lymphoma younger than 45 years old, all in remission for at least 24 months after completion of therapy [7]. Only 21% of men treated for NHL showed signs of gonadal dysfunction, compared with 65% of those with Hodgkin's lymphoma, as assessed by FSH levels. Interestingly, the chemotherapy regimens in both the Hodgkin's and NHL groups included similar cumulative doses of cyclophosphamide, vincristine, and doxorubicin. The difference between the groups lay in the use of procarbazine. Hodgkin's patients received a median cumulative dose of 13.3 g of procarbazine, while NHL patients received no procarbazine. Currently, procarbazine is almost never given as a part of front-line therapy in NHL, and male infertility after chemotherapy is rare.

Leukemia

There is a paucity of data investigating fertility in patients who have undergone therapy for acute leukemias. Induction agents and maintenance agents that are used to treat acute myeloid leukemias tend not to affect fertility to a great extent. For example, in a study of 10 men treated with induction and maintenance chemotherapy for acute leukemia, all of the patients recovered spermatogenesis by the second year of their treatment [8]. The main induction agents used to treat acute myeloid leukemias, the anthracycline daunorubicin and the antimetabolite cytarabine, are not alkylating agents and hence would not be predicted to have a profound effect on fertility.

In a recent case report a boy treated with imatinib for chronic myeloid leukemia since age nine was noted, once postpubertal, to have severe oligospermia [9]. The connection between tyrosine kinase inhibition and fertility issues has not been evaluated in large groups of patients.

Stem cell transplantation

Stem cell transplantation, either autologous or allogeneic, is used in both leukemia and lymphoma as an aggressive regimen with curative intent. Typically, these regimens use extremely high levels of myeloablative chemotherapy to attempt complete obliteration of the cancer clone. Rescue from hematologic collapse post-chemotherapy is provided by reinfused stem cells collected either from the patient (autologous) or an allogeneic donor. Grigg *et al.* published data on 47 male allogeneic bone marrow transplant recipients treated with busulfan and cyclophosphamide as a conditioning regimen [10]. Of these 47 patients, 21 of 26 with a baseline semen analysis had evidence of return of spermatogenesis; 6 had sperm counts between 1 and 20 million/mL, while 20 had sperm counts greater than 20 million/mL. Six of the remaining patients, with only FSH levels drawn but without semen analysis, were able to father children without the use of assisted reproductive technologies. The authors of the study concluded that a conditioning regimen with busulfan and cyclophosphamide resulted in 27 of 32 males showing at least some level of spermatogenesis. In general, however, it is widely assumed that patients will have a significant decrease in their ability to produce offspring after stem cell transplantation, and because of this fertility preservation is often sought.

An alternative to myeloablative conditioning is reduced dose intensity (RDI) transplant. This technique is becoming increasingly used in both indolent and aggressive lymphomas with curative intent. As the chemotherapy given is not directed at the underlying malignancy, but is merely immunosuppressive enough to allow engraftment, relatively little alkylator is used in comparison to myeloablative transplant. In theory, RDI should have a low impact on fertility; however, many of these patients are already heavily pre-treated. The impact of this preparative regimen in RDI has not been explored.

Conclusion

As increasingly effective therapies have been developed for hematologic malignancies, the goal of many clinical trials has been to find chemotherapies with less toxicity and equivalent efficacy. Many of these trials have shown the effectiveness of less toxic chemotherapeutic agents and dosing schedules. With less toxicity has come preservation of fertility in the majority of male patients after treatment. As biological targeted therapies are being developed and increasingly used to treat lymphomas and leukemias in lieu of and in combination with cytotoxic agents, the number of men with decreased fertility levels after therapy may decrease further. Ultimately, nearly all young men with hematologic malignancy are likely to remain fertile once their treatment is completed and disease cured.

References

1. Meistrich ML. Male gonadal toxicity. *Pediatr Blood Cancer* 2009; 53: 261–6.

2. Chapman RM, Sutcliffe SB, Malpas JS. Male gonadal dysfunction in Hodgkin's disease: a prospective study. *JAMA* 1981; 245: 1323–8.

3. Sieniawski M, Reineke T, Nogova L, *et al.* Fertility in male patients with advanced Hodgkin lymphoma treated with BEACOPP: a report of the German Hodgkin Study Group (GHSG). *Blood* 2008; 111: 71–6.

4. Sieniawski M, Reineke T, Josting A, *et al.*, Assessment of male fertility in patients with Hodgkin's lymphoma treated in the German Hodgkin Study Group (GHSG) clinical trials. *Ann Oncol* 2008; 19: 1795–801.

5. van der Kaaij MA, Heutte N, Le Stang N, *et al.* Gonadal function in males after chemotherapy for early-stage Hodgkin's lymphoma treated in four subsequent trials by the European Organisation for Research and Treatment of Cancer: EORTC Lymphoma Group and the Groupe d'Etude des Lymphomes de l'Adulte. *J Clin Oncol* 2007; 25: 2825–32.

6. Pryzant RM, Meistrich ML, Wilson G, Brown B, McLaughlin P. Long-term reduction in sperm count after chemotherapy with and without radiation therapy for non-Hodgkin's lymphomas. *J Clin Oncol* 1993; 11: 239–47.

7. Bokemeyer C, Schmoll HJ, van Rhee J, *et al.* Long-term gonadal toxicity after therapy for Hodgkin's and non-Hodgkin's lymphoma. *Ann Hematol* 1994; 68: 105–10.

8. Kreuser ED, Hetzel WD, Heit W, *et al.* Reproductive and endocrine gonadal functions in adults following multidrug chemotherapy for acute lymphoblastic or undifferentiated leukemia. *J Clin Oncol* 1988; 6: 588–95.

9. Mariani S, Basciani S, Fabbri A, *et al.*, Severe oligozoospermia in a young man with chronic myeloid leukemia on long-term treatment with imatinib started before puberty. *Fertil Steril* 2011; 95: 1120.e15–17.

10. Grigg AP, Stone J, Milner AD, *et al.* Phase II study of autologous stem cell transplant using busulfan-melphalan chemotherapy-only conditioning followed by interferon for relapsed poor prognosis follicular non-Hodgkin lymphoma. *Leuk Lymphoma* 2010; 51: 641–9.

Chapter

16

Stem cell transplantation

Ann A. Jakubowski

Introduction

Hematopoietic stem cell transplantation (HSCT) has become a curative treatment modality for benign and malignant hematologic diseases, and is currently being extended to increasing populations of patients. It has been shown to be of benefit in only a few non-hematologic diseases such as relapsed testicular cancer and neuroendocrine tumors, though it has been studied investigationally in a variety of others such as renal cell carcinoma, melanoma, and breast cancer. Unfortunately, it has not demonstrated significant efficacy in the latter malignancies. Classical HSCT utilizes high doses of chemotherapy and/or radiotherapy for tumors that have demonstrated chemotherapy or radiation sensitivity. It is a treatment that is used after at least one, and often many, courses of standard therapy for the disease. Historically, HSCT was often used as a final option when it became apparent that choices for salvage therapy were limited. Hence a large proportion of patients were very heavily pre-treated by the time they were evaluated for transplant.

Recently, however, genetic markers and clinical parameters at the time of diagnosis have been identified that can assist oncologists with prognosis for cure using standard therapy. Furthermore, the improvement in outcomes of transplantation, the variety of types of transplants available, and better supportive care have led to greater numbers of patients being considered for transplant. Currently, therefore, HSCT is being moved to an earlier point in the course of treatment for some diseases. Patients may enter transplant now with a history of as little as 1–2 courses of therapy, with others having received only "targeted therapy" which has a very focused activity on the hematologic disorder.

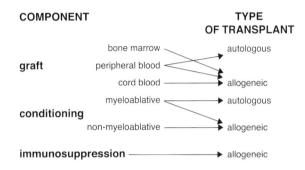

Figure 16.1. Hematopoietic stem cell transplantation.

Even the spectrum of diseases for which transplant is performed has changed over the last decade. Chronic myelogenous leukemia (CML) has become a disease which infrequently requires transplant, although previously it was one of the most common diagnoses for transplant patients. Greater numbers of patients, over a wide range of ages, are undergoing transplantation, and more of these patients are becoming survivors of their cancer. As the number of survivors increases, attention is being focused on the long-term complications of HSCT.

The process of HSCT

To understand the influence of HSCT on fertility, it is necessary to understand the process of transplantation. HSCT can be broken down into three components: (1) the graft, (2) the conditioning, and in some types of transplant (3) the immunosuppression (Fig. 16.1). There are two general categories of HSCT, based on the source of the graft. The first is autologous, when the stem cells are harvested from a patient at the time of blood count recovery after chemotherapy

Fertility Preservation in Male Cancer Patients, ed. John P. Mulhall, Linda D. Applegarth, Robert D. Oates and Peter N. Schlegel.
Published by Cambridge University Press. © Cambridge University Press 2013.

for the tumor, or after receiving granulocyte colony-stimulating factor (G-CSF), a white blood cell growth factor that mobilizes stem cells from the bone marrow to the peripheral blood. The second category is allogeneic HSCT, which utilizes stem cells donated from a family member or from an unrelated donor.

When derived from a donor, the stem cells are preferentially matched. Matching is determined by human leukocyte antigen (HLA) typing, the major histocompatibility complex (MHC) in humans, a group of genes located on chromosome 6 that are related to the immune system function. These genes encode cell-surface antigen-presenting proteins that contribute to defining the cellular identity of an individual. Because of limited availability of donors in some populations, a well-matched donor may not be available and it may be necessary to use stem cells from a mismatched donor. The stem cells can be obtained directly from the bone marrow by performing aspirations from the iliac crest under general anesthesia; by mobilizing the stem cells from the bone marrow into the peripheral blood using G-CSF and harvesting by leukopheresis; or in the form of cord blood stem cells which were harvested from the placenta at the time of a birth.

In an autologous transplant, the stem cells are used to rescue the bone marrow from the damage caused by the chemo-, radio-, and/or antibody therapy given to treat any residual tumor just prior to the stem cell infusion. In an allogeneic HSCT, the stem cells rescue the bone marrow from treatment damage, but in addition they also provide a new immune system, which may produce a biologic effect (allo-effect) against the tumor.

The second component of a transplant is the conditioning, which generally includes chemo-, radio-, and/or antibody therapy. The conditioning is administered to treat any disease that may remain after the standard chemotherapy used by the oncologist as primary treatment of the disease. There are at least two forms of conditioning regimens. Myeloablative is the classical form in both allogeneic and autologous transplants. The intensity of this conditioning is such that the hematopoietic system would not be expected to recover, or would take a very long time to recover without stem cell rescue. This would obviously place the pancytopenic patient at risk of life-threatening infections or bleeding and likely death, without rescuing the patient's bone marrow with the stem cells.

A newer type of allogeneic transplant, developed over the past decade, utilizes non-myeloablative conditioning. This conditioning is not expected to destroy the bone marrow, but rather to provide some treatment of the tumor, to make space in the marrow for the new stem cells, and to suppress the patient's immune system so that the stem cells and new immune system from the donor will be able to develop. This non-myeloablative type of transplant is used to a greater degree for the immunologic/biologic effect of the allogeneic HSCT. The intensity of this conditioning can be much milder than that of the myeloablative transplant, and the patient's marrow would be expected to recover even if the transplant failed. Due to the less intense nature of this conditioning, it has allowed older patients who could not tolerate myeloablative conditioning to become candidates for allogeneic HSCT. Often the conditioning regimens include alkylating agents and/or lower doses of radiotherapy.

The third component of an allogeneic HSCT is the immunosuppression. Since the patient is receiving both new bone marrow stem cells and cells to generate a new immune system, the latter cells from the donor must be kept under control with immunosuppressive drugs until they become tolerant of the patient. The immunosuppression is most often provided by lymphocytotoxic drugs, such as calcineurin inhibitors (cyclosporine, tacrolimus) and methotrexate. Obviously, immune suppression is not an issue for patients receiving an autologous transplant, since they are being transplanted with their own stem cells.

In summary, HSCT involves the use of chemo-, radio-, or biologic therapy known as conditioning, followed by infusion of stem cells, (1) to rescue the bone marrow from the consequences of the therapy and (2), in the case of allogeneic HSCT, to rescue the bone marrow and provide a new immune system, hence a biologic effect against any residual disease.

The introduction of a new immune system with an allogeneic HSCT sets the stage for one of the major complications of such transplants, which is graft versus host disease (GVHD). This disorder develops when the donor's immune cells in the stem cell donation see a patient's organ, such as the skin, liver, or intestinal tract, as foreign and the donor's cells infiltrate that organ in an effort to destroy it. This can result in tissue injury, which ranges from a simple rash to a lethal condition such as large-volume bloody diarrhea. The less well-matched the donor's cells are to the patient (HLA typing), the higher the risk of developing GVHD. GVHD is treated by increasing the immunosuppressive medications. In addition to the calcineurin inhibitor drugs used for prophylaxis of GVHD, corticosteroids, monoclonal antibodies that target specific cytokines or cytokine receptors associated with the damage caused in GVHD such as etanercept or infliximab, or broader-acting cytolytic agents such as antithymocyte globulin, may be added as treatment. All of these agents act by destroying lymphocytes (the cells responsible for GVHD), or attempt to block the inflammatory proteins driving the lymphocytes or the cytokines produced by the lymphocytes which contribute to tissue damage.

HSCT and fertility

One late complication of HSCT is infertility due to premature gonadal failure. This may be caused directly by the toxic effects of the medications used to treat the tumor or as part of the pre-transplant conditioning (see below), or secondarily as a consequence of the disruption of the hypothalamic–pituitary–gonadal (HPG) axis. Surveys have shown that infertility developing as a consequence of HSCT can impose a major negative impact on survivors' quality of life, and for some it has been viewed as equal to or worse than the diagnosis of cancer [1].

Until recently, limited attention has been paid to the incidence and impact of infertility after transplantation. The National Marrow Donor Program/Center for International Blood and Marrow Transplant Research (NMDP/CIBMTR) has now made it a focus of retrospective reviews and a part of their clinical database to assist in reevaluating the old assumptions that fertility was universally lost during transplant (www.cibmtr.org/Data/Available/pages).

The incidence of most hematologic malignancies increases with age in the adult population and, for most diseases, the median age is >50 years, often in the seventh decade of life. The expectation of the Leukemia and Lymphoma Society was that ~140 000 new blood cancers would be diagnosed in 2010 in the USA, which represents < 10% of all new cases of cancer. Approximately 15 000 autologous or allogeneic stem cell transplants were performed in 2009. Thus, while gonadal failure can impact all men undergoing stem cell transplantation, infertility remains an issue for a much smaller population. Nevertheless, even if only for a subpopulation, its effect on quality of life can be very significant for those survivors. Additionally, as the number of survivors increases, the number potentially affected may also increase.

Testes tend to suffer less damage from irradiation and chemotherapy than ovaries, and within the testis, Leydig cells are more resistant to treatment injury than the spermatogonial germ cells. Extensive clinical data have been published and included in reviews that describe the loss of spermatogenesis after therapy for cancer, and after conditioning for HSCT [2–15]. Despite the relatively high incidence of reduced or absent spermatogenesis, however, sex-hormone replacement is often not necessary, being indicated primarily in patients with severe hypogonadism.

The true incidence of infertility after stem cell transplantation is difficult to assess because of the lack of a formal database. Records on the status of fertility pre- and post-transplant are lacking, as are actual birth rates, and a method of tracking the desire of patients to become parents. Fear of relapse and death from the cancer is often difficult to overcome, even among survivors, and contributes to decisions about becoming a parent. Patients often raise concerns about genetic transmission of cancer, or damage to sperm, caused by treatment, potentially producing an abnormal child. Most of the available data, derived from the limited number of studies, are obtained from patients with cancer who received autologous or myeloablative allogeneic HSCTs using the more intensive conditioning regimens [4,16–21]. A smaller proportion of patients in the allogeneic HSCT groups received their transplants for aplastic anemia (a benign hematologic disease). This latter group had not received any significant chemotherapy prior to the transplant, and their conditioning for the transplant was often not myeloablative [18,21,22].

The largest retrospective study was that of Salooja and the Late Effects Working Party of the European Group for Blood and Marrow Transplantation (EBMT) [2]. Two hundred and thirty-two patients from 229 transplant centers and > 37 000 patients who had undergone autologous or allogeneic transplant prior to 1995 reported pregnancies by questionnaire. One hundred and nineteen were partners of male HSCT patients. The distribution of the male patients between allografts and autografts was 93 and 26, respectively. The median age of both groups was approximately 25 years, with a median time from transplant to pregnancy of 65 and 45 months, respectively. A larger proportion of men had received chemotherapy alone than irradiation or a combination of chemotherapy plus irradiation. In the small allograft group (11%) that received irradiation (median dose 10 Gy), 90% conceived naturally. All autograft patients were transplanted for malignant disease, and 81% were <30 years old. The rate of miscarriages and stillbirths was similar to or lower than the England and Wales national average. Furthermore, the rates of congenital anomalies, developmental delay, and malignant disease in the offspring were not higher than that in the general population.

Three recent publications on the incidence of pregnancies are that of the Bone Marrow Transplant Survivor Study (BMTSS), which utilized a mailed survey [3], Hammond et al., a single-center study of patients transplanted between 1987 and 1990 who survived 10 years after a myeloablative transplant [1], and Loren et al., which summarized pregnancies reported to the CIBMTR [4]. There was obvious overlap between the three studies, but the largest cohort of 178 pregnancies (83 pregnancies in female HSCT recipients and 95 in female partners of male HSCT recipients) was described by Loren et al. This study included reports to the CIBMTR from 2002, when a formal request was made to transplant centers to report pregnancies, until 2007. The majority of patients had undergone autologous or myeloablative allogeneic HSCT. Due to the time span of the study and the more recent development of non-myeloablative transplants, the latter group comprised a much smaller number. Information on the use of assisted conception was generally not collected, but a very small number of unassisted conceptions were reported. Interestingly, the BMTSS noted findings similar to those of Salooja et al. [2]: although the incidence of pregnancy in the patient group was lower than that in the sibling control group, survivors did not report any higher incidence of miscarriage or stillbirth than the control group. This again suggested that if conception could be achieved, it generally resulted in a positive outcome.

Fertility in the male patient following HSCT is impacted upon by a variety of factors throughout the phases of diagnosis and treatment. At least two publications have described abnormal semen characteristics in male patients with cancer even prior to receiving therapy for their disease. A single institution's experience in evaluating semen samples in 164 men pre- and post-treatment for lymphoma and leukemia was published by Chung et al. [5]. They found oligospermia in 25% to >50% of men. Van Casteren et al. reported that in 764 men with cancer in the Netherlands, >60% referred for semen cryopreservation prior to

cancer therapy already exhibited abnormal semen characteristics, and in > 10% azoospermia existed [6]. Although the pathophysiology is not well understood, this disruption in spermatogenesis by the cancer is felt to be multifactorial [7], and it certainly may influence the fertility of men undergoing HSCT.

Treatment for the most common diseases for which HSCTs are performed also impact the risk of infertility. The risk from chemotherapy and/or radiation is generally dose-dependent. In the spectrum of chemotherapeutic agents, alkylating agents, commonly used in standard treatment regimens, as well as the conditioning of HSCT, pose the greatest risk of infertility. Two published reviews have developed tables of various groups of chemotherapeutic agents with their potential risk for azoospermia, which can be used as guides in predicting the risk [8,9]. In the majority of patients receiving chemotherapy, however, their regimens include combinations of drugs, and even for a specific disease, different combination regimens may be more or less gonadotoxic. The classic treatment regimen for Hodgkin's disease, for example, which includes mechlorethamine, vinblastine or vincristine, procarbazine, and prednisone (MOPP and MVPP) has been reported in a small group of patients to induce azoospermia in > 85% of men and recovery in less than 25%. On the other hand, the more alternative regimen of doxorubicin, bleomycin, vinblastine, and dacarbazine (ABVD) is less gonadotoxic, with only about a third of patients developing azoospermia and full recovery observed in the majority [10]. For non-Hodgkin's lymphoma, one of the most common treatment regimens is CHOP (cyclophosphamide, doxorubicin, vincristine, and prednisone). This produces a relatively high rate of azoospermia over the first year, but a reported > 65% of patients demonstrate normal sperm counts by five years and > 70% show at least some improvement in sperm count over time [11].

Data relating to the treatment for acute leukemia are generally derived from reports on long-term follow-up of children, with many publications more than a decade old [12]. Very little published information exists for adult patients [13,14]. Several of the reports on children considered therapy for leukemia less gonadotoxic than that for lymphoma, reporting vincristine–prednisone-based regimens for acute lymphocytic leukemia causing a < 20% incidence of gonadal damage [15] and anthracycline-based regimens for acute myeloid leukemia (AML) producing 10% [12,16]. Bahadur et al., however, found even the chemotherapy regimens for leukemia gonadotoxic [14]. Notably, the influence on gonadal function has not been defined for the newer oncologic agents such as fludarabine, monoclonal antibodies, and tyrosine kinase inhibitors.

The association between azoospermia, infertility, and increasing doses of radiation, both local/regional and total-body, has been well known for many years [17]. Many of the factors that impact fertility in the oncology patient receiving therapy are applicable to the HSCT setting. Transplant combines the influence on fertility of chemotherapy and/or radiation and a variety of other pre-transplant and transplant-related factors, often with some controversy due to the limited number of publications and reliable data. Patient and transplant aspects that have been evaluated and shown to be associated with fertility include the patient's age at transplant (< 30 years old has been associated with a greater chance of regaining fertility [18]); the type of disease for which the transplant is performed (patients with non-malignant disease are more likely to recover gonadal function than those transplanted for a malignancy [4,19]); the history of treatment for the disease/tumor prior to transplant (alkylating agents tend to be more toxic to the gonads); the total dose, administration rate, and duration of chemotherapy [9,17]; and the type of transplant, which includes the intensity of the conditioning (myeloablative with total-body irradiation [TBI] produces a higher incidence of permanent infertility [18,20–23]).

Factors such as the source of the graft (autologous vs. allogeneic) and the degree of match of donor stem cells, which determines the need for immunosuppressive medications and the risk of GVHD, remain controversial and are not supported by any definitive clinical reports [18,23,24]. Although the majority of publications find the recovery of spermatogenesis low following a myeloablative transplant, one study, which evaluated it after the classic chemotherapy conditioning of busulfan plus cyclophosphamide in 26 adult men, reported an 80% recovery at a median of five years post-transplant [24]. Melphalan alone or associated with etoposide or cyclophosphamide in HSCT conditioning is compatible with return of fertility in up to 50% of female patients [25], but the effect of high-dose melphalan in the male patient has only been assessed by elevated levels of follicle-stimulating hormone [17]. In autologous HSCT using BEAM (bischlorethylnitrosourea, a.k.a. carmustine, etoposide, cytarabine, melphalan)

conditioning for non-Hodgkin's lymphoma, azoospermia is almost always the rule [21,26,27]. Recovery of spermatogenesis from TBI conditioning regimens has remained no better than ~25%, more often observed in the patients who were younger at the time of transplant and with little previous therapy [18,23]. Nakayama et al. published a clear definition of the development of azoospermia and potential for recovery based on increasing doses of radiation [9]. Interestingly, only three studies have addressed patients treated with a non-myeloablative HSCT for malignant disease, which might have been expected to produce less risk of infertility, given the less intensive conditioning. Two of these publications included only two patients each: the Savani et al. study [28], with near normal sperm counts at the 5–7-year follow-up, who had not demonstrated fertility at the time of reporting, and two male patients in the Loren study [4] who produced pregnancies. A third study evaluated germ cell damage and Leydig cell injury in 32 male recipients (age 23–55 years) of a non-myeloablative transplant using a conditioning of fludarabine, melphalan, and CAMPATH-1H. Measurements of follicle-stimulating hormone, luteinizing hormone, and testosterone levels were obtained pre-transplant and up to 24 months post-transplant [29]. As a group, these patients were felt to have sustained severe damage to the germ cell compartment which was similar to that experienced by patients receiving a myeloablative, autologous transplant with the BEAM regimen.

Summary

In summary, based on the available medical literature today, HSCT can impact on the biologic and psychological aspects of fertility and parenting for the male patient. The severity of this impact to individuals remains somewhat of an open question, which cannot be easily answered because of the lack of quality information that is currently available. Retrospective studies, while providing some statistical information, must be interpreted carefully. Recovery of fertility, measured by parenting, can take several years; it includes recovery of spermatogenesis, psychological aspects of survivorship, desire to be a parent, and partner fertility potential issues. Most studies have suggested that the longer the time that has elapsed from transplant before the analysis is performed, the better the numbers will be.

Since cancer diagnostics, therapy, and approaches to HSCT can change significantly in as little as a few years, results from such retrospective studies may not be applicable to the management of patients at the time of the publication. As an example, there are insufficient follow-up data on patients who have received non-myeloablative transplant regimens, a common form of transplant today, to determine if it will preserve fertility better than myeloablative regimens, if parenting is used as the measure of fertility. Biologic evaluation of patients as well as evaluation of patients' understanding of the counseling and educational materials provided on this aspect of care should be included in clinical trials, prospectively. In this way the impact of current practice can be evaluated in a more useful time frame. Based on the variability of information in the literature regarding the impact of chemotherapies and combination regimens, patients who have received treatment for their cancer and are proceeding to transplant should not necessarily be considered infertile. Whenever possible, consideration should be given to counseling and collection of sperm for cryopreservation in all appropriate cases prior to initiating anticancer therapy. When delaying therapy may risk a poor outcome for the patient, counseling should still be provided, but collection of sperm should be entertained when the patient is in remission prior to transplant. For those patients from whom sperm cannot be obtained, newer urologic techniques may provide an option for parenting.

References

1. Hammond C, Abrams JR, Syrjala KL. Fertility and risk factors for elevated infertility concern in 10-year hematopoietic cell transplant survivors and case-matched controls. *J Clin Oncol* 2007; 25: 3511–7.

2. Salooja N. Pregnancy outcomes after peripheral blood or bone marrow transplantation: a retrospective survey. *Lancet* 2001; 358: 271–6.

3. Carter A. Prevalence of conception and pregnancy outcomes after hematopoietic cell transplantation: report from the Bone Marrow Transplant Survivor Study. *Bone Marrow Transplant* 2006; 37: 1023–9.

4. Loren A, Chow E, Jacobsohn D, *et al.* Pregnancy after hematopoietic cell transplantation: a report from the late effects working committee of the Center for International Blood and Marrow Transplant Research (CIBMTR). *Biol Blood Marrow Transplant* 2011; 17: 157–66.

5. Chung K, Irani J, Knee G, *et al.* Sperm cryopreservation for male patients with cancer: an epidemiological analysis at the University of Pennsylvania. *Eur J Obst Gynecol Reprod Biol* 2004; 113: S7–S11.

6. van Casteren N, Boellaard W, Romijn J, Dohle GR. Gonadal dysfunction in male cancer patients before cytotoxic treatment. *Int J Androl* 2010; 33: 73–9.

7. Agarwal A, Allamaneni SSR. Disruption of spermatogenesis by the cancer disease process. *J Natl Cancer Inst Monogr* 2005; 34: 9–12.

8. Trottmann M, Becker AJ, Stadler T, *et al.* Semen quality in men with malignant diseases before and after therapy and the role of cryopreservation. *Eur Urol* 2007; 52: 355–67.

9. Nakayama K, Milbourne A, Schover L, Champlin R, Ueno N. Gonadal failure after treatment of hematologic malignancies: from recognition to management for health-care providers. *Nat Clin Pract Oncol* 2008; 5: 78–89.

10. Viviani S. Gonadal toxicity after combination chemotherapy for Hodgkin's disease. Comparative results of MOPP vs ABVD. *Eur J Cancer Clin Oncol* 1985; 21: 601–5.

11. Pryzant RM. Long-term reduction in sperm count after chemotherapy with and without radiation therapy for non-Hodgkin's lymphomas. *J Clin Oncol* 1993; 11: 239–47.

12. Leung W. Late effects of treatment in survivors of childhood acute myeloid leukemia. *J Clin Oncol* 2000; 18: 3273–9.

13. Lemez P, Urbnek V. Chemotherapy for acute myeloid leukemias with cytosine arabinoside, daunorubicin, etoposide, and mitoxantrone may cause permanent oligoasthenozoospermia or amenorrhea in middle-aged patients. *Neoplasma* 2005; 52: 398–401.

14. Bahadur G, Ozturk O, Muneer A, *et al.* Semen quality before and after gonadotoxic treatment. *Hum Reprod* 2005; 20: 774–81.

15. Wallace WH. Male fertility in long-term survivors of childhood acute lymphoblastic leukaemia. *Int J Androl* 1991; 14: 312–9.

16. Waxman J. Gonadal function in men treated for acute leukaemia. *Br Med J* (Clin Res Ed) 1983; 287: 1093–4.

17. Howell S, Shalet S. Spermatogenesis after cancer treatment: damage and recovery. *J Natl Cancer Inst Monogr* 2005; 34: 12–17.

18. Rovo A, Tichelli A, Passweg JR, *et al.* Spermatogenesis in long-term survivors after allogeneic hematopoietic stem cell transplantation is associated with age, time interval since transplantation, and apparently absence of chronic GvHD. *Blood* 2006; 108: 1100–5.

19. Sanders J, Hawley J, Levy W, *et al.* Pregnancies following high-dose cyclophosphamide with or without high dose busulfan or total-body irradiation

and bone marrow transplantation. *Blood* 1996; 87: 3045–52.

20. Sanders JE. Late effects on gonadal function of cyclophosphamide, total-body irradiation, and marrow transplantation. *Transplantation* 1983; 36: 252–5.

21. Jacob A. Recovery of spermatogenesis following bone marrow transplantation. *Bone Marrow Transplant* 1998; 22: 277–9.

22. Anserini P, Chiodi S, Spinelli S, *et al.* Semen analysis following allogeneic bone marrow transplantation. Additional data for evidence-based counselling. *Bone Marrow Transplant* 2002; 30: 447–51.

23. Savani BN, Kozanas E, Shenoy A, *et al.* Recovery of spermatogenesis after total-body irradiation. *Blood* 2006; 108: 4292–4.

24. Grigg AP, McLachlan R, Zaja J, Szer J. Reproductive status in long-term bone marrow transplant survivors receiving busulfan-cyclophosphamide (120 mg/kg). *Bone Marrow Transplant* 2000; 26: 1089–95.

25. Jackson GH, Wood A, Taylor PR, *et al.* Early high dose chemotherapy intensification with autologous bone marrow transplantation in lymphoma associated with retention of fertility and normal pregnancies in females. Scotland and Newcastle Lymphoma Group, UK. *Leuk Lymphoma* 1997; 28: 127–32.

26. Socie G, Salooja N, Cohen A, *et al.* Nonmalignant late effects after allogeneic stem cell transplantation. *Blood* 2003; 101: 3373–85.

27. Chatterjee R, Mills W, Katz M, McGarrigle HH, Goldstone AH. Germ cell failure and Leydig cell insufficiency in post-pubertal males after autologous bone marrow transplantation with BEAM for lymphoma. *Bone Marrow Transplant* 1994; 13: 519–22.

28. Savani B, Kozanas E, Shenoy A, Barrett AJ. Recovery of spermatogenesis after total-body irradiation. *Blood* 2006; 108: 4292–3.

29. Kyriacou C, Kottaridis PD, Eliahoo J, *et al.* Germ cell damage and Leydig cell insufficiency in recipients of nonmyeloablative transplantation for haematological malignancies. *Bone Marrow Transplant* 2003; 31: 45–50.

Chapter

17

Fertility preservation in men with germ cell tumors

Matthew T. Roberts and Keith Jarvi

Introduction

The vast majority of testicular cancers are germ cell tumors (GCTs), with approximately half being seminomas (SGCTs) and the remainder being non-seminomatous germ cell tumors (NSGCTs) [1]. Testicular cancer overall is an uncommon malignancy and accounts for only 1–2% of all cancer diagnoses [2]. It is, however, the most common solid malignancy in men aged 15–34 years, and its incidence is increasing worldwide [1]. Thus, testicular cancer affects men during their prime reproductive years, and both the disease and its treatment have important implications for a man's fertility. Cancer survivors have reported that loss of fertility can be as disturbing as facing the original cancer diagnosis, and both men and women suffer a great deal of stress when dealing with infertility following cancer treatment [3]. With overall survival exceeding 90% [4], the impacts of treatment on the future health and quality of life of patients with testicular cancer has become increasingly important, and many men may wish to become fathers after successful treatment.

It has long been recognized that men presenting with testicular GCTs often have abnormal semen parameters and compromised fertility, even prior to initiation of cytotoxic therapy [5]. Of all malignancies, testicular cancer appears to have the most profound negative effect on semen quality, with over 50% of men with GCTs possessing semen parameters that fall below the WHO reference standards [6]. In addition, men seeking evaluation for infertility are at higher risk of subsequently developing testicular cancer, with men possessing a "male factor" for infertility having three times the risk of developing cancer when compared to age-matched controls [7].

How is testicular cancer related to male infertility? This could be due to:

(1) a common etiology for both cancer and infertility,
(2) the negative impact of testis cancer itself on fertility, and/or
(3) the negative effect of cancer therapy on fertility.

The association between infertility and testicular cancer may be due to a common etiology. Congenital conditions such as cryptorchidism or the testicular dysgenesis syndrome [8] are associated with both infertility and testicular cancer, and exposure to gonadal toxins and trauma can lead to both altered spermatogenesis and tumorigenesis [5].

In addition to a common etiology, it has also been well described that testicular cancer itself may have a negative impact on semen parameters and male fertility. Tumors can have local effects within the testicle that impair spermatogenesis, likely through disruption of local testicular architecture and possibly local effects (increased heat and local hormone effects); higher-stage GCTs (locally within the testicle) are associated with worse semen quality then lower-stage GCTs [9], and spermatogenesis seems to be most impaired in the testicular tissue that is adjacent to the tumor itself [10]. Malignancy in general, and testicular cancer in particular, could have systemic effects mediated through cytokines and metabolic derangements. These systemic derangements can have negative impacts on spermatogenesis, and the negative impact seems to be greater with higher clinical stages of cancer [11]. Finally, many GCTs are hormonally active and produce beta-human chorionic gonadotropin (β-hCG) and alpha-fetoprotein (AFP). These substances can disrupt spermatogenesis both through paracrine mechanisms

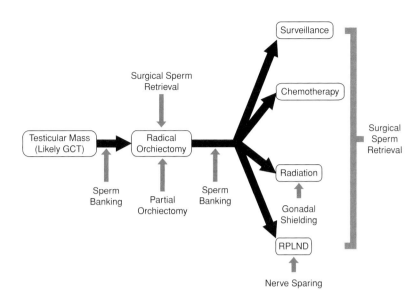

Figure 17.1. Strategies for fertility preservation along the continuum of care of the testicular cancer patient. GCT, germ cell tumor; RPLND, retroperitoneal lymph node dissection.

at the testicular level and by altering the function of the hypothalamic–pituitary–gonadal (HPG) axis, resulting in reduced spermatogenesis [12,13].

In addition, the treatments for testicular cancer could have negative impacts on future fertility. Initial treatment of a suspected GCT is radical orchiectomy, which is often followed by chemotherapy, radiation, retroperitoneal lymph node dissection (RPLND), or a combination of the above. All of these therapies, as described below, can temporarily or permanently affect a man's fertility.

Fertility preservation in patients with testicular cancer

The cornerstone of fertility preservation in male cancer patients remains cryopreservation of sperm prior to the institution of cytotoxic therapy. In testicular cancer, treatment often occurs in multiple stages with different potential impacts on fertility, and thus there are multiple time points at which fertility preservation can be pursued during the therapeutic process. The multiple stages of treatment of testicular cancer, and the methods through which fertility preservation can be achieved, are depicted in Fig. 17.1.

In addition, modifications to some of the treatment modalities, such as orchiectomy and RPLND, may be made in order to minimize the impact of treatment on fertility.

Sperm banking prior to cancer therapy

Cryopreservation of sperm remains the mainstay of fertility preservation in men with cancer. The American Society of Clinical Oncology recommends that sperm banking be offered to all male cancer patients prior to the initiation of cancer therapy [14]. With advances in assisted reproductive technologies (ART) such as in-vitro fertilization with intracytoplasmic sperm injection (IVF-ICSI), even low numbers of cryopreserved sperm may be used to establish pregnancies, and although some sperm may not survive the freezing and thawing process, long-term survival and recovery of sperm function has been reported [15]. With IVF-ICSI, a single sperm can be injected into an egg to produce a viable embryo. Furthermore, IVF-ICSI cycles using post-thawed sperm have been proven to be safe and effective [16].

There are many options to obtain sperm from men with cancer:

(1) Masturbation. The most common method to provide a semen specimen is by masturbation into a sterile container. Typically three semen collections are recommended, with 24–48 hours of abstinence between collections if feasible. However, in men with very low sperm counts, or in whom multiple collections are not possible due to urgent initiation of cancer treatment, collecting and preserving even a single semen sample is still important.

(2) Semen collection devices. In men whose semen cannot be obtained by masturbation, a seminal collection device can be used to collect sperm during sexual intercourse. This is a special condom without spermicidal agents, which men may use if they are unable or unwilling to provide a semen specimen by masturbation.

(3) Vibrostimulation or electroejaculation. For patients with anejaculation due to neurogenic (spinal cord injury) or psychogenic etiologies, penile vibratory stimulation (PVS) and/or electroejaculation (EEJ) may be used to obtain sperm [17].

(4) Treatment of retrograde ejaculation. In men with retrograde ejaculation, medical therapy (sympathomimetics such as pseudoephedrine) may be used to induce antegrade ejaculation, or sperm could be isolated from the bladder with previously alkalinized urine.

(5) Failure of emission. As above, medical therapy may be used to induce antegrade ejaculation or convert a failure of emission into retrograde ejaculation. If this fails, sperm may be retrieved from the testicles or epididymis.

(6) Finally, for men with obstructive azoospermia or where all of the above techniques have failed, sperm may be retrieved surgically from the testicle or epididymis by either a percutaneous or an open sperm aspiration or testicular biopsy prior to cancer treatment [18].

Utilization of sperm banking by men with testicular cancer

Recent reports suggest that only 40% of eligible patients bank sperm prior to therapy for testicular cancer [19]. While sperm banking for most men is a relatively simple process, various factors may influence a patient's decision to store sperm. Younger men, and those without children at the time of testicular cancer diagnosis, are more likely to bank sperm [20]. Some men are not aware of the potential impact of the therapy on their fertility, or they may not believe that their particular type of therapy will have an adverse impact on fertility [21]. Storage fees for cryopreservation are often not covered by health insurance plans, and the cost burden often lies with the patient to bear. Also, it has been reported that only 10% of men who have banked sperm prior to cancer treatment ever use it in the future [22–25]. Finally, some men are unable or unwilling to produce samples for various reasons.

Use of cryopreserved sperm

Numerous studies have been published concerning fertility rates with the usage of cryopreserved sperm in cancer patients. A recent Canadian study demonstrated a 20% pregnancy rate per cycle of intrauterine insemination (IUI) and 50% pregnancy rate per cycle of IVF-ICSI using cryopreserved sperm from cancer patients [26]. Testicular cancer patients had similar pregnancy rates as compared to patients with all other types of cancer. Thus, sperm cryopreservation should be offered to testicular cancer patients prior to initiation of treatment. Cancer patients who eventually use cryopreserved sperm to establish a pregnancy have fertility outcomes comparable to other patients who make use of ART.

Partial orchiectomy: fertility-sparing approaches

The standard initial therapy for testicular masses consistent with testicular GCT is radical orchiectomy. This provides histological confirmation of malignancy and subtype as well as local therapy for the primary tumor. However, in patients with a tumor in a solitary testicle or who present with bilateral testicular tumors, radical orchiectomy results in anorchia and obviously prevents future fertility. In addition, it has now become clear that many small testicular masses (typically < 1 cm, non-palpable, incidentally detected) are benign and do not require radical treatment [27]. As a result, partial orchiectomy has been proposed as an alternative to radical orchiectomy in situations where radical orchiectomy would lead to anorchia or where there is a high likelihood of a benign lesion.

There are several concerns regarding the risks of partial orchiectomy in men with GCTs. Intratubular germ cell neoplasia (ITGCN) is a premalignant lesion of the testicle, and is much more common in men with testicular GCTs, particularly in the testicle affected by the primary tumor [28]. There is a 50–70% risk of progression to invasive GCT within 5–7 years of diagnosis of ITGCN [29]. In addition, testicular GCTs (particularly seminomas) may be multifocal in up to 63% of cases [30]. Thus, leaving a portion of the affected testicle in situ after partial orchiectomy may put patients at risk of future local recurrence of disease. However, a large series of 73 patients undergoing partial orchiectomy for GCT in a solitary testicle or bilateral GCTs demonstrated that 98.6% remained disease-free at a mean of 91 months following surgery [31]. Some have advocated adjuvant radiation or chemotherapy following partial orchiectomy, particularly in patients with ITGCN present in the affected testicle. However, both radiation and chemotherapy could impact spermatogenesis and androgen production within the testicle and thus may compromise the fertility-preserving goals of partial orchiectomy.

Current guidelines recommend that partial orchiectomy be reserved for suspected GCTs in a solitary testicle, or bilateral GCTs [32]. In addition, the tumors most amenable are small (< 2 cm) and polar in location. Partial orchiectomy should not be performed if a normal contralateral testicle is present.

Another application of partial orchiectomy is in the setting of small, sub-centimetre, non-palpable testicular masses. While reports now support that the majority of these lesions are benign and can safely be followed with ultrasound after initial evaluation with serum tumor markers [27], excision is often performed because of concerns regarding malignancy and patient/surgeon anxiety.

In either case (GCT or small testis mass), standard oncologic principles should be followed [32]. The testicle is delivered through an inguinal incision as in a radical orchiectomy. The spermatic cord is clamped or occluded and the testicle is cooled. The tumor is then excised with a margin of healthy tissue. The mass is sent for frozen section examination (FSE), and multiple biopsies of the remaining testicular parenchyma are also taken to exclude residual tumor or ITGCN. If the surgical margins are negative for malignancy, the tunica albuginea is closed and the testicle is returned to the scrotum. Final pathology must be reviewed to determine whether to provide adjuvant treatment with radiation, chemotherapy, or completion orchiectomy, since FSE is unreliable for the detection of ITGCN [33].

For elective partial orchiectomy in small, likely benign masses, the same principles are followed. Intra-operative ultrasound, with or without needle localization, can be used if the lesion is not palpable. In addition, use of the operating microscope has been described in order to aid the dissection and preserve maximum amounts of healthy tissue [34]. The lesion is sent for FSE. If benign then the testicle can be closed and returned to the scrotum, and if malignant then radical orchiectomy should be performed if there is a normal contralateral testicle. If the patient has presented with azoospermia in conjunction with the testis mass then concurrent surgical sperm retrieval through testicular sperm extraction (TESE) or microTESE can be performed on the testicle undergoing partial orchiectomy (see detailed description in subsequent section).

Thus, partial orchiectomy is a viable method for fertility preservation in selected patients with GCTs or small testis masses, particularly when radical orchiectomy would result in anorchia. The benefits must be weighed against the risks of tumor recurrence, and treatment should be individualized after a detailed discussion with the patient.

Sperm retrieval at the time of orchiectomy

It is estimated that up to 50% of men with testicular cancer have abnormal semen parameters prior to any treatment [6], and 10–15% may be completely azoospermic at presentation [35,36]. In men with azoospermia, sperm banking from an ejaculated sample (or from PVS or EEJ) is obviously not possible. Traditionally, men with testicular cancer and azoospermia have undergone radical orchiectomy and subsequent chemo- or radiotherapy without any option for fertility preservation. However, since the introduction of IVF-ICSI, these men do now have the option of undergoing a surgical sperm retrieval at the time of radical orchiectomy and cryopreservation of sperm for later use with IVF-ICSI.

Delouya et al. demonstrated that mature sperm are present in the testicular tissue of radical orchiectomy specimens in up to 80% of cases, and are present in the epididymis in 50% of cases [37]. This study, however, did not correlate these findings with semen parameters, and the likelihood of finding sperm in the cancerous testicle of men with azoospermia is unknown.

Several case reports have demonstrated successful sperm retrieval from the cancerous testicle in men with azoospermia at the time of radical orchiectomy [38–41]. In this setting, sperm retrieval has been most widely reported through multiple microsurgical biopsies (microTESE) of the testicular tissue surrounding the tumor. This can be done with the spermatic cord clamped and the testicle cooled prior to excision of the testicle, although most authorities utilize a sterile "back-bench" immediately following radical orchiectomy in an effort to avoid in-vivo tumor spillage. Attempts to retrieve sperm from the epididymis and vas deferens of the orchiectomy specimen in azoospermic men have also been successful [39]. Finally, live births using cryopreserved sperm from orchiectomy specimens in conjunction with IVF-ICSI have been reported [41].

Sperm may also be retrieved from the contralateral, non-cancerous testicle at the time of orchiectomy. Six of fourteen azoospermic patients undergoing routine contralateral testis biopsy to exclude ITGCN had sperm identified and cryopreserved for later use with ICSI [18]. The need for contralateral testicular biopsy to exclude ITGCN in men with unilateral testis cancer is controversial, and carries with it risks of testicular damage as well as potential tumor seeding and violation of lymphatic drainage planes. While microTESE of the non-cancerous testicle either at the time of radical orchiectomy or prior to adjuvant chemo- or radiotherapy is an option for some men, a number of these men will note an improvement in semen parameters after orchiectomy, and thus (if time permits) observation with repeat semen analysis is an alternative option.

Thus, surgical sperm retrieval and cryopreservation in men presenting with azoospermia is feasible at the time of radical orchiectomy and has yielded successful live births after ICSI. Currently there are no known predictors of successful sperm retrieval in this setting. Furthermore, it has been shown that some men with azoospermia and unilateral testicular cancer will have a return of sperm to the ejaculate following radical orchiectomy [42]. Thus, when counseling azoospermic men with testicular cancer, the advantages of sperm retrieval at the time of radical orchiectomy (avoiding the need for future sperm retrieval procedures, cryopreserving sperm prior to cytotoxic therapy) must be weighed against the disadvantages (financial cost, risks of contralateral testicular biopsy, chance of spontaneous return of sperm to the ejaculate). Finally, these men should be investigated with hormonal and genetic evaluations to detect alternative causes of azoospermia.

Fertility preservation following radical orchiectomy

If possible, men should cryopreserve ejaculated sperm prior to radical orchiectomy, or if they are azoospermic consider surgical sperm retrieval at the time of orchiectomy. However, the timeline from diagnosis of a testicular mass to radical orchiectomy is often short, and patients with metastases may be systemically unwell. Patients may thus not have sufficient time prior to radical orchiectomy to cryopreserve sperm, or may not be psychologically prepared to contemplate sperm banking while coping with a new cancer diagnosis.

Following radical orchiectomy there are four general treatment options for patients, depending on tumor type (seminoma versus NSGCT) and stage: surveillance, radiation therapy, chemotherapy, or RPLND. Radiation, chemotherapy, and RPLND can all negatively affect fertility, and fertility preservation, ideally through sperm cryopreservation, should be offered prior to the institution of these treatments.

Surveillance

Surveillance following radical orchiectomy for GCT is an option for patients with stage 1 disease who have a low risk of metastases. The rationale for this approach comes from the findings that (1) many patients will never have a cancer recurrence following orchiectomy alone, (2) all adjuvant treatments (radiation, chemotherapy, and RPLND) have potential short- and long-term toxicities including negative impacts on fertility, and (3) patients who do have cancer recurrence while on surveillance may be salvaged with delayed treatment [5].

Surveillance itself does not pose any threat to fertility, and in patients who do not have cancer recurrence semen parameters may actually improve following orchiectomy. It has been estimated that up to 50% of men with abnormal semen parameters prior to orchiectomy will become normospermic following orchiectomy [43], and some patients with azoospermia may have return of sperm to the ejaculate [42].

Radiation

Radiation therapy is indicated for the treatment of patients with low-stage seminoma who are not candidates for surveillance or who have low-volume retroperitoneal metastases. As with chemotherapy, radiation can have both short- and long-term impacts on fertility. Spermatogenesis is exquisitely sensitive to radiation, and impairment of spermatogenesis is thought to occur with testicular doses as low as 10 cGy [44]. Typical testicular doses received during infradiaphragmatic radiation for seminoma can range from

28 to 90 cGy [45], and thus transient declines in sperm counts are typically seen immediately following radiotherapy. Most patients recover by 2–3 years following radiation, with 56% of men having normal sperm counts [45,46]. Poor pre-treatment semen parameters are associated with less chance of recovery following radiation [46], but cumulative dose does not seem to be a major factor in contemporary series [47].

The main methods used to reduce the toxicity of radiation on the remaining testicle are gonadal shielding and reduction of radiation field size. Currently, for stage 1 seminoma, radiation is delivered to the para-aortic region only, without pelvic extension. All patients, regardless of radiation field, receive gonadal shielding unless the testicle is purposely being radiated due to the presence of ITGCN. While these methods do reduce the radiation dose to the testicle, some radiation is still absorbed by the testicle, and this can affect spermatogenesis [5]. Thus, all patients should be offered sperm cryopreservation prior to radiation therapy for testicular cancer.

Chemotherapy

Chemotherapy is administered to patients with NSGCTs who are at high risk of retroperitoneal metastases despite organ-confined disease, and to patients with seminoma and NSGCTs who have bulky retroperitoneal metastases or distant metastases. The most common chemotherapy regimens are EP or the combination bleomycin–etoposide–cisplatin (BEP), and its use has led to significant improvements in survival as compared to older regimens. However, BEP can affect fertility potential in the short and long term following administration. Endocrine dysfunction, as evidenced by elevated levels of follicle-stimulating hormone (FSH) and luteinizing hormone (LH), occurs in up to 89% of men with NSGCT following BEP and can persist for up to two years and beyond [48]. Spermatogenesis is also significantly affected by BEP. Abnormal semen parameters are present in 35–50% of men at 1–2 years following conventional BEP chemotherapy [4,49], and azoospermia is present in approximately 20% at 2 years following BEP [4]. Despite these short-term impacts of BEP on spermatogenesis, up to 80% of men will have an improvement in semen parameters five years following therapy, and 58% will have completely normal semen parameters [4]. However, higher rates of permanent azoospermia and oligospermia are seen in patients with lower pre-treatment sperm concentration, age over 30, and

those receiving higher-dose chemotherapy, cisplatin rather than carboplatin, or combination chemotherapy and radiotherapy [4,48]. The paternity rate in men receiving chemotherapy has been reported as 67%, compared to 85% in men on surveillance alone [50].

Thus, despite the fact that the majority of men do not have permanent azoospermia following chemotherapy, many can have temporary or permanent impairment in spermatogenesis, and paternity rates are lower than among testicular cancer patients who never received chemotherapy. In addition, while there is no proof of higher rates of birth defects in the offspring of men treated with chemotherapy, there is concern of higher rates of sperm aneuploidy in the first 1–2 years following treatment [51], and men are often counseled not to establish a pregnancy during this time period. For these reasons, all men should be offered sperm cryopreservation prior to chemotherapy. Chemotherapy regimens are typically not altered in order to reduce the impacts on spermatogenesis (such as by substituting carboplatin for cisplatin) since efficacy may be compromised, and thus the focus must be on preserving fertility prior to chemotherapy treatment.

Are there any effective methods to protect the testis from the gonadotoxic effects of chemotherapy? Gonadal protection with hormonal suppression has been proposed as one method of preserving fertility during chemotherapy. Various methods of suppressing the HPG axis have been attempted, and the concept is to induce a quiescent state in the testes (i.e., prevent spermatogenesis temporarily) in order to protect these rapidly dividing cells from the effects of chemotherapy. Small trials using luteinizing hormone-releasing hormone (LHRH) agonists, testosterone, or a combination have been conducted in patients receiving chemotherapy for Hodgkin's disease and GCTs, and radiation for seminoma [52,53]. While in most cases successful suppression of the HPG axis was achieved, there is no convincing evidence of benefit in terms of overall recovery or time to recovery of hormonal function or spermatogenesis compared to control patients. Therefore, gonadal suppression is not routinely used.

Retroperitoneal lymph node dissection

Retroperitoneal lymph node dissection (RPLND) is indicated following orchiectomy in patients with NSGCTs who (1) have low-volume retroperitoneal nodal metastases or (2) are at high risk of metastases despite a clinically localized primary tumor (termed "primary RPLND"). In addition, RPLND can be performed to resect residual retroperitoneal masses following chemotherapy for metastatic NSGCTs and occasionally seminomas (termed "post-chemotherapy RPLND"). RPLND involves complete removal of the lymph node tissue surrounding the aorta and vena cava, and this is the same region where the postganglionic sympathetic nerve fibers that control ejaculation are located. Thus, undergoing RPLND puts the man at risk of developing ejaculatory dysfunction postoperatively. Ejaculatory dysfunction following RPLND can be in the form of retrograde ejaculation or complete failure of emission, and is usually permanent if it occurs [54]. Ejaculatory dysfunction alone can impair future fertility, or can further compound the effects of preexisting spermatogenetic dysfunction and the cytotoxic effects of previous chemotherapy and radiation.

Traditional RPLND, which involves complete resection of all retroperitoneal lymphatic tissue including the postganglionic sympathetic nerves, results in ejaculatory dysfunction in nearly 100% of patients [55]. Patients with low-stage NSGCTs undergoing RPLND, and even those treated successfully with chemotherapy prior to RPLND, have survival rates in excess of 90%. Thus, efforts have been made to minimize the impact of RPLND on ejaculatory dysfunction and subsequent fertility. Two main modifications to the surgical technique have been described in order to achieve this goal: modified-template RPLND and nerve-sparing RPLND.

Modified-template RPLND involves modifying the boundaries of the surgical dissection in order to avoid the region where the sympathetic nerves controlling ejaculation travel [56]. Modified-template RPLND can result in preservation of ejaculation in 51–88% of patients. Higher rates of preservation of ejaculation likely occur for right-sided dissections, and for primary versus post-chemotherapy RPLND.

The most recent modification to the RPLND procedure involves prospectively identifying and preserving the postganglionic nerve fibers in the retroperitoneum, so-called "nerve-sparing RPLND" [57]. In nerve-sparing RPLND the borders of dissection may be wide and include all of the retroperitoneal lymphatic tissue surrounding the sympathetic nerves, but the nerves themselves are not cut. This procedure can be performed during both primary and post-chemotherapy RPLND. Most modern series demonstrate high rates of preservation of antegrade ejaculation when nerve sparing is performed, with some authors reporting preservation of antegrade ejaculation in 99% of patients [57].

Thus, modification to the surgical technique of RPLND can result in successful preservation of ejaculation, and should be considered in all men undergoing RPLND who wish to preserve their future fertility. In the setting of primary nerve-sparing RPLND, where patients have not received prior chemotherapy, paternity rates with natural intercourse have been reported to be as high as 73% [57], and a smaller percentage of men may require the use of assisted reproductive technologies (ART) such as intrauterine insemination (IUI) or in-vitro fertilization with intracytoplasmic sperm injection (IVF-ICSI).

A detailed description of the management of retrograde ejaculation or anejaculation is beyond the scope of this chapter. However, conversion of retrograde ejaculation to antegrade ejaculation following RPLND has been reported with the use of imipramine [56]. Patients with retrograde ejaculation may also have sperm retrieved from the urine following oral alkalinization for use with IUI or IVF-ICSI. Finally, when failure of emission occurs and does not respond to pharmacotherapy (sympathomimetics: see below), surgical sperm retrieval through percutaneous epididymal sperm extraction (PESA) or testicular sperm extraction (TESE) can be performed in conjunction with IVF-ICSI.

Re-establishing fertility following cytotoxic treatment

While fertility preservation should be offered to patients prior to the institution of cytotoxic treatment, some patients do not have the time or opportunity to take advantage of it, and in many cases the option is never discussed by the treating physician [14]. As described in previous sections, most men do recover spermatogenesis following chemotherapy and radiation, but due to uncertainties about persistent effects on sperm DNA and ploidy, paternity should be delayed for 1–2 years following cytotoxic therapy.

In the past, patients who remained azoospermic following treatment and did not have any sperm cryopreserved were unable to have biologically related children. However, the newest technologies allow us to offer even these men reproductive choices.

With modern sperm retrieval techniques such as micro-testicular sperm extraction (microTESE), several authors have demonstrated successful sperm retrieval and subsequent pregnancy via ICSI from men who have had chemotherapy. Sperm retrieval rates in this setting are approximately 50% [58–60]. However, the long-term outcomes and health of children born through this method are not known.

Men with ejaculatory dysfunction following RPLND who have not cryopreserved sperm have several options in order to restore fertility. Sympathomimetics such as pseudoephedrine and imipramine can be utilized [61] (see Chapter 9). When oral agents are unsuccessful, electroejaculation can lead to successful semen collection in up to 70% of men following RPLND [17]. Finally, surgical sperm retrieval with testicular sperm extraction (TESE) can be employed in order to obtain sufficient sperm for IVF-ICSI [61].

Conclusion

Men with testicular cancer may suffer from infertility as a consequence of both the disease and its treatment. There are multiple options for fertility preservation in men with testicular cancer, and all clinicians who treat men with testicular cancer should be aware of these methods in order to provide appropriate counseling to patients. In complex cases where sperm banking is not possible, the involvement of a male fertility specialist/urologist is critical in order to provide advanced fertility preservation options.

References

1. Manecksha RP, Fitzpatrick JM. Epidemiology of testicular cancer. *BJU Int* 2009; 104: 1329–33.

2. Bosl GJ, Motzer RJ. Testicular germ-cell cancer. *N Engl J Med* 1997; 337: 242–53.

3. Schover LR. Motivation for parenthood after cancer: a review. *J Natl Cancer Inst Monogr* 2005; 34: 2–5.

4. Lampe H, Horwich A, Norman A, Nicholls J, Dearnaley DP. Fertility after chemotherapy for testicular germ cell cancers. *J Clin Oncol* 1997; 15: 239–45.

5. Lambert SM, Fisch H. Infertility and testis cancer. *Urol Clin North Am* 2007; 34: 269–77, xi.

6. Williams DH, Karpman E, Sander JC, *et al.* Pretreatment semen parameters in men with cancer. *J Urol* 2009; 181: 736–40.

7. Walsh TJ, Croughan MS, Schembri M, Chan JM, Turek PJ. Increased risk of testicular germ cell cancer among infertile men. *Arch Intern Med* 2009; 169: 351–6.

8. Wohlfahrt-Veje C, Main KM, Skakkebaek NE. Testicular dysgenesis syndrome: foetal origin of adult reproductive problems. *Clin Endocrinol* 2009; 71: 459–65.

9. Agarwal A, Tolentino MV, Sidhu RS, *et al.* Effect of cryopreservation on semen quality in patients with testicular cancer. *Urology* 1995; 46: 382–9.

10. Ho GT, Gardner H, Mostofi K, *et al.* The effect of testicular nongerm cell tumors on local spermatogenesis. *Fertil Steril* 1994; 62: 162–6.

11. Rueffer U, Breuer K, Josting A, *et al.* Male gonadal dysfunction in patients with Hodgkin's disease prior to treatment. *Ann Oncol* 2001; 12: 1307–11.

12. Hayashi T, Arai G, Hyochi N, *et al.* Suppression of spermatogenesis in ipsilateral and contralateral testicular tissues in patients with seminoma by human chorionic gonadotropin beta subunit. *Urology* 2001; 58: 251–7.

13. Hansen PV, Trykker H, Andersen J, Helkjaer PE. Germ cell function and hormonal status in patients with testicular cancer. *Cancer* 1989; 64: 956–61.

14. Lee SJ, Schover LR, Partridge AH, *et al.* American Society of Clinical Oncology recommendations on fertility preservation in cancer patients. *J Clin Oncol* 2006; 24: 2917–31.

15. Clarke GN, Liu de Y, Baker HW. Recovery of human sperm motility and ability to interact with the human zona pellucida after more than 28 years of storage in liquid nitrogen. *Fertil Steril* 2006; 86: 721–2.

16. Kuczynski W, Dhont M, Grygoruk C, *et al.* The outcome of intracytoplasmic injection of fresh and cryopreserved ejaculated spermatozoa: a prospective randomized study. *Hum Reprod* 2001; 16: 2109–13.

17. Ohl DA, Denil J, Bennett CJ, *et al.* Electroejaculation following retroperitoneal lymphadenectomy. *J Urol* 1991; 145: 980–3.

18. Schrader M, Muller M, Sofikitis N, *et al.* "Onco-tese": testicular sperm extraction in azoospermic cancer patients before chemotherapy-new guidelines? *Urology* 2003; 61: 421–5.

19. Magelssen H, Haugen TB, von During V, *et al.* Twenty years experience with semen cryopreservation in testicular cancer patients: who needs it? *Eur Urol* 2005; 48: 779–85.

20. Girasole CR, Cookson MS, Smith JA, Jr., *et al.* Sperm banking: use and outcomes in patients treated for testicular cancer. *BJU Int* 2007; 99: 33–6.

21. Achille MA, Rosberger Z, Robitaille R, *et al.* Facilitators and obstacles to sperm banking in young

men receiving gonadotoxic chemotherapy for cancer: the perspective of survivors and health care professionals. *Hum Reprod* 2006; 21: 3206–16.

22. Sanger WG, Olson JH, Sherman JK. Semen cryobanking for men with cancer: criteria change. *Fertil Steril* 1992; 58: 1024–7.

23. Audrins P, Holden CA, McLachlan RI, Kovacs GT. Semen storage for special purposes at Monash IVF from 1977 to 1997. *Fertil Steril* 1999; 72: 179–81.

24. Blackhall FH, Atkinson AD, Maaya MB, *et al.* Semen cryopreservation, utilisation and reproductive outcome in men treated for Hodgkin's disease. *Br J Cancer* 2002; 87: 381–4.

25. Agarwal A, Ranganathan P, Kattal N, *et al.* Fertility after cancer: a prospective review of assisted reproductive outcome with banked semen specimens. *Fertil Steril* 2004; 81: 342–8.

26. Selk A, Belej-Rak T, Shapiro H, Greenblatt E. Use of an oncology sperm bank: a Canadian experience. *Can Urol Assoc J* 2009; 3: 219–22.

27. Toren PJ, Roberts M, Lecker I, *et al.* Small incidentally discovered testicular masses in infertile men–is active surveillance the new standard of care? *J Urol* 183: 1373–7.

28. Dieckmann KP, Skakkebaek NE. Carcinoma in situ of the testis: review of biological and clinical features. *Int J Cancer* 1999; 83: 815–22.

29. Hoei-Hansen CE, Rajpert-De Meyts E, Daugaard G, Skakkebaek NE. Carcinoma in situ testis, the progenitor of testicular germ cell tumours: a clinical review. *Ann Oncol* 2005; 16: 863–8.

30. Ehrlich Y, Konichezky M, Yossepowitch O, Baniel J. Multifocality in testicular germ cell tumors. *J Urol* 2009; 181: 1114–19.

31. Heidenreich A, Weissbach L, Holtl W, *et al.* Organ sparing surgery for malignant germ cell tumor of the testis. *J Urol* 2001; 166: 2161–5.

32. Zuniga A, Lawrentschuk N, Jewett MA. Organ-sparing approaches for testicular masses. *Nat Rev Urol* 2010; 7(8): 454–64.

33. Berney DM. Staging and classification of testicular tumours: pitfalls from macroscopy to diagnosis. *J Clin Pathol* 2008; 61: 20–4.

34. Hopps CV, Goldstein M. Ultrasound guided needle localization and microsurgical exploration for incidental nonpalpable testicular tumors. *J Urol* 2002; 168: 1084–7.

35. Ragni G, Somigliana E, Restelli L, *et al.* Sperm banking and rate of assisted reproduction treatment: insights from a 15-year cryopreservation program for male cancer patients. *Cancer* 2003; 97: 1624–9.

36. Lass A, Akagbosu F, Abusheikha N, *et al.* A programme of semen cryopreservation for patients with malignant disease in a tertiary infertility centre: lessons from 8 years' experience. *Hum Reprod* 1998; 13: 3256–61.

37. Delouya G, Baazeem A, Boman JM, *et al.* Identification of spermatozoa in archived testicular cancer specimens: implications for bench side sperm retrieval at orchiectomy. *Urology* 75: 1436–40.

38. Carmignani L, Gadda F, Gazzano G, *et al.* Testicular sperm extraction in cancerous testicle in patients with azoospermia: a case report. *Hum Reprod* 2007; 22: 1068–72.

39. Baniel J, Sella A. Sperm extraction at orchiectomy for testis cancer. *Fertil Steril* 2001; 75: 260–2.

40. Binsaleh S, Sircar K, Chan PT. Feasibility of simultaneous testicular microdissection for sperm retrieval and ipsilateral testicular tumor resection in azoospermic men. *J Androl* 2004; 25: 867–71.

41. Choi BB, Goldstein M, Moomjy M, *et al.* Births using sperm retrieved via immediate microdissection of a solitary testis with cancer. *Fertil Steril* 2005; 84: 1508.

42. Carmignani L, Gadda F, Paffoni A, *et al.* Azoospermia and severe oligospermia in testicular cancer. *Arch Ital Urol Androl* 2009; 81: 21–3.

43. Carroll PR, Morse MJ, Whitmore WF, Jr., *et al.* Fertility status of patients with clinical stage I testis tumors on a surveillance protocol. *J Urol* 1987; 138: 70–2.

44. Rowley MJ, Leach DR, Warner GA, Heller CG. Effect of graded doses of ionizing radiation on the human testis. *Radiat Res* 1974; 59: 665–78.

45. Centola GM, Keller JW, Henzler M, Rubin P. Effect of low-dose testicular irradiation on sperm count and fertility in patients with testicular seminoma. *J Androl* 1994; 15: 608–13.

46. Fossa SD, Abyholm T, Normann N, Jetne V. Post-treatment fertility in patients with testicular cancer. III. Influence of radiotherapy in seminoma patients. *Br J Urol* 1986; 58: 315–19.

47. Nalesnik JG, Sabanegh ES, Jr., Eng TY, Buchholz TA. Fertility in men after treatment for stage 1 and 2A seminoma. *Am J Clin Oncol* 2004; 27: 584–8.

48. Pilarchopoulou K, Pectasides D. Late complications of chemotherapy in testicular cancer. *Cancer Treat Rev* 2010; 36: 262–7.

49. Stephenson WT, Poirier SM, Rubin L, Einhorn LH. Evaluation of reproductive capacity in germ cell tumor patients following treatment with cisplatin, etoposide, and bleomycin. *J Clin Oncol* 1995; 13: 2278–80.

50. Huddart RA, Norman A, Moynihan C, *et al.* Fertility, gonadal and sexual function in survivors of testicular cancer. *Br J Cancer* 2005; 93: 200–7.

51. Burrello N, Vicari E, La Vignera S, *et al.* Effects of anti-neoplastic treatment on sperm aneuploidy rate in patients with testicular tumor: a longitudinal study. *J Endocrinol Invest* 2011; 34: e121–5.

52. Johnson DH, Linde R, Hainsworth JD, *et al.* Effect of a luteinizing hormone releasing hormone agonist given during combination chemotherapy on posttherapy fertility in male patients with lymphoma: preliminary observations. *Blood* 1985; 65: 832–6.

53. Kreuser ED, Hetzel WD, Hautmann R, Pfeiffer EF. Reproductive toxicity with and without LHRHA administration during adjuvant chemotherapy in patients with germ cell tumors. *Horm Metab Res* 1990; 22: 494–8.

54. Kaufman MR, Chang SS. Short- and long-term complications of therapy for testicular cancer. *Urol Clin North Am* 2007; 34: 259–68, xi.

55. Sheinfeld J, Bartsch G, Bosl GJ. Surgery of testicular tumors. In Wein AJ, Kavoussi LR, Novick AC, Partin AW, Peters CA, eds. *Campbell–Walsh Urology*, 9th edn. Philadelphia, PA: Saunders, 2007.

56. Narayan P, Lange PH, Fraley EE. Ejaculation and fertility after extended retroperitoneal lymph node dissection for testicular cancer. *J Urol* 1982; 127: 685–8.

57. Beck SD, Bey AL, Bihrle R, Foster RS. Ejaculatory status and fertility rates after primary retroperitoneal lymph node dissection. *J Urol* 2010; 184: 2078–80.

58. Chan PT, Palermo GD, Veeck LL, Rosenwaks Z, Schlegel PN. Testicular sperm extraction combined with intracytoplasmic sperm injection in the treatment of men with persistent azoospermia postchemotherapy. *Cancer* 2001; 92: 1632–7.

59. Meseguer M, Garrido N, Remohi J, *et al.* Testicular sperm extraction (TESE) and ICSI in patients with permanent azoospermia after chemotherapy. *Hum Reprod* 2003; 18: 1281–5.

60. Damani MN, Master V, Meng MV, *et al.* Postchemotherapy ejaculatory azoospermia: fatherhood with sperm from testis tissue with intracytoplasmic sperm injection. *J Clin Oncol* 2002; 20: 930–6.

61. Shin D, Lo KC, Lipshultz LI. Treatment options for the infertile male with cancer. *J Natl Cancer Inst Monogr* 2005; 34: 48–50.

Chapter

18

Effects of therapy for brain cancer

Elena Pentsova and Andrew B. Lassman

Introduction

Around the world, approximately 200 000 people develop primary brain tumors per year [1], with a rising incidence for the last three decades [2], currently 24.35 per 100 000 person-years for adults age $\geq$ 20 [1]. In addition to primary brain tumors, metastases to the brain are also a frequent complication of systemic malignancies, most commonly in patients with lung and breast cancers [2]. Brain metastases comprise over 50% of all intracranial tumors [2].

The median survival of the most aggressive primary malignant brain tumor, the glioblastoma, is 1–2 years despite aggressive therapy [3]. In addition, most patients with primary malignant tumors are over age 50 at diagnosis. Consequently, questions focusing on treatment efficacy and survival are typically given highest priority, with a discussion of fertility often avoided entirely or answered inadequately. Time constraints, perceptions about prognosis, and physician discomfort also hinder the discussion [4,5]. Although quality-of-life measures are increasingly incorporated into clinical trials, they usually focus on neurocognitive and related effects without capturing or reporting data related to fertility or sexual function.

However, the median age of patients diagnosed with brain tumors varies greatly by histology. For example, low-grade gliomas, which may have an indolent course associated with survival of over 10 years, disproportionately affect young adults when issues of family planning are most pressing. In addition, almost all primary brain tumors occur more frequently in men than women, with the notable exception of meningiomas and pituitary tumors [1]. Therefore, the effect of therapy for brain cancer on fertility, especially in men, is an understudied area of neuro-oncology.

Table 18.1. Treatment for central nervous system tumors that can affect fertility

Symptomatic	Corticosteroids
	Anticonvulsants
Definitive	Surgery
	Radiotherapy
	Chemotherapy

Brain tumors are unique in several ways. For example, patients with primary brain tumors or brain metastases almost always receive corticosteroids at some point during their disease course, and patients with seizures also receive anticonvulsants (Table 18.1). In addition, tumor location can have a direct effect on libido from involvement of the frontal lobes, sexual dysfunction from tumors of the spinal cord, or from mass effect on the pituitary and surrounding structures causing endocrinopathies. Cranial radiotherapy can also injure or permanently damage pituitary function. Finally, some of the chemotherapies differ from those used in the treatment of other malignancies. All of these factors can affect fertility (Table 18.2).

Supportive treatment for patients with brain tumors

Antiepileptic drugs

Seizures occur in 20–40% of brain tumor patients [2]. They are more common in patients with low-grade gliomas and tumors of oligodendroglial histology. Libido is reduced in men with seizures, as is sexual confidence [6,7]. Seizure disorders, especially from an epileptogenic focus in the temporal lobe, are also associated with reduced testosterone [7,8].

Fertility Preservation in Male Cancer Patients, ed. John P. Mulhall, Linda D. Applegarth, Robert D. Oates and Peter N. Schlegel.
Published by Cambridge University Press. © Cambridge University Press 2013.

Table 18.2. Mechanism of impaired fertility in patients with central nervous system tumors

Category	Mechanism
Endocrine dysfunction	Tumor directly affecting hypothalamic–pituitary axis
	Damage to hypothalamic–pituitary axis following cranial radiotherapy
	Antiepileptic drugs
	Epilepsy
Sexual dysfunction	Corticosteroids
	Epilepsy
	Antiepileptic drugs
	Chemotherapy
	Frontal lobe tumor or edema
	Spinal cord tumor
	Spinal cord injury
	Antiepileptic drugs
	Epilepsy
Impaired spermatogenesis or DNA mutation	Chemotherapy
	Antiepileptic drugs
	Damage to testicles from spine radiotherapy

For patients without a history of seizures, current guidelines do not recommend prophylactic antiepileptic drugs (AEDs) except during the perioperative period for tumor biopsy or resection [9]. Patients with a history of seizures are generally treated with one or more AEDs, which may also be associated with reduced libido, sexual dysfunction, and reduced testosterone levels [6,10,11]. They can also interfere with levels of follicle-stimulating hormone (FSH) and luteinizing hormone (LH), and affect the testosterone/LH ratio which may indicate the level of testicular dysfunction [12].

It is also now widely recognized that some AEDs activate the hepatic cytochrome P450 (CYP) enzyme system, which can increase metabolism and decrease efficacy of various chemotherapies and oral contraceptives. CYP enzyme-inducing AEDs (EIAEDs) such as carbamazepine, barbiturates, and phenytoin increase production of sex-hormone binding globulin (SHBG), which reduces the level of free testosterone [8,10,13], although the physiologic significance may be muted by equilibrating feedback loops. In addition, carbamazepine and phenytoin are associated with reduced testosterone and increased LH levels, resulting in a significantly lower testosterone/LH ratio [8]. Patients taking primidone had reduced libido compared to patients taking other EIAEDs [11]. Valproic acid is an enzyme inhibitor which is distinct from other AEDs, and it can also affect testosterone and gonadotropin levels [10]. It suppresses enzymatic metabolism of

estradiol and subsequently elevates estradiol level, which may impact on sexual and reproductive function [14]. In addition, valproic acid has been associated with reduced testicular volume [14].

Carbamazepine, oxcarbamazepine, and valproic acid are associated with abnormalities of sperm count and morphology [14], although one study suggests that oxcarbamazepine may modulate sex hormone levels to a lesser degree than carbamazepine [10]. Effects of valproic acid may be of particular importance in the brain tumor population, because it is under investigation in clinical trials as an agent that may have efficacy for gliomas.

Among the non-EIAED agents, lamotrigine (Lamictal) does not appear to influence sexual function or testosterone levels [7]. However, lamotrigine is not frequently used in brain tumor patients at this time, as a complicated titration schedule is required and patients are at risk of Stevens–Johnson syndrome of the skin, which can be fatal.

The most widely used AED in patients with brain tumors is levetiracetam (Keppra), in part because it is a non-EIAED, and because it does not typically require monitoring of serum levels. Although it can cause mood alteration, with the potential to modify libido, there is no indication from preclinical studies that it adversely effects fertility, at least in women [15].

Corticosteroids

Corticosteroids are widely used to control cerebral edema. They can rapidly improve symptoms and reduce life-threatening intracranial pressure elevations. They can exert an oncolytic effect in lymphoma but probably not to a medically significant degree in other tumors. Dexamethasone is the corticosteroid most commonly used, in part because it has almost no mineralocorticoid effect relative to other corticosteroids. Typical dexamethasone doses are 4–10 mg per day divided 2–4 times daily, although doses ranging from less than 1 mg (in patients who cannot wean completely) to 100 mg (for emergent treatment of high intracranial pressure or spinal cord compression) are occasionally used. Almost all patients with brain tumors receive corticosteroids at some point during their illness, and they are used routinely during the perioperative period and as antiemetic prophylaxis for some chemotherapies.

There are very limited data on the effects of glucocorticoids on fertility in men. They can cause behavioral problems, typically at high doses given over long periods, that can include mania, euphoria, or psychosis with hypersexuality; less commonly they can cause depression and reduced libido. Extrapolating from effects of increased endogenous glucocorticoid secretion during a stress response, stressed animals demonstrated reduced inhibition of the hypothalamic–pituitary–gonadal (HPG) axis, erectile dysfunction, and behavioral alterations [16]. However, not all human studies have demonstrated that administration of glucocorticoids suppresses gonadotropin secretion even when it is used at clinically meaningful doses (100–300 mg of hydrocortisone, equivalent to approximately 4–11 mg dexamethasone) [17].

Primary brain tumors

Like most tumors, brain tumors are classified histologically according to their presumed cell of origin. "Primary" tumors, such as the gliomas, are those that arise within the central nervous system. Distinct from other tumors, the TNM classification scheme does not apply, because primary brain tumors almost never involve lymph nodes (N), nor do they typically metastasize (M) to other body organs. Rather, the histologic tumor *type* and *grade* are of paramount importance in determining both treatment and prognosis.

Gliomas

Approximately 50% of all primary tumors of the brain are gliomas (Table 18.3) [1]. Approximately 75% of these are astrocytomas [1]. Glioblastomas (WHO grade IV tumors, typically astrocytomas) are the most common (54% of all gliomas) and most aggressive [1]. Oligodendrogliomas are rare gliomas (5–10%), including both low-grade (WHO grade II) and anaplastic (WHO grade III) variants [1]. However, oligodendrogliomas are generally more responsive to treatment than astrocytomas of the same histologic grade, and are associated with a better prognosis.

The low-grade (WHO grade II) gliomas are often called "benign," although they do not behave in a benign fashion. They are almost never cured by surgery because tumor cells invade surrounding brain tissue, thus precluding complete resection with a "clean margin." Median survival for patients with low-grade astrocytomas is about 5 years, and 10 years for patients with oligodendrogliomas [1]. Following maximal surgical resection, most patients with low-grade

Table 18.3. Common intracranial tumors in adults

Category	Major subtypes

Gliomas	WHO grade II
	  Astrocytoma
	  Oligodendroglioma
	  Oligoastrocytoma
	  Ependymoma
	WHO grade III
	  Anaplastic astrocytoma
	  Anaplastic oligodendroglioma
	  Anaplastic oligoastrocytoma
	WHO grade IV
	  Glioblastoma

Meningiomas	WHO grade I
	  Meningioma
	WHO grade II
	  Atypical meningioma
	  Clear cell meningioma
	  Choroid meningioma
	WHO grade III
	  Anaplastic meningioma
	  Papillary meningioma
	  Rhabdoid meningioma

Primary central nervous system lymphoma	
Pituitary adenomas	
Central nervous system metastases	Brain Spinal cord Leptomeningeal

gliomas receive fractionated external beam radiotherapy of approximately 50 Gy at some point during the course of their disease, However, the timing of radiotherapy remains controversial, because it appears to delay tumor progression without prolonging survival [18]. The use of chemotherapy is more controversial, as low-grade gliomas typically exhibit low mitotic activity and an indolent growth rate that has led to their characterization as chemo-resistant. When chemotherapy is used, temozolomide (DNA alkylator, Table 18.4) is the most common agent.

The high-grade (WHO grade III and IV) tumors are called "malignant" although they almost never metastasize to lymph nodes or other organs as other malignancies can. Rather, they are malignant because they can enlarge rapidly and quickly become refractory to treatment. Median survival for patients with anaplastic (WHO grade III) astrocytomas is about 2–3 years, and for anaplastic oligodendrogliomas about 5 years [1]. Survival for aggressively treated glioblastoma is 1–2 years [3]. Standard therapy for glioblastoma is the most well established, comprising maximal surgical resection (with or without locally implanted carmustine-eluting wafers, reviewed

Table 18.4. Common chemotherapies used in central nervous system tumors

Category	Agent(s)
Alkylator	Temozolomide Procarbazine Nitrosoureas Carbo/cisplatin
Topoisomerase inhibitor	Etoposide
Tyrosine kinase inhibitor	Erlotinib
Antibody	Rituximab Bevacizumab
Vinca alkyloids	Vincristine
Antimetabolite	Methotrexate Cytarabine

elsewhere [2]), followed by 60 Gy of fractionated cranial radiotherapy over six weeks administered concurrently with temozolomide chemotherapy (75 mg/m^2 daily), followed by $\geq$ six monthly cycles of adjuvant temozolomide (150–200 mg/m^2 for five days) [3]. However, many neuro-oncologists advise continuing temozolomide for $\geq$ 12 cycles, or indefinitely, resulting in prolonged exposure that may potentiate effects on fertility. Standard treatment for anaplastic astrocytomas is more controversial, with many neuro-oncologists advocating treatment analogous to glioblastomas. There is no clear standard of care for newly diagnosed anaplastic oligodendrogliomas, with radiotherapy alone, chemotherapy (typically temozolomide) alone, and combined-modality therapy all used commonly [19].

Temozolomide chemotherapy

The type, dose, and duration of chemotherapy can influence fertility following transient or permanent damage to developing spermatogonial stem cells, along with at least a theoretical risk of teratogenicity from germ line mutagenesis. Many of the agents used against brain tumors are in the same class or classes as those which treat other cancers. For example, the effects of DNA alkylators are well known, and some, like nitrogen mustard derivatives, have been used for over 60 years against tumors of multiple histologies, including gliomas, and are associated with the highest risks of permanent testicular damage [4,20]. Other chapters in this book provide a detailed discussion of the deleterious effects on fertility of various chemotherapies used for solid tumors and hematologic malignancies. Therefore, this chapter will focus on the specific agents used most frequently in patients

with central nervous system tumors today, such as temozolomide.

It is well established that the DNA alkylating chemotherapies pose a high risk of infertility by affecting sperm-forming germ cells and causing azoospermia [4,5,20]. Temozolomide is an oral cytotoxic alkylating agent which was initially Food and Drug Administration (FDA)-approved for the treatment of recurrent anaplastic astrocytomas [21] and then approved for newly diagnosed glioblastoma [3]. However, the ease of administration and low toxicity profile have led to temozolomide replacing other cytotoxic regimens. As a consequence, temozolomide has become the de facto first-line chemotherapy for patients with astrocytic and oligodendroglial tumors, regardless of grade, although evidence of superior or even equivalent efficacy to other regimens is often lacking [22].

Extrapolating from experience with other alkylators such as ntirosoureas, temozolomide almost certainly has analogous detrimental effects. For example, temozolomide can reduce formation of mature sperm and cause testicular atrophy in animals [23]. Activity of the repair enzyme O6-methylguanine (O6-MG)-DNA-methyltransferase (MGMT) appears to reduce efficacy of temozolomide. O6-benzylguanine inhibits MGMT activity and is under investigation in clinical trials for gliomas as a method to enhance nitrosourea or temozolomide efficacy. Animals treated with O6-benzylguanine concurrently with nitrosourea demonstrate changes in seminiferous epithelium and increased apoptosis of immature sperm but with recovery after the nadir [24]. These effects were not seen with either nitrosourea or O6-benzylguanine monotherapy [24]. However, it is unknown whether similar effects would occur during concurrent O6-benzylguanine with temozolomide in humans.

Like other alkylators, another concern with temozolomide is the potential for teratogenicity, but there is a paucity of human data and published reports are anecdotal. For example, a 30-year-old man with a right frontal lobe anaplastic astrocytoma underwent concurrent radiotherapy and daily temozolomide followed by six adjuvant cycles of temozolomide. Thirteen months after completing treatment he reportedly fathered a healthy child [25].

At our institution we have also identified men who fathered healthy children after receiving temozolomide. In one case, 27 months after completing cranial radiotherapy and temozolomide, a man fathered a

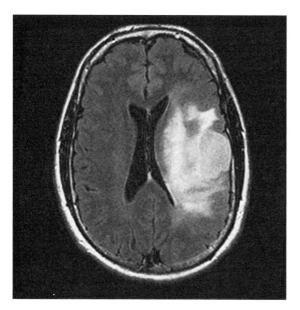

Figure 18.1. Anaplastic astrocytoma. Extensive non-enhancing tumor (anaplastic astrocytoma) in a 39-year-old man treated with cranial radiotherapy as well as chemotherapy with the DNA alkylator temozolomide. He naturally fathered a healthy child following treatment, but subsequently developed low testosterone, presumably a late consequence of radiotherapy-induced hypopituitarism as the radiotherapy port encompassed a large area, seizures, the use of antiepileptic drugs, or a combination.

naturally conceived healthy baby. However, he then developed symptomatic low serum testosterone, likely from either cranial radiotherapy discussed further below (Fig. 18.1), seizures, AED, or a combination of these etiologies.

In summary, the limited available evidence suggests that any effect on spermatogenesis appears temporary, and men are not rendered permanently infertile by treatment with temozolomide. Robust data are lacking regarding the duration of the risk of teratogenecity following treatment with temozolomide. However, delaying attempts to father children until at least six months have passed since taking temozolomide is typically recommended. Certainly conception during treatment is absolutely contraindicated, with a high risk of birth defects. For example, our colleagues cared for a 32-year-old woman with a right frontal anaplastic oligodendroglioma harboring 1p and 19q co-deletion treated with neo adjuvant temozolomide. During her third cycle, she discovered she was seven weeks pregnant, and she elected against terminating the pregnancy. Temozolomide was immediately discontinued, and she underwent radiotherapy with

abdominal shielding following completion of the first trimester. She delivered a full-term boy with spina bifida, cleft foot, and hydrocephalus (Terri S. Armstrong and Mark R. Gilbert, UT MD Anderson Cancer Center, personal communication).

Despite reports of success in conceiving a child after treatment with temozolomide, all men planning to father children should bank sperm prior to treatment. In addition, we strongly suggest using at least two forms of contraception while on temozolomide to avoid conception during treatment, including condoms to avoid exposing their sexual partners to the potential existence of temozolomide metabolites in semen.

Bevacizumab

Bevacizumab is a humanized monoclonal antibody against vascular endothelial growth factor (VEGF) thought to act as an antiangiogenic agent. It received accelerated FDA approval for recurrent glioblastoma in May 2009 [26]. Dosing for glioblastoma is typically 10 mg/kg every two weeks or 15 mg/kg every three weeks. Two phase III trials are accruing for patients with newly diagnosed glioblastoma. Animal studies of angiogenesis inhibitors demonstrated negative effects on normal angiogenesis such as in the female reproductive system [27], but data in men are limited [5].

Effects of cranial radiotherapy on pituitary function

Although the testes are not harmed directly by cranial radiotherapy, injury to the hypothalamic–pituitary axis can disrupt fertility. Such abnormalities can occur following pituitary radiotherapy [28], but patients who receive cranial radiotherapy for primary brain tumors distant from the pituitary may also develop pituitary dysfunction (hypogonadotropic hypogonadism).

Low serum testosterone with inappropriately low gonadotropin levels is a potential late complication. In one study of 56 patients (28 men) treated with cranial radiotherapy for non-pituitary tumors (including gliomas and meningiomas), 41% had at least some form of hypopituitarism, with gonadotropin abnormalities in 27% of patients tested more than one year after radiotherapy [29]. The effect was both time- and dose-dependent, becoming more apparent after longer latency and with radiotherapy dosing above 44 Gy. Cranial radiotherapy doses used for gliomas generally exceed this threshold. Moreover, whole-brain radiotherapy (WBRT) at doses over 30 Gy has been shown to cause hypopituitarism [30]. Others reported an incidence of gonadotropin impairment in 22–71% of patients treated with cranial radiotherapy for non-pituitary tumors [30–32], with the range likely dependent on differences in both dose and follow-up duration.

Radiation can also induce hyperprolactinemia. Hyperprolactinemia has been described in both genders but is most frequently seen in women. Occasionally, it can be severe enough to impair gonadotropin secretion and cause decreased libido and erectile dysfunction in men. One study showed that hyperprolactinemia was more common in adults (75%) than in children (30%) but was unrelated to radiotherapy dose or latency. Asymptomatic decreased serum testosterone was observed in 30% of postpubertal men treated with cranial or craniospinal radiotherapy, but semen analysis was not performed in this study [32].

The frequencies cited above may represent an underestimate of the true incidence, because pituitary and testicular function are not routinely tested in asymptomatic patients. In addition, many patients with high-grade gliomas succumb to their tumor before late toxicities occur. Moreover, patients who do develop symptoms often have them attributed to other comorbidities as potential etiologies, such as age or concurrent medications, leading the clinician away from an endocrine evaluation. However, symptomatic patients should have their sex hormone concentrations (total and free testosterone, SHBG and estradiol) tested, including gonadotropin-releasing hormone (GnRH), LH, and FSH. Effects may occur over a decade later. Regular assessment of anterior pituitary function may be important for all patients receiving cranial radiation, with the possibility of introducing hormone replacement therapy to improve sexual function if indicated.

Effect of systemic therapy for erectile dysfunction on glioma growth rate

Use of the cyclic guanosine monophosphate (cGMP)-specific phosphodiesterase (PDE) inhibitors such as sidenafil and vardenafil in glioma patients with erectile dysfunction is infrequent, with few data to guide safety. One concern is whether the vasodilation they induce could increase glioma growth. Of note, to the contrary, these agents increased permeability across the blood–brain barrier in a rat glioma model, and enhanced the antineoplastic effects of chemotherapy

with adriamycin [33]. Therefore, clinical trials may be warranted to determine potential benefit in humans.

Meningiomas

Meningiomas are tumors of the membranous covering of the brain and spinal cord. Therefore, they are not technically "brain" tumors, but they are the most common primary intracranial tumor (34%) [1]. The prevalence of meningiomas in the population remains uncertain because many are clinically silent, discovered incidentally at autopsy or during brain imaging performed for another reason (head trauma or stroke). Sporadic meningiomas occur in men approximately one-third as frequently as in women [1].

Approximately 90% of meningiomas are WHO grade I tumors that either grow very slowly or not at all, although more aggressive variants exist (Table 18.3) [1]. Median survival for patients with benign meningiomas is over 10 years. The relatively long survival puts patients at risk for late toxicities, including impaired fertility.

Location of the tumor, as well as consequences of treatment, especially radiotherapy, may directly influence sexual function in men. Bilateral frontal lobe lesions (Fig. 18.2) can cause apathy, emotional sluggishness, and "abulia" as well as other symptoms. Abulia is the concomitant reduction in speech, movements, and ideation, which may include loss of libido.

In asymptomatic meningiomas, observation with surveillance MRI scans is reasonable. For symptomatic patients or those with enlarging tumors, surgery is frequently recommended. WHO grade III tumors are treated with postoperative radiotherapy, as are most incompletely removed grade II tumors, and this can also cause hypopituitarism (Fig. 18.2). There is no established role for chemotherapy, although several agents are under investigation including various receptor tyrosine kinase and angiogenesis inhibitors.

Pituitary tumors

Pituitary tumors can impair fertility directly through effects of hormones on sexual function and spermatogenesis. Therefore, they are discussed in brief here. Pituitary adenomas represent approximately 15% of intracranial tumors, the third most common intracranial neoplasm after gliomas and meningiomas [1], although, like meningiomas, they are not technically tumors of the "brain." Autopsy series suggest the

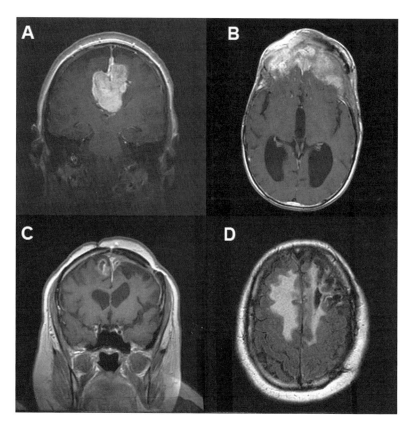

Figure 18.2. Meningiomas. (A) Coronal T1 post-contrast MRI of a 42-year-old man with a bifrontal meningioma who experienced reduced libido, likely from injury to the frontal lobes from the tumor. (B) Axial T1 post-contrast MRI of a 39-year-old man with an atypical bifrontal meningioma who complained of decreased sexual desire and difficulty with erections six months after receiving radiation therapy. In addition to direct effects on the frontal lobes from the tumor as one potential cause of decreased libido, he also had low testosterone, likely from radiotherapy-induced hypopituitarism. (C and D) Coronal T1 post-contrast images of a 64-year-old man with recurrent meningiomas who developed decreased libido and erectile dysfunction six months after radiotherapy. He was also found to have a low testosterone, likely as a consequence of radiotherapy-induced hypopituitarism. Additional imaging demonstrated substantial injury to both frontal lobes that did not enhance with contrast (D).

prevalence may be as high as 25% when incidental tumors are included [34]. Clinically, pituitary adenomas usually present with neurological symptoms such as headaches and visual field loss, endocrine symptoms, or both. Occasionally hemorrhage (pituitary apoplexy) causes abrupt symptoms [35].

Prolactin-secreting tumors are the most common hormone-secreting adenomas, accounting for about one-third of symptomatic tumors and 40% of all pituitary adenomas [36]. They can become large enough to compress normal anterior pituitary cells, causing reduced LH and FSH secretion. Excess prolactin can also reduce hypothalamic secretion of GnRH via feedback loops [37]. In men, symptoms of hyperprolactinemia can include erectile dysfunction and decreased libido despite normal testosterone [38]. Men do not typically seek medical attention for prolactinomas until neurological symptoms develop, although 78% can have erectile dysfunction [36]. Pharmacological treatment with dopamine agonists (bromocriptine, cabergoline) can induce dramatic and rapid responses, avoiding surgery and radiotherapy.

Gonadotropic adenomas secrete LH, FSH, and the alpha subunit of the pituitary glycoprotein hormone. They account for 10–15% of pituitary adenomas. They induce loss of libido in 65% of men, erectile dysfunction in 50%, and testicular atrophy in 35%, with low testosterone in 78% [39].

Transphenoidal surgery followed by radiation therapy has been a common treatment of pituitary adenomas refractory to medical therapy. Hypopituitarism is the most frequent long-term complication of radiation therapy and has been confirmed by multiple studies, with gonadotropin deficiencies in 100% of patients and hyperprolactinemia in 73% in one series [28]. The effects may be more pronounced in patients who undergo both surgery and radiotherapy compared to either modality alone [40].

Primary central nervous system lymphoma

Primary central nervous system lymphoma (PCNSL) is exceedingly rare, representing approximately 2% of all brain tumors, with a peak incidence at age 50–70 years and a slight male predominance [1]. It is a typical non-Hodgkin's lymphoma most commonly originating anywhere in the brain, but it can also affect the eyes, spinal cord, and leptomeninges. Although median survival is approximately three years, some patients are effectively cured, making them vulnerable to late toxicities of treatment.

PCNSL is typically treated first with high-dose methotrexate (MTX)-based chemotherapy. Controversies surround the optimal dose of MTX, efficacy of adding other cytotoxic agents, and the ability to reduce WBRT dosing below the typical 45 Gy, or to avoid WBRT altogether among patients with a complete response to chemotherapy.

A commonly used initial chemotherapy regimen is five cycles of MVP (methotrexate 3.5 g/m^2, procarabazine 100 mg/m^2 daily for seven days on alternate cycles, vincristine 1.4 mg/m^2) followed by WBRT and consolidation with high-dose cytarabine (3 g/m^2 per day for two days, repeated one month later) [41]. Ritixumab (approximately 500 mg/m^2) may be incorporated into the regimen (typically the day before MTX as R-MPV) for patients with CD20-expressing disease [41]. Other regimens include methotrexate combined with ritixumab and temozolomide ("MR. T"; Tracy T. Batchelor, Massachusetts General Hospital, Harvard Medical School, personal communication). The effects of these agents on fertility are described below, but it should be noted that attribution to single agents is difficult to discern when most data are drawn from combinations used for other malignancies such as systemic (non-CNS) lymphomas.

Methotrexate

MTX causes sperm abnormalities but the effect appears temporary with almost no risk of permanent infertility [4,42]. Examinations of semen, testicular histology, and spermatogenic function demonstrated no irreversibly unfavorable effects on male fertility [43]. However, severe oligospermia was found in men who received a combination of high-dose MTX and vincristine and were evaluated during and immediately after treatment. Only 50% of the men developed transient testicular failure associated with a significant increase in serum FSH but not LH levels. Sperm concentration and serum FSH levels typically return to normal after completion of therapy [44]. High-dose MTX can also cause renal insufficiency or renal failure, and chronic renal failure can also contribute to reduced libido.

Vincristine

Vincristine is a vinca alkaloid that inhibits mitosis via inhibition of microtubule formation. This agent has been the cause of arrest in spermatogenesis and decreased motility of spermatozoids [45]. When used alone, these effects are not necessarily irreversible [4].

Procarbazine

Procarbazine is an alkylating agent that can cause significant gonadal damage [5]. In adult men, the effect is not age-related, but severity depends on intensity and dose. Procarbazine-containing regimens used for treatment of systemic lymphomas (MOPP) are associated with a high risk of prolonged if not irreversible azoospermia [46]. Whether this effect is lasting in the regimens for PCNSL such as MVP is less well established. However, extrapolation would suggest there is at least a moderate risk of permanent infertility, as azoospermia associated with cumulative doses above 4g/m^2 can be prolonged [4].

Rituximab

To our knowledge there are no data on effects on fertility or gonadal function of the anti-CD20 monoclonal antibody rituximab.

Cytarabine

Cytarabine is gonadotoxic [20], with significant damage to the testis and sperm number and integrity observed in combination regimens for other cancers that incorporate doses at or exceeding those used in PCNSL [47,48]. When used alone, effects are likely temporary [4].

Tumors of the spinal cord and associated structures

In contrast to intracranial tumors, spinal cord tumors can directly affect sexual function. They are rare tumors and occur either within the substance of the spinal cord itself (intramedullary) or outside of the spinal cord (extramedullary). Primary intramedullary tumors are histologically equivalent to those arising in the brain: ependymomas and gliomas, most frequently astrocytomas. The most common primary extramedullary tumors are meningiomas and neurofibromas. The most rostral section of the spinal cord is the conus medullaris, and the cauda equina contains the spinal nerve roots exiting from the cord. Erection and ejaculation are frequently impaired in conus medullaris abnormalities rather than cauda equina compression. However, severe sexual dysfunction was reported by 35% of men with cauda equina lesions, and only 15% of patients reported normal sexual function [49]. In addition, surgery and spinal radiotherapy can directly injure pathways controlling sexual function.

Central nervous system metastases

Central nervous system metastases can also impair fertility. In addition to direct effects of tumor mass from brain metastases on the frontal lobes described above, they are often treated with WBRT, especially when there is more than one lesion. WBRT can cause dementia [50], with resulting abnormalities of libido and sexual function. As above, WBRT at clinically relevant doses (such as 30 Gy) can induce hypopituitarism. Leptomeningeal metastases are an infrequent complication of systemic cancer, occurring in 5–10% of patients [50]. When they occur around the spinal cord, conus medullaris, or cauda equina, they can disrupt normal sexual function, as can injury from spinal radiotherapy.

Cytotoxic chemotherapies have limited efficacy for brain or leptomeningeal metastases, with small cell lung cancer and lymphoma as notable exceptions. Temozolomide is used most commonly for lung cancers and melanoma. High-dose intravenous MTX is used occasionally for brain or leptomeningeal metastases from breast cancer. Effects of these agents on fertility are discussed above. CNS metastases from non-small cell lung cancer harboring mutations in epidermal growth factor receptor (EGFR) can respond to the EGFR inhibitor erlotinib, but the effect on fertility of this and other receptor tyrosine kinase inhibitors is unknown [5].

Conclusion

Brain tumors (primary and metastatic) can disrupt fertility, as can treatment. Older age and poor prognosis for many patients often makes discussion of fertility a low priority for the neuro-oncologist. However, for some, especially young patients with meningiomas or low-grade gliomas, family planning is of paramount importance. Increased attention to the issues of fertility is merited.

Acknowledgments

We thank Dr. Lisa M. DeAngelis for her thoughtful input and review of the manuscript, and Judith Lampron for her expert editorial assistance.

References

1. Central Brain Tumor Registry of the United States statistical report: primary brain and central nervous system tumors diagnosed in the United States 2004–2006. CBTRUS, 2010. www.cbtrus.org (accessed January 2012).

2. DeAngelis LM, Gutin PH, Leibel SA, *et al. Intracranial Tumors: Diagnosis and Treatment*. London: Martin Duntz, 2002.

3. Stupp R, Mason WP, van den Bent MJ, *et al.* Radiotherapy plus concomitant and adjuvant temozolomide for glioblastoma. *N Engl J Med* 2005; 352: 987–96.

4. Lee SJ, Schover LR, Partridge AH, *et al.* American Society of Clinical Oncology recommendations on fertility preservation in cancer patients. *J Clin Oncol* 2006; 24: 2917–31.

5. Levine J, Canada A, Stern CJ. Fertility preservation in adolescents and young adults with cancer. *J Clin Oncol* 2010; 28: 4831–41.

6. Talbot JA, Sheldrick R, Caswell H, *et al.* Sexual function in men with epilepsy: how important is testosterone? *Neurology* 2008; 70: 1346–52.

7. Herzog AG, Drislane FW, Schomer DL, *et al.* Differential effects of antiepileptic drugs on sexual function and hormones in men with epilepsy. *Neurology* 2005; 65: 1016–20.

8. Bauer J, Blumenthal S, Reuber M, *et al.* Epilepsy syndrome, focus location, and treatment choice affect testicular function in men with epilepsy. *Neurology* 2004; 62: 243–6.

9. Glantz MJ, Cole BF, Forsyth PA, *et al.* Practice parameter: anticonvulsant prophylaxis in patients with newly diagnosed brain tumors. Report of the Quality Standards Subcommittee of the American Academy of Neurology. *Neurology* 2000; 54: 1886–93.

10. Rattya J, Turkka J, Pakarinen AJ, *et al.* Reproductive effects of valproate, carbamazepine, and oxcarbazepine in men with epilepsy. *Neurology* 2001; 56: 31–6.

11. Mattson RH, Cramer JA, Collins JF, *et al.* Comparison of carbamazepine, phenobarbital, phenytoin, and primidone in partial and secondarily generalized tonic-clonic seizures. *N Engl J Med* 1985; 313: 145–51.

12. Giagulli VA, Vermeulen A. Leydig cell function in infertile men with idiopathic oligospermic infertility. *J Clin Endocrinol Metab* 1988; 66: 62–7.

13. Stoffel-Wagner B, Bauer J, Flugel D, *et al.* Serum sex hormones are altered in patients with chronic temporal lobe epilepsy receiving anticonvulsant medication. *Epilepsia* 1998; 39: 1164–73.

14. Isojarvi JI, Lofgren E, Juntunen KS, *et al.* Effect of epilepsy and antiepileptic drugs on male reproductive health. *Neurology* 2004; 62: 247–53.

15. French J. Use of levetiracetam in special populations. *Epilepsia* 2001; 42 (Suppl 4): 40–3.

16. Wingfield JC, Sapolsky RM. Reproduction and resistance to stress: when and how. *J Neuroendocrinol* 2003; 15: 711–24.

17. Samuels MH, Luther M, Henry P, *et al.* Effects of hydrocortisone on pulsatile pituitary glycoprotein secretion. *J Clin Endocrinol Metab* 1994; 78: 211–15.

18. van den Bent MJ, Afra D, de Witte O, *et al.* Long-term efficacy of early versus delayed radiotherapy for low-grade astrocytoma and oligodendroglioma in adults: the EORTC 22845 randomised trial. *Lancet* 2005; 366: 985–90.

19. Abrey LE, Louis DN, Paleologos N, *et al.* Survey of treatment recommendations for anaplastic oligodendroglioma. *Neuro Oncol* 2007; 9: 314–18.

20. Howell S, Shalet S. Gonadal damage from chemotherapy and radiotherapy. *Endocrinol Metab Clin North Am* 1998; 27: 927–43.

21. Yung WK, Prados MD, Yaya-Tur R, *et al.* Multicenter phase II trial of temozolomide in patients with anaplastic astrocytoma or anaplastic oligoastrocytoma at first relapse. Temodal Brain Tumor Group. *J Clin Oncol* 1999; 17: 2762–71.

22. Gibson NW, Hickman JA, Erickson LC. DNA cross-linking and cytotoxicity in normal and transformed human cells treated in vitro with 8-carbamoyl-3-(2-chloroethyl) imidazo[5,1-d]-1,2,3,5-tetrazin-4(3H)-one. *Cancer Res* 1984; 44: 1772–5.

23. Temodar prescribing information. Last updated November 2011. www.spfiles.com/pitemodar.pdf (accessed Januaray 2012).

24. Thompson MJ, Abdul-Rahman S, Baker TG, *et al.* Role of O6-alkylguanine-DNA alkyltransferase in the resistance of mouse spermatogenic cells to O6-alkylating agents. *J Reprod Fertil* 2000; 119: 339–46.

25. Palmieri C, Brock C, Newlands ES. Maintenance of fertility following treatment with temozolomide for a high grade astrocytoma. *J Neurooncol* 2005; 73: 185.

26. Cohen MH, Shen YL, Keegan P, *et al.* FDA drug approval summary: bevacizumab (Avastin) as treatment of recurrent glioblastoma multiforme. *Oncologist* 2009; 14: 1131–8.

27. Kruger EA, Figg WD. TNP-470: an angiogenesis inhibitor in clinical development for cancer. *Expert Opin Investig Drugs* 2000; 9: 1383–96.

28. Littley MD, Shalet SM, Beardwell CG, *et al.* Hypopituitarism following external radiotherapy for pituitary tumours in adults. *Q J Med* 1989; 70: 145–60.

29. Agha A, Sherlock M, Brennan S, *et al.* Hypothalamic-pituitary dysfunction after irradiation of nonpituitary brain tumors in adults. *J Clin Endocrinol Metab* 2005; 90: 6355–60.

30. Littley MD, Shalet SM, Beardwell CG, *et al.* Radiation-induced hypopituitarism is dose-dependent. *Clin Endocrinol (Oxf)* 1989; 31: 363–73.

31. Harrop JS, Davies TJ, Capra LG, *et al.* Hypothalamic-pituitary function following successful treatment of intracranial tumours. *Clin Endocrinol (Oxf)* 1976; 5: 313–21.

32. Constine LS, Woolf PD, Cann D, *et al.* Hypothalamic–pituitary dysfunction after radiation for brain tumors. *N Engl J Med* 1993; 328: 87–94.

33. Black KL, Yin D, Ong JM, *et al.* PDE5 inhibitors enhance tumor permeability and efficacy of chemotherapy in a rat brain tumor model. *Brain Res* 2008; 1230: 290–302.

34. Burrow GN, Wortzman G, Rewcastle NB, *et al.* Microadenomas of the pituitary and abnormal sellar tomograms in an unselected autopsy series. *N Engl J Med* 1981; 304: 156–8.

35. Dulipsingh L, Lassman MN. Images in clinical medicine. Pituitary apoplexy. *N Engl J Med* 2000; 342: 550.

36. Gillam MP, Molitch ME, Lombardi G, *et al.* Advances in the treatment of prolactinomas. *Endocr Rev* 2006; 27: 485–534.

37. Prescott RW, Johnston DG, Kendall-Taylor P, *et al.* Hyperprolactinaemia in men-response to bromocriptine therapy. *Lancet* 1982; 1: 245–8.

38. Buvat J, Lemaire A, Buvat-Herbaut M, *et al.* Hyperprolactinemia and sexual function in men. *Horm Res* 1985; 22: 196–203.

39. Young WF, Jr., Scheithauer BW, Kovacs KT, *et al.* Gonadotroph adenoma of the pituitary gland: a clinicopathologic analysis of 100 cases. *Mayo Clin Proc* 1996; 71: 649–56.

40. Snyder PJ, Fowble BF, Schatz NJ, *et al.* Hypopituitarism following radiation therapy of pituitary adenomas. *Am J Med* 1986; 81: 457–62.

41. Shah GD, Yahalom J, Correa DD, *et al.* Combined immunochemotherapy with reduced whole-brain

radiotherapy for newly diagnosed primary CNS lymphoma. *J Clin Oncol* 2007; 25: 4730–5.

42. Morris LF, Harrod MJ, Menter MA, *et al.* Methotrexate and reproduction in men: case report and recommendations. *J Am Acad Dermatol* 1993; 29: 913–16.

43. El-Beheiry A, El-Mansy E, Kamel N, *et al.* Methotrexate and fertility in men. *Arch Androl* 1979; 3: 177–9.

44. Shamberger RC, Rosenberg SA, Seipp CA, *et al.* Effects of high-dose methotrexate and vincristine on ovarian and testicular functions in patients undergoing postoperative adjuvant treatment of osteosarcoma. *Cancer Treat Rep* 1981; 65: 739–46.

45. Arnon J, Meirow D, Lewis-Roness H, *et al.* Genetic and teratogenic effects of cancer treatments on gametes and embryos. *Hum Reprod Update* 2001; 7: 394–403.

46. Viviani S, Santoro A, Ragni G, *et al.* Gonadal toxicity after combination chemotherapy for Hodgkin's disease. Comparative results of MOPP vs ABVD. *Eur J Cancer Clin Oncol* 1985; 21: 601–5.

47. Lendon M, Hann IM, Palmer MK, *et al.* Testicular histology after combination chemotherapy in childhood for acute lymphoblastic leukaemia. *Lancet* 1978; 2: 439–41.

48. Lemez P, Urbanek V. Chemotherapy for acute myeloid leukemias with cytosine arabinoside, daunorubicin, etoposide, and mitoxantrone may cause permanent oligoasthenozoospermia or amenorrhea in middle-aged patients. *Neoplasma* 2005; 52: 398–401.

49. Podnar S, Oblak C, Vodusek DB. Sexual function in men with cauda equina lesions: a clinical and electromyographic study. *J Neurol Neurosurg Psychiatry* 2002; 73: 715–20.

50. DeAngelis LM, Posner JB. *Neurological Complication of Cancer*, 2nd edn. New York, NY: Oxford University Press, 2009.

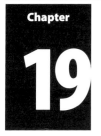

Male infertility following childhood cancer: special considerations for fertility preservation in children

Mark F. H. Brougham and W. Hamish B. Wallace

Introduction

Survival from childhood cancer has markedly improved over recent decades, following advances in treatment and supportive care, such that over 80% of children with cancer now achieve long-term cure [1]. The number of long-term survivors is therefore increasing, and as a result it is estimated that approximately 1 in 715 of the young adult population is a survivor of childhood cancer [2]. However, this improved survival comes at a cost, in terms of long-term adverse effects of cytotoxic treatment. Adverse late effects of childhood cancer treatment are diverse, and include disorders of the endocrine system, cardiac and pulmonary dysfunction, renal and hepatic impairment, secondary malignancies and psychosocial difficulties. Such late effects can have significant implications for survivors, who must live with the cost of cure. In view of this, quality of life after treatment has become a prominent consideration in the management of childhood cancer. Thus, while continuing to strive for improved survival, attention is increasingly directed towards minimizing the late effects of treatment.

Although problems with fertility do not become apparent until after puberty, it is clear that many treatments for childhood cancer can lead to infertility and subfertility in later life [3]. This can have a particularly devastating impact as the patient enters adulthood. Having survived cancer as a child, it can be very difficult for many patients to accept that they cannot produce their own children because of the treatment they received earlier in their life. Indeed, the impact of such treatment on future fertility is of significant concern to both patients and parents at the time of diagnosis [4], regardless of the risk of subsequent infertility.

It is therefore imperative to consider, at an early stage, strategies that may protect or restore fertility in later life.

This chapter will discuss the etiology of reduced fertility following treatment for childhood cancer in the male, and the ability to predict future fertility potential after particular treatment regimens. Strategies to protect or restore fertility will then be discussed, including novel experimental options, which are currently generating much interest within the scientific community.

Gonadal toxicity following childhood cancer treatment

Subfertility in boys treated for cancer can result from either systemic chemotherapy or radiotherapy involving the gonads. This damage may involve the somatic cells of the testis, the Sertoli and Leydig cells, and the germ cells.

Cytotoxic treatment, in general, targets rapidly dividing cells, and it is therefore not surprising that spermatogenesis can be impaired after treatment for cancer. The exact mechanism of this damage is uncertain but appears to involve depletion of the proliferating germ cell pool, by killing cells not only at the stage of differentiating spermatogonia [5] but also stem cells themselves [6]. The prepubertal testis does not complete spermatogenesis and produce mature spermatozoa, and therefore one may assume that cytotoxic treatment would not affect future fertility. However, it is clear that prepubertal boys treated for cancer can exhibit impaired fertility in later life [7], indicating that the testis is susceptible to such damage in this age group. In fact, there is evidence that far from being

Fertility Preservation in Male Cancer Patients, ed. John P. Mulhall, Linda D. Applegarth, Robert D. Oates and Peter N. Schlegel. Published by Cambridge University Press. © Cambridge University Press 2013.

a quiescent organ, the prepubertal testis demonstrates significant cellular activity, including a steady turnover of early germ cells, which undergo spontaneous degeneration before the haploid stage [8]. It is postulated that this activity is essential for normal adult function [9], accounting for the effect on fertility as a consequence of cytotoxic treatment in childhood.

The effects of chemotherapy

The nature and extent of gonadal damage due to cytotoxic chemotherapy is predominantly dependent upon the agent administered and its cumulative dose [10,11]. A number of commonly used chemotherapeutic agents have been identified as causing long-lasting or permanent gonadotoxicity. Those particularly implicated are the alkylating agents such as cyclophosphamide, thiotepa, and melphalan, but also include platinum agents such as cis platin, and others including procarbazine.

Within the testes, the seminiferous epithelium is the area most sensitive to the detrimental effects of chemotherapy. Therefore, after receiving gonadotoxic agents, patients may be rendered oligospermic or azoospermic, but testosterone production by the Leydig cell is usually unaffected, and thus secondary sexual characteristics develop normally [12]. Despite this, testes will be small and atrophied following such treatment, suggestive of reduced sperm production [13]. On clinical examination, using the Prader orchidometer, a testicular volume of 12 mL or less in a postpubertal male is likely to be associated with azoospermia. Following higher cumulative doses of gonadotoxic chemotherapy, Leydig cell dysfunction may also become apparent [14].

The effects of radiotherapy

The gonads are exquisitely sensitive to radiotherapy, with resultant damage depending on the field of treatment, total dose, and fractionation schedule [15,16]. Fractionation usually improves the therapeutic margin, but there is evidence to suggest that the gonads are an exception [17], and that fractionation may be more harmful to testicular function by reducing the time available for repair.

It has been demonstrated that doses as low as 0.1–1.2 Gy can have detectable effects on spermatogenesis in adult men, with doses over 4 Gy causing a more permanent detrimental effect [15]. As with chemotherapy, somatic cells are more resistant to radiation-induced damage than germ cells. Indeed, Leydig cell dysfunction is not observed until doses of around 20 Gy are administered to the prepubertal boy, and up to 30 Gy in sexually mature males [18,19]. Testosterone production is therefore relatively preserved below these doses, and thus many patients will develop normal secondary sexual characteristics, despite severe impairment of spermatogenesis.

Because of the significant adverse long-term consequences of radiotherapy, this treatment modality is used sparingly within pediatric oncology. However, it is unavoidable in certain circumstances. Radiation-induced gonadal damage may be encountered following direct testicular irradiation, as used for management of testicular relapse of leukemia, following total-body irradiation (TBI) given prior to bone marrow transplantation (BMT), pelvic radiotherapy, or scatter radiotherapy from treatment involving the spine.

Radiation doses of 24 Gy are used to treat leukemic involvement of the testes, and this results in permanent azoospermia [19]. The effects of TBI on gonadal function can be difficult to elucidate as this is usually given with other treatment modalities, including high-dose chemotherapy. However, doses of 9–10 Gy have been associated with subsequent gonadal failure [20].

Tumors of the central nervous system are the commonest solid malignancy seen in the pediatric population. These tumors are often less sensitive to chemotherapy than other pediatric malignancies, and therefore cranial and craniospinal irradiation is frequently required. Although cranial irradiation does not harm the gonads directly, fertility can be affected by disruption to the hypothalamic–pituitary–gonadal (HPG) axis. Indeed, patients receiving radiation doses of 35–45 Gy have demonstrated subsequent deficiencies in follicle-stimulating hormone (FSH) and luteinizing hormone (LH) [21]. The clinical sequelae of gonadotropin deficiency exhibit a broad spectrum of severity, from subclinical abnormalities detectable only by gonadotropin-releasing hormone (GnRH) testing, to a significant reduction in circulating sex hormone levels and delayed puberty. In the latter, exogenous GnRH can be used as replacement therapy in order to restore gonadal function and fertility. Radiotherapy involving the spine may also affect gonadal function due to scatter from the target radiation field [22], although the relative contribution of this may be difficult to determine due to the administration of concurrent gonadotoxic chemotherapy.

The effects of disease

Although many aspects of cancer treatment may affect fertility, it is important to note that the disease itself may contribute to male gonadal dysfunction. Indeed, it has been demonstrated that up to 70% of patients with Hodgkin's disease assessed prior to commencing treatment have impaired semen quality [23], and this has also been shown with other malignancies [24]. In addition to the disease itself, other non-specific conditions commonly observed at presentation, such as fever, anorexia, and pain, can impair semen quality [25]. Although these findings relate to adult patients, as semen analysis is not possible in prepubertal boys, these studies may have implications when options for preserving fertility in this patient group become technically and clinically feasible.

The potential for fertility following childhood cancer treatment

Because of the varied nature of the gonadal insult following chemotherapy or radiotherapy, and the uncertain baseline fertility status in prepubertal boys, it can be very difficult to predict whether a child undergoing cancer treatment will subsequently have impaired fertility as an adult. The risk of subfertility can be categorized according to the type of malignancy and associated treatment, as demonstrated in Table 19.1, which describes the subfertility risk based on current treatment protocols [26]. Such guides are based on cumulative doses of gonadotoxic drugs, particularly alkylating agents, and treatment requiring radiotherapy involving the gonads. Thus treatment for Hodgkin's disease with alkylating agent-based therapy is profoundly gonadotoxic, as is conditioning prior to bone marrow transplantation with high-dose chemotherapy and TBI. In contrast, acute lymphoblastic leukemia (ALL), which is the commonest childhood malignancy accounting for approximately one-third of all cancers in this age group, is associated with a relatively low risk of subsequent infertility.

However, this best assessment of risk only represents an approximate guide, and thus providing children and their families with accurate information regarding future fertility is very difficult. In addition treatment protocols are continually evolving, in order to improve survival and reduce adverse effects. Thus adult survivors who can now have their fertility accurately assessed may have been treated many years ago

Table 19.1. Risk of subfertility in male patients following treatment for cancer: assessment based on current treatment protocols as per CCLG consensus document [26]

Low risk ($\leq$ 10%)	Acute lymphoblastic leukemia Acute myeloid leukemia Non-Hodgkin's lymphoma • Anaplastic large cell lymphoma • T-cell lymphoma • B-cell lymphoma: cyclophosphamide < 3.3 g/m^2 Hodgkin's lymphoma stage I: no alkylating agents Brain tumors: 24 Gy radiotherapy dose to the pituitary Soft tissue sarcomas • Rhabdomyosarcoma: ifosfamide < 30 g/m^2 • Synovial sarcoma: ifosfamide < 36 g/m^2 Infant neuroblastoma: cyclophosphamide 3 g/m^2 Wilms' tumor: no gonadotoxic drugs Retinoblastoma: no gonadotoxic drugs Germ cell tumors: no gonadotoxic drugs
Medium risk (10–80%)	Relapsed acute lymphoblastic leukemia Non-Hodgkin's lymphoma • B-cell: cyclophosphamide 6.8 g/m^2 Hodgkin's lymphoma stage II and III treatment with alkylating agents Brain tumors: 24–55 Gy radiotherapy dose to the pituitary Bone tumors • Osteogenic sarcoma Soft tissue sarcoma • Rhabdomyosarcoma: ifosfamide 54g/m^2 • Malignant mesenchymal tumors: ifosfamide 54g/m^2 • Synovial sarcoma: ifosfamide 48g/m^2 Infant neuroblastoma: cyclophosphamide < 6g/m^2 Wilms' tumor: cyclophosphamide < 8.1 g/m^2 Hepatoblastoma Retinoblastoma: cranial radiation Relapsed and refractory germ cells tumors
High risk ($\geq$ 80%)	Total body irradiation: 12–14.4 Gy in 6–8 fractions Localized radiotherapy: pelvic or testicular Brain tumors: > 55 Gy radiotherapy dose to the pituitary Chemotherapy conditioning for bone marrow transplant Hodgkin's lymphoma: any stage that requires radiation to the pelvis Bone tumors • Ewing sarcoma Neuroblastoma stage IV Relapsed and refractory Wilms' tumor

with treatment combinations very different from those utilized in the present day. To complicate matters further, there are reports of patients having received sterilizing treatment who have subsequently demonstrated recovery of spermatogenesis [27]. This not only has implications for counseling with regards to infertility, but also demonstrates the importance of discussing contraception with adult patients whose fertility status is uncertain.

Determining the impact of cancer treatment on gonadal function currently involves clinical assessment of pubertal status, biochemical assessment of plasma gonadotropins and testosterone, and semen analysis. However, in prepubertal children, clinical assessment such as this is non-contributory and biochemical assessment is unreliable because the HPG axis is relatively quiescent in this age group. Thus it is currently not possible to detect gonadal damage early, due to the lack of a sensitive marker of gonadal function in prepubertal children.

Inhibin B is a dimeric glycoprotein secreted predominantly from the Sertoli cells, and is involved in negative feedback regulation of FSH; it is also a good indicator of the status of spermatogenesis in adulthood [28]. There is some evidence to suggest that gonadotoxic chemotherapy is associated with a reduction in inhibin B levels in adults [29], presumably indicating reduced sperm production [28]. However, this relationship has not been clearly demonstrated in prepubertal boys [30], perhaps because spermatogenesis has not yet been initiated, although studies are ongoing to investigate the role of inhibin B, and whether it could function as a marker of gonadotoxicity in this patient group in the future.

Options for fertility preservation

Established methods: semen cryopreservation

Currently the only established option to preserve fertility following gonadotoxic therapy is cryopreservation of spermatozoa prior to commencing treatment. Patients for whom this procedure is suitable must be peri- or postpubertal and sexually mature. In addition they must be able to give consent for the storage of gametes.

Although semen cryopreservation in adult patients is standard practice, within the pediatric population this process can be problematic. Sperm banking is not universally offered in pediatric oncology centers, although this situation has improved in recent years [31]. In addition, there are few suitable "adolescent-friendly" facilities. In most circumstances treatment

of the cancer needs to start promptly following confirmation of the diagnosis. However, semen must be obtained for storage prior to starting any cytotoxic treatment. After receiving such devastating news regarding the diagnosis, it can be very difficult for teenagers to then discuss fertility and future children and subsequently go on to produce a semen specimen. On the positive side, however, many patients and their families derive benefit from open discussion regarding fertility, particularly as this places emphasis on looking to the future and provides reassurance that curative treatment is the aim [32].

The semen specimen is ideally produced by masturbation. Discussions regarding this process can be difficult to develop with younger teenagers, particularly with the knowledge that their parents are aware of the issues being raised. It is imperative that the specimen is not produced within the ward area, but instead in appropriate, and ideally dedicated, facilities. Alternatives to masturbation include rectal electrostimulation, epididymal aspiration, or testicular biopsy, but these are invasive procedures requiring general anesthesia.

The specimens produced in these circumstances are often of poor quality [33]. Many adolescent patients may have only recently commenced spermarche, which may partially explain this. In addition the effects of disease, as previously discussed, and psychological stress, often observed at this difficult time, can also impair semen quality [34].

Despite these difficulties, semen cryopreservation should be offered to all suitable patients prior to commencing treatment. However, this option is clearly not applicable to the prepubertal boy. At present there are no established methods of fertility preservation in this age group, and therefore options for these patients currently remain entirely experimental.

Experimental techniques

Testicular tissue harvesting

The prepubertal testis does not complete spermatogenesis and therefore does not produce mature spermatozoa. However, diploid stem germ cells are present from which haploid spermatozoa will ultimately be derived. Testicular tissue could therefore theoretically be harvested from a biopsy and stored, either as a segment of tissue or as isolated germ cells, prior to gonadotoxic treatment. Following cure and on entering adulthood, this tissue could be thawed and used in one of two ways

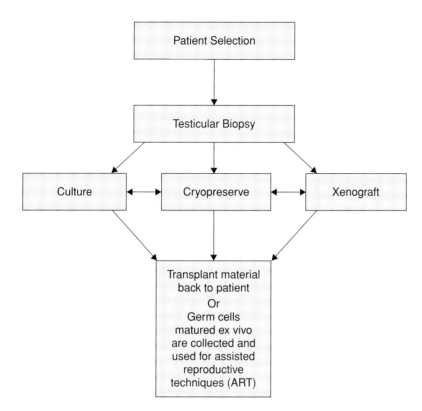

Figure 19.1. Potential scenario for preserving fertility in young males. Patients due to receive high-risk gonadotoxic treatment could be given the option of a testicular biopsy to retrieve tissue containing spermatogonial stem cells for storage. If consent is given, some of the material can be used for research into the development of potential methods of fertility preservation. A patient's fertility could be restored by transplanting their tissue back, allowing the spermatogonial stem cells to repopulate the testes. Alternatively germ cells matured in vitro are collected and used for assisted reproductive techniques (ART).

in order to produce offspring. Firstly, the stored germ cells could be re-implanted into the patient's own testes in order to restore natural fertility, a procedure known as germ cell transplantation. Alternatively, the stored stem cells could be matured in vitro until they are able to achieve fertilization using procedures such as intra-cytoplasmic sperm injection (ICSI). These options are shown in Fig. 19.1.

Germ cell transplantation

Germ cell transplantation was pioneered by Brinster and colleagues in 1994 [35]. Following the injection of germ cell suspensions from donor mice into genetically sterile mice, restoration of spermatogenesis was observed from the donor stem cells. Alternative techniques for restoring spermatogenesis following germ cell transplantation have also been developed, including xenografting of testicular tissue from mice, pigs, and goats into castrated immunodeficient mice [36]. More recently, primate studies have demonstrated restoration of spermatogenesis following autologous grafting of testicular tissue [37].

The technique of germ cell transplantation is clearly of relevance to prepubertal boys requiring treatment for cancer, offering hope to those patients at risk of subsequent infertility. Prior to starting gonadotoxic therapy testicular tissue could be harvested and stored in order to restore fertility in the future. However, these procedures are associated with a number of problems that must first be overcome before routine clinical application.

Firstly, obtaining testicular tissue would require an additional surgical procedure following confirmation of the diagnosis and before cytotoxic treatment commenced. Testicular biopsy within the prepubertal period is not without risk, particularly in view of the small size of the testis at this age. This procedure could result in damage to the testis, thus compromising future testicular function. Although this technique has been performed, with apparent acceptability and minimal complications [38], it remains difficult to justify until the potential advantages have been more clearly demonstrated.

Secondly, there remain uncertainties regarding the optimal cryopreservation process. Although cryopreservation of mature, haploid spermatozoa is well established there are substantial biological differences between these cells and undifferentiated, diploid stem cell spermatogonia, and thus the requirements for successful freezing and thawing differ considerably. Glycerol is used as the preservative of choice for ejaculated spermatozoa. However, dimethylsulfoxide (DMSO) may represent a more suitable cryoprotectant for earlier germ cells [39], which have proportionately larger amounts of cytoplasm. Despite this potential, the safety of DMSO in clinical use requires further evaluation before human application.

Thirdly, and of more concern, autologous germ cell transplantation requires tissue that was removed from a patient with cancer prior to treatment to be returned to the patient following cure. There is, therefore, a genuine risk of reintroducing malignant cells, with potentially fatal consequences. This is unlikely to occur with malignancies such as Hodgkin's disease, which is often localized at presentation, but the risk would be substantial with hematological malignancies [40], where the testes can act as sanctuary sites for leukemic cells. Indeed, any theoretical risk of returning cancer cells following treatment, however small, would not be acceptable. Although xenografting tissue using nude mice would circumvent this risk, it is unlikely that this process would become accepted for clinical use.

In order to alleviate this problem the germ cells, and in particular the stem cells, from the testicular biopsy would need to be isolated prior to transplantation. However, the reliable identification and isolation of stem cells is difficult because of the lack of specific cell surface markers. Stem cells express alpha-6 and beta-1 integrins [41], but other progenitor cells, including hematopoietic cells, also express these antigens, and thus these markers do not have sufficient specificity to exclude malignant cells. More recently, glial cell-derived neurotrophic factor receptor alpha-1 has been demonstrated on spermatogonia from rodents and primates, and offers potential for purification via magnetic cell sorting [42].

For germ cell transplantation to be successful, sufficient numbers of stem cells must be injected into the testes. Due to the paucity of stem cells, particularly within the prepubertal testis, there is a need to develop an in-vitro enrichment system that will safely augment stem cell numbers following harvesting and isolation. Nagano et al. have demonstrated the feasibility of enrichment of mouse stem germ cells [43].

However, because of the low numbers of stem cells that are likely to be returned, it may be that patients in whom germ cell transplantation is successful will still only be oligospermic rather than having normal sperm counts. They will therefore still require assisted reproduction in order to produce offspring.

Following harvest, stem cell isolation, cryopreservation, and enrichment, the cells then need to be returned to the testes. Although this has been successfully performed in animal models, the procedure for transplantation into the human testis remains unclear. The most effective method of reinfusion in larger testes, including humans, is likely to be injection into the rete testis under ultrasound guidance [44], as this allows a much larger volume to be infused. This technique is particularly successful in immature or regressed testes because of the lower intratubular fluid pressure, and therefore has potential for patients treated for cancer, as the testes can be regressed secondary to cytotoxic treatment.

In-vitro maturation

As an alternative to autologous transplant, maturing germ cells in vitro, stimulating their differentiation into spermatozoa, would circumvent the risk of reintroducing malignant cells. In addition, this technique could be particularly useful in patients who have received such profoundly gonadotoxic therapy that the supporting Sertoli cells would be unable to support spermatogenesis. Tesarik et al. reported the restoration of fertility following in-vitro spermatogenesis [45]. However, this process involved in-vitro maturation of the later stages of spermatogenesis rather than development from stem cells. In-vitro maturation of diploid stem cells into haploid spermatozoa is much more difficult to achieve, although Sato et al. have recently developed a culture system that supports the complete process of spermatogenesis within a mouse model [46]. This is an extremely exciting development, and offers promise for this approach in the future (Fig. 19.2).

Hormonal manipulation

Cytotoxic treatment, as mentioned previously, acts principally on rapidly dividing cells. The testis is vulnerable to this damage as it demonstrates significant cellular activity. Inducing testicular quiescence could therefore theoretically prevent gonadal toxicity, by making germ cells less susceptible to cytotoxic effects.

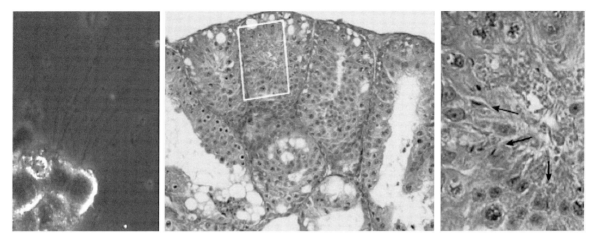

Figure 19.2. Completion of spermatogenesis in the mouse within an in-vitro culture system. Left: flagellated sperm. Centre: section of testis tissue after 38 days in culture shows well-developed seminiferous tubules and spermatogenesis. Right: white box has been enlarged, and arrows point out sperm formation (Reproduced from Sato *et al.* 2011 [46], with permission from Nature Publishing Group). *See color plate section.*

Studies investigating this technique using rodent models have produced very encouraging results. Ward *et al.* induced suppression of the HPG axis using a GnRH agonist [47]. This was administered to rats before treatment with procarbazine, and subsequently enhanced recovery of spermatogenesis was demonstrated, as compared to control animals. Similar protection of spermatogenesis has also been demonstrated using other methods of suppressing the reproductive axis, and following other gonadotoxic agents.

Although this technique is clearly of interest, these studies involve hormonal manipulation for several weeks prior to administration of the cytotoxic agent. There is an obvious urgency in starting cancer treatment as soon as possible following confirmation of the diagnosis, and therefore this delay would not be acceptable, either to patients or to professionals. However, Meistrich and Kangasniemi demonstrated that hormonal manipulation with a GnRH antagonist or testosterone led to the successful recovery of spermatogenesis in rats even when given *after* sterilizing treatment [48]. While this would circumvent the concerns regarding the delay in cancer treatment, this finding questions the hypothesis of gonadal protection simply involving a reduction in the susceptibility of germ cells.

Rodent models have demonstrated that azoospermia following cytotoxic therapy does not necessarily result from complete depletion of spermatogonia, but is secondary to failure of surviving spermatogonia

to replicate and differentiate [49]. In view of this it has been postulated that recovery of spermatogenesis following hormonal treatment is due to the stimulation of differentiation of surviving spermatogonia.

Despite the success of these techniques in rodent models, clinical trials of hormonal manipulation in patients receiving gonadotoxic therapy have thus far failed to demonstrate any benefit. Administration of a GnRH analog prior to and during treatment for lymphoma has been ineffective in conserving fertility [50]. In addition, attempts have been made to stimulate differentiation using hormonal manipulation. Thomson *et al.* treated seven men rendered azoospermic following treatment for childhood cancer with testosterone and medroxyprogesterone acetate [51]. However, after suppression of the HPG axis the men remained azoospermic. Testicular biopsy demonstrated a complete lack of germ cells. Perhaps in this study the hormonal treatment was initiated too long after the cytotoxic therapy. In addition, the lack of success may be because the initial testicular insult was too severe, and this technique may be more beneficial in patients with less severe gonadal damage, in whom some spermatogonial stem cells are preserved following cytotoxic treatment. However, it is difficult to justify further clinical trials in this area until the mechanism of gonadal "protection" is better understood. Indeed, extrapolating evidence from rodent models to clinical trials assumes that both the physiology of spermatogenesis and the mechanisms of gonadotoxic damage are similar in both species. However, there is evidence to suggest that significant inter-species differences do exist. Other primates, for example the common marmoset (*Callithrix jacchus*), which demonstrates similar phases of testicular development and displays similarities in its organization of spermatogenesis to the human, would represent a more appropriate model in which to study spermatogenesis in this regard [52].

Kelnar *et al*. investigated this phase of development using immunoexpression studies of marmoset testes [53]. Functional development of both Sertoli cells, based on the expression of sulfated glycoprotein-2 and androgen receptor, and of Leydig cell activity, based on the expression of 3β-hydroxysteroid dehydrogenase, was demonstrated prepubertally. In addition, proliferation of germ cells was noted at this age, indicated by the immunoexpression of proliferating cell nuclear antigen (PCNA). This provides further evidence that the prepubertal testis is not quiescent, and improves our understanding of why the testis is susceptible to cytotoxic damage in this age group.

However, studies of GnRH antagonist treatment in this marmoset model demonstrated no effect on germ cell proliferation, suggesting that this process in prepubertal primates is in fact gonadotropin-*independent*. Thus hormone manipulation based on suppression of the HPG axis is unlikely to be successful in alleviating cytotoxic damage within the testes in primates. It is therefore essential to improve our understanding of human spermatogenesis before this approach becomes a realistic option.

Ethical and legal issues

Harvesting gonadal tissue for future use, and hormonal manipulation to improve future spermatogenesis, are both exciting prospects that provide hope for children with cancer. Although there are still many scientific and technical issues to resolve, this technology also raises a number of important ethical and legal issues, which must be addressed before these procedures are utilized in a clinical setting.

Of prime importance when considering options for future fertility following childhood cancer treatment must be that any decision is taken in the child's best interests. Thus the advantages of any intervention, or of an active decision not to intervene, must outweigh any disadvantages, both in the short and long term. Attempts to preserve fertility must not raise

unrealistic expectations, and must not have undue adverse effects in either the patient or any subsequent offspring.

Comparing potential benefits with long-term risks is particularly problematic in this situation. The effectiveness of therapeutic intervention is still unknown at present, and it will be many years until expertise has improved sufficiently to assess it realistically. However, unless these techniques are considered and appropriate methods offered now, the opportunity for fertility preservation will be missed. Deleterious effects will also take many years to fully evaluate, particularly with respect to future progeny. Thus fertility preservation must be considered in the context of clinical benefit within the management of childhood cancer, but also in the context of ongoing research. Clearly, valid consent to perform these procedures is both a legal and ethical requirement.

For consent to be valid it must be informed, obtained voluntarily, and given by a competent person. Legal competence to consent requires that the individual giving it is able to understand the information given, believes it applies to them, retains it, and uses it to make an informed choice. In view of the complexity of the issues surrounding fertility preservation, the anxieties of both patients and their families at the time of diagnosis, and the limited time for discussion due to the urgency of commencing treatment, the validity of such consent may be impaired.

The issue of valid consent is further complicated by the age of the patients involved and their degree of understanding of the issues being discussed. In the UK, young persons may consent to treatment under the Family Law Reform Act (1969), specifically over the age of 16 years in Scotland and 18 years in England. Otherwise consent is obtained by proxy, from a parent or legal guardian. Younger children may give valid consent if they demonstrate sufficient understanding and intelligence to enable them to make an informed decision, so-called "Gillick competence" [54]. However, with respect to the storage and future use of gametes, consent by proxy is specifically excluded by the Human Fertilisation and Embryology Act [55]. Thus parents, or legal guardians, cannot give consent on behalf of the child. However, immature germ cells are not within the HFEA definition of a gamete, as they are unable to take part in fertilization. Therefore these cells could be harvested with parental consent, if the procedure was in the child's best interests. If this immature material were subsequently matured to produce gametes, this tissue would then fall under the jurisdiction of the HFEA.

Consent in situations such as this would be best viewed as a dynamic, continual process that is adapted as new information becomes available. Indeed, many of the difficulties discussed above may be alleviated by obtaining consent in different stages [56]. The first stage of consent would be for the harvest and storage of the gonadal tissue. The second stage, at a later date, would involve consent for the use of stored germ cell material for both fertilization and research. In addition, it is essential to discuss what should happen to gonadal tissue in the event of the child's death, and whether in this circumstance the material should be destroyed, or alternatively consent obtained for the tissue to be used for research purposes. Clearly discussions regarding this must be handled delicately and sensitively with both the patient and his family.

These issues must be addressed in order that new techniques are adequately regulated. Following extensive, collaborative discussion within a multidisciplinary setting, a number of recommendations have been suggested [57]. These include ongoing, structured research with centralization of data and rapid dissemination of results, a rigorous review of procedures, and development of the process of obtaining informed consent. This will ensure that children with cancer have a realistic and safe prospect for fertility in the future.

Conclusion

Infertility can be a major long-term side effect following treatment for childhood cancer, and will become increasingly important as greater numbers of children survive into adulthood. It is therefore imperative to consider ways of protecting or restoring fertility at an early stage.

Infertility is associated with a number of chemotherapeutic agents and with radiotherapy. Treatments for certain cancers are more likely to result in subsequent infertility than others. However, it can be very difficult to predict which children will be affected in later life.

At present there is nothing to offer the prepubertal boy at risk of infertility, and indeed the provision for postpubertal boys is inadequate. However, there are a number of potential therapeutic interventions that may be of benefit. Although many scientific, technical, legal, and ethical issues need to be addressed before

these techniques become part of the routine management of these patients, there exists genuine hope for childhood cancer survivors at risk of infertility in the future.

References

1. Mertens AC, Yasui Y, Neglia JP, *et al.* Late mortality experience in five-year survivors of childhood and adolescent cancer: the Childhood Cancer Survivor Study. *J Clin Oncol* 2001; 19: 3163–72.

2. Campbell J, Wallace WH, Bhatti LA *et al.* Cancer in Scotland: trends in incidence, mortality, and survival 1975–1999. Edinburgh 2003: Information and Statistics Division. www.isdscotland.org/cancer_information (accessed January 2012).

3. Brougham MFH, Wallace WHB. Subfertility in children and young people treated for solid and haematological malignancies. *Br J Haematol* 2005; 131: 143–55.

4. Oosterhuis BE, Goodwin T, Kiernan M, *et al.* Concerns about infertility risks among pediatric oncology patients and their parents. *Pediatr Blood Cancer* 2008; 50: 85–9.

5. Meistrich ML, Finch M, da Cunha MF, *et al.* Damaging effects of fourteen chemotherapeutic drugs on mouse testis cells. *Cancer Res* 1982; 42: 122–31.

6. Bucci LR, Meistrich ML. Effects of busulfan on murine spermatogenesis: cytotoxicity, sterility, sperm abnormalities, and dominant lethal mutations. *Mutat Res* 1987; 176: 259–68.

7. Whitehead E, Shalet SM, Jones PH, *et al.* Gonadal function after combination chemotherapy for Hodgkin's disease in childhood. *Arch Dis Child* 1982; 57: 287–91.

8. Rey RA, Campo SM, Bedecarras P, *et al.* Is infancy a quiescent period of testicular development? Histological, morphometric, and functional study of the seminiferous tubules of the cebus monkey from birth to the end of puberty. *J Clin Endocrinol Metab* 1993; 76: 1325–31.

9. Chemes HE. Infancy is not a quiescent period of testicular development. *Int J Androl* 2001; 24: 2–7.

10. Mackie EJ, Radford M, Shalet SM. Gonadal function following chemotherapy for childhood Hodgkin's disease. *Med Pediatr Oncol* 1996; 27: 74–8.

11. Wallace WH, Shalet SM, Crowne EC, *et al.* Gonadal dysfunction due to cis-platinum. *Med Pediatr Oncol* 1989; 17: 409–13.

12. Kreuser ED, Xiros N, Hetzel WD, Heimpel H. Reproductive and endocrine gonadal capacity in patients treated with COPP chemotherapy for

Hodgkin's disease. *J Cancer Res Clin Oncol* 1987; 113: 260–6.

13. Siimes MA, Rautonen J. Small testicles with impaired production of sperm in adult male survivors of childhood malignancies. *Cancer* 1990; 65: 1303–6.

14. Gerl A, Muhlbayer D, Hansmann G, *et al*. The impact of chemotherapy on Leydig cell function in long term survivors of germ cell tumors. *Cancer* 2001; 91: 1297–303.

15. Centola GM, Keller JW, Henzler M, Rubin P. Effect of low-dose testicular irradiation on sperm count and fertility in patients with testicular seminoma. *J Androl* 1994; 15: 608–13.

16. Rowley MJ, Leach DR, Warner GA, Heller CG. Effect of graded doses of ionizing radiation on the human testis. *Radiat Res* 1974; 59: 665–78.

17. Ash P. The influence of radiation on fertility in man. *Br J Radiol* 1980; 53: 271–8.

18. Shalet SM, Tsatsoulis A, Whitehead E, Read G. Vulnerability of the human Leydig cell to radiation damage is dependent upon age. *J Endocrinol* 1989; 120: 161–5.

19. Castillo LA, Craft AW, Kernahan J, *et al*. Gonadal function after 12-Gy testicular irradiation in childhood acute lymphoblastic leukaemia. *Med Pediatr Oncol* 1990; 18: 185–9.

20. Leiper AD, Stanhope R, Lau T, *et al*. The effect of total body irradiation and bone marrow transplantation during childhood and adolescence on growth and endocrine function. *Br J Haematol* 1987; 67: 419–26.

21. Littley MD, Shalet SM, Beardwell CG, *et al*. Radiation-induced hypopituitarism is dose-dependent. *Clin Endocrinol (Oxf)* 1989; 31: 363–73.

22. Schmiegelow M, Lassen S, Poulsen HS, *et al*. Gonadal status in male survivors following childhood brain tumors. *J Clin Endocrinol Metab* 2001; 86: 2446–52.

23. Rueffer U, Breuer K, Josting A, *et al*. Male gonadal dysfunction in patients with Hodgkin's disease prior to treatment. *Ann Oncol* 2001; 12: 1307–11.

24. Hallak J, Mahran A, Chae J, Agarwal A. The effects of cryopreservation on semen from men with sarcoma or carcinoma. *J Assist Reprod Genet* 2000; 17: 218–21.

25. Agarwal A, Shekarriz M, Sidhu RK, Thomas AJ. Value of clinical diagnosis in predicting the quality of cryopreserved sperm from cancer patients. *J Urol* 1996; 155: 934–8.

26. Brougham MFH, Levitt G on behalf of the Children's Cancer and Leukaemia Group, Late Effects Working Group. Subfertility Risk Consensus Document: Update 2010. www.cclg.org.uk (accessed January 2012).

27. Marmor D, Duyck F. Male reproductive potential after MOPP therapy for Hodgkin's disease: a long-term survey. *Andrologia* 1995; 27: 99–106.

28. Anderson RA, Sharpe RM. Regulation of inhibin production in the human male and its clinical applications. *Int J Androl* 2000; 23: 136–44.

29. Wallace EM, Groome NP, Riley SC, *et al*. Effects of chemotherapy-induced testicular damage on inhibin, gonadotropin, and testosterone secretion: a prospective longitudinal study. *J Clin Endocrinol Metab* 1997; 82: 3111–15.

30. Crofton PM, Thomson AB, Evans AEM, *et al*. Is inhibin B a potential marker of gonadotoxicity in prepubertal children treated for cancer? *Clin Endocrinol (Oxf)* 2003; 58: 296–301.

31. Anderson RA, Weddell A, Spoudeas HA, *et al*. Do doctors discuss fertility issues before they treat young patients with cancer? *Hum Reprod* 2008; 23: 2246–51.

32. Wallace WHB, Thomson AB. Preservation of fertility in children treated for cancer. *Arch Dis Child* 2003; 88: 493–6.

33. Postovsky S, Lightman A, Aminpour D, *et al*. Sperm cryopreservation in adolescents with newly diagnosed cancer. *Med Pediatr Oncol* 2003; 40: 355–9.

34. Clarke RN, Klock SC, Geoghegan A, Travassos DE. Relationship between psychological stress and semen quality among in-vitro fertilization patients. *Hum Reprod* 1999; 14: 753–8.

35. Brinster RL, Zimmermann JW. Spermatogenesis following male germ-cell transplantation. *Proc Natl Acad Sci U S A* 1994; 91: 11298–302.

36. Honaramooz A, Snedaker A, Boiani M, *et al*. Sperm from neonatal mammalian testes grafted in mice. *Nature* 2002; 418: 778–81.

37. Luetjens CM, Stukenborg JB, Nieschlag E, *et al*. Complete spermatogenesis in orthotopic but not in ectopic transplants of autologously grafted marmoset testicular tissue. *Endocrinology* 2008; 149: 1736–47.

38. Ginsberg JP, Carlson CA, Lin K, *et al*. An experimental protocol for fertility preservation in prepubertal boys recently diagnosed with cancer: a report on acceptability and safety. *Hum Reprod* 2010; 25: 37–41.

39. Goossens E, Frederickx V, Geens M, *et al*. Cryosurvival and spermatogenesis after allografting prepubertal mouse tissue: comparison of two cryopreservation protocols. *Fertil Steril* 2008; 89: 725–7.

40. Jahnukainen K, Hou M, Petersen C, *et al*. Intratesticular transplantation of testicular cells from leukemic rats causes transmission of leukemia. *Cancer Res* 2001; 61: 706–10.

41. Shinohara T, Avarbock MR, Brinster RL. Beta 1 and alpha 6-integrin are surface markers on mouse spermatogonial stem cells. *Proc Natl Acad Sci U S A* 1999; 96: 5504–9.

42. Gassei K, Ehmcke J, Dhir R, Schlatt S. Magnetic activated cell sorting allows isolation of spermatogonia from adult primate testes and reveals distinct GFRα1-positive subpopulations in men. *J Med Primatol* 2010; 39: 83–91.

43. Nagano M, Avarbock MR, Leonida EB, *et al.* Culture of mouse spermatogonial stem cells. *Tissue Cell* 1998; 30: 389–97.

44. Schlatt S, Rosiepen G, Weinbauer GF, *et al.* Germ cell transfer into rat, bovine, monkey and human testes. *Hum Reprod* 1999; 14: 144–50.

45. Tesarik J, Bahceci M, Ozcan C, *et al.* Restoration of fertility by in-vitro spermatogenesis. *Lancet* 1999; 353: 555–6.

46. Sato T, Katagiri K, Gohbara A, *et al.* In vitro production of functional sperm in cultured neonatal mouse testes. *Nature* 2011; 471: 504–7.

47. Ward JA, Robinson J, Furr BJ, *et al.* Protection of spermatogenesis in rats from the cytotoxic procarbazine by the depot formulation of Zoladex, a gonadotropin-releasing hormone agonist. *Cancer Res* 1990; 50: 568–74.

48. Meistrich ML, Kangasniemi M. Hormone treatment after irradiation stimulates recovery of rat spermatogenesis from surviving spermatogonia. *J Androl* 1997; 18: 80–7.

49. Kangasniemi M, Huhtaniemi I, Meistrich ML. Failure of spermatogenesis to recover despite the presence of A spermatogonia in the irradiated LBNF1 rat. *Biol Reprod* 1996; 54: 1200–8.

50. Johnson DH, Linde R, Hainsworth JD, *et al.* Effect of a luteinizing hormone releasing hormone agonist given during combination chemotherapy on posttherapy fertility in male patients with lymphoma: preliminary observations. *Blood* 1985; 65: 832–6.

51. Thomson AB, Anderson RA, Irvine DS, *et al.* Investigation of suppression of the hypothalamic-pituitary-gonadal axis to restore spermatogenesis in azoospermic men treated for childhood cancer. *Hum Reprod* 2002; 17: 1715–23.

52. Sharpe RM, Walker M, Millar MR, *et al.* Effect of neonatal gonadotropin-releasing hormone antagonist administration on sertoli cell number and testicular development in the marmoset: comparison with the rat. *Biol Reprod* 2000; 62: 1685–93.

53. Kelnar CJ, McKinnell C, Walker M, *et al.* Testicular changes during infantile "quiescence" in the marmoset and their gonadotrophin dependence: a model for investigating susceptibility of the prepubertal human testis to cancer therapy? *Hum Reprod* 2002; 17: 1367–78.

54 Gillick *v* West Norfolk and Wisbech Area Authority. *All England Law Reports* 1985; 402.

55. Human Fertilisation and Embryology Act 1990. Chapter 37. London: HMSO.

56. Grundy R, Larcher V, Gosden RG, *et al.* Fertility preservation for children treated for cancer (2): ethics of consent for gamete storage and experimentation. *Arch Dis Child* 2001; 84: 360–2.

57. Wallace WH, Walker DA. Conference consensus statement: ethical and research dilemmas for fertility preservation in children treated for cancer. *Hum Fertil (Camb)* 2001; 4: 69–76.

Chapter

20

Facilitating discussion about fertility preservation

Gwendolyn P. Quinn and Susan T. Vadaparampil

Introduction

Men with a cancer diagnosis are at risk for infertility. The level of risk depends on many factors, including the cancer site and stage, the type of treatment, and the age of the patient. Men of reproductive age are most commonly diagnosed with leukemia, Hodgkin's lymphoma, and testicular tumors [1]. The physiology of male infertility due to cancer is discussed in detail elsewhere. In general, male risk of infertility from cancer may be manifested not only in poor sperm quality but also in the prevention of natural conception due to problems with arousal and ejaculation. Males who undergo surgery for genitourinary, prostate, testicular, penile, or bladder cancers may also have higher rates of sexual dysfunction, which may in turn impact fertility [2].

Men of reproductive age diagnosed with cancer have one established option for fertility preservation: sperm cryopreservation [3]. There are additional experimental options available for males, and these are discussed later in the book. The American Society of Clinical Oncology (ASCO) recommends that oncologists discuss the risks of infertility with patients prior to cancer treatment. ASCO further recommends that patients interested in fertility preservation be referred to a reproductive endocrinologist/infertility specialist [3].

Interest in fertility preservation among men

Multiple studies with cancer survivors indicate that men are interested in having biological children in the future. Recent reviews of the literature confirm that as many as 75% of young men diagnosed with cancer did not have any children at the time of diagnosis but hoped to in the future [4]. The act of sperm banking, irrespective of subsequent decisions to use stored sperm, has been shown to have positive psychological effects for men, who perceive banking sperm as hope for the future. A study of 776 men referred for sperm banking prior to cancer treatment found that 80% opted to cryopreserve. Of those men, 12% were unable to bank due to existing azoospermia. Among the men who chose to bank sperm and were able to, 80% reported the act of sperm banking helped them psychologically in their battle against cancer. These men reported that the recommendation to bank was encouraging, and the majority said they would suggest sperm cryopreservation to other cancer patients [5].

Barriers to discussing fertility preservation with men

Studies reporting on the use of sperm banking among men diagnosed with cancer are quite varied. The rate varies from as low as 6% [6] to 50% [5,7], with the average rate around 24% [3,8]. Most studies attribute the low rates of banked sperm to lack of awareness among males about the potential for sterility after cancer treatment and the availability of fertility preservation.

A study of testicular cancer survivors referred for infertility treatment post-cancer treatment showed that the majority were unaware of their current fertility status at that time as well as their potential fertility status at the time of diagnosis [9]. Similar studies with testicular cancer survivors showed that the majority had received information or communicated with their oncologist about the possibility of sperm banking but

Fertility Preservation in Male Cancer Patients, ed. John P. Mulhall, Linda D. Applegarth, Robert D. Oates and Peter N. Schlegel.
Published by Cambridge University Press. © Cambridge University Press 2013.

less than half had elected to pursue fertility preservation [10].

ASCO guidelines suggest it is the role of the oncologist to inform men about potential infertility and refer for sperm banking [3]. A recent study of US oncologists showed that less than 38% were aware of the ASCO guidelines and less than 47% routinely referred patients for fertility preservation [11]. The reasons for not discussing or referring patients were attributed to: patient's inability to delay treatment to pursue fertility preservation; patients diagnosed with late-stage disease or with a poor prognosis may not be suitable for fertility preservation; physician attitudes towards the unacceptability or lack of awareness of posthumous reproduction; financial costs involved in sperm banking; and lack of knowledge of local or national sperm banking facilities [11].

Other single-institution studies have reported that as many as 90% of oncologists agree that sperm banking should be offered to all men at risk of infertility but 50% never bring up the topic to eligible men [12]. Among the respondents in this study, the likelihood of discussion was not dependent on knowledge or seeing large numbers of eligible men, as physicians who had high rates of knowledge and saw a large volume of patients were just as unlikely to discuss sperm banking as those with low knowledge or a low patient volume. The primary barriers reported among this physician group were lack of time for the discussion, perceived costs of fertility preservation and patient inability to afford costs, and lack of convenient sperm banking facilities [12]. This study also identified additional unique patient barriers; oncologists who knew their patient was HIV-positive or self-reported as homosexual were less likely to refer these men. Further, this group of physicians were more likely to over-estimate the costs of sperm banking and the number of samples needed for successful cryopreservation [12].

In contrast, other single-institution studies have shown that physician knowledge of fertility preservation and having a high patient volume can increase the likelihood of referral [8]. A survey of ASCO members in one state (Minnesota) showed that oncologists were more likely to refer younger patients for fertility preservation. This same group of physicians estimated that less than 30% of their male patients opted for sperm banking, and the majority (89%) were aware of facilities to refer patients to. This physician group reported that in addition to the age of the patient, patients diagnosed with lymphoma, leukemia, or testicular carcinomas were of greatest risk for impaired fertility [13].

Another barrier to the discussion of fertility preservation between healthcare providers and male cancer patients may be low rates of use of banked sperm and low levels of knowledge about recent advances in assisted reproductive technology (ART), such as intracytoplasmic sperm injection (ICSI), that require only a few sperm for successful fertilization when used in combination with in-vitro fertilization (IVF). Physicians may be reluctant to refer a patient for sperm banking when there is the perception that sperm quality is poor due to disease or the fact that treatment has begun.

Studies examining the use of banked sperm among cancer survivors show rates varying from as low as 5% [14] to as high as 27% [7]. It is not known if the banked sperm is unused because of lack of interest in parenthood or because fertility was not compromised and successful pregnancy was achieved through natural conception. The highest rates of use of stored sperm appear to be among survivors of Hodgkin's lymphoma, perhaps because this cancer is most highly associated with permanent sterility [14]. In a large-scale survey of male cancer survivors in the United Kingdom, only 139 men from a sample of 2219 returned to use their stored sperm [12]. A recent study conducted among US cancer survivors estimates the rates of use to be ~5% [15].

Despite reports of low rates of use of banked sperm, the success rates for pregnancy achieved through ART are moderate. Several studies report a live birth rate from cryopreserved sperm ranging from 27% to 33% [7,15,16]. The length of time for which sperm can be successfully cryopreserved and still remain viable is unknown. One case reported in the literature is that of a successful pregnancy achieved after more than 21 years of storage [17]. It is also suggested that any decline in the quality of semen from pre-freeze to post-thaw among cancer patients is similar to that of healthy donors [18].

Patient barriers

While some communication barriers about discussing and referring for male fertility preservation may be specific to the healthcare providers, others may fall in the patient domain. It is understood that among men who are not informed about fertility issues at or near the time of their diagnosis, use of fertility preservation will be low. However, it is unclear why men who are informed about potential infertility as a result of cancer treatment have low rates of uptake of fertility preservation. There are three predominant hypotheses for low uptakes rates among this group. The first is that men, like women, are overwhelmed with their cancer diagnosis and want to focus exclusively on treating the disease. The news of a cancer diagnosis can be devastating and patients may be unable to process additional information, particularly news that relates to future quality of life and survivorship issues such as parenthood. Patients may also misunderstand the limited window of opportunity that exists for sperm banking. While the recommendation is that sperm be cryopreserved prior to the initiation of treatment, some men may be able to bank sperm after one or two cancer treatments. However, waiting until treatments are complete in most cases is not an option for a quality sperm sample.

The second hypothesis is that patients diagnosed with cancer may actually fear having a biological child because of perceived transmission of the disease or potential birth defects to offspring. Schover's 1998 study showed that male cancer survivors perceived their future offspring had a high risk for birth defects [19]. Another study conducted by Schover *et al.* indicated that 19% of male survivors had "significant anxiety" that their cancer treatment could negatively impact their future children's health [6].

Several recent and large-scale longitudinal studies have shown that the rates of poor birth outcomes, birth defects, or impaired health among the children of cancer survivors are similar to those of the general population. While there is increased risk among those with a hereditary cancer to transmit the genetic mutation to future offspring, rates of hereditary cancer account for less ~5–10% of all cancers in the USA. Furthermore, recent advances in reproductive technology have resulted in the availability of pre-implantation genetic diagnosis (PGD) to identify embryos which have a genetic mutation associated with a hereditary cancer predisposition syndrome.

PGD is not well known among the general populations and is awash in ethical and moral dilemmas. A recent study of high-risk men (men who either were aware of a personal susceptibility for hereditary cancer or had a partner with risk) showed that less than 30% were also aware of PGD [20]. Patients who are concerned about the transmission of risk of hereditary cancer to future offspring should be informed

about the availability of PGD, and the benefits, costs, and potential harm of such a procedure should be discussed with a genetic counselor or infertility specialist.

The third hypothesis as to why more men do not participate in sperm banking relates to financial barriers. The costs associated with sperm banking range from $100 to $500 for the collection and from $250 to $1000 for yearly storage fees. Most fertility preservation procedures are not covered by insurance. Several studies report that financial barriers may prevent men from considering sperm banking. Currently, no state laws or regulations address insurance coverage for males diagnosed with cancer and the unique medical needs of these patients both for immediate storage of sperm and for the possibility of future need for ART to achieve successful pregnancy. There is one known national program, Fertile Hope/Livestrong Foundation (www.fertilehope.org), that provides financial assistance to men diagnosed with cancer to pursue sperm banking.

Facilitating provider discussion

The American Society of Clinical Oncology (ASCO) and the American Society for Reproductive Medicine (ASRM) guidelines, as well as advocacy organizations such as the American Cancer Society (ACS) and Fertile Hope (now part of Livestrong Foundation), recommends that newly diagnosed cancer patients receive risk information and a referral to a fertility specialist. Fertility specialists offer counseling and fertility preservation services tailored to the individual patient. Thus, general risk factors such as age, cancer type and stage, and the therapeutic agent recommended for treatment will be considered. These specialists also assess the patient's risk for infertility, reproductive capacity, and physical health in order to determine which fertility preservation options are available and likely to be successful for that individual patient. Studies of pediatric and adult oncologists examining referral practice patterns to fertility specialists have found that a lack of resources providing information about where or how to refer is a significant barrier and deterrent to discussion [21]. In addition, a 2008 national study of oncologists in the USA showed that fewer than 50% routinely refer patients to a reproductive endocrinologist/infertility specialist [11]. Likelihood of providing routine referrals was predicated on patients' request for information and the physician having a positive attitude about fertility preservation.

Educational materials may be one way to promote patient – provider discussion. There are several options for obtaining educational materials. For example, Fertile Hope provides information on the impact of cancer on fertility, possible fertility preservation options, and resources related to fertility preservation, and has a set of tools tailored for healthcare professionals [22]. The Oncofertility Consortium has developed a smart-phone application for oncology healthcare professionals which is available as a free download or may be viewed on a micro-website [23]. However, educational materials are not well disseminated. In a national study of 511 oncologists, only 13.5% ($n = 69$) reported "always or often" giving their patients educational materials about fertility preservation. Among those who reported ever distributing materials, 39.5% used American Cancer Society materials, 11.0% used Fertile Hope, 6.4% used Livestrong Foundation, and 11.8% used "other." Among those who provided materials, only 27.4% believed the fertility preservation materials they provided were "relevant to patient's specific cancer diagnosis" [24].

Perceived physician endorsement has been shown to play a significant role in patient uptake across a range of supportive services. The process of referrals for supportive care services within the healthcare system is largely dependent upon healthcare provider knowledge, availability of services, and perception of patient need [25,26]. Several large studies have found that physicians are more likely to make appropriate referrals (e.g., for palliative care) when they practice within a system that has established guidelines and processes for referrals [27–31]. Patients report higher levels of satisfaction with referrals when there is a system in place for receiving referrals and services as well as the perception that such services are endorsed by their treating physician [32]. The vast body of work on clinical trial accrual also indicates that a patient's perception that his or her physician supports consideration of the trial is a key factor in decision making [33]. For some patients, receiving tailored information about cancer-related support services has been shown to help them and their families recognize that the service provided is endorsed by their physician [34]. In contrast, patients who receive information from national organizations may perceive the information to be a resource but not necessarily a course of action suggested for their

situation [35]. For example, patients who received generic information about genetic counseling for hereditary cancer syndromes tended to perceive this as information provided to all patients and not unique to their personal and family history [36,37]. Similar research with referrals for depression indicates that the provision of educational information without a referral causes patients to perceive the information as simply educational and not indicative of need [38]. Thus, the benefits of a referral system and process that are integrated into oncology patients' course of care, combined with receipt of this information by their physician, may increase the likelihood that a patient will view the information as personally relevant and consider uptake of the service.

As more oncology care providers become aware of the importance of fertility preservation discussions with cancer patients, improved communication methods have been developed to aid in incorporating this important information into discussions in the treatment setting. For example, the Fertile Hope organization has a national "Centers of Excellence" program that offers guidelines for cancer centers. In addition to the suggestion that the cancer center have a hospital-wide policy of informing all patients of reproductive age about the risk of infertility due to cancer treatment prior to the administration of treatment, the program also suggests providing written educational materials. Many cancer centers that have received this Center of Excellence award have developed systems that are institutionally based and supported. Some of these systems include: having a nurse specialist who provides information about fertility preservation to patients; having a social worker or psychologist who serves as a patient navigator; having a staff fertility specialist who assesses individual risk; identifying fertility preservation providers in the community setting; and developing educational materials that are unique to their healthcare setting or specific cancer site. Some of these strategies can be readily incorporated into a variety of academic and community-based practice settings.

Conclusion

Healthcare providers are in a unique position to identify and refer men at risk for impaired or loss of fertility associated with cancer. Despite guidelines from ASCO stating that all cancer patients should be provided with information about risk of infertility, provider discussion of fertility preservation remains suboptimal.

Based on the available literature, it appears that there are both healthcare-provider and patient factors associated with discussion about fertility preservation options for men. From a healthcare provider perspective, the primary barriers associated with lack of discussion include misperceptions about the process and cost of sperm banking, limited understanding of newer options related to fertility preservation options for men such as ICSI, personal attitudes or beliefs, and the perception that patients are not concerned with fertility. While there is evidence to suggest that providers are discussing fertility with their male patients at increased rates, the rates of uptake of sperm banking remain low. The decision to engage in any clinical service or procedure is ultimately up to a patient, but there is some evidence to suggest that these decisions may be based on psychological status, misperceptions, and/or financial constraints. Thus discussions between healthcare providers and newly diagnosed cancer patients related to fertility preservation may need to probe deeper to ensure that these factors are considered. By identifying and discussing each of these key areas, providers may increase the likelihood that patients are making informed decisions related to fertility preservation.

References

1. Dohle GR. Male infertility in cancer patients: review of the literature. *Int J Urol* 2010; 17: 327–31.

2. Ofman US. Preservation of function in genitourinary cancers: psychosexual and psychosocial issues. *Cancer Invest* 1995; 13: 125–31.

3. Lee SJ, Schover LR, Partridge AH, *et al*. American Society of Clinical Oncology recommendations on fertility preservation in cancer patients. *J Clin Oncol* 2006; 24: 2917–31.

4. Schover LR. Patient attitudes toward fertility preservation. *Pediatr Blood Cancer* 2009; 53: 281–4.

5. Saito K, Suzuki K, Iwasaki A, Yumura Y, Kubota Y. Sperm cryopreservation before cancer chemotherapy helps in the emotional battle against cancer. *Cancer* 2005; 104: 521–4.

6. Schover LR, Rybicki LA, Martin BA, Bringelsen KA. Having children after cancer: a pilot survey of survivors' attitudes and experiences. *Cancer* 1999; 86: 697–709.

7. Blackhall FH, Atkinson AD, Maaya MB, *et al*. Semen cryopreservation, utilisation and reproductive outcome in men treated for Hodgkin's disease. *Br J Cancer* 2002; 87: 381–4.

8. Schover LR, Brey K, Lichtin A, Lipshultz LI, Jeha S. Knowledge and experience regarding cancer, infertility, and sperm banking in younger male survivors. *J Clin Oncol* 2002; 20: 1880–9.

9. Fraietta R, Spaine DM, Bertolla RP, Ortiz V, Cedenho AP. Individual and seminal characteristics of patients with testicular germ cell tumors. *Fertil Steril* 2010; 94: 2107–12.

10. Gritz ER, Wellisch DK, Wang HJ, *et al*. Long-term effects of testicular cancer on sexual functioning in married couples. *Cancer* 1989; 64: 1560–7.

11. Quinn GP, Vadaparampil ST, Lee JH, *et al*. Physician referral for fertility preservation in oncology patients: a national study of practice behaviors. *J Clin Oncol* 2009; 27: 5952–7.

12. Schover LR, Brey K, Lichtin A, Lipshultz LI, Jeha S. Oncologists' attitudes and practices regarding banking sperm before cancer treatment. *J Clin Oncol* 2002; 20: 1890–7.

13. Zapzalka DM, Redmon JB, Pryor JL. A survey of oncologists regarding sperm cryopreservation and assisted reproductive techniques for male cancer patients. *Cancer* 1999; 86: 1812–17.

14. Ragni G, Somigliana E, Restelli L, *et al*. Sperm banking and rate of assisted reproduction treatment. *Cancer* 2003; 97: 1624–9.

15. Chung K, Irani J, Knee G, *et al*. Sperm cryopreservation for male patients with cancer: an epidemiological analysis at the university of Pennsylvania. *Eur J Obstet Gynecol Reprod Biol* 2004; 113: S7–11.

16. Audrins P, Holden CA, McLachlan RI, Kovacs GT. Semen storage for special purposes at Monash IVF from 1977 to 1997. *Fertil Steril* 1999; 72: 179–81.

17. Horne G, Atkinson AD, Pease EHE, *et al*. Live birth with sperm cryopreserved for 21 years prior to cancer treatment: case report. *Hum Reprod* 2004; 19: 1448–9.

18. Agarwal A. Semen banking in patients with cancer: 20-year experience. *Int J Androl* 2000; 23 (Suppl 2): 16–19.

19. Schover LR. Motivation for parenthood after cancer: a review. *J Natl Cancer Inst Monogr* 2005; 34: 2–5.

20. Quinn GP, Vadaparampil ST, Miree CA, *et al*. High risk men's perceptions of pre-implantation genetic diagnosis for hereditary breast and ovarian cancer. *Hum Reprod* 2010; 25: 2543–50.

21. Goodwin T, Oosterhuis BE, Kiernan M, Hudson MM, Dahl GV. Attitudes and practices of pediatric oncology providers regarding fertility issues. *Pediatr Blood Cancer* 2007; 48: 80–5.

22. FertileHope website. www.fertilehope.org/healthcare-professionals (accessed January 2012).

23. Save My Fertility. www.savemyfertility.org (accessed January 2012).

24. Quinn GP, Vadaparampil ST, Malo T, *et al*. Oncologists' use of patient educational materials about cancer and fertility preservation. *Psychooncology* 2011. doi: 10.1002/pon.2022 [epub ahead of print].

25. Gershenson D. Why American women are not receiving state-of-the-art gynecologic cancer care. *Cancer J* 2001; 7: 450–7.

26. Johnson CE, Girgis A, Paul CL, Currow DC. Cancer specialists' palliative care referral practices and perceptions: results of a national survey. *Palliat Med* 2008; 22: 51–7.

27. Borg W, Gall M. *Educational Research*, 5th edn. New York, NY: Longman, 1989.

28. Webb C, Kever J. Focus groups as a research method: a critique of some aspects of their use in nursing research. *J Adv Nurs* 2001; 33: 798–805.

29. Morgan D. *The Focus Group Guidebook*. Thousand Oaks, CA: Sage, 1988.

30. McGrath P, Holewa H. Missed opportunities: nursing insights on end-of-life care for haematology patients. *Int J Nurs Pract* 2006; 12: 295–301.

31. Lorenz KA, Lynn J, Dy SM, *et al*. Evidence for improving palliative care at the end of life: a systematic review. *Ann Intern Med* 2008; 148: 147–59.

32. Koithan M, Bell IR, Caspi O, Ferro L, Brown V. Patients' experiences and perceptions of a consultative model integrative medicine clinic: a qualitative study. *Integr Cancer Ther* 2007; 6: 174–84.

33. Mannel RS, Walker JL, Gould N, *et al*. Impact of individual physicians on enrollment of patients into clinical trials. *Am J Clin Oncol* 2003; 26: 171–3.

34. McPherson CJ, Higginson IJ, Hearn J. Effective methods of giving information in cancer: a systematic literature review of randomized controlled trials. *J Public Health Med* 2001; 23: 227–34.

35. Bryant CA, Forthofer MS, McCormack Brown KR, Alfonso ML, Quinn G. A social marketing approach to increasing breast cancer screening. *J Health Educ* 2000; 31: 320–8.

36. McCann S, MacAuley D, Barnett Y, *et al*. Cancer genetics: consultants' perceptions of their roles, confidence and satisfaction with knowledge. *J Eval Clin Pract* 2007; 13: 276–86.

37. Grande GE, Hyland F, Walter FM, Kinmonth AL. Women's views of consultations about familial risk of breast cancer in primary care. *Patient Educ Couns* 2002; 48: 275–82.

38. Lloyd-Williams M, Payne S. Nurse specialist assessment and management of palliative care patients who are depressed: a study of perceptions and attitudes. *J Palliat Care* 2002; 18: 270–4.

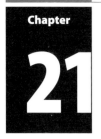

Development of a program to address fertility preservation and parenthood after cancer treatment

Joanne Frankel Kelvin

Introduction

Advances in cancer treatment have resulted in increasing numbers of long-term cancer survivors, many of whom are of childbearing age and want to be parents [1–3]. Unfortunately, many cancer treatments impair fertility, reducing the likelihood that these men and women will be able to have children naturally. Infertility can affect self-esteem, identity, and body image; create difficulties in forming or maintaining intimate relationships; destroy hopes for parenthood; and cause considerable distress [3–6].

Recognizing the significance of these concerns for cancer survivors, the American Society for Reproductive Medicine (ASRM), the American Society of Clinical Oncology (ASCO), the American Academy of Pediatrics (AAP), and the European Society for Medical Oncology (ESMO) have published guidelines addressing fertility issues. They all highlight the need for oncology clinicians to inform patients about risks of infertility from treatment, discuss options for fertility preservation, and refer interested patients to reproductive specialists before treatment begins [7–10].

Patients want and are able to cope with information about fertility preservation [11–13]. However, oncology clinicians do not routinely discuss this with patients at the start of their cancer treatment [14–19]. Many patients do not recall being told about the impact of treatment on fertility [6], and in a survey of male survivors, only 50% were offered sperm banking, a well-established and effective method for preserving fertility in postpubertal males. Of those offered sperm banking, only half actually collected sperm before treatment, with a lack of information as the most common reason given by those men who chose not to [3].

Patients are strongly influenced by the messages they receive from their healthcare providers, and they may be more likely to sperm bank before treatment if the provider is clear about the potential for infertility from treatment, encourages sperm banking, and introduces it as standard care [20,21]. The challenge is to identify strategies to enhance clinicians' ability and willingness to incorporate these discussions into their practices.

The Memorial Sloan–Kettering Cancer Center program

In 2003, Memorial Sloan–Kettering Cancer Center (MSKCC) established a Survivorship Initiative that included the development of programs and services to address the needs of patients who have completed treatment for adult-onset cancer and are free of disease. As part of the planning process to identify strategic goals for the initiative, patients were surveyed about services they wished had been provided to them at diagnosis and during treatment, but had not been offered. A number of patients reported that they had not received adequate education about the effects of treatment on their fertility or about options for preserving fertility before their treatment. Thus, establishing information and services related to reproductive health as well as access to specialists who offer fertility preservation became part of the initiative's strategic plan.

In January 2009, the organization created a position for a clinical nurse specialist (CNS) to address this gap in care through the introduction of a new program, Cancer and Fertility. Development of the program has been guided by an advisory committee, with clinical

Table 21.1. Fertility goals of the MSKCC program

Provide clinicians caring for patients of reproductive potential with:
- Information about effects of treatment on fertility, options for fertility preservation, and reproductive services where they can refer patients
- Resources to educate patients
- Access to consult service to assist patients wanting a referral to explore fertility preservation options

Provide patients of reproductive potential with:
- Information about effects of treatment on fertility
- Information about options for fertility preservation
- Referrals to a reproductive specialist if they are interested in exploring these options
- Information about other options for parenthood if they are not able to have a biologic child

Table 21.2. Fertility components of the MSKCC program

Assessment
- Patient volume
- Clinician survey
- Patient survey

Resources for patients
- Booklets
- Internet
- Live and online classes
- Financial assistance

Resources for clinicians
- Defined referral process
- Intranet
- Electronic orders

Education of clinicians
- Instructional presentations
- Continuing education

Clinical expertise
- Consultation
- Education and counseling
- Liaison with reproductive specialists and resources for financial assistance

Implementation and evaluation
- Policies, procedures, guidelines
- Monitoring of referrals
- Monitoring use of resources

Clinical research
- Multiple collaborative projects in development

representatives from services that treat high volumes of patients with reproductive potential, as well as two former patients who underwent fertility preservation prior to their treatment.

Specific goals of the program are listed in Table 21.1. The program infrastructure comprises seven components, illustrated in Fig. 21.1 and described in detail in Table 21.2. The program provides clinicians with the information, resources, and assistance they need to inform their patients about the effects of treatment on fertility and the options available to them for fertility preservation, and to make referrals to reproductive specialists. The program infrastructure can be used as a model within any cancer setting seeking to improve how fertility is addressed with their patients.

Developing a program based on the MSKCC infrastructure

Bring together clinicians with a shared interest and commitment to the issue of fertility preservation. Reach out to colleagues in medical, surgical, and

Figure 21.1. MSKCC program: Fertility.

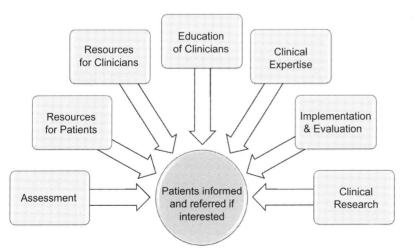

radiation oncology; survivorship; general gynecology and urology; and reproductive medicine. Work together to identify opportunities and challenges unique to the organization. This group will also be key as the program is rolled out. Individuals championing this day-to-day effort in the clinical setting and providing feedback for improvements and enhancements needed are essential to successful implementation.

Assessment

An important first step in developing a program is to collect baseline data about the organization, clinicians, and patients. These data will guide efforts in building the program.

There are a number of areas to assess within the healthcare organization. These include the number of patients of reproductive potential started on treatment each year, as well as their most common diagnoses. It is also critical to the program development to (1) consider the different providers (e.g., attending physician, nurse, fellow, social worker) who see the patient prior to initiation of treatment and the roles of each; (2) identify what resources, if any, are already available to help clinicians address fertility; (3) determine if there are reproductive specialists in the region to whom clinicians already refer their patients; (4) determine how much time generally elapses between consultation and the start of gonadotoxic treatment; and (5) learn if electronic systems are used for entering orders and/or documenting clinical notes. Finally, it is also necessary to understand the culture of the organization. Is it one of shared decision making, or is it more hierarchical? Is wide variation in practice common, or are there centralized efforts in place to reduce variation?

To assess clinicians, if feasible, it may be useful to conduct a survey to evaluate the knowledge, attitudes, and practices of nurses and physicians related to the effects of treatment on fertility and options for fertility preservation. However, a formal study is not essential. Initiate discussions among different clinician groups, ask how they address fertility in their practice, and what things make it easier or more difficult to address these issues. In addition, it is important to learn what they perceive to be the major barriers to discussing fertility with their patients.

To assess patient perspectives, if feasible, conduct a survey of patients of reproductive potential to determine what information they recall receiving about the effects of cancer treatment on fertility and options for fertility preservation, as well as their satisfaction with and preferences for receiving this information. Again, a formal study is not essential. Contact long-term follow-up patients. Ask what they remember being told about fertility and their options for fertility preservation. Probe to learn what was helpful and what was not adequately discussed with them prior to beginning treatment.

Resources for patients

To ensure that patients are adequately informed, it is important to have educational materials available that provide more in-depth information than oncology clinicians might have the knowledge or time to discuss. Create booklets or cards that address such issues as the effects of treatment on fertility and options for fertility preservation; how to select a sperm bank or reproductive endocrinologist; and options for parenthood after completing treatment. However, it is not essential to develop new materials. Explore what is available from other organizations focused on cancer and fertility. Fertile Hope/LIVE**STRONG** provides reproductive information and support to cancer patients and survivors whose medical treatments present the risk of infertility. The website (www.fertilehope.org) has a wealth of resources, including a pamphlet *Fertility Resources for Cancer Patients and Survivors* available free of charge. The Oncofertility Consortium is a national interdisciplinary initiative supported by the National Institutes of Health through the NIH Roadmap for Medical Research/Common Fund. One offering of the consortium, *MyOncoFertility* (myoncofertility.org), provides information for patients whose fertility will be or may have been impaired by treatment.

If the organization or practice has an external website, post information about fertility for patients to access. Add links to other resources for education and support. Table 21.3 lists a variety of Internet resources to which patients can be directed.

The costs of fertility preservation present a significant barrier for many patients. Provide clinicians with access to *Fertile Hope* applications they can give to their patients. This LIVE**STRONG** program provides

Table 21.3. Internet resources on cancer and fertility

Sites on fertility for patients with cancer

Fertile Hope (www.fertilehope.org)
- A non-profit organization, incorporated as a Livestrong initiative, dedicated to providing reproductive information, support, and hope to cancer patients and survivors whose medical treatments present the risk of infertility

MyOncoFertility (myoncofertility.org)
- An informational resource developed by the Oncofertility Consortium, a national interdisciplinary initiative to explore the reproductive options for patients diagnosed with cancer or other serious diseases

Sites on fertility for teens with cancer

Cancer Net (www.cancer.net)
- An informational resource for patients and families, developed by the American Society of Clinical Oncology (ASCO) [search *fertility and teens*]

Cure Search (www.curesearch.org)
- A professional organization of the Children's Oncology Group and the National Childhood Cancer Foundation with health information resources for patients [search *male fertility* or *female fertility*]

Sites on fertility as a general issue

Reproductive Facts (www.reproductive.facts.org)
- A site developed by the American Society for Reproductive Medicine with information on a variety of fertility-related topics

Resolve (www.resolve.org)
- A community offering information and support to women and men with infertility, developed by the National Infertility Association

Society for Assisted Reproductive Technology (www.sart.org)
- A professional organization for specialists in assisted reproductive technologies (ART) which provides information on IVF success rates of fertility centers throughout the United States

International Council on Infertility Information and Dissemination (www.inciid.org)
- A non-profit organization that helps individuals and couples explore their family-building options

Table 21.4. Resources for identifying local reproductive specialists

Sperm banks
American Association of Tissue Banks (www.aatb.org)
Sperm Center (www.spermcenter.com)

Reproductive urologists
Society for Male Reproduction and Urology (www.smru.org)

Reproductive endocrinologists
American Society for Reproductive Medicine (www.asrm.org)
Society for Assisted Reproductive Technology (www.sart.org)

For all reproductive services
FertileHope/Livestrong's *Fertility Resource Guide* (www.fertilehope.org/tool-bar/referral-guide.cfm)

and learn about the services the center can provide. Establish a simple method for referring patients to them, ideally with a single point of contact. It can be very useful to outline a process to ensure that patients are seen quickly, relevant medical information is shared, and fertility preservation efforts are coordinated with the planned timing for initiation of the patient's cancer treatment.

In addition, it is recommended that clinicians be provided with access to resources at the time they encounter patients who need fertility-related information and referrals. This can include the creation of paper packets, or if the organization or practice has an internal website, the creation of fertility-related web pages with relevant information, including steps for making referrals, printable resources for patients, references, clinical algorithms, and other related tools. The benefit of creating a website is that it is accessible from any workstation, at any location throughout the organization, and documents can be updated in real time, without concern about having outdated materials stocked in the clinical setting. For example, the home page of the MSKCC site is illustrated in Fig. 21.2.

If the organization or practice has computerized order entry, it is suggested that fertility-related order sets for such services as sperm banking, semen analysis, or referral to a reproductive specialist be created. Depending on the IT system, these can generate either direct referrals or referral prescriptions.

financial assistance to eligible patients undertaking fertility preservation at a participating center.

Resources for clinicians

For oncology clinicians to be able to initiate discussions about fertility with their patients, they need to know where and how to refer interested patients to reproductive specialists and identify sperm banks, reproductive urologists, and reproductive endocrinologists in the region. Table 21.4 lists Internet resources to assist with this. Meet with the staff at each of the centers to discuss the unique needs of oncology patients

Education of clinicians

For oncology clinicians to be able to initiate discussions about fertility with their patients, they must

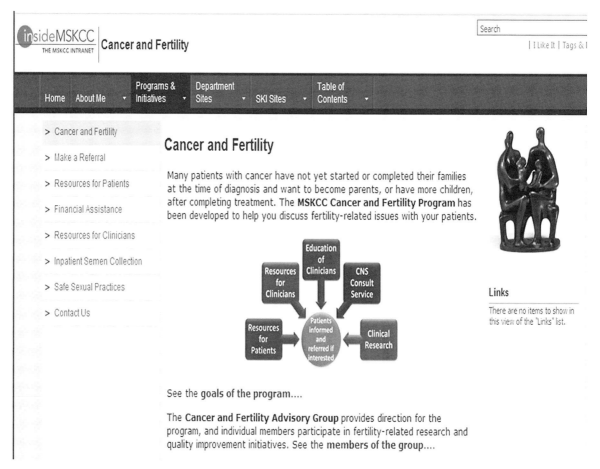

Figure 21.2. MSKCC intranet site.

be knowledgeable about the effects of treatment on fertility and the options for fertility preservation. A variety of methods to provide this information can be employed. Examples of this include posting relevant articles in the clinical area, selecting an article on fertility preservation for a journal club, or presenting a patient who is requesting fertility preservation at a case conference. Inviting local reproductive specialists to present updates on the technology available to help patients desiring fertility preservation or having difficulty conceiving after treatment can be very effective as well.

Clinical expertise

Some patients will desire more information than their oncology clinicians can provide. If there is a team of individuals with expertise in fertility within the oncology group, a member of the team can provide consultation to answer complex questions, or can see patients themselves for more in-depth education and counseling. The team can also serve as a liaison with the reproductive specialists to coordinate care. If an individual or team with this expertise is not available internally, referring patients directly to the reproductive specialists will ensure that patients are fully informed of their options.

Implementation and evaluation

Instituting a policy or standard mandating that clinicians discuss fertility with all patients of reproductive age and referring those interested in fertility preservation when appropriate makes a strong statement about the organization's commitment to this issue. However, it is important to recognize that this will probably not be sufficient to change practice. A systematic approach to developing and implementing a program is needed.

Initially, time and effort should be spent on developing or attaining basic resources and on building relationships with reproductive specialists in the region. It may be best to roll out the program gradually, and focus first where there is a high volume of young adult patients and where there is interest. The program can be presented at medical service conferences and meetings. Begin by asking questions that trigger discussion about variations in practice, and in particular about barriers. It is important to acknowledge and respect these difficulties, but this will also create an opportunity to challenge assumptions about what is important to patients and what is feasible, and then to explain how the program can help clinicians personally in their practice.

Nurses, residents, fellows, and mental health professionals should be included in all educational efforts. They can be extremely influential because of the roles they play in clinic daily. They can assess patients' interest in future parenting, and for interested patients they can advocate to ensure the attending physician initiates discussion about fertility. In addition, they can provide educational materials and make referrals for interested patients.

The practice might also consider inserting reminders into standard processes or workflows to prompt clinicians prior to scheduling procedures or ordering treatments that may affect fertility. These can be in the form of paper checklists, or they can be computer-based alerts or hard stops if a required step is not followed. If the organization or practice has computerized documentation, consider embedding a field for clinicians to document if fertility discussions were held and if referrals were made.

Evaluation of the program can be challenging. If the workflow requires electronic documentation or order entry for most clinical activity, the practice can liaise with the systems staff to create reports indicating what percentage of all patients of reproductive potential is receiving information about fertility. Alternatively, the organization can perform chart audits, although this can be very labor-intensive. Examples of other strategies to evaluate the program include monitoring the number of educational materials distributed and the number of referrals made to reproductive specialists, or the utilization of internal or external

Table 21.5. Criteria for Fertile Hope/LIVESTRONG's Centers of Excellence Program

Hospital-wide policy stating commitment to addressing the cancer-related fertility needs of patients
Notification procedures to ensure a systematic approach to informing patients verbally and in writing about their risks and options
Professional education
Resources for patient education
A process for making referrals to reproductive specialists

websites. If a formal survey of clinicians or patients is conducted, repeat the survey at intervals after the program has launched to monitor the impact of the program.

Clinical research

If a large number of patients with reproductive potential are treated within the organization or practice, the infrastructure of a cancer and fertility program can create a mechanism to bring together clinicians from multiple services to collaborate in researching specific fertility-related issues. Such an infrastructure can, in turn, assist all of these entities to learn more about cancer treatment and reproductive health. The possibilities are unlimited.

Developing a program based on Fertile Hope's Centers of Excellence program

Another model for developing a program is Fertile Hope's Centers of Excellence program, created in 2005. This voluntary, merit-based designation recognized cancer centers that addressed fertility in a comprehensive, timely, and systematic way. Table 21.5 lists specific criteria of success. There were no particular requirements for how to meet these criteria; each center could develop strategies based on its unique characteristics. Examples of strategies used by different centers include: posters and brochures to inform patients of available fertility services; manual and electronic intake forms to indicate patient interest in learning about fertility; review of daily clinic lists to identify eligible patients; incorporation of reproductive risks in consent forms; electronic best-practice alerts triggered by patient age at time of visit; use of educational brochures; and "fertility kits" stocked in the clinical areas with materials for both clinicians and patients (Reinecke, Kelvin, 2012). These strategies can be incorporated in many practice settings.

Conclusion

The existence of professional guidelines and a body of evidence highlighting the importance of fertility to cancer survivors have not been adequate to ensure that clinicians incorporate discussion about fertility preservation into their practices. The question remains as to how best to enhance clinicians' ability and willingness to speak with patients about the risk of infertility from treatment, options for fertility preservation, and parenthood after cancer. No single approach is right for every center, but there are a number of strategies that can move everyone closer to achieving these goals.

References

1. Schover LR, Rybicki LA, Martin BA, Bringelsen KA. Having children after cancer. A pilot survey of survivors' attitudes and experiences. *Cancer* 1999; 86: 697–709.

2. Schover LR. Motivation for parenthood after cancer: a review. *J Natl Cancer Inst Monogr* 2005; 34: 2–5.

3. Schover LR, Brey K, Lichtin A, Lipshultz LI, Jeha S. Knowledge and experience regarding cancer, infertility, and sperm banking in younger male survivors. *J Clin Oncol* 2002; 20: 1880–9.

4. Schover LR. Psychosocial aspects of infertility and decisions about reproduction in young cancer survivors: a review. *Med Pediatr Oncol* 1999; 33: 53–9.

5. Crawshaw M, Sloper P. 'Swimming against the tide'-the influence of fertility matters on the transition to adulthood or survivorship following adolescent cancer. *Eur J Cancer Care* 2010; 19: 610–20.

6. Tschudin S, Bitzer J. Psychological aspects of fertility preservation in men and women affected by cancer and other life-threatening diseases. *Hum Reprod Update* 2009; 15: 587–97.

7. Lee SJ, Schover LR, Partridge AH, *et al.* American Society of Clinical Oncology recommendations on fertility preservation in cancer patients. *J Clin Oncol* 2006; 24: 2917–31.

8. Pentheroudakis G, Orecchia R, Hoekstra HJ, Pavlidis N; ESMO Guidelines Working Group. Cancer, fertility and pregnancy: ESMO Clinical Practice Guidelines for diagnosis, treatment and follow-up. *Annals Oncology* 2010; 21 (Suppl 5): v266–73.

9. Ethics Committee of the American Society for Reproductive Medicine. Fertility preservation and reproduction in cancer patients. *Fertil Steril* 2005; 83: 1622–8.

10. Fallat ME, Hutter J; Committee on Bioethics SoHO, Section on Surgery. Preservation of fertility in pediatric and adolescent patients with cancer. *Pediatrics* 2008; 121: e1461–9.

11. Crawshaw MA, Glaser AW, Hale JP, Sloper P. Male and female experiences of having fertility matters raised alongside a cancer diagnosis during the teenage and young adult years. *Eur J Cancer Care* 2009; 18: 381–90.

12. Thewes B, Meiser B, Taylor A, *et al.* Fertility and menopause-related information needs of younger women with a diagnosis of early breast cancer. *J Clin Oncol* 2005; 23: 5155–65.

13. Peate M, Meiser B, Hickey M, Friedlander M. The fertility-related concerns, needs and preferences of younger women with breast cancer: a systematic review. *Breast Cancer Res Treat* 2009; 116: 215–23.

14. Kotronoulas G, Papadopoulou C, Patiraki E. Nurses' knowledge, attitudes, and practices regarding provision of sexual health care in patients with cancer: critical review of the evidence. *Support Care Cancer* 2009; 17: 479–501.

15. Schover LR, Brey K, Lichtin A, Lipshultz LI, Jeha S. Oncologists' attitudes and practices regarding banking sperm before cancer treatment. *J Clin Oncol* 2002; 20: 1890–7.

16. Quinn G, Vadaparampil S, Gwede C, *et al.* Discussion of fertility preservation with newly diagnosed patients: oncologists' views. *J Cancer Surviv* 2007; 1: 146–55.

17. King L, Quinn G, Vadaparampil S, *et al.* Oncology nurses' perceptions of barriers to discussion of fertility preservation with patients with cancer. *Clin J Oncol Nurs* 2008; 12: 467–76.

18. Vadaparampil ST, Clayton H, Quinn GP, *et al.* Pediatric oncology nurses' attitudes related to discussing fertility preservation with pediatric cancer patients and their families. *J Pediatr Oncol Nurs* 2007; 24: 255–63.

19. Quinn GP, Vadaparampil ST, Lee JH, *et al.* Physician referral for fertility preservation in oncology patients: a national study of practice behaviors. *J Clin Oncol* 2009; 27: 5952–7.

20. Achille MA, Rosberger Z, Robitaille R, *et al.* Facilitators and obstacles to sperm banking in young

men receiving gonadotoxic chemotherapy for cancer: the perspective of survivors and health care professionals. *Hum Reprod* 2006; 21: 3206–16.

21. Crawshaw M, Glaser A, Hale J, Sloper P. Male and female experiences of having fertility matters raised alongside a cancer diagnosis during the teenage and young adult years. *Eur J Cancer Care* 2009; 18: 381–90.

22. Reinecke JD, Kelvin JF, *et al.* Implementing a systematic approach to meeting patient's cancer and fertility needs: a review of the Fertile Hope Centers of Excellence Program. *J Oncol Pract* 2012; 8(5): 303–8.

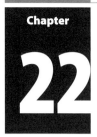

Psychological consultation and assessment

Linda D. Applegarth

Introduction

Advances in reproductive medicine and greater knowledge regarding male infertility have provided us with technologies that can assist male cancer patients who wish to preserve their potential for paternity. Similarly, significant improvements in cancer treatments have translated into a growing number of young men with cancer experiencing long-term survival. Although men with cancer are a relatively small percentage of the infertile population, the treatment options now available make parenthood possible for more men who might otherwise have been unable to procreate. Nonetheless, these two discrete medical conditions – cancer and infertility – mean that many patients must also confront complex psychological issues. Decision-making challenges regarding cancer and infertility treatment protocols, sperm accessibility and cryopreservation, as well as plans for future gamete disposition, are all issues that impact a man's psychological status and sense of emotional well-being.

The aim of this chapter is to describe the psychological and counseling issues that may arise for men who are dealing with fertility preservation before, during, and after cancer treatment. In addition, the mental health professional's role in working with this special population is addressed, particularly with respect to medical team collaboration. This chapter also provides psychological education, consultation, and assessment protocols that are appropriate for this treatment group.

Background

Formal studies that address the psychological aspects of cancer and fertility preservation in men are sparse. Nonetheless, the significant emotional and psycho-

logical consequences of gonadal damage and "functional castration" associated with high-dose chemotherapy and radiotherapy have been recognized for many years [1]. Tschudin and Bitzer recently reviewed the limited literature investigating the psychological aspects of fertility preservation in both men and women affected by cancer as well as other life-threatening diseases [2]. They found that fertility is an important issue for cancer patients. Although health professionals along with patients and parents consider fertility preservation as an important option, the authors also note that there are notable "knowledge and information deficits," and obtaining counseling and information for at-risk patients on this issue is selective and not offered on a global basis [2]. A recent study by Schover also supported the idea that the ability to have children after cancer is very important to most survivors [3].

Oppenheim and colleagues write that sperm preservation should be offered to all adolescents undergoing cancer treatment because "fertility is a major desire of young adults cured of a cancer" [4]. They add that this sperm preservation can, however, lead to psychological problems for these young patients. The authors indicate that such patients need a positive environment in which their feelings and behaviors are fully understood. They may worry about their body, their appearance, their sexuality, their parental and peer relationships, their positive sense of self, and their identity. They may also be anxious, pessimistic about the future, and disillusioned. Oppenheim et al. further suggest that it is important to find a balance between over-respecting a patient's superficial opposition to fertility preservation and coercing him to make a decision that he does not truly support. Lastly, the authors also propose that there

Fertility Preservation in Male Cancer Patients, ed. John P. Mulhall, Linda D. Applegarth, Robert D. Oates and Peter N. Schlegel. Published by Cambridge University Press. © Cambridge University Press 2013.

be improved relationships between sperm banks and oncology departments, adolescent-friendly informational materials, and a greater knowledge of adolescent psychology in working with this population [4].

Rosen *et al.* report that psychological distress may precede, exacerbate, or follow the diagnosis of cancer [5]. They point out that more research is needed to clarify the complex interactions, but state that many cancer patients suffer significant emotional distress. Such distress is clearly exacerbated in those cancer patients who are also of reproductive age and for whom dreams of having biological offspring are potentially thwarted. Bloch and colleagues also note that the psychosocial needs of men with cancer have been studied less than those of women [6], and other researchers have found that the diagnosis of cancer is distressing for both men and women [2,7] and that all of these patients benefit from social support. Green *et al.* studied the psychological reactions of young men who were rendered infertile by cancer therapy [8]. These men described not only depression, but also anger about their cancer diagnosis and treatment. Notably, younger men who had not known that cancer treatment would negatively affect their ability to parent a biological child and who wished to have a child reported the most powerful reactions. They were angry that they had been denied such an important life choice, expressed rage at the injustice of human suffering, and were also angry that they had not been informed about the treatment side effect of infertility [8]. It should be pointed out, however, that with the advent of improved reproductive technologies for male-factor infertility, such as intracytoplasmic sperm injection (ICSI), most medical researchers and clinicians now clearly recommend that fertility preservation be made available to men and boys with cancer [9–12].

In considering the psychosocial components of fertility preservation in men with cancer, Hubner and Glazer have described with sensitivity the "existential intertwining of two profoundly related themes...the longing for biologic continuity and the longing for survival" [13]. These patients are thus confronted with a "double blow" [13]. Cancer has threatened not only their normal life expectancy, but also their opportunity for biological continuity.

Psychosocial and emotional factors

Historically, we know that men and women tend to respond differently to stress and crisis [13]. This may

have to do with biology and anatomy as well as with cultural factors. In any case, men with cancer tend to experience the potential loss of their reproductive ability in ways that may be very different than women. We know that fatherhood is often assumed but may not be a life goal [13–15]. By contrast, women have been reminded of their reproductive organs and reproductive capacity since puberty. Most men simply assume that their sperm are capable of impregnation. Ironically, the ability to procreate, which men often seem to pay little attention to, is also closely tied to self-esteem. Men equate fertility with virility and masculinity [13]. At the same time, the greater availability, lower cost, and success of sperm banking (as opposed to oocyte or ovarian tissue banking) makes it easier for men to father children at a time when they are functionally sterile. This means that men, more often than women, are able to preserve and sacrifice fertility at the same time.

Lee's work on counseling in male infertility also offers insights into the psychology of men that can also be useful in understanding the additional psychosocial and emotional issues that arise in men with cancer [14]. For example, he points to Hite's description of male ideology, which posits that men traditionally have tended to perceive female roles or behavior as "inferior" – i.e., men do not cry, they are not likely to love or express love as women do, and they do not display their emotions in private and certainly not in public [16]. Male ideology, in Hite's opinion, dictates that men are responsible, capable, brave, virile, and macho; they do not need help, they are rational, logical, scientific, and objective. Thus, men do not let their guards down and usually strive to keep control of all situations [16]. These biopsychosocial and cultural factors, in turn, have definite implications in our understanding of as well as in our clinical work with men with cancer who also wish to procreate in the future.

In any case, adolescent boys and young men with cancer are most certainly in a state of psychological crisis. Although we know that a crisis can ultimately be an opportunity for emotional growth and the development of new coping skills, it is also important to recognize that this situation can lead to emotional distress and psychological deterioration. Such deterioration is often characterized by depression, hopelessness, poor judgment, and over-reactivity. These patients are usually in a state of shock, and may have difficulty articulating their feelings, fears, and needs. It is helpful for both health and mental health professionals to know the range of feelings that men experience at this difficult time. In addition to anxiety, depression, and loss of self-esteem, there may also be feelings of self-blame, guilt, and self-punishment. It should be noted, however, that these feelings and responses might not be overtly expressed or immediately evident. All men affected very much wish to regain some sense of control. Lee has commented, however, that in his work with infertile men he has "rarely found a man who is capable of positively re-appraising his life effectively whilst he is still held thrall by uncertainties in his life" [14]. Decision making at such a time can be difficult when issues of survival seem paramount and may overshadow thoughts and concerns about future fertility and parenthood. Parents of child or adolescent males (as well as adolescent patients themselves) are also likely to have similar feelings and responses, and may be focused solely on the cancer diagnosis [17]. Ginsberg *et al.* also point out that parents appear to play an important role in the decision to bank sperm, and these as well as other researchers recommend that sperm banking be offered to all eligible patients [18–20].

Theories, as well as data, about stress and coping are also worthwhile in our understanding of the emotional and psychosocial factors that exist when considering fertility preservation in men with cancer [21–23]. *Stress* is defined by events in which demands of the internal or external environment challenge or exceed a person's adaptive resources [22]. Tunks and Bellissimo state that an individual's behavior or response to illness or a health condition is mediated by such factors as the medical condition itself, individual personality characteristics, and cultural beliefs about health and/or illness [22]. The authors also point out that most of the important factors that determine one's status of being ill appear to be cognitive and sociological. Thus, both acute and chronic health disorders may be modified by emotions and beliefs [22]. *Coping* on the other hand refers to the process by which a person takes some action to manage external or internal demands that cause stress and tax the individual's inner resources [21]. Although the focus of her research is primarily on the infertility experience, Stanton succinctly outlines a number of strategies that are used when coping with a life crisis (Table 22.1), including confrontation (fighting for what is desired), distancing (denial), self-control (keeping feelings

Table 22.1. Coping strategies

Confrontational
Distancing
Self-control
Seeking support
Accepting responsibility
Escape/avoidance
Problem-solving
Positive reappraisal

internalized), seeking support, accepting responsibility (I brought this problem on myself – which may be entirely not relevant to men with cancer), avoidance (hoping for miracles), problem-solving, positive reappraisal [24].

These coping strategies may be adaptive or maladaptive, and those that are maladaptive are deemed so because they actually can cause or increase distress. A number of researchers report that men in crisis generally seem to adopt coping strategies such as denial, distancing, avoidance, and withdrawal, and are less likely to seek social support, counseling, or discussions with professional caregivers as a way of managing stress and crisis [14,15,24,25]. Men's tendencies to use the above-mentioned strategies may therefore be creating more personal distress at a time that is already uncertain and stressful. Understanding these specific coping strategies as they pertain to the diagnosis of cancer and subsequent decisions about fertility preservation can be important in the medical team's (including the mental health professional's) approach to supporting and assisting these men.

Psychological consultation and assessment

Psychological consultation at the time of the cancer diagnosis is critical and can be an excellent time to provide these patients with an opportunity to deal with issues and problems in a safe and confidential setting. Psychological consultation and assessment should not only be seen as providing additional clinical information that can be helpful to physicians and the medical staff in treating the patient, but also must be considered to be an important and effective way of supporting and assisting the patient and his family. The long-term goal, ultimately, is to help improve the patient's decision-making abilities as well as his overall quality of life. Psychological consultation and assessment may therefore evolve into ongoing supportive counseling or psychotherapy, depending on the emotional needs, issues, and motivations of the patient.

Although referrals to a mental health professional usually come from physicians and nursing staff, it should be clear that sharing of information with the medical team about the patient is done only with the express permission of the patient, *or*, the patient is informed (and consents) in advance as to what specific kind of information is shared (often as part of program policy). This type of shared information is quite general and speaks to the overall psychological well-being of the patient, recommends additional psychological and social support (if needed), and clarifies decisions regarding fertility preservation, as well as decisions about future disposition of sperm (or possible embryos), if applicable.

In most cases, psychological assessment and consultation are considered as two separate entities. Each usually has a separate format and purpose. Although the establishment of a positive and caring working relationship between patient and mental health professional is important at any point, the *psychological assessment* is time-limited and structured. In the case of fertility preservation, it aims to rule out significant psychopathology and/or substance abuse prior to moving forward. The assessment also can provide significant information about the patient's family and personal background, relationship history, and so forth that may, in turn, assist the medical team in treating the patient in a more sensitive and understanding manner. *Psychological consultation*, on the other hand, is often less structured, more open-ended, and aimed at meeting the patient "where he is" emotionally. Although the psychological consultation often includes an assessment of the patient and his response to his current circumstance, it is an opportunity to educate the patient and assist him in better understanding his feelings, fears, and emotions. Additionally, the psychological consultation can be informational and may improve the patient's ability to make appropriate decisions that can have a far-reaching impact on his sense of well-being, as well as upon those close to him.

Psychosocial assessment for fertility preservation

The psychological assessment gathers information to diagnose or rule out any mental disorder that a

Table 22.2. Information to be sought during psychological assessment

Demographic information
Information regarding the cancer diagnosis
Past medical history
Personal and sexual history
Family history
History of substance abuse
Current medications
Feelings about future parenthood
Feelings about fertility preservation prior to cancer therapy
Available social support system

person may have. In the case of fertility preservation, it is also intended to ascertain the capacity of the patient to understand his current situation and make appropriate decisions. If the patient is an adolescent male, it may also be necessary to meet with him and his parents, as well as with him alone. Coercion, whether direct or indirect, on the part of the patient's parents must also be carefully assessed and addressed – especially at a time of crisis.

The psychosocial assessment should include the following pieces of information (Table 22.2): (1) identifying demographic information such as name, age, education, occupation, religion, marital status, and number of children; (2) gaining information regarding the cancer diagnosis, including the patient's understanding of severity of the illness and treatment success rates; (3) past medical history, including treatment(s); (4) personal and sexual histories, including information about past and/or present marital/partner relationships; (5) family history, including relationships with family members, presence of dysfunction, and history of familial losses; (6) history of substance abuse (if any); (7) current medications, including psychotropic medications; (8) thoughts and feelings about future parenthood and its meaning to the patient; (9) thoughts, feelings, and understanding about fertility preservation prior to cancer therapy; (10) available social support system.

The psychosocial assessment is not intended to rule out candidates for fertility preservation; rather, it is meant to provide useful clinical information as well as a framework for assisting the patient as well as healthcare providers in managing expectations and developing strategies for care and support.

Psychological consultation for fertility preservation

The psychological assessment also becomes the basis for the consultation, as well as for any ongoing psychotherapeutic treatment. As a result, assessment and consultation ultimately go "hand in glove." Having a solid clinical understanding of the patient, his family and marital relationships, and his cultural and religious milieu will naturally provide an important framework for psycho-education and consultation. Psychological consultation, in fact, can provide the patient with much-needed emotional support during a time of uncertainty. In addition, the establishment of a therapeutic alliance (i.e., a positive, working relationship between the healthcare professional and the patient) even over the short term can be critical in assisting the patient (and his family) with decision making for fertility preservation. To this end, Hershberger and Pierce provide an excellent conceptual framework for both healthcare and mental health professionals regarding the process involved in decision making [26]. Although their work focuses on decision making in pre-implantation genetic diagnosis (PGD), there are also many useful applications to decision making in fertility preservation. Specifically, they describe three "critical dimensions" of decision making: *cognitive appraisals*, *emotional responses*, and *moral judgments*. The authors are quick to point out, however, that these dimensions are "not mutually exclusive and fixed but rather are iterative and dynamic" [26, p. 55].

Cognitive appraisals refers to the cognitive information that is provided regarding procedures and facilities, success rates, time, and financial costs. The ability of the individual, the couple, or the family to consider and evaluate this information can be difficult and stressful. Patients can often feel overwhelmed and may have difficulty listening to and interpreting this information. Again, decisions based on cognitive or procedural aspects of fertility preservation usually come at a time when anxious patients are also considering cancer treatment protocols and options. However, spending sufficient time with patients and guiding them through this decision-making component is critical in order to avoid patients' regret or feeling that they were not fully advised about possible measures to spare their fertility.

Emotional responses refers to ways in which decision making may be impacted upon by feelings of pain (anxiety, fear, ambivalence) or happiness (excitement and hopefulness). One can surmise that the primary reason that men undergo fertility preservation is to avoid or reduce the likelihood of future pain or suffering by being deprived of parenthood. The notion that a man (with his current or potential partner) can survive cancer to raise a healthy biological child and experience parenthood during the rearing of his own prodigy is a powerful one. Thus, emotions have a major impact on decision making in the context of fertility preservation.

For men with cancer, *moral judgments* may also play a role in decision making. As such, they comprise the third component of this process and focus on the patient's moral evaluations related to fertility preservation and assisted reproductive technology (ART). Moral judgments may be especially compelling when human embryos are to be created. Many individuals have strong feelings and clear ideas about the moral status of the embryo, and must potentially grapple with the possibility that these embryos may never be used. The future disposition of embryos is seldom easy for most couples, and when the decision also implies that a man may not survive his illness, it is especially troubling and emotionally painful. Is it, in fact, morally acceptable to use available technology over naturally occurring reproduction? In making a decision not to cryopreserve sperm or create human embryos, for example, a couple may be faced with sperm donation, or – if the female partner has aged beyond her reproductive years – oocyte donation, or both. These options, too, can have significant emotional, moral, and religious implications. Future donation of cryopreserved embryos to another infertile couple in this case is also problematic, because they may not meet governmental requirements for donation, and many potential recipients might be fearful of accepting the embryos of a cancer victim.

Decision making and education is ultimately an intrinsic part of the psychological consultation when assisting men and adolescent males who are dealing with cancer and fertility preservation. The goals of psychological consultation and assessment are: (1) to understand the patient and his emotional needs; (2) to clarify issues and concerns that may exist for the patient, his partner, and/or his family; (3) to assist with decision making; and (4) to provide emotional support to the patient. Patient support can be multifaceted, and can be brief or longer term. It may include helping the patient advocate for himself during all phases of cancer therapy and fertility preservation, assisting the patient and his partner and/or family develop more positive and productive working relationships with healthcare professionals, or assisting the patient in dealing with his hopes and fears about cancer survival, or possibly, his anticipatory grief and feelings of loss about his future as a biological parent. Importantly, the mental health professional must be a well-trained clinician who understands gender-specific responses to crisis. He or she must also make it a priority to be well versed in the medical aspects of cancer therapy and success rates. In addition, it is critical that the mental health professional have a solid knowledge about fertility preservation options as well as available assisted reproductive technologies.

The treatment team: the collaborative role of the mental health professional

In essence, the mental health professional can play an important role in assisting adolescents and men who wish to preserve their fertility following a cancer diagnosis. For the childless male who is likely to be left sterile as a result of treatment, the option of sperm banking or other measures is of great significance in that it represents his only hope for biologic parenthood. Yet some men may not be fully informed of the availability (and limitations) of sperm banking. For others, the information comes at a time of crisis, when fecundity is not foremost in their minds, and patients may not be able to comprehend its significance. Still others may struggle with moral or legal implications of fertility preservation. Consultation with the mental health professional at this time can afford these men the opportunity to absorb information and consider thoughtfully their options regarding future parenthood. This is also a time when feelings and fears can be examined in a supportive, objective, caring, and confidential environment.

In addition, the mental health professional should be considered a part of the medical treatment team – whether it be in urology, oncology, or reproductive medicine. Although most healthcare providers, including physicians, nurses, technicians, and administrative personnel, often provide counsel, comfort, and guidance to cancer patients (regardless of fertility status), increased specialization and collaboration in all fields of healthcare practice point to the need for formalized psychological services [27]. This

Table 22.3. Ten-step circular process [27,28]

Step 1	Introduction and initiation of a working alliance
Step 2	Problem assessment and monitoring
Step 3	Clarification about problem definition and negotiation about objectives and priorities
Step 4	Exchange of hypotheses and decision making concerning diagnostic procedures
Step 5	Investigations, diagnostic procedures
Step 6	Information giving about results
Step 7	Elaboration of options to resolve infertility problem
Step 8	Decision making about specific options
Step 9	Treatment procedures
Step 10	Evaluation of outcome

is particularly true for cancer patients who want to preserve their fertility at a time when they are also confronted with important decisions regarding specific cancer therapies along with potential, albeit well-meaning, pressures from family members and healthcare providers. Technological advances in cancer treatment as well as male-factor fertility treatments can lead to complex psychosocial issues and stressors for the patient. Ideally, the mental health professional becomes part of a collaborative team that works to "treat the patient, not the disease" [27, p. 493].

A collaborative treatment model that is perhaps most appropriate to a medical situation that involves both cancer therapy and fertility preservation is Johannes Bitzer's "ten-step circular process model" (Table 22.3) [28]. Although this is an integrative model that was developed to focus on different critical points during the infertility diagnosis and treatment process, it also seems particularly applicable to maximizing effective collaboration between the patient and two potentially different or discrete medical teams. Importantly, Bitzer's model therefore provides a framework for integrating psychological counseling and assessment within the medical environment (as presented in the *Guidelines for Counselling in Infertility* of the European Society of Human Reproduction and Embryology [ESHRE]) [28].

Again, it should be stressed that this model was intended for infertility patients; however, mental health professionals can easily extrapolate those areas that may be especially helpful in collaborating with cancer patients wanting to preserve their fertility and the medical team(s). In this model, Covington suggests that "psychosocial needs and counseling are identified and addressed in terms of purpose (i.e., why it is necessary); objective (i.e., what is to be achieved); typical issues (i.e., potential problem areas); and communication skills (i.e., attitude and knowledge needed for success)" [27]. She notes that "it is a fluid model in which the cycle may restart at different points or terminate at any step." Covington goes on to state that step 1 is the *introduction and initiation of a working alliance*, which lays the groundwork for the helping relationship. Step 2 involves *problem assessment and monitoring* where information is gathered about the patients' psychosocial experience and history. Step 3 is *clarification about the problem definition and negotiation about objectives and priorities*, where the patient's problems are summarized and possible limitations to treatment can be discussed. During step 4, in the case of fertility preservation, there is an *exchange of hypotheses and decision making* that takes place regarding diagnostic plans, if needed. Step 5 concerns *investigations and diagnostic procedures* that allow for more patient information, and step 6 allows the team to do *information giving about results* to the patient and discuss their implications. Step 7 provides the *elaboration of options to resolve (future) fertility problem*, which is presented and processed with the patient based on information and diagnosis. During step 8, the team and patient discuss *decision making about specific options* including advantages, disadvantages, and possible outcomes. Step 9, *treatment procedures*, when applicable, occurs when patients and the medical team take action with further diagnostic tests and/or treatments. Lastly, the cycle is completed with step 10, the *evaluation of outcome*, when the medical team and patient access information from previous steps, and may eventually re-enter the cycle at a previous step, if appropriate or necessary.

As Covington points out, this model presents a "biopsychosocial approach" that allows for the involvement and input of all members of the treatment team and in turn addresses the emotional and psychosocial needs of the patient [27]. In addition, this model need not be strictly formalized, but instead is an approach that allows for the ongoing involvement of the mental health professional when needed. This collaborative approach also permits patients to have more access to the mental health professional (if so desired) than simply a single-session consultation and/or assessment.

As mentioned above, this model may have some limitations in its applicability to men with cancer who wish to preserve their fertility. However, the notion of collaboration between the patient, medical personnel, and mental health professional is one that can most effectively address the numerous emotional and medical concerns with which our patients must cope.

Countertransference issues in cancer and fertility preservation

It is important that health and mental health professionals are aware of their personal feelings about fertility preservation in patients with cancer. Countertransference has to do with both the conscious and unconscious awareness of thoughts, feelings, and reactions that one displaces onto the patient within the context of the treating relationship. Goodheart and Lansing point to two dimensions of induced countertransference responses that are relevant to working with cancer patients: (1) responses to the disease impact and its usual course, and (2) responses to the individual patient's characterological reactions to the disease [29].

Not all patients are likeable or easy to work with. Some are angry, needy, demanding, and manipulative. Not all patients will choose fertility preservation even when they are excellent candidates for this option. Some patients' helplessness, anxiety, fear, and/or the prognosis for survival from their cancer will impact the ways in which caregivers respond to them. It is therefore important that healthcare and mental health professionals be aware of their own feelings, anxieties, defenses, and other responses to each patient. As Maier and colleagues indicate, helplessness is a very difficult feeling for most healthcare providers. Preoccupation with, or persistent, intense feelings concerning the patient outside the clinical setting is often a sign of prominent countertransference issues that should be addressed with peers or other professionals. It is important in these situations to turn to others who can assist us in effectively managing these challenging patients [30]. Only by doing so can we, as caregivers, provide the best-quality care.

Summary

Many exciting medical possibilities now exist for cancer survivors to have children after treatment, and it is now widely recommended that all patients of reproductive age (and younger) be afforded the opportunity to preserve their fertility prior to cancer therapy. Mental health professionals can play a vital role in assisting men with cancer who also must address fertility preservation and future biologic parenthood. Male patients (and their families) who have been diagnosed with cancer are often dealing with complex emotional and psychosocial issues and concerns as they confront their immediate illness as well as their desire to survive and move forward in their lives. Although fertility preservation offers hope and opportunity for many men with cancer, there is no guarantee that these treatments will be successful, and some come with substantial limitations.

Not only is it important to understand some of the gender-specific emotional responses of men to the immediate crisis of their cancer diagnoses, it is also especially helpful to know more about how they cope with the stresses that this challenging experience engenders. Feelings of anxiety, depression, fear, loss, grief, and anger are common. A knowledge and understanding of these responses can, in turn, assist all helping professionals in their work with this population. Unlike the general infertile population, these men are also confronted with issues of mortality and survival. Therefore, a thorough discussion of fertility preservation signals a sense of hopefulness about the future, and also helps these patients avoid future regret.

The mental health professional plays a significant role in this process. Psychological assessment and consultation protocols included in this chapter can be important in assuring that each patient is given individualized care, and that decision making occurs with full knowledge of the patient's psychological and emotional strengths and weaknesses. Including family members at various points in discussions of fertility preservation often must be a part of the psychological consultation. Included in the psychological consultation is the necessity of assisting the patient with complex and difficult decisions, not only about cancer therapy and fertility preservation, but also about future disposition of gametes or embryos should the patient not survive. As a member of the treatment team, the mental health professional should be called upon to collaborate with other healthcare professionals, and can also provide ongoing psychological and emotional support to the patient throughout every aspect of this process. As result, mental health professionals must be not only clinically competent, but also well educated on the medical aspects of cancer therapies as well as fertility preservation and ART techniques.

Lastly, the powerful needs and issues that men with cancer experience as they also consider or undergo fertility preservation can often lead to countertransference feelings on the part of helping professionals. Recognition of these feelings, and addressing them appropriately, can ultimately better serve this special patient population.

References

1. Chatterjee R, Goldstone AH. Gonadal damage and effects on fertility in adult patients with hematological malignancy undergoing stem cell transplantation. *Bone Marrow Transplant* 1996; 17: 5–11.

2. Tschudin S, Bitzer J. Psychological aspects of fertility preservation in men and women affected by cancer and other life-threatening diseases. *Hum Reprod Update* 2009; 15: 587–97.

3. Schover LR. Patient attitudes toward fertility preservation. *Pediatr Blood Cancer* 2009; 53: 281–4.

4. Oppenheim D, Brugieres L, Hartmann O. Adolescents treated for cancer and fertility preservation: psychological aspects. *Gynecol Obstet Fertil* 2005; 33: 627–31.

5. Rosen A, Rodriguez-Wallberg K, Oktay K. Psychological issues of cancer survivors. In Donnez J, Kim SS, eds. *Principles and Practice of Fertility Preservation*. Cambridge: Cambridge University Press, 2011; pp. 473–84.

6. Bloch S, Love A, Macvean M, *et al*. Psychological adjustment of men with prostate cancer: a review of the literature. *Biopsychosoc Med* 2007; 1: 2.

7. Kiss A, Meryn S. Effect of sex and gender on psychosocial aspects of prostate and breast cancer. *BMJ* 2001; 323: 1055–8.

8. Green BL, Galvin H, Horne B. The psychosocial impact of infertility on young male cancer survivors: a qualitative investigation. *Psychooncology* 2003; 18: 1084–93.

9. Tournaye H, Goossens E, Verheyen G, *et al*. Preserving the reproductive potential of men and boys with cancer: current concepts and future prospects. *Hum Reprod Update* 2004; 10: 525–32.

10. Shin D, Lo KC, Lipshultz LI. Treatment options for the infertile male with cancer. *J Natl Cancer Inst Monogr* 2005; 34: 48–50.

11. Williams DH. Sperm banking and the cancer patient. *Ther Adv Urol* 2010; 2: 19–34.

12. Jeruss JS, Woodruff TK. Preservation of fertility in patients with cancer. *N Engl J Med* 2009; 360: 902–11.

13. Hubner MK, Glazer ES. Now on common ground: cancer and infertility in the 1990s. *Infertil Reprod Med Clin North Am* 1993; 3: 581–97.

14. Lee S. *Counselling in Male Infertility*. Oxford: Blackwell, 1996.

15. Nachtigall RD, Becker G, Wozny M. The effects of gender-specific diagnosis on men's and women's response to infertility. *Fertil Steril* 1992; 57: 113–21

16. Hite S. *The Hite Report on Love, Passion and Emotional Violence*. London: MacDonald Optima, 1991.

17. Quinn GP, Vadaparampil ST. Fertility preservation and adolescent/young adult patients: physician communication challenges. *J Adol Health* 2009; 44: 394–400.

18. Ginsberg JP, Ogle SK, Tuchman LK, *et al*. Sperm banking for adolescent and young adult cancer patients: sperm quality, patient, and parent perspectives. *Pediatr Blood Cancer* 2008; 50: 594–8.

19. Williams DH. Sperm banking and the cancer patient: barriers to sperm banking. *Ther Adv Urol* 2010; 2: 19–34.

20. Gilbert E, Adams A, Mehanna H, Harrison B, Hartshorne GM. Who should be offered sperm banking for fertility preservation? A survey of UK oncologists and hematologists. *Ann Oncol* 2011; 22: 1209–14.

21. Verhaak C, Burns LH. Behavioral medicine approaches to infertility counseling. In Covington SN, Burns LH, eds. *Infertility Counseling: A Comprehensive Handbook for Clinicians*, 2nd edn. New York, NY: Cambridge University Press, 2006.

22. Tunks E, Bellissimo A. *Behavioral Medicine: Concepts and Procedures*. New York, NY: Pergamon Press, 1991.

23. Lazarus RS, Folkman S. *Stress, Appraisal, and Coping*. New York, NY: Springer, 1984.

24. Stanton AL. Cognitive appraisals, coping processes and adjustment to infertility. In Stanton AL, Dunkel-Schetter, eds. *Infertility Perspectives from Stress and Coping Research*. New York, NY: Plenum Press, 1991.

25. Mason MC. *Male Infertility: Men Talking*. London: Routledge, 1993.

26. Hershberger PE, Pierce PF. Conceptualizing couples' decision-making in PGD: emerging cognitive, emotional, and moral dimensions. *Patient Educ Couns* 2010; 81: 53–62.

27. Covington SN. Infertility counseling in practice: a collaborative reproductive healthcare model. In Covington SN, Burns LH, eds. *Infertility Counseling: A Comprehensive Handbook for Clinicians*, 2nd edn. New York, NY: Cambridge University Press, 2006.

28. Bitzer J. The ten-step circular process model. In Boivin J, Kenenich H, eds. *Guidelines for Counselling in Infertility*. ESHRE Monographs. Oxford: Oxford University Press, 2002.

29. Goodheart CD, Lansing MH. *Treating People with Chronic Disease: A Psychological Guide*. Washington, DC: American Psychological Association, 1996.

30. Maier DB, Covington SN, Maier LU. Patients with medically complicating conditions. In Covington SN, Burns LH, eds. *Infertility Counseling: A Comprehensive Handbook for Clinicians*, 2nd edn. New York, NY: Cambridge University Press, 2006.

Chapter

23 Nutraceuticals in fertility preservation

Mark A. Moyad

Lifestyle changes

It is imperative that clinicians never gloss over the importance of lifestyle changes for overall health and male fertility. It is interesting that most heart-unhealthy behaviors also negatively impact almost all other areas of male health [1], including fertility [2], and that improving heart health or encouraging heart-healthy changes in patients may improve overall mental health and quality of life [3]. Heart-healthy recommendations are arguably the most logical suggestions that simultaneously can also improve quality and perhaps quantity of life for cancer patients [4]. Thus, spending time reviewing the impact of obesity, high cholesterol and blood pressure, lack of exercise, improper diet, stress, depression, and multiple other cardiovascular risk factors that increase oxidative stress, which all have some minor or major impact on fertility, is arguably the most holistic approach to changing patients' lives and improving overall outcomes [3–6]. In other words, it is the ultimate 2-for-1 beneficial impact on your patients. Heart health is tantamount to male fertility health, and this is the theme of this chapter, which also includes nutraceutical recommendations. In addition, clinicians need to keep in mind that lifestyle changes can immediately increase nutrient levels before supplementation with an antioxidant pill is recommended, because obesity, substance abuse, and other heart-unhealthy changes accelerate the depletion or dilution of a variety of antioxidants in the serum [1]. Lifestyle changes and minimal supplement dosages are more logical, practical, safe, and heart-healthy than high doses of antioxidants from pills in the absence of lifestyle alterations.

Nutraceuticals/dietary supplements

Past authoritative medical reviews have suggested that antioxidant supplement treatment could be considered a primary treatment for some male fertility issues [7]. Additionally, a recently released Cochrane review is arguably one of the most extensive ever published in male fertility and dietary supplements, as it reviewed 34 clinical trials with 2876 couples in total [8]. The overall findings continue to surprise a number of clinicians and patients, in my opinion, by concluding that antioxidant supplementation in males appears to have a positive role in improving the outcomes of live birth and pregnancy rates in couples participating in assisted reproductive technologies (ART). In fact, for live births the p-value was 0.0008 and for pregnancy rates it was $p < 0.00001$. Critics of this analysis on "live births" will also perhaps point toward the small number of such events ($n = 20$) that occurred from a total of 214 couples in only three studies that were used in this part of the analysis, or the "pregnancy rate," which actually was derived from 96 pregnancies in 15 trials that included 964 couples. However, it is still remarkable that this is a viable minimal or moderate option for some men, given the low cost of most "antioxidants" utilized in these studies. Additionally, acute side effects were similar to a placebo, with no serious adverse events reported in any trial.

The common question that will arise from this or any other positive analysis for male fertility and antioxidants is, which specific dietary supplements and at what dosage and frequency? Interestingly, this extensive Cochrane review considered all supplement interventions in a pooled analysis, so it could not identify one superior individual antioxidant or combination product from these trials [8]. Readers are therefore left without a defined approach to supplement intervention for patients interested in enhancing fertility. Thus, an overview of antioxidant supplements used in past well-designed placebo-controlled trials is needed with an overall cost, safety, and health perspective to determine which products should be recommended and perhaps avoided by patients. This was the weakness of the Cochrane review and other reviews in male fertility [8], the overall lack of specific recommendations based on overall safety and efficacy of these agents long term for overall health and fertility maintenance. This chapter will attempt to provide clarity on the issue of which supplements to recommend and which ones should be avoided, based on heart-healthy recommendations.

Coenzyme Q_{10} (CoQ_{10})

CoQ_{10} appears to be a safe agent that requires a low dose for male fertility preservation. CoQ_{10} (also known as ubiquinone) supplements have an excellent overall safety profile, and actually have some clinical data to suggest that they may reduce blood pressure, decrease myalgias from statin therapy, and improve some symptoms of Parkinson's disease [9]. The role of CoQ_{10} in the respiratory pathway as a method to improve energy production and reduce oxidative stress is well known in the physiologic sciences. It is for this reason that there should be some interest in utilizing these agents for the reduction of oxidative stress. Additionally, a recent randomized study demonstrated a potential benefit for 200 mg a day of CoQ_{10} on Peyronie's disease [10].

Seminal fluid also contains a measurable quantity of CoQ_{10}, which appears to correlate with sperm count and motility. Patients with idiopathic asthenospermia might benefit in terms of spermatozoa motility when consuming 200 mg/day of CoQ_{10} for six months [11]. Another study of 212 infertile men taking 300 mg over 26 weeks found significant improvements in multiple parameters including sperm density, motility, and acrosome reaction [12]. Serum levels of follicle-stimulating hormone (FSH) and luteinizing hormone (LH) were significantly reduced by the supplement by the end of the study. CoQ_{10} can be a costly supplement, so patients should be encouraged to compare prices from multiple commercial resources to determine the most cost-effective product. CoQ_{10} appears to be a heart-healthy or safe supplement [9], except

that it does have the potential to reduce the impact of warfarin because it has vitamin K-like properties [13]. Regardless, it is a supplement that could be encouraged for fertility preservation in most men with cancer at a dosage of 200–300 mg per day.

Folic acid

Folic acid is not an ideal antioxidant for male fertility, and should not be used at this time in cancer patients. Folate is a water-soluble B-vitamin, which is also known as vitamin B_9, and it occurs naturally in many healthy foods and multiple diverse beverages [14]. Folic acid is the synthetic, human-produced, or manufactured form of folate that is found in dietary supplements and added to a variety of grain products, which are also known as "fortified foods." Folate from foods and folic acid both assist in the production of DNA, RNA, and other items that are critical for the production and maintenance of cells, especially ones involved in rapid cell division and growth such as in pregnancy and infancy [15]. Humans of all ages need folate to produce normal red blood cells and to prevent macrocytic anemia. Folate is also critical for metabolizing the amino acid homocysteine, which may cause cellular damage in abnormally high amounts and is important for the synthesis of methionine. Folate has multiple roles in human development, which is why this compound is probably best known for preventing neural tube defects (NTDs) [14].

Green leafy vegetables, fruits, legumes, and peas are just some of the natural sources of folate. Still, due to the importance of folate in the prevention of NTDs, the US Food and Drug Administration (FDA) required the addition of folic acid to grain products such as breads, cereals, corn, flours, meals, pastas, and rice. In 1998, the USA and Canada officially began fortifying grain products with folic acid [14]. The recommended daily allowance (RDA) is only 400 µg a day [16]. Table 23.1 is a partial listing of food and other sources of folate and folic acid in order of highest to lowest concentrations [16]. It is important to keep in mind that folic acid is generally added to foods that are labeled "enriched" and/or "fortified" in the USA and other countries.

Synthetic folic acid was believed to be more bioavailable compared to dietary sources of folate, which may have been one of the many reasons to fortify foods around the world. However, recent research has suggested that folate from foods may be only

Table 23.1. A selected list of beverage/food and other sources of folate and folic acid

Food/beverage or other	Micrograms (µg)
100% Fortified breakfast cereals	400
Multivitamin (on average, 1 pill)	400
B-complex vitamin (on average, 1 pill)	400–800
Brewer's yeast (1 tablespoon)	250
Beef liver (cooked, 3 ounces)	185
Spinach (cooked, $\frac{1}{2}$ cup)	100
Asparagus (4 spears)	85
Rice (white, enriched, $\frac{1}{2}$ cup)	65
Beans (baked, 1 cup)	60
Green peas (boiled, $\frac{1}{2}$ cup)	50
Avocado ($\frac{1}{2}$ cup)	45
Broccoli (2 spears)	45
Lettuce ($\frac{1}{2}$ cup)	40
Peanuts (dry roasted, 1 ounce)	40
Orange or orange juice (6 ounces)	30–35
Tomato juice (6 ounces)	35
Bread (white, whole wheat, enriched, 1 slice)	25
Egg (whole)	25
Banana (medium)	20
Wheat germ (1 tablespoon)	20
Rice (brown, $\frac{1}{2}$ cup)	5–10

slightly less absorbable (about 20%) than synthetic folic acid [17]. Other recent issues with the overall safety and impact of folic acid on male health abound. A recent large-scale meta-analysis has reviewed all of the randomized trial data on folic acid and other B-vitamin supplementation to reduce the risk of cardiovascular disease, cancer, or all-cause mortality [18]. It concluded that there was minimal to no impact of these supplements in reducing the risk of these conditions. In other words, currently it does not seem to impact the risk of most chronic diseases, despite the fact that it can reduce blood homocysteine levels by at least 25%. However, folic acid supplements may increase or encourage the growth of a variety of common tumors [19], including prostate cancer [20,21]. Serum levels of folic acid also appear to be increasing dramatically, such that unmetabolized folic acid (UMFA) has become a concern in men of all ages [22]. Thus, clinicians should not encourage supplemental folic acid use in men with a history of cancer who are concerned about fertility, despite some minimal positive data in the area of fertility itself [23], because other supplements are safer, just as effective, and do not appear to require mega-dosage (like folic acid) for a clinical impact. Food sources of folate can be recommended, but not the concentrated nutraceuticals.

L-carnitine

L-carnitine is a potential supplement for male fertility, but large dosages may be needed, and it is not a low-cost product. L-carnitine transports fatty acids from the cytosol to the mitochondria for energy production in each cell of the body [24]. There is some preliminary research that it may slightly reduce fatigue in some cancer patients. It is of interest that vitamin C (ascorbic acid) is needed to synthesize carnitine in the human body. The highest concentration of carnitine, apart from supplements, occurs in red meat and dairy products, so vegetarians who are trying to maintain fertility would potentially be better candidates for this supplement. There are several minimally different forms of L-carnitine available for purchase that have been used in clinical trials, including L-carnitine itself, acetyl-L-carnitine, and propionyl-L-carnitine. These other types of L-carnitine have been tested because L-carnitine itself tends to be unstable. Yet these other forms of L-carnitine do not necessarily have better fertility data, although they are more costly for the patient. Multiple clinical trials have demonstrated the ability of L-carnitine or other forms of carnitine to improve sperm kinetic characteristics and potentially pregnancy rates [25–29]. Adverse events using L-carnitine, or serious drug interactions, have not been identified. Doses of 2–3 g per day on average have been used in clinical trials.

Omega-3 fatty acids

Omega-3 fatty acid supplements should not be recommended to maintain fertility, but dietary sources of omega-3 should be encouraged in most individuals. Numerous fish contain high levels of omega-3 fatty acids, vitamin D, protein, and selenium, including salmon, tuna, sardines, and a variety of other baked, broiled, raw, but not fried fish are potentially beneficial [30]. Variety should be encouraged to increase compliance and exposure. The data to support the benefit of fish consumption to reduce the risk or progression of cancer are preliminary, but its positive

Table 23.2. Commercially available seafood that has demonstrated minimal levels of mercury

Anchovies
Catfish
Cod
Crab
Flounder/sole
Haddock
Herring
Lobster
Mahi-mahi
Ocean perch
Oysters
Rainbow trout
Salmon (farmed and wild)
Sardines
Scallops
Shrimp
Spiny lobster
Tilapia
Trout (farmed)

role in reducing the risk of a cardiovascular event or impacting all-cause mortality is a more definitive conclusion from clinical trials encouraging fish [31] or fish-oil consumption [32,33] in patients with a history of heart disease. Thus, fish-oil supplements should probably be reserved for patients concerned about heart health, because they are high-risk, or for those who want to reduce triglycerides. The data on fish oil for fertility maintenance is minimal and controversial because there have not been enough studies [34,35]. Again, dietary sources of healthy fish can be encouraged.

Mercury concentrations in specific fish have been reported by the FDA and in the general medical literature, but the preliminary data are controversial and it is not known at this time what kind of clinical impact these mercury levels may have on the individual [30]. Four types of larger predatory fish have been most concerning because these fish (king mackerel, shark, swordfish, and tilefish) have the ability to retain greater amounts of methyl mercury. Moderate consumption (2–3 times per week) of most fish should have minimal impact on overall human mercury serum levels, but more ongoing research in this area should soon provide better clarity. The positive impact of consuming fish seems to outweigh the negative impact in the majority of individuals, with the exception of women considering pregnancy or who are pregnant. Table 23.2 is a summary of a variety of fish that have consistently demonstrated low levels of mercury, and this table should also teach patients that a variety of fish and shellfish are healthy [30]. It

should be kept in mind that approximately two servings per week of fatty, oily, low-mercury fish is equivalent to ingesting approximately one 500 mg fish-oil pill per day. Clinicians who recommend high dosages of fish-oil supplements must keep in mind that these supplements could increase the risk of internal bleeding at higher dosages and in combination with other anticoagulants [13].

Some fish are low in mercury levels but also low in omega-3 fatty acid concentration, and tilapia is a classic example of this problem. On the other hand, I find it interesting that low-cost fish such as anchovies and sardines are low in mercury, and have some of the highest concentrations of omega-3 oils, and are used more than any other fish in the manufacturing of fish-oil pills to be utilized by the public and in clinical trials [30]. Patients who cannot eat fish or do not want to utilize fish oil because of an allergy or a personal belief could be recommended the newer algae-based omega-3 oils or regularly consume the largest plant-based sources of omega-3 fatty acids, which are found in plant oils (canola and soy), flaxseed, and chia seed. It should also be kept in mind that there is some interest in investigating the potential positive role of vitamin D for maintaining fertility, and currently the highest natural sources of vitamin D are from fish that are also high in omega-3 fatty acids, such as salmon [36].

Selenium and vitamin E

It is my opinion that selenium or vitamin E supplements should not be recommended to maintain fertility in men with cancer. Safety and efficacy issues abound with these specific nutraceuticals for overall health and wellness. For example, the initiation, and even the final results of the SELECT trial of selenium and/or vitamin E were concerning for a multitude of reasons [37]. Both agents failed to prevent prostate cancer, and there were multiple past and current safety issues with these nutritional supplement agents. Selenium had a history of potentially increasing the risk of skin cancer recurrence [38], and there were concerns over an increased risk of type 2 diabetes [39]. Interestingly, SELECT observed a non-significant increased risk of type 2 diabetes when the trial was halted [37].

Vitamin E supplements were also replete with some similar but even more concerning issues before the SELECT trial. Past meta-analysis of other clinical trials found a potential increased risk of all-cause mortality with higher doses of vitamin E supplements [40]. It is also of interest that a significantly increased risk of hemorrhagic stroke was found for subjects receiving vitamin E supplements in another major chemoprevention trial of healthy physicians (Physicians' Health Study II) that was conducted concurrently with SELECT [41]. SELECT also found a non-significant ($p = 0.06$) increased risk of prostate cancer in the vitamin E arm when the study was terminated [37]. Thus there needs to be more clinician and patient awareness over the multiple serious safety issues with vitamin E and selenium [42], and these supplements should not be encouraged for an individual with cancer attempting to maintain fertility, despite past trials in infertility suggesting some benefit to supplementation with these agents[43,44].

Vitamin C

There is enough indirect information on the use and long-term safety of vitamin C in cancer that this is a supplement that can be encouraged in maintaining fertility [30,45]. Some positive preliminary data exist for improving fertility in men consuming 500–1000 mg of vitamin C supplements per day in combination with other antioxidants [7,8]. Whether or not vitamin C alone can perform as well as the combination supplement treatments is not known.

Some of the best dietary sources of vitamin C are listed in Table 23.3 [30,46], but keep in mind that although these foods are healthy, one should be careful about getting an excessive amount of calories from them. It is also possible that with the growing popularity of the low-carbohydrate dietary programs for weight loss, a consequence of this behavioral change may be a lower intake of citrus fruits, which could lead to a lower blood level of vitamin C. Regardless, being able to achieve vitamin C concentrations from diet that are similar to the dosage utilized in clinical trials of supplementation is simply unrealistic. Still, a combination of regular vitamin C intake from food and daily nutraceutical consumption may be one of the best methods of maintaining adequate ascorbic acid and antioxidant blood levels that could maintain fertility. There is some concern about oxalate increases with plain vitamin C supplements, but it has recently been preliminarily demonstrated that buffered vitamin C or

Table 23.3. Sources of vitamin C (foods and beverages)

Fruit	Portion size	Vitamin C content (mg)
Guava	1 (medium)	100
Strawberries	1 cup	95
Papaya	1 cup	85
Kiwi	1 (medium)	75
Orange	1 (medium)	70
Cantaloupe	¼ (medium)	60
Mango	1 cup	45
Cantaloupe melon	1 cup	40
Grapefruit	½ fruit	40
Honeydew melon	1/8 medium	40
Lemon	1 medium	40
Tangerines or tangelos	1 medium	25
Watermelon	1 cup	15
Apple	1 medium	10
Avocado	1 medium	10
Apricot	1 medium	10
Banana	1 medium	10
Blueberry	1 cup	10
Crabapple	1 medium	10
Grape	1 cup	10
Pawpaw	1 medium	10
Pineapple	1 cup	10
Plum	1 medium	10
Grape juice	½ cup	120
Apple juice	½ cup	50
Orange juice (fortified)	½ cup	50
Cranberry juice	½ cup	45
Grapefruit juice	½ cup	35
Tomato juice	6 ounces	35
Pepper (red or green, raw)	½ cup	65
Broccoli (cooked)	½ cup	60
Kale (cooked)	1 cup	55
Brussels sprouts (cooked)	½ cup	50
Snow peas (fresh, cooked)	½ cup	40
Mustard greens (cooked)	1 cup	35
Potato (sweet or regular, baked)	1 medium	25–30
Cauliflower (raw or cooked)	½ cup	25

(cont.)

Table 23.3. (cont.)

Fruit	Portion size	Vitamin C content (mg)
Cabbage (red, raw or cooked)	$\frac{1}{2}$ cup	20–25
Plantains (sliced and cooked)	1 cup	15
Tomato (raw)	$\frac{1}{2}$ cup	15
Cabbage (raw or cooked)	$\frac{1}{2}$ cup	10–15
Asparagus (cooked)	$\frac{1}{2}$ cup	10

calcium ascorbate may be a safer alternative for these specific patients [47].

Other supplements

Other supplements, such as magnesium [48], simply have shown no benefit or should not be recommended because of their health concerns for men with a history of cancer, despite some initial positive preliminary data with fertility parameters [49]. For example, zinc supplementation has potentially negative effects for patients concerned about heart health and cancer, especially at the high dosages that have been utilized in past fertility studies [49,50].

Conclusion

It is time to view fertility nutraceuticals from a wider perspective, because a plethora of research has been performed on numerous antioxidants. Large and authoritative meta-analyses actually endorse the utilization of multiple products for men attempting to maintain or improve fertility [8]. However, before endorsement of a specific supplement becomes logical it would seem imperative to teach clinicians and patients about the overall safety and efficacy of these interventions outside of fertility. What is the impact of these agents on general health, and on the specific conditions that bring the largest toll of morbidity and mortality both in men and in women, such as heart disease and cancer? When this is kept in mind, the "forest over the tree" approach that benefits all our patients will have been exercised.

References

1. Moyad MA, Lowe FC. Educating patients about lifestyle modifications for prostate health. *Am J Med* 2008; 121 (8 Suppl 2): S34–42.
2. Cabler S, Agarwal A, Flint M, du Plessis SS. Obesity: modern man's fertility nemesis. *Asian J Androl* 2010; 12: 480–9.
3. Yusuf S, Hawken S, Ounpuu S, et al. Effect of potentially modifiable risk factors associated with myocardial infarction in 52 countries (the INTERHEART study): case-control study. *Lancet* 2004; 364: 937–52.
4. Eyre H, Kahn R, Robertson RM; ACS/ADA/AHA Collaborative Writing Committee. Preventing cancer, cardiovascular disease, and diabetes: a common agenda for the American Cancer Society, the American Diabetes Association, and the American Heart Association. *CA Cancer J Clin* 2004; 54: 190–207.
5. Kasturi SS, Tannir J, Brannigan RE. The metabolic syndrome and male infertility. *J Androl* 2008; 29: 251–9.
6. Campagne DM. Should fertilization treatment start with reducing stress? *Hum Reprod* 2006; 21: 1651–8.
7. Agarwal A, Sekhon LH. The role of antioxidant therapy in the treatment of male infertility. *Hum Fertil* 2010; 13: 217–25.
8. Showell MG, Brown J, Yazdani A, Stankiewicz MT, Hart RJ. Antioxidants for male subfertility. *Cochrane Database Syst Rev* 2011; (1): CD007411.
9. Littarru GP, Tiano L. Clinical aspects of coenzyme Q_{10}: an update. *Nutrition* 2010; 26: 250–4.
10. Safarinejad MR. Safety and efficacy of coenzyme Q_{10} supplementation in early chronic Peyronie's disease: a double-blind, placebo-controlled randomized study. *Int J Impot Res* 2010; 22: 298–309.
11. Balercia G, Buldreghini E, Vignini A, et al. Coenzyme Q_{10} treatment in infertile men with idiopathic asthenozoospermia: a placebo-controlled randomized trial. *Fertil Steril* 2009; 91: 1785–92.
12. Safarinejad ME. Efficacy of coenzyme Q_{10} on semen parameters, sperm function and reproductive hormones in infertile men. *J Urol* 2009; 182: 237–48.
13. Mousa SA. Antithrombotic effects of naturally derived products on coagulation and platelet function. *Methods Mol Biol* 2010; 663: 229–40.
14. Obican SG, Finnell RH, Mills JL, Shaw GM, Scialli AR. Folic acid in early pregnancy: a public health success story. *FASEB J* 2010; 24: 4167–74.
15. Zeisel SH. Importance of methyl donors during reproduction. *Am J Clin Nutr* 2009; 89: 673S–677S.
16. Institute of Medicine. Food and Nutrition Board. Folate. *Dietary Reference Intakes for Thiamin, Riboflavin, Niacin, Vitamin B6, Folate, Vitamin B12, Pantothenic Acid, Biotin, and Choline*. Washington, DC: National Academy Press, 2000; pp. 196–305.

17. Winkels RM, Brouwer IA, Siebelink E, Katan MB, Verhoef P. Bioavailability of food folates is 80% of that of folic acid. *Am J Clin Nutr* 2007; 85: 465–73.

18. Clarke R, Halsey J, Lewington S, *et al.*; B-vitamin Treatment Trialists' Collaboration. Effects of lowering homocysteine levels with B vitamins on cardiovascular disease, cancer, and cause-specific mortality. Meta-analysis of 8 randomized trials involving 37,485 individuals. *Arch Intern Med* 2010; 170: 1622–31.

19. Cole BF, Baron JA, Sandler RS, *et al.*; Polyp Prevention Study Group. Folic acid for the prevention of colorectal adenomas: a randomized clinical trial. *JAMA* 2007; 297: 2351–9.

20. Figueiredo JC, Grau MV, Haile RW, *et al.* Folic acid and risk of prostate cancer: results from a randomized clinical trial. *J Natl Cancer Inst* 2009; 101: 432–5.

21. Collin SM, Metcalfe C, Refsum H, *et al.* Circulating folate, vitamin B12, homocysteine, vitamin B12 transport proteins, and risk of prostate cancer: a case-control study, systematic review, and meta-analysis. *Cancer Epidemiol Biomarkers Prev* 2010; 19: 1632–42.

22. Bailey RL, Mills JL, Yetley EA, *et al.* Unmetabolized serum folic acid and its relation to folic acid intake from diet and supplements in a nationally representative sample of adults aged ≥60 y in the United States. *Am J Clin Nutr* 2010; 92: 383–9.

23. Wong WY, Merkus HM, Thomas CM, *et al.* Effects of folic acid and zinc sulfate on male factor subfertility: a double-blind, randomized, placebo-controlled trial. *Fertil Steril* 2002; 77: 491–8.

24. Acetyl-L-carnitine. Monograph. *Altern Med Rev* 2010; 15: 76–83.

25. Balercia G, Regoli F, Armeni T, *et al.* Placebo-controlled double-blind randomized trial on the use of L-carnitine, L-acetylcarnitine, or combined L-carnitine and L-acetylcarnitine in men with idiopathic asthenozoospermia. *Fertil Steril* 2005; 84: 662–71.

26. Lenzi A, Lombardo F, Sgro P, *et al.* Use of carnitine therapy in selected cases of male factor infertility: a double-blind crossover trial. *Fertil Steril* 2003; 79: 292–300.

27. Li Z, Chen GW, Shang XJ, *et al.* A controlled randomized trial of the use of combined L-carnitine and acetyl-L-carnitine treatment in men with oligoasthenozoospermia. *Zhong Hua Nan Ke Xue* 2005; 11: 761–4.

28. Peivandi S, Abasali K, Narges M. Effects of L-carnitine on infertile men's spermogram: a randomized clinical trial. *J Reprod Infertil* 2010; 10: 331.

29. Lombardo F, Gandini L, Agarwal A, *et al.* A prospective double blind placebo controlled cross over trial of carnitine therapy in selected cases of male infertility. *Fertil Steril* 2002; 78 (Suppl 1): 68–9.

30. Moyad MA. *Dr. Moyad's No Bogus Science Health Advice.* Ann Arbor, MI: Ann Arbor Editions, 2009.

31. Burr ML, Fehily AM, Gilbert JF, *et al.* Effects of changes in fat, fish, and fibre intakes on death and myocardial reinfarction: Diet and Reinfarction Trial (DART). *Lancet* 1989; 2: 757–61.

32. Marchioli R, Barzi F, Bomba E, *et al.* Early protection against sudden cardiac death by n-3 polyunsaturated fatty acids after myocardial infarction: time-course analysis of the results of the Gruppo Italiano per lo Studio della Sopravvivenza nell'Infarto Miocardico (GISSI)-Prevenzione. *Circulation* 2002; 105: 1897–903.

33. Matsuzaki M, Yokoyama M, Saito Y, *et al.* Incremental effects of eicosapentaenoic acid on cardiovascular events in statin-treated patients with coronary artery disease. *Circ J* 2009; 73: 1283–90.

34. Conquer JA, Martin JB, Tummon I, Watson L, Tekpetey F. Effect of DHA supplementation on DHA status and sperm motility in asthenozoospermic males. *Lipids* 2000; 35: 149–54.

35. Safarinejad MR. Effect of omega-3 polyunsaturated fatty acid supplementation on semen profile and enzymatic anti-oxidant capacity of seminal plasma in infertile men with idiopathic oligoasthenoteratospermia: a double-blind, placebo-controlled, randomized study. *Andrologia* 2011; 43: 38–47.

36. Corbett ST, Hill O, Nangia AK. Vitamin D receptor found in human sperm. *Urology* 2006; 68: 1345–9.

37. Lippman SM, Klein EA, Goodman PJ, *et al.* Effect of selenium and vitamin E on risk of prostate cancer and other cancers: the Selenium and Vitamin E Cancer Prevention Trial (SELECT). *JAMA* 2009; 301: 39–51.

38. Duffield-Lillico AJ, Slate EH, Reid ME, *et al.* Selenium supplementation and secondary prevention of nonmelanoma skin cancer in a randomized trial. *J Natl Cancer Inst* 2003; 95: 1477–81.

39. Stranges S, Marshall JR, Natarajan R, *et al.* Effects of long-term selenium supplementation on the incidence of type 2 diabetes: a randomized trial. *Ann Intern Med* 2007; 147: 217–23.

40. Miller ER, Pastor-Barriuso R, Dalal D, *et al.* Meta-analysis: high-dosage vitamin E supplementation may increase all-cause mortality. *Ann Intern Med* 2005; 142: 37–46.

41. Sesso HD, Buring JE, Christen WG, *et al.* Vitamins E and C in the prevention of cardiovascular disease in

men: the Physicians' Health Study II randomized controlled trial. *JAMA* 2008; 300: 2123–33.

42. Moyad MA. Selenium and vitamin E supplements for prostate cancer: evidence or embellishment? *Urology* 2002; 59 (4 Suppl 1): 9–19.

43. Keskes-Ammar L, Feki-Chakroun N, Rebai T, *et al.* Sperm oxidative stress and the effect of an oral vitamin E and selenium supplement on semen quality in infertile men. *Arch Androl* 2003; 49: 83–94.

44. Kessopoulou E, Powers HJ, Sharma KK, *et al.* A double-blind randomized placebo cross-over controlled trial using the antioxidant vitamin E to treat reactive oxygen species associated with male infertility. *Fertil Steril* 1995; 64: 825–31.

45. Colagar AH, Marzony ET. Ascorbic acid in human seminal plasma: determination and its relationship to sperm quality. *J Clin Biochem Nutr* 2009; 45: 144–9.

46. 6. Vitamin C content in foods. www. vitamincfoundation.org/usda.html (accessed March 20, 2011).

47. Moyad MA, Combs MA, Baisley JE, Evans M. Vitamin C with metabolites: additional analysis suggests favorable changes in oxalate. *Urol Nurs* 2009; 29: 383–5.

48. Zavaczki Z, Szollosi J, Kiss S, *et al.* Magnesium-orotate supplementation for idiopathic infertile male patients: a randomized, placebo-controlled clinical pilot study. *Magnesium Res* 2003; 16: 131–6.

49. Omu AE, Dashti H, Al-Othman S. Treatment of asthenozoospermia with zinc sulphate: andrological, immunological and obstetric oucome. *Eur J Obstet Gynecol Reprod Biol* 1998; 79: 179–84.

50. Moyad MA. Zinc for prostate disease and other conditions: a little evidence, a lot of hype, and a significant potential problem. *Urol Nurs* 2004; 24: 49–52.

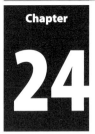

Section 4 Preservation strategies

Chapter 24

Application of spermatogenesis suppression therapies for fertility preservation

Rian J. Dickstein, Gunapala Shetty, and Marvin L. Meistrich

Introduction

The lifetime risk of development of cancer for individuals in the United States is 40%, and treatment commonly involves the use of chemotherapy and/or radiotherapy. These cytotoxic cancer treatments have a significant impact on a patient's future fertility status, which is of particular concern to cancer patients of childbearing age. The ability to achieve a pregnancy may be temporarily diminished, forcing the patient to delay parenthood, or infertility may become permanent. Loss of potential fertility can be an especially devastating consequence to a patient, in light of other physical and emotional turmoil entailed in cancer treatment.

Clinical manifestations of male infertility as a result of chemotherapy or radiotherapy include potential oligo/azoospermia and occasionally androgen insufficiency. There is a significant effort to enhance patients' awareness of these sequelae and to ensure that physicians are adequately informing patients of the consequences. In addition, efforts are ongoing to investigate strategies for preventing loss of gonadal function before and restoring gonadal function after cytotoxic treatment. Various therapeutic interventions have been studied in both animal models and humans; in particular, researchers' focus has centered on hormonal modulation [1]. Manipulation of the endocrine system to prevent or reverse damage to male germline cells is the focus of this chapter.

Gonadal toxicity

The general model for male gonadal toxicity resulting from antineoplastic therapies is based on observations that actively dividing spermatogonia are the testicular cells most sensitive to treatment. The loss of

dividing spermatogonia leads to depletion of maturing germ cells and a reduction in sperm count. If the stem spermatogonia are not killed, there is usually a return of normal sperm count and potential fertility in most patients after three months [2]. In reality, stem spermatogonia are killed by some cytotoxic agents, such as radiation and alkylating agents [3,4]. When only some of the stem cells are killed, recovery of sperm count often occurs but it is very gradual, usually over a period of 2–5 years [5]. If all stem cells are killed by the antineoplastic agents, permanent azoospermia results.

After cytotoxic therapy in a mouse model, surviving spermatogonia usually initiate cell division and differentiation [6], but in the rat (particularly in sensitive strains) spermatogonia often fail to differentiate and remain in the testicular tubules for prolonged periods of time [7] (Fig. 24.1). Spermatogonial transplantation experiments have demonstrated that rat spermatogonia are capable of differentiating in a suitable environment, but that the irradiated rat testes are not capable of supporting differentiation, even of healthy spermatogonia [8]. Thus, damage from toxic antineoplastic agents also involves the somatic environment, as well as the spermatogonia. For the production of sperm, the milieu surrounding progenitor stem cells is therefore just as important as, if not in some cases more important than, the cells themselves, but we have yet to understand the nature of the interaction between the two.

History of the suppression hypothesis

Chemotherapy- and radiotherapy-induced cell death is based on the destruction/alteration of normal cellular machinery involved in cell replication, thus targeting rapidly dividing cells such as those that

Fertility Preservation in Male Cancer Patients, ed. John P. Mulhall, Linda D. Applegarth, Robert D. Oates and Peter N. Schlegel.
Published by Cambridge University Press. © Cambridge University Press 2013.

203

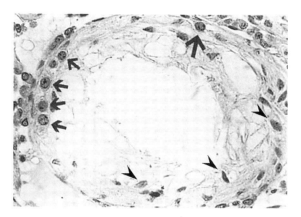

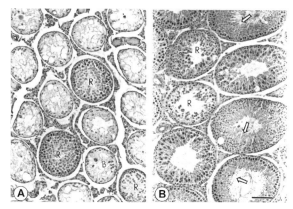

Figure 24.1. Block in differentiation of type A spermatogonia in a seminiferous tubule of a rat (sensitive strain) irradiated with 4 Gy 25 weeks previously. A single type A spermatogonium (potentially a stem cell) is indicated by the large arrow. A chain-like colony of type A spermatogonia is indicated by small arrows. No cells at more advanced stages of differentiation were observed. A few of the Sertoli cell nuclei in the tubule are indicated by arrowheads. (Reprinted with permission from Kangasniemi *et al., Biol Reprod* 1996; 54: 1200–8 [7].)

Figure 24.2. Protection of the recovery of spermatogenesis from chemotherapy in rats by pre-treatment hormonal suppression. Testis of rats at 10 weeks after a single dose of procarbazine either (A) without any hormonal suppression or (B) with treatment with low-dose testosterone plus estradiol for the five weeks up to the time of procarbazine injection. Note that after procarbazine injection (panel A) most tubule cross-sections contain only Sertoli cells. Active spermatogenic recovery is observed in only about 30% of tubules with development either to the B spermatogonial stage, "B," or the round spermatid stage, "R." When the rats were given hormonal suppression therapy (panel B), recovery of spermatogenesis is observed in all tubules, most showing complete spermatogenesis and sperm being produced (open arrows). Bar = 100 μm. (Reprinted with permission from Parchuri *et al., J Androl* 1993; 14: 257–66 [13].)

are neoplastic. It was originally observed that non-dividing cells are more resistant to cell death induced by antineoplastic agents than rapidly proliferating cells. Male germ line cells, in addition to the target neoplastic cells, fall into the category of rapidly dividing cells. Based on this concept, the hypothesis was developed that interruption of the hypothalamic–pituitary–gonadal (HPG) axis, which inhibits spermatogenesis, would arrest the proliferation of these rapidly dividing testicular progenitor cells, and render the spermatogonia resistant to chemotherapy [9].

Initially, it was claimed that spermatogenesis in mice receiving cyclophosphamide was successfully protected using a gonadotropin-releasing hormone (GnRH) agonist to suppress the HPG axis; however, this analysis utilized a qualitative histological endpoint as the outcome [9]. A subsequent attempt to repeat these experiments using quantitative assays failed to show any protective effects in this mouse model [10]. In fact, deprivation of gonadotropins or androgen action does not arrest the development of spermatogonia in rodent models, indicating that the original hypothesis was wrong [11].

However, numerous studies in rat models have shown that blockade of the HPG axis prior to or during exposure to chemotherapy or radiotherapy appears to protect spermatogenesis, as it markedly enhances subsequent recovery of spermatogenesis [12,13]

(Fig. 24.2). Again, it was clearly shown that the hormone suppression resulting in this apparent protection did not alter the kinetics of spermatogonial proliferation [14]. Since suppression of proliferation of spermatogonia is not involved in this phenomenon, investigators have since begun to suspect alternative mechanisms by which HPG suppression results in enhanced recovery of spermatogenesis.

One study utilizing a GnRH antagonist to induce protection of rat spermatogenic recovery from chemotherapy-induced damage made the interesting observation that additional treatment with exogenous testosterone, which suppresses luteinizing hormone (LH) and intratesticular testosterone, after chemotherapy further stimulated recovery of spermatogenesis [15]. Investigators then began to study the effect of HPG interruption with GnRH agonists or antagonists given only after the cytotoxic therapy [16]. Hormone-suppressive treatments with either exogenous testosterone or GnRH agonists given after irradiation dramatically stimulate the recovery of spermatogenesis from surviving spermatogonia (Fig. 24.3).

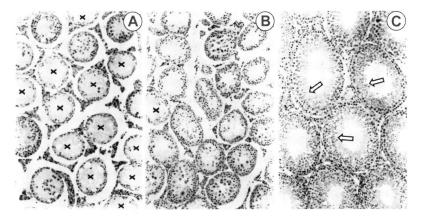

Figure 24.3. Stimulation of spermatogenesis recovery by hormonal suppression after irradiation with 3.5 Gy. (A) 10 weeks after irradiation: most of the tubules show no recovery of spermatogenesis (x). (B) 10 weeks after irradiation with continuous hormonal suppression treatment: nearly all of the tubules (except one marked with x) show recovery of spermatogenesis to the spermatocyte or occasionally the round spermatid stage. (C) 16.5 weeks after irradiation (6.5 weeks after cessation of the hormone treatment): all tubules show active spermatogenesis and many show sperm being produced (open arrows). (Reprinted with permission from Meistrich and Kangasniemi, *J Androl* 1997; 18: 80–7 [16].)

Experimental studies in the rat

Hormonal suppression *prior to* antineoplastic treatment has repeatedly been shown to protect the recovery of spermatogenesis in rats against damage from irradiation (with both gamma rays and neutrons) and chemotherapy (procarbazine and doxorubicin) [17–19]. Initial studies employed exogenous testosterone prior to toxic therapy, which suppressed intratesticular testosterone; later studies have shown that GnRH agonists and particularly GnRH antagonists are more effective, especially when combined with an antiandrogen such as flutamide [20]. Addition of estradiol to the suppression regimen also enhances the subsequent recovery of spermatogenesis from antineoplastic therapy [13].

Since kinetic changes were not involved, several studies have examined alternative mechanisms by which protection might occur. One possibility was that hormonal suppression altered intratesticular toxic drug delivery and/or metabolism. However, the HPG-suppressive treatment that enhanced spermatogonial stem cell recovery after toxic therapies did not increase the survival of neighboring germ cells, thereby disproving this hypothesis [21]. Furthermore, spermatogonial counts indicate that HPG suppression did not appear to protect stem cells from destruction by cytotoxic agents [22]. This led to the conclusion that the hormonal suppression acted by enhancing spermatogenic recovery from surviving stem cells, and the suggestion that this resulted from prevention of

injury to the testicular environment. Although the factor in the microenvironment that induces blockade in the differentiation of surviving stem cells after cytotoxic injury is not yet known, the HPG suppression prevents the induction of this blockade, forming the basis for the prevailing explanation of the protection.

Several studies have now shown that hormonal suppression *after* radiation or chemotherapy stimulates the recovery of spermatogenesis [16,23,24]. During the course of these hormone-suppressive treatments, there was a dramatic stimulation in the development of surviving spermatogonia to spermatocytes, but mature sperm could not be formed because of the absence of high levels of testosterone (Fig. 24.3). However, after suppression ceased, complete spermatogenesis was restored; the rats then regained nearly full fertility [25].

More recent work has focused on the mechanisms causing the block in stem cell differentiation and how it could be reversed by the hormonal suppression after antineoplastic therapy. The hormone primarily responsible for inhibition of spermatogonial differentiation in toxin-treated rats is testosterone; however, follicle-stimulating hormone (FSH) does exert some inhibitory effect as well [26]. The blockade of spermatogonial differentiation in rats treated with cytotoxic therapy also seems to be associated with interstitial edema, but the mechanism is unclear [27]. Although low-dose testosterone can stimulate recovery of stem cell differentiation by suppressing intratesticular testosterone and FSH, GnRH agonists and especially GnRH antagonists are more effective; the addition of an antiandrogen such as flutamide further enhances recovery [25,28]. Whereas addition of estrogen treatment to the GnRH antagonist further stimulated recovery, a progestin, with weak androgenic activity, somewhat inhibited the recovery [29,30]. Currently, factors produced by Leydig cells are being studied as potential effectors of the testosterone-induced inhibition of spermatogonial differentiation. Despite the active work in this field, the true underlying mechanism for damage protection or maintenance of germ cell differentiation in the testis with HPG suppression is not known.

Experimental studies in other species

After the initial conflicting studies in mice, several subsequent reports have showed lack of success in protecting or enhancing the recovery of spermatogenesis from antineoplastic treatments in this species [6,31,32]. Only recently has stimulation of spermatogenic recovery in mice been reported by HPG suppression given after radiation therapy, but the degree of stimulation was much smaller than that observed in the rat [33].

Furthermore, there has been no reliable success in other animal species, including dogs and monkeys. Two studies in dogs yielded conflicting results, one indicating a more rapid recovery and the other indicating potentiation of damage when GnRH agonists were given concomitantly with the antineoplastic agent [34,35]. Similarly, one study suggested that HPG suppression protected spermatogenesis in primates from cyclophosphamide-induced gonadal damage, based on results from a single animal [36], while larger studies showed neither protection nor stimulation of spermatogenic recovery from radiation with HPG suppression [37,38].

The question remains as to why there are conflicting results in each of the different animal models. Various explanations have been proposed, including differences in the relative importance of stem cell killing compared to loss of ability of stem cell differentiation secondary to somatic damage, differences in degree of spermatogenic suppression from various methods designed to disrupt the HPG, and differences in the regulation of recovery from surviving stem cells.

Human clinical trials

In addition to the research attempting to understand the basic mechanisms of fertility preservation in animal models, there have been ongoing trials in humans. Seven clinical trials have been performed, attempting to demonstrate protection of spermatogenesis with hormonal suppression before and during cytotoxic therapy, and six have indicated no benefit (Table 24.1). Three studies used HPG suppression to protect the testis from procarbazine-containing chemotherapy regimens for Hodgkin's lymphoma. Two employed GnRH agonist for suppression. In one of these, the suppressive treatment resulted in only 20% of patients recovering their sperm counts after cessation of therapy, but there was no matched control group for comparison [39]. In the second trial there was no recovery in either the hormonally suppressed or control group [40,41]. A third study utilized testosterone injections and found that 70% of patients in both the treatment and control group had spermatogenic recovery at three years [42]. Three other studies examined protection from cytotoxic damage in testicular cancer patients. HPG suppression with a progestin, medroxyprogesterone acetate, resulted in poorer recovery of sperm count or normalization of FSH levels than in the control group [43]. Two studies employing GnRH agonist showed recovery of sperm counts at two years, with a similar time course between the hormone-suppressed and non-suppressed groups [44,45].

The one study that did demonstrate preservation of sperm production used testosterone therapy in men receiving cyclophosphamide as an immunosuppressive for nephritic syndrome [46]. All but one man remained azoospermic six months after the completion of cyclophosphamide therapy in the control group (no testosterone therapy), but sperm concentrations returned to normal in all five patients treated with testosterone. Although this encouraging study was published in 1997, as of 2012 we are not aware of any subsequent studies repeating a similar experimental design.

In addition to the protection studies, there was one attempt to restore spermatogenesis with hormonal suppression utilized after cytotoxic therapy. None of seven men treated with medroxyprogesterone acetate and testosterone after chemotherapy and/or radiation recovered any sperm production over a 24-week follow-up period [47]. This is not surprising, as very high doses of gonadal radiation and

Table 24.1. Results of hormone suppression treatments given before and during cytotoxic therapy on spermatogenic recovery in humans

Study	Disease	Antineoplastic therapy[a]	Hormonal suppression	Recovery after hormonal suppression[b]	Recovery in control group[b]
Johnson et al. 1985 [39]	Hodgkin's lymphoma	MOPP × 3 or 6 cycles	GnRH agonist	1 of 5	--
Waxman et al. 1987 [40,41]	Hodgkin's lymphoma	MVPP, ChlVPP	GnRH agonist + testosterone	0 of 20	0 of 10
Redman & Bajorunas, 1987 [42]	Hodgkin's lymphoma	MOPP × ~4 cycles	Testosterone	≈70% of 23[c]	≈70% of 22[c]
Fossa et al. 1988 [43]	Testis cancer	PVB, ADR/CY, XRT	Medroxy-progesterone	0 of 4 (2 of 12)[d]	2 of 3 (7 of 13)[d]
Kreuser et al. 1990 [44]	Testis cancer	PVB	GnRH agonist	6 of 6	8 of 8
Brennemann et al. 1994 [45]	Testis cancer (seminoma)	XRT	GnRH agonist + antiandrogen	12 of 12	8 of 8
Masala et al. 1997 [46]	Glomerulonephritis	Cyclophosphamide	Testosterone	5 of 5	1 of 5

[a] Radio-chemotherapy regimens: MOPP, mechlorethamine, vincristine, procarbazine, prednisone; MVPP, mechlorethamine, vinblastine, procarbazine, prednisone; ChlVPP, chlorambucil, vinblastine, procarbazine, prednisone; PVB, cisplatin, vinblastine, bleomycin; ADR/CY, adriamycin, cyclophosphamide; XRT, radiation therapy.
[b] Fraction of men recovering testicular function as assessed by restoration of sperm counts to normospermic levels unless otherwise noted.
[c] Actuarial recovery calculated by Kaplan–Meier analysis.
[d] Recovery assessed by restoration of FSH levels to within the normal control range.

cytotoxic chemotherapy were used, likely killing all of the stem cells. Furthermore, previous studies using HPG suppression with medroxyprogesterone acetate failed to show improved recovery of spermatogenesis after cytotoxic therapy [30,43].

Although the clinical trial results seem to indicate either that the application of hormone-suppressive therapies does not enhance the recovery of spermatogenesis in humans or that we have not yet found the appropriate treatment conditions to effect a response, we believe that we should not yet abandon this approach in humans. There are several alternative explanations for failures of these trials that may open avenues to future studies. First, humans have higher intratesticular androgen levels than other animals and the regimens that were utilized may not have resulted in adequate androgen suppression to elicit an effect [48]. Second, the numbers of patients accrued have led to a power insufficient to tease out a modest statistical difference. Finally, some of the treatment regimens were not sufficiently gonadotoxic to cause prolonged sterility [45,49] and others delivered doses that likely destroyed all spermatogonial stem cells [39,41,47], indicating that hormonal manipulation management

strategies may need to be selectively applied based on type of disease and differing toxic treatment regimens.

Comparisons can be drawn amongst the studies in an attempt to determine factors that may be more predictive of treatment success. First, it may be appropriate to exclude cases involving cancer of the testes, as there may be an underlying derangement of spermatogenesis making it susceptible to additional associated toxicities. Second, the studies utilized different hormonal agents, which do not completely suppress the HPG axis; newer agents able to suppress testosterone levels and their action on androgen receptors to an even lower level than before will make this question worth revisiting. In this context, however, it is not apparent why testosterone appeared to stimulate spermatogenesis better, as it does not completely reduce intratesticular testosterone and it also seemed to suppress FSH as much as GnRH agonists did [45]. A third variable is the duration of chemotherapy and hormonal treatment: prolonged hormonal treatment, which was given during the long cyclophosphamide treatment for glomerulonephritis, may be more beneficial. The last issue with the trials relates to the different mechanisms by which

Table 24.2. Summary of effects of hormone-suppressive therapies on recovery of spermatogenesis in experimental models and humans, and relationship to recovery patterns (recovery patterns based on given single doses of radiation as an example)

Species	Recovery pattern after moderate cytotoxic damage (4–7 Gy irradiation)	Presence of A spermatogonia in atrophic tubules	Protective effects of HPG suppression before and/or during cytotoxic therapy	Stimulatory effects of HPG suppression after cytotoxic therapy
Mouse	Gradual recovery (70% sperm count) after 6 months (6 Gy)	Infrequently observed	No protection of spermatogenesis	Slight stimulation of recovery from surviving stem cells
Rat	Resistant strains – similar to but less recovery than in mouse Sensitive strains – no recovery	Frequently observed in sensitive and resistant strains	Marked stimulation of spermatogenic recovery	Marked stimulation of spermatogenic recovery
Non-human primate	Recovery (40% sperm count) in 12–18 months (4 Gy) No recovery in 18 months (7 Gy)	Not observed	No enhancement of spermatogenic recovery after irradiation	No enhancement of spermatogenic recovery after irradiation
Human	Azoospermia for 2 years; recovery (<10% sperm count) by 3 years (6 Gy)	Rarely observed	(6 studies) No spermatogenic protection from procarbazine or cisplatin chemotherapy or radiation (1 study) Testosterone offers some protection to spermatogenesis from cyclophosphamide	No restoration of spermatogenesis from delayed treatment

the chemotherapeutic agents damage cells. For example, cyclophosphamide is known to be less effective than other alkylating agents or radiation with respect to killing stem cells in rodents [50,51]. Thus, cyclophosphamide might induce less stem spermatogonial death but more somatic damage than other agents, and hence be more susceptible to hormonal modulations.

Relationship of experimental to human studies

As the vast majority of our knowledge base is derived from animal models, it is important to consider what the limitations for extrapolation to humans are and what may be applicable to humans. Experimental studies, particularly in rodents, are highly controlled, have larger sample sizes, and can be used to optimize treatments and elucidate mechanisms. Studies with non-human primates, which are evolutionarily closer to humans, have greater variability and uncertainties in addition to having limited sample sizes. Because of differences between species, one must be careful not to extrapolate all data directly. However, we can compare the general effects of treatments across species in order to elucidate basic concepts and their applicability to the question of whether hormonal suppression could protect spermatogenesis and/or stimulate its recovery from cytotoxic exposures.

It is most useful to compare the response amongst species to an agent such a radiation, in which the dose is delivered directly to the target and pharmacological differences can be ignored (Table 24.2). Although the short-term response of the testis to cytotoxic injury is similar amongst species, there are inter-species differences in the long-term recovery of spermatogenesis, due to differences either in stem cell survival or in the ability of the testis to support recovery from surviving stem cells. The recovery of spermatogenesis is greatest in mice, in which stem cell survival is relatively high and nearly all surviving stem cells undergo differentiation. Although stem cell survival in rats also appears to be high, a block in spermatogonial differentiation is induced and is the principal cause of prolonged oligospermia or azoospermia.

In contrast, in both human and non-human primates, the sensitivity of spermatogenesis to long-term injury seems to be largely a result of the greater sensitivity to stem cell killing. In humans, there also appears to be some block in spermatogonial differentiation, though it is not as common as in rats. In most cases, seminiferous tubules in men assessed after chemotherapy or radiotherapy contain only Sertoli cells without spermatogonia [52]; only occasionally are isolated spermatogonia observed after treatment [53] (Fig. 24.4). However, the spontaneous recovery of spermatogenesis observed in men more than a year

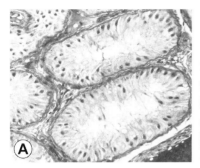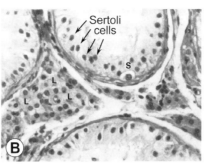

Figure 24.4. Spermatogenesis in human testes after chemotherapy. (A) Biopsy from a patient taken three years after receiving MOPP (mechlorethamine, vincristine, procarbazine, prednisone) for Hodgkin's lymphoma. Tubules are lined only with Sertoli cells; no germ cells are observed. (Reprinted with permission from Van Thiel *et al., J Clin Invest* 1972; 51: 1009–19 [52].) (B) Biopsy from a patient treated with four cycles of a cisplatin-based regimen for testicular cancer. Spermatogonia (one shown, labeled S), but no differentiated germ cells are observed in the tubules amongst the Sertoli cells. L, Leydig cells (Reprinted with permission from Kreuser *et al., Klin Wochenschr* 1989; 67: 367–78 [53].)

after radiation or chemotherapy also implies that there is a block in the differentiation of germ cells derived from the spermatogonia that survive the toxic exposure [5]. This suggests that after some cytotoxic therapy, there is a potentially reversible block to germ cell differentiation in humans. Since the reversal of this block in spermatogonial differentiation appears to be the mechanism by which hormonal suppression protects or restores spermatogenesis in toxicant-exposed rats [22], this indicates that hormonal treatment might do the same in humans, under specific conditions.

There are also inter-species differences in the degree to which HPG suppression reduces the levels of intratesticular testosterone [28,54,55] and the stage at which spermatogenic differentiation is inhibited. In particular, even after hormone suppression, spermatogenesis progresses to the round spermatid stage in rats but to only the B spermatogonial stage in primates [20,55]. It is possible that the re-stimulation of spermatogonial differentiation by hormonal suppression in rats is dependent upon the ability of germ cells to continue to develop through to the spermatocyte stage during testosterone suppression. Further germ cell differentiation in the presence of suppressed testosterone can be induced in human testes by treatment with FSH [56], and this treatment might improve the ability of HPG suppression, specifically of LH/testosterone, to protect or stimulate human spermatogenesis.

Spermatogonial transplantation

For those extremely toxic chemotherapeutic regimens that completely destroy spermatogonial stem cells, hormonal suppression alone will not offer improved

recovery of spermatogenesis. However, spermatogonial transplantation is a potential method for restoring spermatogenesis and rescuing fertility when all stem cells are killed [57]. Spermatogonial transplantation has been shown to restore spermatogenesis and in many cases fertility after sterilizing doses of chemotherapy or radiotherapy in mice, rats, and in five different farm and domestic animal species [58]. Despite these achievements, there are not yet any published reports of success in primates. Since the success of spermatogonial transplantation depends upon the ability of a depleted testis to support the differentiation of introduced spermatogonia, it is likely that the protection or restoration of the somatic environment by hormonal suppression will promote the ability of transplanted stem cells to develop in the testis treated with a cytotoxic agent. Indeed, there is a significant increase in colonization of transplanted stem spermatogonia and restoration of fertility if mice are subjected to HPG suppression after radiation and during the time of transplantation [33]. In rats, HPG suppression even more markedly enhances the differentiation of the transplanted stem cells and recovery of fertility, particularly when adults are used as recipients [8]. Thus, the use of hormonal suppression on the recipient combined with spermatogonial transplantation can potentially be applied to fertility preservation in humans.

Conclusion

In male rats, HPG suppression reliably stimulates recovery of spermatogenesis from surviving stem cells after cytotoxic therapy by reversing the block in spermatogonial differentiation induced by the cytotoxic therapy itself. There is strong evidence to support this mechanism in rats and some supporting data in the mouse, but it is not as robust as in the rat. In human males, clinical data to support the use of HPG suppression to prevent loss and enhance recovery after gonadotoxic therapy are very limited; the method may only be applicable to particular cytotoxic regimens. Current investigations have focused on a novel approach using stem cell transplantation combined with HPG suppression to recover testicular function after aggressive chemotherapy or radiation regimens, and we eagerly await further results of these studies.

Although two published studies using HPG suppression in monkeys [37,38] failed to show stimulation of spermatogenic recovery, our recent study (G. Shetty, unpublished data) indicates that HPG suppression, with a lower dose of GnRH-antagonist appears to accelerate recovery of spermatogenesis from endogenous surviving stem cells and even more significantly enhances recovery from transplanted spermatogonial stem cells in cynomolgus macaques.

We have become aware that the group who reported protection of spermatogenesis with HPG-suppressive testosterone therapy in glomerulonephritis patients treated with cyclophosphamide [46], published another paper, (A. Cigni, *et al.*, *Am J Kidney Dis* 1977; 52: 887–96) in which they reported (without concurrent controls) that nine out of ten additional patients treated with a similar dose of cyclophosphamide and testosterone as used in the initial study also recovered normal sperm counts within 1 year.

These two results taken together provide additional encouragement that appropriate HPG suppression might enhance recovery of spermatogenesis in primates after certain cytotoxic regimens.

References

1. Meistrich ML, Zhang Z, Porter KL, *et al.* Prevention of adverse effects of cancer treatment on the germline. In Anderson D, Brinkworth MH, eds. *Male-Mediated Developmental Toxicity*. Cambridge: Royal Society of Chemistry, 2007; pp. 114–23.

2. da Cunha MF, Meistrich ML, Haq MM, *et al.* Temporary effects of AMSA [4'(9-acridinylamino) methanesulfon-m-anisidide] chemotherapy on spermatogenesis. *Cancer* 1982; 49: 2459–62.

3. Meistrich ML, Finch M, da Cunha MF, *et al.* Damaging effects of fourteen chemotherapeutic drugs on mouse testis cells. *Cancer Res* 1982; 42: 122–31.

4. Meistrich ML, Vassilopoulou-Sellin R, Lipshultz LI. Gonadal dysfunction. In DeVita VT, Hellman S, Rosenberg SA, eds. *Cancer: Principles and Practice of Oncology*, 7th edn. Philadelphia, PA: Lippincott Williams & Wilkins, 2005; pp. 2560–74.

5. Meistrich ML, Chawla SP, da Cunha MF, *et al.* Recovery of sperm production after chemotherapy for osteosarcoma. *Cancer* 1989; 63: 2115–23.

6. Kangasniemi M, Dodge K, Pemberton AE, *et al.* Suppression of mouse spermatogenesis by a gonadotropin-releasing hormone antagonist and antiandrogen: failure to protect against radiation-induced gonadal damage. *Endocrinology* 1996; 137: 949–55.

7. Kangasniemi M, Huhtaniemi I, Meistrich ML. Failure of spermatogenesis to recover despite the presence of A spermatogonia in the irradiated LBNF1 rat. *Biol Reprod* 1996; 54: 1200–8.

8. Zhang Z, Shao S, Meistrich M. The radiation-induced block in spermatogonial differentiation is due to damage to the somatic environment, not the germ cells. *J Cell Physiol* 2007; 211: 149–58.

9. Glode LM, Robinson J, Gould SF. Protection from cyclophosphamide-induced testicular damage with an analogue of gonadotropin-releasing hormone. *Lancet* 1981; 1: 1132–4.

10. da Cunha MF, Meistrich ML, Nader S. Absence of testicular protection by a gonadotropin releasing hormone analog against cyclophosphamide-induced testicular cytotoxicity in the mouse. *Cancer Res* 1987; 47: 1093–7.

11. Cattanach BM, Iddon CA, Charlton HM, *et al.* Gonadotrophin-releasing hormone deficiency in a mutant mouse with hypogonadism. *Nature* 1977; 269: 338–40.

12. Delic JI, Bush C, Peckham MJ. Protection from procarbazine-induced damage of spermatogenesis in the rat by androgen. *Cancer Res* 1986; 46: 1909–14.

13. Parchuri N, Wilson G, Meistrich ML. Protection by gonadal steroid hormones against procarbazine-induced damage to spermatogenic function in LBNF1 hybrid rats. *J Androl* 1993; 14: 257–66.

14. Meistrich ML, Wilson G, Zhang Y, *et al.* Protection from procarbazine-induced testicular damage by hormonal pretreatment does not involve arrest of spermatogonial proliferation. *Cancer Res* 1997; 57: 1091–7.

15. Pogach LM, Lee Y, Gould S, *et al.* Partial prevention of procarbazine induced germinal cell aplasia in rats by sequential GnRH antagonist and testosterone administration. *Cancer Res* 1988; 48: 4354–60.

16. Meistrich ML, Kangasniemi M. Hormone treatment after irradiation stimulates recovery of rat spermatogenesis from surviving spermatogonia. *J Androl* 1997; 18: 80–7.

17. Morris ID. Protection against cytotoxic-induced testis damage – Experimental approaches. *Eur Urol* 1993; 23: 143–7.

18. Manabe F, Takeshima H, Akaza H. Protecting spermatogenesis from damage induced by doxorubicin using the luteinizing hormone-releasing hormone agonist leuprorelin: an image analysis study of a rat experimental model. *Cancer* 1997; 79: 1014–21.

19. Meistrich ML, Shetty G. Inhibition of spermatogonial differentiation by testosterone. *J Androl* 2003; 24: 135–48.

20. Kangasniemi M, Wilson G, Parchuri N, *et al.* Rapid protection of rat spermatogenic stem cells against procarbazine by treatment with a gonadotropin-releasing hormone antagonist (Nal-Glu) and an antiandrogen (flutamide). *Endocrinology* 1995; 136: 2881–8.

21. Meistrich ML, Wilson G, Ye W-S, *et al.* Hormonal protection from procarbazine-induced testicular damage is selective for survival and recovery of stem spermatogonia. *Cancer Res* 1994; 54: 1027–34.

22. Meistrich ML, Wilson G, Kangasniemi M, *et al.* Mechanism of protection of rat spermatogenesis by hormonal pretreatment: stimulation of spermatogonial differentiation after irradiation. *J Androl* 2000; 21: 464–9.

23. Meistrich ML. Restoration of spermatogenesis by hormone treatment after cytotoxic therapy. *Acta Paediatr Scand* 1999; 88: 19–22.

24. Udagawa K, Ogawa T, Watanabe T, *et al.* GnRH analog, leuprorelin acetate, promotes regeneration of rat spermatogenesis after severe chemical damage. *Int J Urol* 2001; 8: 615–22.

25. Meistrich ML, Wilson G, Shuttlesworth G, *et al.* GnRH agonists and antagonists stimulate recovery of fertility in irradiated LBNF1 rats. *J Androl* 2001; 22: 809–17.

26. Shetty G, Weng CC, Meachem SJ, *et al.* Both testosterone and FSH independently inhibit spermatogonial differentiation in irradiated rats. *Endocrinology* 2006; 147: 472–82.

27. Porter KL, Shetty G, Meistrich ML. Testicular edema is associated with spermatogonial arrest in irradiated rats. *Endocrinology* 2006; 147: 1297–305.

28. Shetty G, Wilson G, Huhtaniemi I, *et al.* Gonadotropin-releasing hormone analogs stimulate and testosterone inhibits the recovery of spermatogenesis in irradiated rats. *Endocrinology* 2000; 141: 1735–45.

29. Porter KL, Shetty G, Shuttlesworth G, *et al.* Estrogen enhances recovery from radiation-induced spermatogonial arrest in rat testes. *J Androl* 2009; 30: 440–51.

30. Shetty G, Weng CCY, Bolden-Tiller OU, *et al.* Effects of medroxyprogesterone and estradiol on the recovery of spermatogenesis in irradiated rats. *Endocrinology* 2004; 145: 4461–9.

31. Nonomura M, Okada K, Hida S, *et al.* Does a gonadotropin-releasing hormone analogue prevent cisplatin-induced spermatogenic impairment? An experimental study in the mouse. *Urol Res* 1991; 19: 135–40.

32. Crawford BA, Spaliviero JA, Simpson JM, *et al.* Testing the gonadal regression-cytoprotection hypothesis. *Cancer Res* 1998; 58: 5105–9.

33. Wang G, Shao SH, Weng CC, *et al.* Hormonal suppression restores fertility in irradiated mice from both endogenous and donor-derived stem spermatogonia. *Toxicol Sci* 2010; 117: 225–37.

34. Nseyo UO, Huben RP, Klioze SS, *et al.* Protection of germinal epithelium with luteinizing hormone-releasing hormone analogue. *J Urol* 1985; 134: 187–90.

35. Goodpasture JC, Bergstrom K, Vickery BH. Potentiation of the gonadotoxicity of Cytoxan in the dog by adjuvant treatment with luteinizing hormone-releasing hormone agonist. *Cancer Res* 1988; 48: 2174–8.

36. Lewis RW, Dowling KJ, Schally AV. D-tryptophan-6 analog of luteinizing hormone-releasing hormone as a protective agent against testicular damage caused by cyclophosphamide in baboons. *Proc Natl Acad Sci U S A* 1985; 82: 2975–9.

37. Kamischke A, Kuhlmann M, Weinbauer GF, *et al.* Gonadal protection from radiation by GnRH antagonist or recombinant human FSH: a controlled trial in a male nonhuman primate (*Macaca fascicularis*). *J Endocrinol* 2003; 179: 183–94.

38. Boekelheide K, Schoenfeld H, Hall SJ, *et al.* Gonadotropin-releasing hormone antagonist (cetrorelix) therapy fails to protect non-human primates (*Macaca arctoides*) from radiation-induced spermatogenic failure. *J Androl* 2005; 26: 222–34.

39. Johnson DH, Linde R, Hainsworth JD, *et al.* Effect of a luteinizing hormone releasing hormone agonist given during combination chemotherapy on posttherapy

fertility in male patients with lymphoma: preliminary observations. *Blood* 1985; 65: 832–6.

40. Waxman J, Lowe D, Whitfield HN, *et al.* The effects of a gonadotropin-releasing hormone agonist on testicular histology. *Fertil Steril* 1987; 48: 1067–9.

41. Waxman JH, Ahmed R, Smith D, *et al.* Failure to preserve fertility in patients with Hodgkin's disease. *Cancer Chemother Pharmacol* 1987; 19: 159–62.

42. Redman JR, Bajorunas DR. Suppression of germ cell proliferation to prevent gonadal toxicity associated with cancer treatment. In *Workshop on Psychosexual and Reproductive Issues Affecting Patients with Cancer.* New York, NY: American Cancer Society, 1987; pp. 90–4.

43. Fossa SD, Klepp O, Norman N. Lack of gonadal protection by medroxyprogesterone acetate-induced transient medical castration during chemotherapy for testicular cancer. *Br J Urol* 1988; 62: 449–53.

44. Kreuser ED, Hetzel WD, Hautmann R, *et al.* Reproductive toxicity with and without LHRHA administration during adjuvant chemotherapy in patients with germ cell tumors. *Horm Metab Res* 1990; 22: 494–8.

45. Brennemann W, Brensing KA, Leipner N, *et al.* Attempted protection of spermatogenesis from irradiation in patients with seminoma by D-tryptophan-6 luteinizing hormone releasing hormone. *Clin Investig* 1994; 72: 838–42.

46. Masala A, Faedda R, Alagna S, *et al.* Use of testosterone to prevent cyclophosphamide-induced azoospermia. *Ann Intern Med* 1997; 126: 292–5.

47. Thomson AB, Anderson RA, Irvine DS, *et al.* Investigation of suppression of the hypothalamic-pituitary-gonadal axis to restore spermatogenesis in azoospermic men treated for childhood cancer. *Hum Reprod* 2002; 17: 1715–23.

48. Jarow JP, Chen H, Rosner TW, *et al.* Assessment of the androgen environment within the human testis: minimally invasive method to obtain intratesticular fluid. *J Androl* 2001; 22: 640–5.

49. Kreuser E-D, Hetzel WD, Hautmann R, *et al.* Combination therapy with flutamide and medical (LHRH agonist) or surgical castration in advanced prostate cancer: 7-year clinical experience. *J Steroid Biochem Mol Biol* 1990; 37: 943–50.

50. Lu CC, Meistrich ML. Cytotoxic effects of chemotherapeutic drugs on mouse testis cells. *Cancer Res* 1979; 39: 3575–82.

51. Meistrich ML, Parchuri N, Wilson G, *et al.* Hormonal protection from cyclophosphamide-induced inactivation of rat stem spermatogonia. *J Androl* 1995; 16: 334–41.

52. Van Thiel DH, Sherins RJ, Myers GH, *et al.* Evidence for a specific seminiferous tubular factor affecting follicle-stimulating hormone secretion in man. *J Clin Invest* 1972; 51: 1009–19.

53. Kreuser ED, Kurrle E, Hetzel WD, *et al.* Reversible germ cell toxicity after aggressive chemotherapy in patients with testicular cancer: results of a prospective study. *Klin Wochenschr* 1989; 67: 367–78.

54. Matthiesson KL, Stanton PG, O'Donnell L, *et al.* Effects of testosterone and levonorgestrel combined with a 5alpha-reductase inhibitor or gonadotropin-releasing hormone antagonist on spermatogenesis and intratesticular steroid levels in normal men. *J Clin Endocrinol Metab* 2005; 90: 5647–55.

55. Zhengwei Y, Wreford NG, Schlatt S, *et al.* Acute and specific impairment of spermatogonial development by GnRH antagonist-induced gonadotrophin withdrawal in the adult macaque (*Macaca fascicularis*). *J Reprod Fert* 1998; 112: 139–47.

56. Matthiesson KL, McLachlan RI, O'Donnell L, *et al.* The relative roles of follicle-stimulating hormone and luteinizing hormone in maintaining spermatogonial maturation and spermiation in normal men. *J Clin Endocrinol Metab* 2006; 91: 3962–9.

57. Orwig KE, Schlatt S. Cryopreservation and transplantation of spermatogonia and testicular tissue for preservation of male fertility. *J Natl Cancer Inst Monogr* 2005; 34: 51–6.

58. Honaramooz A, Yang Y. Recent advances in application of male germ cell transplantation in farm animals. *Vet Med Int* 2010; 2011. pii: 657860. www.hindawi.com/journals/vmi/2011/657860 (accessed January 2012).

Chapter 25

Semen cryobiology and sperm banking

Helen R. Levey and Bruce R. Gilbert

Introduction

Semen cryopreservation, also known as sperm bank-ing, is a widely used, safe, effective, and reliable modal-ity for preserving male fertility that has been around for over 50 years. Cryopreservation is the technology whereby cells, whole tissues, or embryos are preserved by cooling to temperatures below the freezing point of water [1]. Cells can endure storage for prolonged periods of time when stored at temperatures below the glass transition point of water (approximately $-132\,^{\circ}$C) [1,2]. The longest period of cryopreservation that has resulted in a live birth is 21 years [3]. However, theoret-ically, sperm should retain fertilizing capability after an indefinite period of cryopreservation. Currently, there are two major techniques for sperm cryopreservation: freeze–thaw processes and vitrification. The develop-ment of cryoprotective agents, semen extenders, and different culture media has dramatically improved the preservation of cells. Additionally, advances in the field of reproductive medicine and assisted reproductive technology (ART) have revolutionized the field, giving hope to men who once had little chance of future fertil-ity [4,5]. Paralleling these developments in ART have been complementary developments in cryobiology which have expanded our indications for sperm bank-ing and optimized gamete survival through extended periods of cryopreservation.

In this chapter we discuss sperm cryobiology and cryopreservation. Starting with the history of cryo-preservation, we continue with the science of cryobi-ology methodologies used and the current indications for sperm cryopreservation, while emphasizing the importance of these methodologies in the male patient with cancer.

History of cryobiology and cryopreservation

The term cryobiology comes from the Greek words *cryos* (cold), *bios* (life), and *logos* (science). Cryobio-logy itself can be traced back to antiquity. As early as 2500 BC, low temperatures were used in Egypt in medicine, and the use of cold was recommended by Hippocrates to stop bleeding and swelling [6,7]. In fact, many living organisms today are able to tolerate prolonged periods at temperatures below the freezing point of water.

The initial interest in storing and cryopreserv-ing sperm dates back to 1776, when Lazzaro Spal-lanzani, an Italian priest and physiologist, first noted that sperm became motionless when cooled by snow [4,8,9]. It is believed that in 1780 he performed the first successful artificial insemination (AI), by impregnat-ing a female dog with semen from a syringe [10]. By the early 1800s the majority of research in the field was being conducted in Europe and Russia, with a focus on veterinary applications [10].

In 1939 the United States formed the American Society of Animal Production, to develop protocols for semen collection from domestic animals in hopes of advancing the dairy and cattle industry [10,11]. Research programs across the country began evaluat-ing sperm biology and fundamental cryobiology [7,8]. By the late 1930s and early 1940s, sperm had been noted to survive freezing to temperatures below $-160\,^{\circ}$C, and shortly thereafter, in 1949, bull sperm was cryopreserved for the first time by Christopher Polge [4,10,12].

However, the preservation of sperm function and survival after freezing was a major problem.

Fertility Preservation in Male Cancer Patients, ed. John P. Mulhall, Linda D. Applegarth, Robert D. Oates and Peter N. Schlegel.
Published by Cambridge University Press. © Cambridge University Press 2013.

Conception rates from thawed sperm averaged 65% in cows [4]. Survival was limited in the absence of a protective agent to prevent cellular damage that occurred during the freeze–thaw process. This cryodamage contributed to a loss of viability in over 50% of cells that underwent cryopreservation. It was not until the 1950s that Polge *et al.* fortuitously discovered the use of glycerol, a cryoprotective agent (CPA) that could protect sperm from damage during the freezing process. This discovery made cryopreservation a viable modality for preservation of cells [10,12]. The fields of animal and veterinary medicine accelerated, and the use of AI for dairy and beef cattle skyrocketed [11,13,14]. It was not long until the first human pregnancy from frozen sperm became a reality in 1953 [4,8]. However, due to moral and legal controversies surrounding AI, it was not until the Eleventh International Congress of Genetics in 1963 that it was reported and a true interest in sperm banking began [4]. Immediately researchers sought to find the best preservation methods possible, and subsequently in 1963 a technique for freezing human semen in liquid nitrogen was discovered, successfully storing sperm at –196 °C. Reports soon followed documenting successful live births from this technique [4].

During the last 30 years advances in sperm cryobanking have continued to occur with the development of CPAs, semen extenders, and different culture media to reduce cryodamage and improve sperm viability following cryopreservation [4,13,14]. Despite these efforts, a considerable loss of viability still occurs with sperm undergoing preservation, and major advances to date have occurred in technique rather than in an improved understanding of cryophysiology [4,13,14]. In order to understand the challenges of sperm cryobiology and the limits of our current preservation methods, it is essential to understand the biological properties and cryophysiology that determine survival and control cryopreservation.

The scientific foundation of cryobiology

Cryobiology as a science is primarily concerned with low-temperature preservation, typically in the range –80 to –196 °C. Generally, for every 10-degree reduction in temperature, there is an accompanying decrease in oxygen consumption by 50% [15]. Maintaining cells at such extreme low temperatures effectively stops all reactions from occurring,

including biochemical reactions that may lead to cell death. The process of cooling cells to reach the low temperatures required to inhibit cellular processes creates cell damage that can hinder cell viability post thaw, or result in cell death. Cryopreservation of cells is guided by the "two-factor hypothesis" of American cryobiologist Peter Mazur, which states that excessively rapid cooling kills cells by intracellular ice formation, and excessively slow cooling kills cells by intracellular solute concentration and the resultant osmotic imbalance [16].

The major objective of cryopreservation protocols and cryopreservation media is thus to ensure the viability and functionality of cells over prolonged periods of cryostorage at liquid nitrogen temperatures (–196 °C). At this temperature neither diffusion nor chemical reactions occur. To ensure cell survival during cryopreservation, damage to the cells during freezing and thawing needs to be mitigated. To expand upon Mazur's two-factor hypothesis, cryodamage results from two complementary events: (1) intracellular ice formation, which is most pronounced with rapid cooling rates once extracellular ice formation has begun, and (2) osmotic stress, which is active at slower cooling rates. During cooling, ice formation results in concentration of the extracellular solutes. This, in turn, causes water to be drawn osmotically out of cells, effectively dehydrating them [4,13,15]. If this process occurs too rapidly, intracellular ice will form, damaging the cell. At lower cooling rates the cell is exposed to high concentrations of solutes for an extended period of time, also resulting in cell damage. During thawing, the osmotic shifts are reversed and cryodamage is now dependent upon the rate of warming.

Therefore, cryopreservation media (CPM) and cryoprotectants (CPA) in particular, together with freezing and thawing protocols, have been developed to ensure optimal preservation and functionality of sperm after prolonged periods of cryostorage. The addition of CPA prior to cooling serves to remove some of the intracellular water, limiting the cellular expansion that occurs as cells freeze. Specific cells even have optimum cooling rates. Cell survival, and consequently the success rate of cryopreservation, is dependent on CPA, sperm extenders, the protective medium in which the cells are frozen, and varying rates of freezing and thawing [4,17,18]. In addition, multiple factors such as plasma membrane damage from free radicals, osmotic changes, and intracellular and extracellular ice formation play a role in sperm integrity during the cryopreservation process [19].

When these variables are not optimized, sperm viability is lost and cell damage occurs. Despite many advances in the cryopreservation methodology, the most common detrimental effect of cryopreservation on human spermatozoa is a decrease in sperm motility [4].

Methodology of cryopreservation

We will now focus on the protective agents used to optimize cell viability and will review the methods of cryopreservation with their relative advantages and disadvantages. The process of cryopreservation begins with the collection of sperm.

Sperm and male gamete collection

Semen samples are typically collected by masturbation into a sterile polypropylene container after a 2–4 day period of abstinence [2,4]. Some studies suggest that abstaining for a period of 24–48 hours is sufficient and results in comparable sperm quality. Specifically, for patients with malignancy or disease, shortening the abstinence period may encourage sperm cryopreservation and minimize the delay in receiving medical therapy [20–22].

In a study by Levitas et al., semen quality was evaluated in a total of 9489 samples grouped into oligospermic and normospermic [22]. In each group mean values of semen volume, sperm concentration, percentage of motile sperm and sperm of normal morphology (according to WHO or Kruger criteria), total sperm count, and total motile sperm count per ejaculate were correlated to different durations of abstinence. In the 3506 oligospermic samples they evaluated, peak mean sperm motility was observed after one day of abstinence and declined with each subsequent day. This was not true for the normospermic samples, which reached their peak motility values after 0–2 days of abstinence. These results challenge the role of abstinence in male infertility treatments and suggest that abstinence recommendations for subfertile men should be different than those for normospermic males [22]. However, current World Health Organization guidelines still recommend abstaining for 2–7 days, based on a series of studies showing improved semen volume and concentration parameters in normal fertile men [20,21,23].

In certain situations, sperm retrieval through the ejaculate is not possible and sperm aspiration/extraction is necessary. The most common predisposing conditions resulting in decreased numbers or absence of viable sperm in the semen are male infertility factors such as ductal obstruction, a blockage in the male reproductive tract (post-vasectomy, congenital absence of the vas deferens); sperm production abnormalities; or necrospermia, immotile, or dead sperm in the ejaculate [4,24].

There are four common procedures for sperm aspiration, which include the percutaneous techniques of epididymal sperm aspiration (PESA) and testicular sperm aspiration (TESA) or open techniques of testicular biopsy, microsurgical epididymal sperm aspiration (MESA), and/or microsurgical testicular sperm extraction (TESE) [4,12,24]. Each has its own unique advantages and disadvantages. Sperm collected from aspiration techniques require intracytoplasmic sperm injection (ICSI), often referred to as single sperm injection, due to low number and/or poor motility of sperm retrieved with these techniques [4,24,25]. However, with ICSI, only one live sperm is needed to fertilize each egg, so no matter how impaired the quality or quantity of ejaculated semen, sperm can usually be retrieved through one of the aspiration methods above and cryopreserved for future use in in-vitro fertilization (IVF) using ICSI [4,12,24,26]. As a result, ICSI has been heralded as the single most important discovery in the field of reproductive medicine, allowing men who make non-motile or very few sperm the ability to fertilize their partner's oocytes and father children of their own [4,12,24]. This single advancement in ART has redefined the definition of sterility.

The success rates of different aspiration techniques with IVF-ICSI have been very encouraging. Studies have demonstrated identical pregnancy rates with IVF-ICSI using freshly aspirated sperm as compared to frozen epididymal sperm [4,26,28]. Similarly, when comparing the results of ICSI cycles with fresh and cryopreserved testicular spermatozoa, no statistically significant differences in fertilization rates, embryo cleavage rates, implantation rates, or clinical pregnancy rates were found [26,28]. Furthermore, studies comparing the use of cryopreserved sperm in patients with obstructive versus non-obstructive azoospermia reported no difference in the outcomes of any IVF-ICSI procedures [12,26,28].

An alternative form of semen collection is electroejaculation. This is used most commonly in men suffering from anejaculation as a result of neurologic disease or traumatic injury, or as a complication of surgery. A specially designed electric probe is inserted into the rectum and a current is applied to stimulate the nerves and produce contraction of the pelvic muscles resulting in an ejaculation [24,25]. The semen specimen is collected and used for intrauterine insemination (IUI) or IVF depending on the sperm quality. When motile sperm are found in the thawed ejaculate, additional electroejaculation can be avoided. In patients who have intact abdominal and perirectal sensation, electroejaculation must be performed under general anesthesia [24,25]. In a study of 25 men suffering from psychogenic anejaculation, fertilization and pregnancy rates with cryopreserved sperm from electroejaculation were found to be equivalent to those of freshly obtained sperm [12]. Success with IUI using fresh sperm has not been encouraging, due primarily to poor sperm motility. Many of these men have required IVF with single sperm injection (ICSI). In addition, when poor sperm number, poor motility, and/or pyospermia are present, sperm can be retrieved successfully from a testicular biopsy [25]. Electroejaculation will be discussed in more detail in later chapters.

Advances in ART have made it possible to collect sperm from almost anyone, using different aspiration procedures or locations from which to draw sperm. Once sperm is collected, the next challenge lies in protecting it through the freeze–thaw process.

Cryoprotective agents (CPA)

When cells are brought to temperatures of between –5 and –15 °C, ice crystals begin to form in the extracellular medium, concentrating the solutes. This creates an osmotic gradient that shifts water from the cytoplasm to the extracellular medium, resulting in cell shrinkage and dehydration [29]. This leaves cells vulnerable to cell death or damage from both the intracellular ice formation and the accumulation of salts inside the cells as they dehydrate [29]. To protect cells from this damage during the freezing and thawing processes, most cryopreservation protocols rely on the use of CPAs. These agents penetrate the cell membrane, stabilizing the intracellular proteins, reducing the temperature at which cells undergo intracellular ice damage, and regulating the concentration of intra- and extracellular electrolytes [30]. CPAs effectively lower the salt concentrations and increase the fraction of

unfrozen water, thereby reducing osmotic stress [31]. The concentration of cryoprotectant used and the rate at which it is added are important in the preservation of sperm motility during the freeze–thaw process [12,32]. Gilmore et al. found that slow addition of CPA showed no significant difference in sperm motility, whereas the abrupt addition of CPA resulted in a significant impairment in sperm motility [12,32]. Additionally, they reported that as CPA concentration increased, sperm motility decreased.

Differences in the relative membrane penetration capability of CPAs are another important factor in cryodamage [33]. Gilmore et al. examined the protective effects of various CPAs on sperm cells during the freeze–thaw process. Comparing dimethylsulfoxide (DMSO), ethylene glycol (EG), and glycerol, they found that EG permeated sperm most rapidly at both higher and lower temperatures and resulted in the least amount of volume excursion during its addition and removal, thereby decreasing cell damage [32]. Sperm that were cryopreserved with EG also resulted in a higher post-thaw motility than those preserved with glycerol [32].

Historically, glycerol has been the CPA of choice, and it is used extensively in sperm banking due to its relative non-toxicity in comparison with other CPAs. However, for tissue preservation, the use of glycerol has been limited due to poor penetration [34]. Therefore, for the preservation of tissues, newer generation CPA such as DMSO, 1,2-propanediol (PROH), and EG have been used (Table 25.1) [35]. These CPAs have high water solubility with rapid penetration and as a result create less osmotic damage during cryopreservation. Their effects on cell viability, however, are still being studied, and glycerol therefore remains the primary CPA used in cellular cryopreservation [29].

While CPAs add tremendous protection to human spermatozoa during the cryopreservation process, they also create dramatic osmotic effects during their addition and removal [13,14]. When cells are exposed to high concentrations of permeating solutes (CPA), they undergo an initial dehydration at freezing, followed by rehydration and gross swelling upon removal. The degree of cell shrinkage and/or swelling propagates the potential for cell damage or death [14,36]. To combat and prevent excessive osmotic swelling, impermeable solutes, such as sugars, are often added to the dilution media [37,38].

The optimal CPA would be one that permeates the cell in the shortest amount of time while causing the

Table 25.1. Cryoprotective agents and their uses in sperm cryopreservation

Preserving tissue	Group characteristics
Dimethylsulfoxide (DMSO) Most toxic, slowest permeability of all CPAs, highest activation energy	Greater permeability Higher water solubility Less osmotic damage at higher concentrations Rapid penetration
Ethylene glycol (EG) Fastest permeability of all CPA, lowest activation energy	
Dimethylacetamide (DMA) Better at higher cooling rates	
1,2-Propanediol	

Preserving cells	Group characteristics
Glycerol Least toxic, most commonly used, requires slow rates of freezing	Low permeability Relatively non-toxic in high concentrations Poor penetration Stabilizes intracellular proteins

Table 25.2. Semen extenders: composition and function

Nutrient (glucose, sucrose)	Provides energy source for sperm
Buffer (sugars)	To balance pH and osmolarity
Cryoprotectant (glycerol, DMSO)	Stabilizes the cell during freezing and thawing
Antibiotic(s)	To control bacterial content that may be present in the raw semen

American Association of Tissue Banks (AATB); New York State Department of Health (NYSDOH); American Society for Reproductive Medicine (ASRM); Food and Drug Administration (FDA); United States Public Health Service (USPHS).

least amount of volume excursion during its addition and removal [32].

Semen extenders

Commercially available solutions have been developed to extend or preserve the fertilizing ability of cryopreserved semen. These solutions are called semen extenders. Typically semen extenders contain a nutrient, a buffer, and an antibiotic. A cryoprotectant is also added if semen is to be cryopreserved (Table 25.2). A typical nutrient used is sugar, such as glucose or sucrose, which serves as an energy source for the sperm, preventing the use of its own intracellular phospholipid. Buffers, which can also be sugars, are added to balance the pH and osmolarity of the solution. The antibiotic serves to protect against bacteria, with the combination ticarcillin and clavulanic acid the most commonly used. Some antibiotics are known to reduce sperm motility; therefore, careful discrimination should be used when deciding which antibiotic to add in the extender [39]. As discussed previously, the cryoprotectant assists in stabilizing the cell during the freezing and thawing process, essentially removing water from the cell and limiting the expansile properties of the cell upon freezing [39].

Egg yolk is a commonly used ingredient in semen extenders because it provides several functions. It has nutrient value for the sperm, acts to some extent as a buffer, and "coats" the sperm, thereby protecting the cell membrane from losses of lipoproteins and hyperosmotic salt solutions that develop during rapid cooling [14,40–42].

Media used in cryopreservation

Media used for sperm cryopreservation are variable. They usually contain an extender and a CPA [43]. However, the individual laboratory decides on what works best for them. TEST yolk buffer (TYB) contains egg yolk combined with TES and Tris buffers [14,44–46]. Tris, short for tris (hydroxymethyl)aminomethane, is an organic compound with basic properties often used as a component in buffer solutions, keeping them in the pH range of 7.0–9.0. TES buffer is composed of Tris, EDTA, and NaCl [47]. Another commonly used medium is human sperm preservation medium (HSPM), which is a HEPES-buffered Tyrode's medium with albumin and glycerol [14].

In studies, TYB has been shown to be superior to HSPM in preserving the chromatin integrity and morphology of sperm, which are directly correlated with fertility potential [14,48,49]. Therefore, TYB is commonly used in the United States for semen cryopreservation in all men [14]. However, there is concern about the possibility of egg yolk introducing microbial agents or unknown infectious disease, since it is of animal origin [50].

Cooling rates in cryopreservation

In addition to incorporating different media, CPA, and semen extenders, improvements in the cryopreservation process have been achieved through studies looking at various cooling rates and their effects on cells [51,52]. There are two basic methods commonly used in freezing sperm. The first, a *rapid freeze cycle*, is employed by placing specimens in liquid nitrogen vapor above the liquid nitrogen level. The second method, a *slow freeze cycle*, uses a programmable freezer designed to freeze cells at a defined rate [4,12]. Studies evaluating optimal rates and temperatures of cooling suggest that overall, to minimize freeze–thaw injury, the cooling rates should be fast enough to minimize cell exposure to the high intracellular solute concentration, yet slow enough to minimize intracellular ice formation [29].

A study by Rofeim *et al.* assessed sperm motility and viability following a series of repetitive freeze–thaw cycles at varying rates [19]. In this study, specimens initially underwent slow freezing, were thawed and subsequently refrozen at varying rates. The authors reported that cells could survive up to seven thaw–refreeze cycles while preserving sperm motility and viability. They concluded that a fast rate of refreezing was significantly better than a slow rate in cryopreserved semen [19].

While the rate of cooling is important in semen cryopreservation, the warming rate has an equally profound effect on cell survival. A standard thaw protocol involves thawing cells for 30 minutes at room temperature, then 10 minutes at 37 °C [19]. However, Calamera *et al.* reported that while there were no significant differences in sperm viability, acrosomal status, adenosine triphosphate (ATP) content, or DNA integrity after thawing cells at 40 °C compared with thawing at temperatures between 20 and 37 °C, they found thawing sperm at 40 °C resulted in statistically significant increases in sperm motility recovery compared with thawing at 20–37 °C [53].

Because of the diversity of protocols and techniques available for sperm cryopreservation, it is imperative that each cryobank determines the optimal rate of freezing and thawing for their preparation of specimens [4,12,54].

Protocols used for cryopreservation

Currently, there is no "gold standard" protocol in place for human sperm cryopreservation, and the techniques used are diverse and varied. Fig. 25.1 illustrates a suggested protocol for sperm cryopreservation.

Prior to processing sperm for cryopreservation, semen analyses are performed to determine the donor quality and quantity of sperm [4,55]. Semen analyses

should be performed on all patients prior to undergoing cryopreservation. Once this is completed, sperm is procured through ejaculated specimens and collected into a sterile polypropylene container, following a 2–4-day period of abstinence [2,4,20]. Collected sperm is processed within one hour and liquefied at room temperature [2,4,12,18]. To protect sperm while freezing and minimize hyperosmolar stress, a cryopreservation medium consisting of TYB with 20% egg yolk and 12% glycerol is added to the semen in a 1 : 1 ratio at room temperature and placed into a 1 mL Nunc Cryotube [2,4]. Semen is then diluted with an extender, consisting of egg yolk in citrate or a physiological salt extender with antibiotics. Specimens are vortexed and divided equally between vials for long-term storage [4]. Different techniques may use plastic straws or vials for specimen containment. For the rapid freeze cycle, aliquots are suspended in liquid nitrogen vapor (10 cm above the level of liquid nitrogen at –180 °C) for 20–30 minutes. Samples are then plunged into liquid nitrogen (–196 °C) and stored until required [2,4]. In this method, samples are suspended vertically on a cane held in liquid nitrogen vapor. Consequently, each vial is subjected to different freezing temperatures since the temperature gradient in the freezer varies. In the slow freeze cycle, programmable controlled-rate freezers are used. These freezers are constructed to accurately and uniformly maintain temperature throughout the chamber and can be used to reproducibly freeze samples [4,8,12]. A three-step programmed freeze is used. Specimens are first cooled to –10 °C at a rate of –1 °C per minute and then lowered to –90 °C at a rate of –10 °C per minute. Then samples are plunged into liquid nitrogen and stored. With this protocol, all specimens are cryopreserved using the exact same technique [2].

After sperm has been cryopreserved, one cryovial, to which a small aliquot of specimen has been added, is routinely set aside and thawed. This allows for the assessment of post-thaw sperm motility without thawing the entire sample, and indicates how well the remaining sperm are expected to survive when thawed at a later time [4]. For men with male-factor infertility, studies have suggested that the optimal time for such a post-thaw analysis is 24 hours post-freezing, to allow adequate freeze time and to assess the response of spermatazoa to cryodamage [20,56].

To do this, the cryovial is first brought to room temperature or 37 °C. It is then diluted with a suitable buffer (human tubal fluid–HEPES) and centrifuged

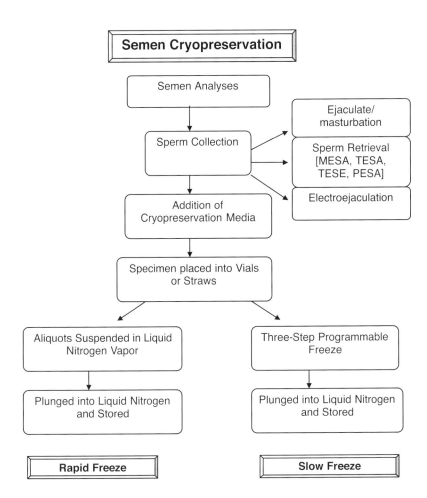

Figure 25.1. Sample protocol for sperm cryopreservation.

slowly (300 *g*) for 8–10 minutes to remove the CPA, leaving a pellet [2,4]. If the sperm are to be used for ICSI, the pellet is re-suspended in a small aliquot of medium. From here, motile or twitching sperm are isolated for the ICSI procedure. Similar procedures are used when cryopreserving testicular tissues, but tissues must be minced or macerated prior to proceeding with the above steps [57].

Vitrification

Vitrification is another method of sperm preservation that provides the benefits of cryopreservation without the damage due to ice crystal formation [1,12]. Vitrification is essentially a super or rapid freeze; it can be defined as the solidification of a solution at low temperatures by extreme elevation of viscosity [12]. At high enough cooling rates, greater than

1000 °C per minute, the extracellular solution does not crystallize. Instead, it forms an amorphous glass-like substance [10,58]. During vitrification, in contrast to the slow-rate freezing protocols presently used for routine cryopreservation, the entire solution remains unchanged and water does not precipitate. Therefore, ice does not form, and little if any cell damage occurs.

This is one of the most appealing cryopreservation protocols, both because of the speed at which freezing can occur and because of the reduction in costs, as no expensive freezer equipment is required [1,10]. Additionally, the faster freeze rates result in improved sperm viability post thaw. The downside to vitrification is that while isotonic saline, essentially the water inside cells, is vitrifiable, the cooling rates needed to achieve this are difficult to attain. In order to vitrify water inside cells, two processes must occur: either the speed of temperature conduction must increase, or the concentration of the cryoprotectant must increase [10].

For the first to occur, the surface-to-volume ratio of the cell suspension must be very high [1,10]. To adjust for this, a device called a "cryo-loop," which maximizes the surface area exposed to liquid nitrogen, and very thin straws with high surface-to-volume ratios have been used [4,10]. The second process is more difficult to address. Cells are frozen most efficiently using small volumes (0.1 mL) of highly concentrated CPA [12]. However, in order to achieve the ultra-rapid cooling rates necessary for vitrification, large volumes of highly concentrated CPA must be used. It is the high molar concentration of the CPA that depresses ice crystal formation during the vitrification process [10]. The addition and removal of CPA results in cellular shrinking and re-swelling. Many cell types have limits to which they can shrink or swell before incurring damage. Thus, one of the difficult compromises faced in vitrification is the balance between limiting the damage produced by the CPA itself and obtaining the desired result [4,56,57]. In contrast to the ice crystal formation damage seen in slow freeze cryopreservation, in vitrification it is the osmotic shock upon thawing that is the major cause of damage to spermatozoa. As a result some authors advocate CPA-free vitrification [12].

Freeze drying

Lastly, freeze drying offers an exciting new potential for the future of sperm banking. As an alternative to sperm preservation, freeze drying offers the advantage of room-temperature storage [12]. In this method, a specimen is diluted with a 0.3 M trehalose solution and then frozen as pellets on dry ice. It is stored in liquid nitrogen for 24 hours prior to freeze drying. The pellets are then transferred to borosilicate glass vials and allowed to dry for 24 hours. Argon gas is then injected and the vial is sealed. The pellets are rehydrated prior to use. With this method, neither liquid nitrogen nor dry ice is needed for the storage or shipment of the preserved spermatozoa [12].

The potential of freeze drying sperm offers several significant advantages. Protocols for cryopreservation could be simplified, and more importantly, if samples were given to the patient himself to store, storage costs would be significantly reduced, if not eliminated [4,12]. The downside to freeze drying is

that the protocols for freeze drying often damage the acrosome and mitochondria of the sperm which are necessary for normal function. As a result, a high percentage of motility is lost and the freeze-dried sperm must be used with ICSI [1,10,59]. Live animals have been derived by ICSI using freeze-dried sperm from the mouse, rat, and rabbit, but presently there has been low evidence of ICSI-derived offspring in larger animals such as pigs [60–63]. Recently, Li *et al.* sought to analyze the health and genetics of three successive generations of freeze-dried ICSI-derived mice [64]. They reported that mice derived by ICSI using freeze-dried mouse sperm were viable, fertile, healthy, and genomically stable, suggesting this as a future safe source of sperm cryopreservation.

However, the viability of the acrosome and mitochondria will need to be evaluated further before this protocol becomes a mainstay for human spermatozoa. Such analyses are necessary, because ICSI essentially bypasses all natural selection barriers to fertilization and genetic defects and/or damaged DNA in sperm may be passed on to progeny and their subsequent generations [64,65]. Further, ethical issues surrounding the use and storage of freeze-dried sperm have been questioned, as it is essentially an imperishable source of genetic material. The implications of this, as well as other issues, will need to be addressed before clinical use is implemented [12].

Semen screening

Once specimens have been cryopreserved, several measures are taken to decrease the potential risk and concerns for contamination in cryopreserved specimens. Foremost, once samples are collected, they are placed in quarantine for a minimum of six months [4,12,23]. This allows for the screening of HIV and other known sexually transmitted diseases. The American Society for Reproductive Medicine (ASRM) recommends screening for HIV, hepatitis B and C, syphilis, human T-lymphotropic virus, cytomegalovirus, chlamydia, and gonorrhea [4]. However, the ASRM is not a regulatory authority as is the Food and Drug Administration (FDA). Several states have also provided legislative requirements for reproductive tissues. These regulations specify the required screening and handling of human cells and tissues that must be complied with in order to operate a licensed tissue or sperm bank. Together these regulatory authorities ensure that sound, high-quality practices are followed to reduce the risk of tissue contamination and of communicable disease transmission to recipients [66].

In May of 2005, the FDA mandated three new regulations concerning the collection and handling of human cells, tissues, and cellular and tissue-based products (HCT/Ps). The first requires that all companies that produce and distribute HCT/Ps register with the FDA. The second is referred to as the "donor eligibility" rule, providing criteria that must be met for donors to be eligible to donate tissues and cells. The third rule, often referred to as the "current good tissue practices" rule, governs the processing and distribution of tissues and cells [66]. An abstract of these regulations, as well as guidelines from other affiliated organizations, can be found in Table 25.3.

Testing is performed on the sperm sample both at the time of collection and six months later, in addition to retesting the donor prior to specimen release for use. If the donor is the husband, quarantine procedures are not required, unless there is concern for contaminating other samples [4]. Adequate vial sealing is critical to prevent the entry and egress of microorganisms into the specimen [56]. Additionally, storing the sample in the vapor phase of liquid nitrogen is another alternative to further decrease the possibility of contamination. It is important to note, however, that this method requires close monitoring to ensure temperatures are maintained at −130 °C, the minimum for long-term sperm storage [4,12].

Tracking

Finally, in any sperm bank, a tracking system must be in place to accurately locate and track cryopreserved specimens from the initial process of collection to the completion of insemination or destruction. Every sperm bank must keep detailed records. In fact, state and federal authorities mandate the tracking of these specimens including documentation of all environmental factors (storage temperature) and reagents (freeze media) that have come into contact with the specimens [4,12,66]. Handwritten notebooks and spreadsheets are most often used, but are cumbersome and highly susceptible to damage or destruction. In addition, looking up specimens or generating required reports from tangible records is often a time-intensive process. Inventory management and report generation can more easily be accomplished through the use of electronic databases and barcode scanners to facilitate data entry and the tracking of specimens [12].

Indications for sperm cryopreservation

Over the past decade, sperm banking has become an essential component of the treatment of the subfertile couple. Sperm cryopreservation has long been a fertility preservation technique for men, but had been limited to those men whose post-thaw specimen after cryopreservation yielded sufficient motile sperm for IUI. New advances in the field of reproductive medicine and ART have greatly expanded the previous indications for sperm cryopreservation, and consequently cryopreservation has become an essential component of fertility treatment for men with oligospermia, cryptospermia, and even azoospermia [4]. ICSI has enabled a single, viable, yet immotile sperm to be used successfully for fertilization of an oocyte. Surgical retrieval of sperm from the testis, epididymis, and/or vas deferens is now standard practice for the patient with cryptospermia or azoospermia, and has become a valuable tool when semen quality declines in the face of standard treatment paradigms or due to disease.

The primary indications for cryopreservation are for donor sperm artificial insemination; preservation of reproductive capacity in men with cancer prior to undergoing treatment; patient convenience (i.e., partner's absence where IUI is performed in the presence of normal sperm parameters); and aiding in the management of infertile men [67]. Common indications for cryopreservation are discussed below (Table 25.4).

Homologous and donor insemination

Cryopreservation of human semen is a standard practice for anonymous, directed donor (known donor), and husband/partner (client depositor) storage of sperm prior to IUI or IVF procedures [4]. Furthermore, regulatory guidelines require that semen be quarantined prior to insemination. While IUI is routinely performed using fresh semen specimens, cryopreserved semen offers the additional benefit of being stored and subsequently used multiple times for artificial inseminations with husband/partner or donor semen. This provides the convenience of being able to time IUI to coincide with a female's cycles or special conditions of the female tract, while maintaining

Table 25.3. Sperm donor guidelines and regulations

Organization	Physical exam	Medical and personal history	Laboratory testing	Additional information
American Association of Tissue Banks (AATB)	Looking for any evidence of high-risk behavior, STDs, signs of HIV, hepatitis infection or any bacterial/viral infection or trauma to retrieval site	Patient is asked a series of questions using the US (USPHS) guidelines for preventing the transmission of HIV through transplantation of human tissue and organs Family history through three generations is collected	HIV-1, HIV-2, HbsAg, HbcB, HCV, HTLV-1 + 2, syphilis, chlamydia, gonorrhea 6-month quarantine of sample with retest prior to release Semen analysis obtained post-thaw	These are only guidelines to be followed in order to be licensed and accredited through the AATB Only if indicated by family, medical, or ethnic background: additional screening for cystic fibrosis, sickle cell trait, Tay–Sachs disease, or thalassemia
New York State Department of Health (NYSDOH)	Exam for signs of injected drug use, infection, or trauma at the retrieval site that may affect tissue quality	Patient is asked a series of questions using the USPHS guidelines for preventing the transmission of HIV through transplantation of human tissue and organs	HIV-1, HIV-2, HbsAg, HbcB, HCV, HTLV-1 + 2, syphilis, chlamydia gonorrhea 6-month quarantine of sample and retest prior to release Semen analysis obtained post-thaw Donor testing: CBC, ABO + Rh, lipid and metabolic panel	These are only guidelines to be followed by sperm banks in the state of NY Only if indicated by family, medical, or ethnic background: additional screening for cystic fibrosis, sickle cell trait, Tay–Sachs disease, or thalassemia
American Society for Reproductive Medicine (ASRM)	Complete exam with evaluation for urethral discharge, genital warts, and genital ulcers with annual follow-up exams	Complete personal and sexual history to exclude donors at high risk for HIV and other STDs	HIV-1, HIV-2, HbsAg, HbcB, HCV, HTLV-1 + 2, syphilis, CMV, chlamydia, gonorrhea with 6-month quarantine and retested CBC, ABO + Rh, S/A with post-thaw, lipid and metabolic panel Minimum genetic testing: karyotype and cystic fibrosis	These are only recommended guidelines to be followed Additional testing if patient is: Jewish (Tay–Sachs + Canavan); African-American (sickle cell trait); South Asian or Mediterranean (thalassemia)
Food and Drug Administration (FDA)	Establish the patient is free from risk factors for, and clinical evidence of, infection due to relevant communicable disease agents and diseases; and communicable disease risks associated with xenotransplantation	Medical records must be reviewed for risk factors for and clinical evidence of infection from relevant communicable diseases of the genitourinary tract in addition to the relevant communicable disease agents and diseases listed under laboratory testing as well as CMV	HIV-1, HIV-2, HbsAg, HbcB, HCV, HTLV-1 + 2, chlamydia, gonorrhea	The FDA does not address genetic testing or karyotyping

comparable numbers of motile sperm as would be found if performed with fresh samples [4]. Moreover, storing, pooling, and concentrating multiple oligospermic samples from one partner can dramatically increase the number of motile cells available for insemination during one setting, improving chances for impregnation. Further, in the unlikely event that the donor is unable to produce a specimen

Table 25.4. Indications for sperm cryopreservation

(1) Patients with cancer in whom the treatment (e.g., chemotherapy, radiation) or the disease itself might impair sperm production or semen quality
(2) Patients undergoing surgery on the testis, prostate, or spinal cord, or retroperitoneal procedures that may disrupt antegrade ejaculation
(3) Patients with severely impaired semen parameters, to preserve future fertility potential
(4) Patients with physical disabilities who may require retrieval of sperm and pooling of specimens and/or timing of insemination with their partner's cycle
(5) Patients involved in hazardous occupations may bank their sperm to preserve their fertility potential
(6) Patients prior to undergoing a vasectomy
(7) Cryopreservation of epididymal or vasal sperm for patients undergoing surgery to reconstruct an obstructed vas deferens or ejaculatory duct, in which specimens are cryopreserved for later use in IVF procedures
(8) Cryopreservation of testicular tissue obtained by testicular biopsy during the diagnostic evaluation of azoospermia
(9) Pooling of cryopreserved specimens for IUI in patients with low sperm counts

on the day of the procedure, sperm preservation can be done prior to IUI or IVF procedures [4].

Preoperative cryopreservation

Prior to undergoing surgical procedures, sperm may be cryopreserved. This serves as an additional protective measure or insurance against postoperative azoospermia resulting from an intraoperative complication or an unforeseen postoperative course. Sperm may also be preserved prior to undergoing surgical infertility treatments such as varicocele ligation, or before a vasectomy, providing the possibility of assisted reproduction in the future if the desire for children changes [4]. Sperm may also be aspirated from the seminal vesicles and cryopreserved during a diagnostic transrectal ultrasound, prior to a planned transurethral resection of the ejaculatory ducts (TURED) [4].

Intraoperative cryopreservation

Often, during primary procedures for refractory cases of obstructive azoospermia (OA), as seen in congenital bilateral absence of the vas deferens, sperm aspiration is performed intraoperatively and sperm is then cryopreserved, retaining the patient's ability to produce offspring [4]. Even during complex surgical reconstructive cases such as vaso-vasostomy (V-V) or vaso-epididymostomy (V-E) procedures, sperm can be collected in case the patient remains azoospermic postoperatively. In men with preserved focal spermatogenesis, despite spermatogenic failure or unreconstructable OA, cryopreservation can be performed during testicular biopsy, obviating the need for further invasive procedures [4]. This also serves to coordinate the ICSI cycle with ovarian stimulation of the female partner, in hopes of avoiding the frustration

and additional expenses that may incur should there be no sperm available on the day of egg retrieval [4,57].

Postoperative cryopreservation

After successful infertility treatments, previously azoospermic men may have their sperm cryopreserved postoperatively to provide additional insurance against a late stricture or re-obstruction forming [4].

Premortem and postmortem cryopreservation

In a donor's absence, whether temporary or permanent, cryopreservation allows for the retention of his fertilizing capability [4]. Sperm may be cryopreserved prior to entry into the military, a long departure, or anticipation of toxin exposure or danger.

The postmortem use of frozen sperm has been an option available to patients with cancer since the introduction of sperm cryopreservation. Before the advent of ICSI, success rates were minimal, but today, with the use of ICSI, pregnancy using sperm from a deceased donor has been achieved [68]. While sperm retrieval can readily be performed on deceased or incapacitated individuals, there are many legal and moral complexities that must be addressed prior to proceeding. Ethical and legal considerations of sperm cryopreservation, including postmortem cryopreservation, will be discussed in further chapters.

Cryopreservation prior to treatment (for non-malignant diseases)

There are many potential threats to spermatogenesis with disease treatment, often resulting in compromised sperm number, motility, morphology, as well as DNA integrity [12]. Many treatment regimens for systemic or non-malignant diseases involve the use of immunosuppressives or cytotoxic therapies, which can result in infertility. Therefore, sperm cryopreservation is recommended in these men prior to the initiation of treatment [4]. This includes men with diseases such as autoimmune disorders, kidney disorders, diabetes, ulcerative colitis, and transplant recipients. Although cryopreservation is often advised when the anticipated treatment regimen is suspected or known to negatively affect spermatogenesis, it should also be considered in reproductive aged men prior to any long-term medical therapy [4]. Often, these men will already have inferior sperm quality prior to the initiation of treatment, as compared to healthy donors. However, with IVF-ICSI, these men still have the potential to fertilize an oocyte [4].

Cryopreservation prior to treatment (for malignancies)

One of the most common indications for preserving sperm is malignant disease. Chemotherapy, radiotherapy, and some surgical treatments are known to cause infertility and can result in testicular failure, ejaculatory dysfunction, or non-reconstructable obstruction [4]. In addition, non-chemotherapeutic drugs, herbal as well as non-herbal supplements, can and do affect sperm quantity, quality, and fertility potential [4]. Therefore, it is paramount that cryopreservation is discussed and offered to all men who may undergo gonadotoxic treatments for cancer [69].

While collection and cryopreservation of sperm is still feasible during chemotherapy, until azoospermia ensues, the effects of chemotherapeutic agents on spermatozoa are not known [70]. Therefore, when possible, it is strongly recommended that patients complete semen cryopreservation before the initiation of chemotherapy.

While this list of indications for sperm cryopreservation is not exhaustive, it is expected that with new discoveries and advances in ART it will only grow larger in the future.

Cryopreservation in the patient with cancer

Cryopreservation is a safe and effective technique utilized by many men for fertility concerns. However, its importance and use in the patient with cancer cannot be emphasized enough. Cancer is a leading cause

of death worldwide, and the second leading cause of death in the USA, with an estimated 1 529 560 new cases diagnosed in 2010 in the United States alone [71,72]. Worldwide cancer rates are predicted to rise, resulting in 15 million new cases by the year 2020 [72]. With advances in medical technology and therapy, we are now able to cure or effectively place into remission many different cancers, with the result that over 11.4 million people were noted to be living cancer survivors in the USA in 2006 [71]. In fact, in a study by Mariotto et al., reviewing data from 1975–2005, over 328 000 of people were survivors of childhood cancers in the USA, with 24% of these people having survived more than 30 years since diagnosis [73]. Despite the many successes medicine has allowed in effectively treating cancers, many survivors are left with often devastating long-term or irreversible sequelae as a result of treatment, one of the most common being infertility [28,73,74]. Chemotherapy, radiation, and some surgeries are all known to negatively impact fertility potential.

Chemo- and radiotherapy disrupt the biochemical processes that occur during spermatogenesis, damage the gonadal tissue, and consequently destroy spermatogenesis in a proportion of young boys and men, resulting in long-lasting or permanent sterility [74,75]. Alkylating and other chemotherapeutic agents cause acute azoospermia in 90–100% of treated men [4]. Although improved chemotherapeutic treatment regimens and lower doses have resulted in increased rates of fertility recovery, the incidence of azoospermia in patients after treatment is still high, with only 20–50% of these men eventually recovering spermatogenesis [4]. Recovery may take years to occur [12,19,70]. Since it is impossible to predict which category of patients with cancer will survive or become sterile after treatment, sperm banking is strongly recommended for all patients with malignant disease who may desire children in the future, even if they eventually decide that the specimens are no longer needed [4].

In addition to the negative spermatogenic effects resulting from cancer treatments, many men with cancer have impaired semen parameters and testicular function even before undergoing treatment [76–80]. Studies report oligospermia and semen abnormalities in 28–67% of cancer patients prior to treatment [81,82]. The exact mechanisms responsible for this are not well understood and are likely multifactorial [78–82]. The most significant factors governing post-treatment semen quality and recovery of spermatogenesis were the type of cancer and the pre-treatment sperm concentration. There appears to be no correlation between semen abnormalities and disease stage or systemic symptoms [82]. The highest percentage of semen abnormalities is found in men with testicular tumors and lymphomas, affecting over half of those diagnosed [2,79,80].

Quite disturbingly, despite the importance of such a treatment to preserve fertility in this population, studies report that on average less than 57% of patients are even made aware that such an opportunity exists, including studies on adolescent cancer patients, where this option assumes an even greater importance [74,77,80]. This was also found to be occurring at tertiary cancer centers in the USA and in centers with their own in-house sperm banks [77]. Even at these centers, men were not consistently provided with information regarding the availability of sperm cryopreservation, the reduction of semen quality and risk of infertility, nor the potential risks to their future children after their cancer treatments [77]. When pre-treatment sperm cryopreservation was offered to young and middle-aged men, almost 50% were interested [79]. The failure of communication has clear consequences.

In a study surveying men diagnosed with cancer, 77% of childless survivors wanted to have children in the future, over 80% felt having had cancer would actually make them better parents, and 66% said they would want to be a parent even if they died prematurely [77,79]. In fact, offering this information and having the ability to assure a patient that his fertility potential is secured by sperm banking could help patients in their emotional battle against cancer when faced with an unpredictable or unfavorable prognosis. In a study by Trottmann et al., 80% of patients who banked their sperm reported a positive psychological effect as a result, offering encouragement to them during treatment. This was regardless of whether they eventually used the specimens or not [79].

The most common reasons cited for physicians not discussing these issues with their patients were lack of time, presumed high cost, limited availability of adequate facilities, and overestimation of the limitations of sperm quality on semen cryopreservation [77,80]. While earlier reports on sperm banking showed few patients with semen samples that were compatible for successful cryopreservation, ICSI has revolutionized the treatment of male infertility, eliminating the former minimal requirements for semen quality [79,80,83]. In the largest series to date, 118 male cancer survivors underwent 169 IVF-ICSI cycles resulting in a clinical pregnancy rate of 56.8%, comparable to the average pregnancy rates seen with male-factor patients in clinics [83]. Other studies have replicated these findings, suggesting that surgically retrieved spermatozoa can be efficiently used for ICSI after freezing and thawing without compromising outcome as compared to fresh spermatozoa [79,84]. While some studies have shown that damage to sperm cryopreserved from cancer patients is more severe than that affecting healthy donors, other studies have shown no difference between these groups [2,79,80]. We do know that pre-treatment sperm quality, the duration and type of chemotherapy used, as well as the specific type of cancer the patient has, all play a role in the quality of sperm in men postcancer treatment [4,61,79,80,85]. In addition, studies have reported an abnormally high percentage of DNA-damaged sperm in samples after chemotherapy, suggesting that sperm quality does not reach normal levels after treatment [85,86]. With the unknown impact cancer therapy ultimately has on the genetic integrity of sperm, it is strongly recommended to preserve semen prior to undergoing any gonadotoxic treatment, if possible.

Potential strategies for the preservation of male fertility are dependent upon the sexual maturity of the patient. Many young pubertal boys may already have spermatozoa in their ejaculate, which can be collected for IVF-ICSI [75]. Cells in meiosis might also be found in testicular biopsy samples. This would allow spermatogenesis to occur in vitro with possible re-implantation at a later date. However, testicular biopsy is an invasive procedure in young boys and is not without possible complications such as bleeding [38]. For prepubertal boys there are currently no options available to preserve fertility, and potential strategies are experimental [75–78].

However, for these boys, advances in assisted reproduction techniques make preserving gonadal tissue and harvesting germ cells for future use a viable option [74,75,78]. Potentially, pieces of whole testicular tissue could be cryobanked prior to gonadotoxic treatment, then the testicular tissue could be re-implanted inside the tunica albuginea of the testis with subsequent spermatogenesis occurring. Alternatively the stored testicular tissue could be used for subsequent culture and in-vitro spermatogenesis.

Testicular germ cell harvesting provides another possible future alternative, where germ cells could be removed and stored during cytotoxic therapy. Later, at the completion of cancer therapy, these germ cells could be autotransplanted or matured in vitro, serving as an alternative way to store immature gametes for infertility treatment in later life [74,75]. Germ cell transplantation has already been successfully accomplished in animals [79]. The achievement of sperm production is the main aim behind these attempts at cryopreservation before chemotherapy, and their potential future use is exciting, with hopes of circumventing the negative effects of cancer therapies in young boys.

There have been reports indicating that the sterilizing effects of cancer treatments may be circumvented by hypogonadotropism [28,29]. These studies showed that treatment with gonadotropin-releasing hormone (GnRH) agonists or antagonists in rats following chemotherapy or radiation treatment restored normal spermatogenesis [74]. However, the evidence for clinical benefit in humans has been inconclusive or non-existent [28]. Currently, sperm cryopreservation represents the only preemptive measure for conserving fertility and is strongly recommended for all patients with cancer, prior to initiation of treatment, to best preserve reproductive capacity [79].

While cryopreservation can be done following cancer treatment initiation, we do not know the full consequences these treatments may have on future progeny. Damage to sperm DNA is seen most commonly post chemotherapy or radiation therapy, and the mutagenic potential of these treatments may confer a potential risk to the fetus conceived posttreatment. Few studies have investigated the effect of these agents on offspring [4,12].

The duration, dosage, and type(s) of drugs used can determine how long it will take before a male's ejaculate and semen parameters return to near baseline (pre-chemotherapy) [12]. Despite recovery of spermatogenesis, the ability for fertilization to take place naturally may still be hindered. Studies such as the Sperm Chromatin Structure Assay (SCSA), terminal deoxynucleotidyl transferase-mediated dUTP nick-end labeling (TUNEL), and the Single Cell Gel Electrophoresis assay (COMET) have been conducted to measure DNA fragmentation and to predict the viability of natural fertilization [27,86,87]. Overall, reports were reassuring that there was no increased incidence

of either congenital abnormalities or childhood malignancies in children born to cancer survivors who received cytotoxic therapy [74]. Other studies such as the Childhood Cancer Survivor Study, a multi-institutional retrospective study started in 1993, which reviewed 4214 live births from childhood cancer survivors, confirmed these findings. They reported no significant differences between childhood cancer survivor offspring in comparison with their siblings' offspring [12]. While encouraging, these findings may be misleading, as all these births resulted from natural conceptions.

Since assisted reproductive procedures, such as ICSI and IVF, bypass the biological control system, effectively circumventing the natural selection processes, there is concern of increased transmission of defective DNA to human offspring. Animal studies looking at the effects of chemotherapeutic agents on offspring have been troubling. One study looking at adult male rats treated with short- and long-term doses of combination chemotherapeutic agents showed embryo loss occurring both pre-implantation and post-implantation [22,27]. Another study by Beiber et al., demonstrated early infant mortality in parent rats that underwent a prolonged course of the combination cancer treatment BEP (bleomycin, etoposide, cisplatin); however, pre- and post-implantation viability were not affected [88].

Further, DNA fragmentation has been found in cancer patients even prior to undergoing treatment. There is the hypothetical possibility of immature spermatogenic cells carrying abnormal genomic DNA with the potential for passing on abnormalities to offspring. We do not know the future consequences, if any, and continued surveillance of the progeny of cancer survivors is essential [75,89].

From these studies and our knowledge of the detrimental effects chemotherapy has on spermatogenesis, combined with the biological two- to three-month cycle of spermatogenesis, patients are recommended to practice reliable contraception from the time of initiation of treatment until 12–18 months after completion of treatment [12,61]. This provides the safest guideline available for patients undergoing cancer treatment.

Another question concerns the safety of collecting sperm from men who have testicular cancer or lymphoma, and the clinical consequences of potentially harboring malignant cells and then re-implanting them into the donor or recipient through fertilization. In a rat model, injection of a minimal number of leukemia cells has resulted in leukemia in the recipient [75]. Unfortunately, there have not been many studies addressing this in humans. However, as discussed earlier, once chemotherapy and/or radiation have occurred, the chance of sperm retrieval is suboptimal. Thus, it is likely best to preserve sperm prior to the onset of treatment. Hopefully, further research will give direction for use of these stored gametes.

As treatment for cancer becomes increasingly successful, with patients surviving their illness and wanting families, adverse effects on reproductive function must be considered in all patients. Chemotherapy, radiotherapy, and other treatments used in cancer treatment have well-known adverse effects on male fertility. At present we do not have an established method to stimulate impaired spermatogenesis after treatment. Therefore it is paramount that all men undergoing potential gonadotoxic therapy are counseled on the effect of their treatment on fertility and offered cryopreservation of sperm before treatment begins. Since semen cryopreservation is an efficacious method for preserving future fertility, cryopreservation should be considered as early as possible during treatment planning, even in cases where an individual's risk of infertility might seem minimal [80].

Increasing awareness and use of ART need to be promoted by an interdisciplinary team of experts caring for adolescent through adult men. While the preservation of fertility in childhood cancers remains a clinical challenge for prepubertal boys, there are many exciting developments and promising advances that are likely to be realized in coming decades.

Future advances in the technology to conserve fertility must rely on an improved understanding of the cryobiology of gametes, further optimization of freezing protocols for each cell type, a new generation of cell culture techniques, and the development of new skills in reproductive surgery [29]. It is hoped that in the coming years, developments in reproductive medicine and assisted reproductive technologies will be able to circumvent the challenges faced today, and provide all men the opportunity to preserve their fertility.

References

1. Bagchi A, Woods EJ, Critser JK. Cryopreservation and vitrification: recent advances in fertility preservation technologies. *Expert Rev Med Devices* 2008; 5: 359–70.

2. Rofeim O, Gilbert BR. Long-term effects of cryopreservation on human spermatozoa. *Fertil Steril* 2005; 84: 536–7.

3. Horne G, Atkinson AD, Pease EHE, *et al.* Live birth with sperm cryopreserved for 21 years prior to cancer treatment: case report. *Hum Reprod* 2004; 19: 1448–9.

4. Anger JT, Gilbert BR, Goldstein M. Cryopreservation of sperm: indications, methods and results. *J Urol* 2003; 170: 1079–84.

5. Ozkavukcu S, Erdemli E, Isik A, *et al.* Effects of cryopreservation on sperm parameters and ultrastructural morphology of human spermatozoa. *J Assist Reprod Genet* 2008; 25: 403–11.

6. Wang H, Olivero W, Wang D, Lanzino G. Cold as a therapeutic agent. *Acta Neurochir (Wien)* 2006; 148: 565–70.

7. Kellogg JH. The therapeutic effects of hydriatic applications. In eds. *Rational Hydrotherapy: A Manual of the Physiological and Therapeutic Effects of Hydriatic Procedures, and the Technique of Their Application in the Treatment of Disease.* Philadelphia, PA: F. A. Davis, 1901.

8. Mahony M C, Morshedi M, Scott RT, *et al.* Role of spermatozoa cryopreservation in assisted reproduction. In Acosta AA, Swanson RJ, Ackerman SB, *et al.*, eds. *Human Spermatozoa in Assisted Reproduction.* Baltimore, MD: Williams & Wilkins, 1990.

9. Triana, V.: Artificial insemination and semen banks in Italy. In David G, Price W, eds. *Human Artificial Insemination and Semen Preservation.* New York, NY: Plenum, 1980.

10. Walters E, Benson J, Woods EJ, *et al.* The history of sperm cryopreservation. In Pacey AA, Tomlinson MJ, eds. *Sperm Banking: Theory and Practice.* Cambridge: Cambridge University Press, 2009.

11. Foote RH. The history of artificial insemination: selected notes and notables. *J Anim Sci* 2002; 80: 1–10.

12. Gilbert, DL, Tash-Anger J, Gilbert BR. Sperm cryopreservation. In Goldstein M, Schlegel P, eds. *Surgical and Medical Management of Male Infertility.* Cambridge: Cambridge University Press, 2012.

13. Woods EJ, Benson JD, Agca Y, Critser JK. Fundamental cryobiology of reproductive cells and tissues. *Cryobiology* 2004; 48: 146–56.

14. Hammadeh ME, Greiner S, Rosenbaum P, Schmidt W. Comparison between human sperm preservation medium and TEST-yolk buffer on protecting

chromatin and morphology integrity of human spermatozoa in fertile and subfertile men after freeze-thaw procedure. *J Androl* 2001; 22: 1012–18.

15. Raison JK. The influence of temperature induced phase changes on the kinetics of respiration and other membrane associated enzyme systems. *J Bioenerg* 1973; 4: 285–309.

16. Mazur P. The role of intracellular freezing in the death of cells cooled at supraoptimal rates. *Cryobiology* 1977; 14: 251–72.

17. Farrant J. General principles of cell preservation. In Ashwood-Smith MJ, Farrant J, eds. *Low Temperature Preservation in Medicine and Biology*. Tunbridge Wells: Pitman Medical, 1980.

18. Holt WV. Basic aspects of frozen storage of semen. *Anim Reprod Sci* 2000; 62: 3–22.

19. Rofeim O, Brown TA, Gilbert BR. Effects of serial thaw-refreeze cycles on human sperm motility and viability. *Fertil Steril* 2001; 75: 1242–3.

20. Agarwal A, Sidhu RK, Shekarriz M, Thomas AJ. Optimum abstinence time for cryopreservation of semen in cancer patients. *J Urol* 1995; 154: 86–8.

21. Lampe EH, Masters WH. Problems of male fertility. II. Effect of frequent ejaculation. *Fertile Steril* 1956; 7: 123–7.

22. Levitas E, Lunenfeld E, Weiss N, *et al*. Relationship between the duration of sexual abstinence and semen quality: analysis of 9,489 semen samples. *Fertil Steril* 2005; 83: 1680–6.

23. World Health Organization. *WHO Laboratory Manual for the Examination and Processing of Human Semen*, 5th edn. Geneva: WHO, 2010.

24. Center for Male Reproductive Medicine (2010) Sperm aspiration. http://malereproduction.com/male-infertility/sperm-aspiration/ (accessed August 15, 2010).

25. Watkins W, Lim T, Bourne H, Baker HW, Wutthiphan B. Testicular aspiration of sperm for intracytoplasmic sperm injection: an alternative treatment to electro-emission: case report. *Spinal Cord* 1996; 34: 696–8.

26. Janzen N, Goldstein M, Schlegel P, *et al*. Use of electively cryopreserved microsurgically aspirated epididymal spermatazoa with in vitro fertilization and intracytoplasmic sperm injection for obstructive azoospermia. *Fertil Steril* 2000; 74: 696–701.

27. Stahl O, Eberhard J, Jepson K, *et al*. Sperm DNA intergrity in testicular cancer patients. *Hum Reprod* 2006; 12: 3199–205.

28. Friedler S, Raziel A, Soffer Y, *et al*. Intracytoplasmic injection of fresh and cryopreserved testicular spermatozoa in patients with nonobstructive

azoospermiaa comparative study. *Fertil Steril* 1997; 68: 892–7.

29. Picton HM, Kim SS, Gosden RG. Cryopreservation of gonadal tissue and cells. *Br Med Bull* 2000; 56: 603–15.

30. Mazur P. Kinetics of water loss from cells at subzero temperatures and the likelihood of intracellular freezing. *J Gen Physiol* 1963; 47: 347–69.

31. Donnelly ET, Steele EK, McClure N, Lewis SE. Assessment of DNA integrity and morphology of ejaculated spermatozoa from fertile and infertile men before and after cryopreservation. *Hum Reprod* 2001; 16: 1191–9.

32. Gilmore JA, Liu J, Woods EJ, Peter AT, Critser JK. Cryoprotective agent and temperature effects on human sperm membrane permeabilities: convergence of theoretical and empirical approaches for optimal cryopreservation methods. *Hum Reprod* 2000; 15: 335–43.

33. Ball BA, Vo A. Osmotic tolerance of equine spermatozoa and the effects of soluble cryoprotectants on equine sperm motility, viability, and mitochondrial membrane potential. *J Androl* 2001; 22: 1061–9.

34. Newton H, Aubard Y, Rutherford A, Sharma V, Gosden R. Low temperature storage and grafting of human ovarian tissue. *Human Reprod* 1996; 11: 1487–91.

35. Prins GS, Weidel L. A comparative study of buffer systems as cryoprotectants for human spermatozoa. *Fertil Steril* 1986; 46: 147–9.

36. Mazur P, Schneider U. Osmotic responses of preimplantation mouse and bovine embryos and their cryobiological implications. *Cell Biophys* 1986; 8: 259–85.

37. Leibo SP. A one step method for direct non-surgical transfer of frozen thawed bovine embryos. *Theriogenology* 1984; 21: 767–90.

38. Diller K, Lynch ME. An irreversible thermodynamic analysis of cell freezing in the presence of membrane permeable additives II transient electrolyte and additive concentrations. *Cryobiology* 1984; 4: 131–44.

39. Mottershead J. Frozen semen preparation and use. www.equine-reproduction.com/articles/FrozenSemen1.htm (accessed September 18, 2010).

40. Newton H, Fisher J, Arnold JRP, *et al*. Permeation of human ovarian tissue with cryoprotective agents in preparation for cryopreservation. *Hum Reprod* 1998; 13: 376–80.

41. Holt WV, Head MF, North RD. Freeze-induced membrane damage in ram spermatozoa is manifested

after thawing: observations with experimental cryomicroscopy. *Biol Reprod* 1992; 46: 1086–94.

42. Katkove II, Gordienko NA, Ostashko FI. Influence of lipid content of cytoplasmic membranes on electro- and cryosurvival of bovine spermatozoa. *Cryobiology* 1996; 33: 681–2.

43. Cellgro Mediatech. Cryopreservation. cellgro.com/media/upload/file/techinfosheets/Cryopreservation_06Jul2010REV03.pdf (accessed January 2012).

44. Prins GS, Weidel L. A comparative study of buffer system as cryoprotectants for human spermatozoa. *Fertil Steril* 1986; 46: 147–9.

45. Weidel L, Prins GS. Cryosurvival of human spermatozoa frozen in eight different buffer systems. *J Androl* 1987; 8: 41–7.

46. Kukis A. Yolk lipids. *Biochim Biophys Acta* 1992; 1124: 205–22.

47. Durst RA, Staples BR. Tris-tris-HCl: a standard buffer for use in the physiologic pH range.*Clin Chem.* 1972; 18: 206–8.

48. Evenson DP, Jost LK, Marshall D, *et al.* Utility of the sperm chromatin structure assay (CASA) as a diagnostic and prognostic tool in the human fertility clinic. *Hum Reprod* 1999; 14: 1039–49.

49. Evenson DP, Thompson L, Jost L. Flow cytometric evaluation of boar semen by the sperm chromatin structure assay as related to cryopreservation and fertility. *Theriogenology* 1994; 41: 637–51.

50. Stacey G. Validation of cell culture media components. *Hum Fertil (Camb)* 2004; 7: 113–18.

51. Gilmore JA, Liu J, Gao DY, Critser JK. Determination of optimal cryoprotectants and procedures for their addition and removal from human spermatozoa. *Hum Reprod* 1997; 12: 112–18.

52. Henry MA, Noiles EE, Gao D, Mazur P, Critser JK. Cryopreservation of human spermatozoa IV. The effects of cooling rate and warming rate on the maintenance of motility, plasma membrane integrity, and mitochondrial function. *Fertil Steril* 1993; 60: 911–18.

53. Calamera JC, Buffone MG, Doncel GF, *et al.* Effect of thawing temperature on the motility recovery of cryopreserved human spermatozoa. *Fertil Steril* 2010; 93: 789–94.

54. Ackerman DR. The effect of cooling and freezing on the aerobic and anaerobic lactic acid production of human semen. *Fertil Steril* 1968; 19: 123–8.

55. Hallak J, Hendin BN, Thomas AJ, Agarwal A. Investigation of fertilizing capacity of cryopreserved spermatozoa from patients with cancer. *J Urol* 1998; 159: 1217–20.

56. Nallella KP, Sharma RK, Said TM, *et al.* Inter-sample variability in post-thaw human spermatazoa. *Cryobiology* 2004; 49: 195–9.

57. Kupker W, Schlegel, PN, Al-Hasani S, *et al.* Use of frozen-thawed testicular sperm for intracytoplasmic sperm injection. *Fertil Steril* 2003; 73: 453–8.

58. Fahy GM, MacFarlane DR, Angell CA, Meryman HT. Vitrification as an approach to cryopreservation. *Cryobiology* 1984; 21: 407–26.

59. Kwon IK, Park KE, Niwa K. Activation, pronuclear formation, and development in vitro of pig oocytes following intracytoplasmic injection of freeze-dried spermatozoa. *Biol Reprod* 2004; 71: 1430–6.

60. Kaneko, T, Whittingham, DG, Overstreet, *et al.* Tolerance of the mouse sperm nuclei to freeze-drying depends on their disulfide status. *Biol Reprod* 2003; 69: 1859–62.

61. Hirabayashi M, Kato M, Ito J, *et al.* Viable rat offspring derived from oocytes intracytoplasmically injected with freeze-dried sperm heads. *Zygote* 2005; 13: 79–85.

62. Hochi S, Watanabe K, Kato M, Hirabayashi M. Live rats resulting from injection of oocytes with spermatozoa freeze-dried and stored for one year. *Mol Reprod Dev* 2008; 75: 890–4.

63. Liu JL, Kusakabe H, Chang CC, *et al.* Freeze-dried sperm fertilization leads to full-term development in rabbits. *Biol Reprod* 2004; 70: 1776–81.

64. Li M, Willis BJ, Griffey SM, *et al.* Assessment of three generations of mice derived by ICSI using freeze-dried sperm. *Zygote* 2009; 17: 239–51.

65. Li MW, Lloyd KCK. Intracytoplasmic sperm injection (ICSI) in the mouse. In Pease S, Lois C, eds. *Principles and Practice: Mammalian and Avian Transgenesis: New Approaches.* Berlin: Springer, 2009; p. 23.

66. Food and Drug Administration. FDA screening, June 03, 2009. www.cdc.gov/ncidod/dhqp/tissueTransplantsFAQ.html#r (accessed September 2010).

67. Oehninger S, Duru NK, Srisombut C, Morshedi M. Assessment of sperm cryodamage and strategies to improve outcome. *Mol Cell Endocrinol* 2000; 169: 3–10.

68. Ahuja KK, Mamiso J, Emmerson G, *et al.* Pregnancy following intracytoplasmic sperm injection treatment with dead husband's spermatozoa: ethical and policy considerations. *Hum Reprod* 1997; 12: 1360–3.

69. Meistrich ML. Potential genetic risks of using semen collected during chemotherapy. *Hum Reprod* 1993; 8: 8–10.

70. Carson SA, Gentry WL, Smith AL, Buster JE. Feasibility of semen collection and cryopreservation during chemotherapy. *Hum Reprod* 1991; 6: 992–4.

71. American Cancer Society. *Cancer Facts and Figures 2010*. Atlanta, GA: American Cancer Society, 2010.

72. World Health Organization. World cancer report. www.who.int/mediacentre/news/releases/2003/pr27/en (accessed January 2012).

73. Mariotto AB, Rowland JH, Yabroff KR, *et al.* Long-term survivors of childhood cancers in the United States. *Cancer Epidemiol Biomarkers Prev* 2009; 18: 1033–40.

74. Thomson AB, Critchley HO, Kelnar CJ, *et al.* Late reproductive sequelae following treatment of childhood cancer and options for fertility preservation. *Best Pract Res Clin Endocrinol Metab* 2002; 16: 311–34.

75. Hovatta O. Cryobiology of ovarian and testicular tissue. *Best Pract Res Clin Obstet Gynaecol* 2003; 17: 331–42.

76. Williams DH, Karpman E, Sander JC, *et al.* Pretreatment semen parameters in men with cancer. *J Urol* 2009; 181: 736–40.

77. Schover LR, Brey K, Lichtin A, *et al.* Knowledge and experience regarding cancer, infertility, and sperm banking in younger male survivors. *J Clin Oncol* 2002; 20: 1880–9.

78. Anderson RA. Fertility preservation techniques: laboratory and clinical progress and current issues. *Reproduction* 2008; 136: 667–9.

79. Trottmann M, Becker AJ, Stadler T, *et al.* Semen quality in men with malignant diseases before and after therapy and the role of cryopreservation. *Eur Urol* 2007; 52: 355–67.

80. Bonetti T, Pasqualotto FF, Queiroz P, *et al.* Sperm banking for male cancer patients: social and semen profiles. *International Braz J Urol* 2009; 35: 190–8.

81. Chung K, Irani J, Efymow B, *et al.* Sperm cryopreservation for male patients with cancer: an epidemiological analysis at the University of Pennsylvania. *Eur J Obstet Gynecol Reprod Biol* 2004; 113: S7–S11.

82. Agarwal A, Allamaneni SS. Disruption of spermatogenesis by the cancer disease process. *J Natl Cancer Inst Monogr* 2005; 34: 9–12.

83. Hourvitz A, Goldschlag DE, Davis OK, *et al.* Intracytoplasmic sperm injection (ICSI) using cryopreserved sperm from men with malignant neoplasm yields high pregnancy rates. *Fertil Steril* 2008; 90: 557–63.

84. van Casteren NJ, van Santbrink EJ, van Inzen W, *et al.* Use rate and assisted reproduction technologies outcome of cryopreserved semen from 629 cancer patients. *Fertil Steril* 2008; 90: 2245–50.

85. Brannigan RE, Sandlow JI. Cryopreservation of sperm after chemotherapy. *J Androl* 2008; 29(3): e1–2.

86. Spermon JR, Ramos L, Wetzels AM, *et al.* Sperm integrity pre- and post- chemotherapy in men with testicular germ cell cancer. *Hum Reprod* 2006; 21: 1781–6.

87. Codrington AM, Hales B, Robaire B. Spermiogenic germ cell phase-specific DNA damage following cyclophosphamide exposure. *J Androl* 2004; 25: 354–62.

88. Beiber A, Marcon L, Hales B, Robaire B. Effects of chemotherapeutic agents for testicular cancer on the male rat reproductive system, spermatozoa, and fertility. *J Androl* 2006; 27: 189–200.

89. Grundy R, Gosden RG, Hewitt M, *et al.* Fertility preservation for children treated with cancer (I): scientific advances and research dilemmas. *Arch Dis Child* 2001: 84: 355–9.

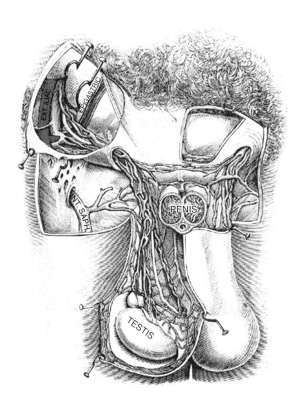

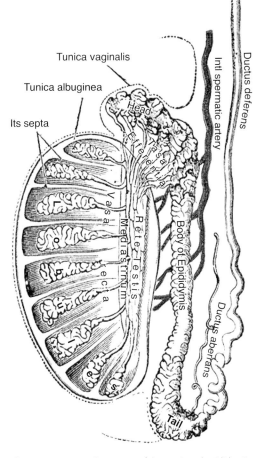

Figure 1.2. Vascular anatomy of the spermatic cord and testis. (Reproduced from Gray H. *Anatomy of the Human Body.* Philadelphia, PA: Lea & Febiger, 1918; Bartleby.com, 2000.)

Figure 1.3. Internal structure of the testis and epididymis. (Reproduced from Gray H. *Anatomy of the Human Body.* Philadelphia, PA: Lea & Febiger, 1918; Bartleby.com, 2000.)

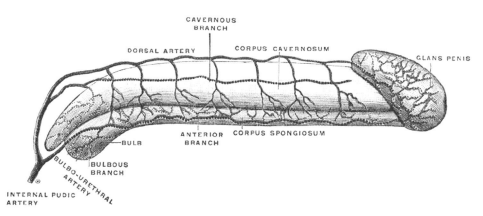

Figure 1.5. Arterial anatomy of the penis. (Reproduced from Gray H. *Anatomy of the Human Body.* Philadelphia, PA: Lea & Febiger, 1918; Bartleby.com, 2000.)

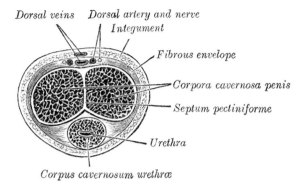

Figure 1.6. Cross-section of the penis. (Reproduced from Gray H. *Anatomy of the Human Body.* Philadelphia, PA: Lea & Febiger, 1918; Bartleby.com, 2000.)

A **Abnormal Spermatogenesis**

ALF	DAZL	SDHA
AP1	MSY2	SOX8
ATM	NLRP14	XRCC1
ATMAC	POLG	XPD
DAX1	PRM1/2	YBX2

Oligozoospermia

ACT	HOMG4	SDHA
ATPase6	KLH10	TSSK4
FASL	PRM1&2	UBE2B
H19&MEST	SHBG	VASA

Acrosome/Fertilization
ERP57

DNA Damage/Infertility

PRM1	GSTM1	IL1
TSSK4	KIT/KITLG	AR USP26
OAZ3	TSPY	MSY2

Azoospermia

ERCC1	RBMY1	APOB
ERCC2	RBMYA1	ACT
FASL	SPATA16	RBMY1F
ACSBGR	FKBP6	SYCP1
ART3	HNRNP	SYCP3
ATM	HSFY TAF7L	TGIFLX
BOULE	KLH10	TSPY
BPY2	MBOAT1	TSSK4
BRCA2	MEI1	UTY
CDY1	MLH1 XPD	XPC
CFTR	MLH3	XRCC1
CREM	MSY2	UBE2B
DAZ	MTR	UPS9Y
DDX25	NYD-SP12	USP26
DDX3Y(DBY)	NLRP14	UTP14c
DRFFY	RBMX YCP1	YBX2
RBMXL9	ZNF230	

Asthenozoospermia

AKAP3	GP130	SNBP
AKAP4	GNA12	SPAG16
CATSPER2	HILS1	POLG
DNMT3b	mtDNA	T mt DNA Haplotypes
DHAH5	MTHFR	TEKT1
DNAH11	ND4	TEKT2
DNAI1	PP1	TPN1
DYN	PRKAR1	TPN2
SHBG	TXNDC3	

Teratozoospermia

AURKC	SPATA16	
NECTIN-2	PRM1	SP1

Oligoasthenozoospermia
JUND mt-ND4   NALP14

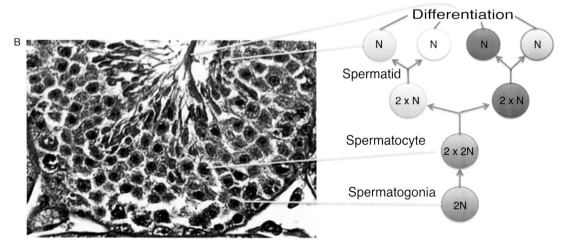

Figure 2.1. (A) Genetic basis of human male infertility defects: spermatogenesis and sperm function. Single nuclear polymorphisms (SNP) shown in blue. (B) Seminiferous tubule, demonstrating spermatogenesis and meiosis.

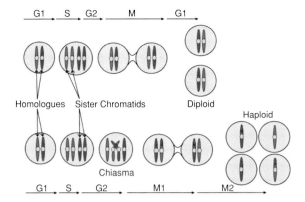

Figure 2.2. Diagrammatic representation of mitosis and meiosis.

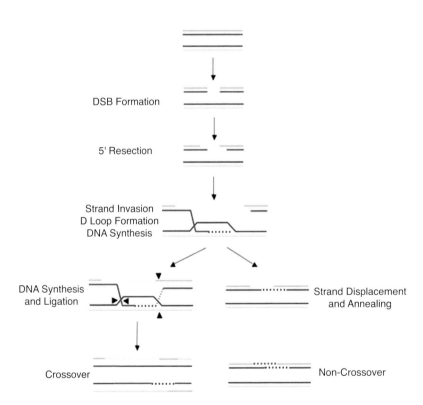

Figure 2.3. Diagrammatic representation of homologous recombination. DSB, double strand break.

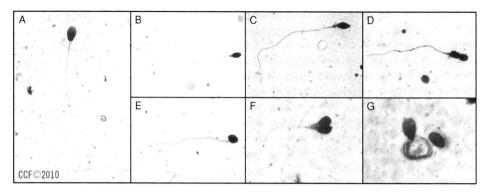

Figure 3.1. (A) Normal sperm; (B) Small head; (C) Tapering head; (D) Pyriform head; (E) Round head; (F) Bicephalic (double head); (G) Coiled tail defect. (Reproduced courtesy of the Cleveland Clinic Foundation.)

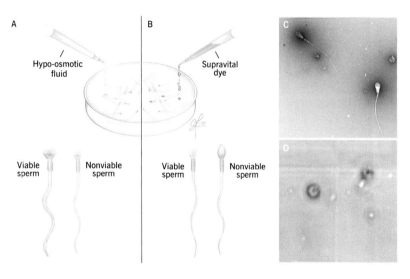

Figure 3.2. (A) Hypo-osmotic sperm swelling test: sperm with an intact cell membrane will swell. (B) Dye exclusion: sperm with an intact cell membrane are able to exclude the dye. (C) Microscopic image of dye exclusion: spermatozoa with dark pink heads are considered dead (membrane-damaged), whereas spermatozoa with white or light pink heads are considered alive (membrane-intact). (D) Endtz test: peroxidase within polymorphonuclear leukocytes is stained, allowing for distinction of seminal leukocytes from immature germ cells.

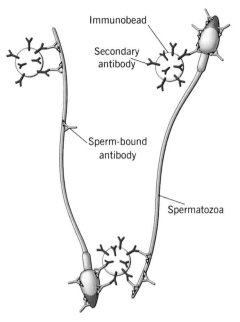

Figure 3.3. Immunobead test for ASA testing. Spermatozoa are mixed with beads that have been coated with IgG class-specific secondary antibodies, and the suspension is observed for agglutination. (Reproduced courtesy of the Cleveland Clinic Foundation.)

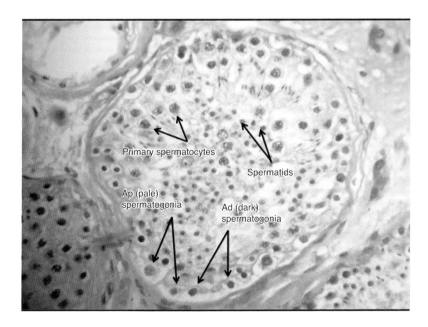

Figure 13.1. Cross-sectional view of a normal seminiferous tubule.

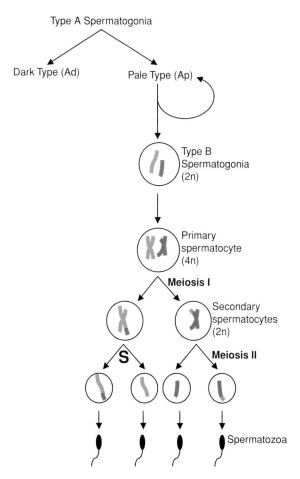

Figure 13.2. Overview of spermatogenesis.

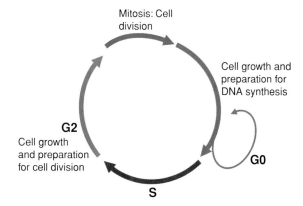

Figure 13.3. Overview of the cell cycle.

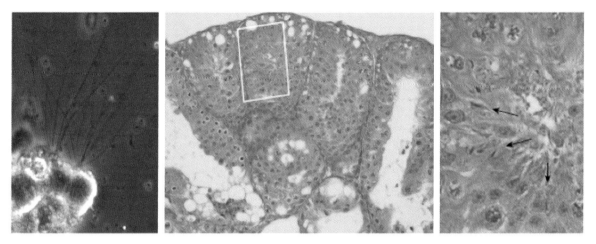

Figure 19.2. Completion of spermatogenesis in the mouse within an in-vitro culture system. Left: flagellated sperm. Centre: section of testis tissue after 38 days in culture shows well-developed seminiferous tubules and spermatogenesis. Right: white box has been enlarged, and arrows point out sperm formation (Reproduced from Sato *et al.* 2011 [46], with permission from Nature Publishing Group).

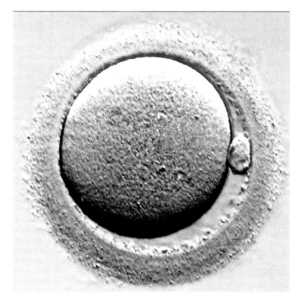

Figure 37.3. A mature oocyte.

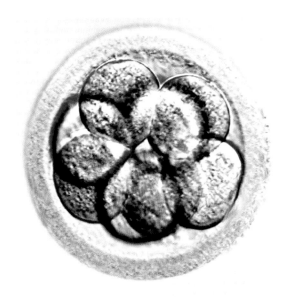

Figure 37.5. A day 3 embryo.

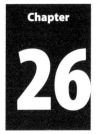

Chapter 26

Ethical and legal considerations of sperm and tissue cryopreservation

Melissa B. Brisman with assistance from Lauren Murray

Introduction

When assisting a patient diagnosed with cancer, very little is simple or straightforward. This is especially true when considering the ethical and legal aspects of a male patient who wishes to cryopreserve his sperm (or embryos created from his sperm) in the hopes that he will be able to parent his biological children once he has defeated the disease. The purpose of this chapter is to identify the most significant ethical and legal issues confronting male cancer patients in a simple, straightforward format and offer advice and guidance to medical professionals in a position to communicate relevant information to their patients. Necessarily, this chapter contemplates the ethical and legal considerations that may arise should the male cancer patient choose to cryopreserve sperm and/or embryos and not survive his treatment. As is the case for a patient making medical decisions, a patient's legal decisions should be made with full knowledge of all legal issues even if this requires contemplation of the worst-case scenario.

This chapter will discuss such topics as: (1) the fertility options for a male cancer patient; (2) how to protect a male patient's right to become a parent posthumously (or protect against becoming a parent posthumously); (3) the legal advantages of freezing sperm rather than embryos; and (4) the eligibility of social security benefits to children conceived and born to a biological father posthumously. Because this chapter is geared toward the male cancer patient, it will not discuss fertility options for female cancer patients or issues specific to them. At the same time, much of what will be discussed applies to both male and female patients. The information provided in this chapter is garnered from a variety of sources including the latest case law in the United States and abroad.

A cancer patient's fertility options and oncologists' responsibilities

First and foremost, an oncologist's goal is to assist the cancer patient in battling cancer into remission. In some ways, when the primary goal was simply to fight the disease itself, an oncologist's job was simpler. With the advances made in the treatment of cancer and a growing population of cancer survivors, oncologists now need to consider not only how to treat the disease itself but how to protect the patient's quality of life during and after treatment. When the cancer patient is diagnosed relatively early in life, preserving the patient's opportunity to reproduce is a significant aspect of maintaining his or her quality of life after cancer.

This is illustrated in a recent New Jersey case, which involved a male plaintiff who was diagnosed with leukemia when he was 16 years old. The plaintiff later sued his oncologist, alleging medical malpractice, for the failure to inform him or his parents: (a) that sterility was a likely consequence of the chemotherapy required to cure his leukemia and (b) as to the availability of sperm banking to preserve his opportunity to procreate children if he became infertile. "During discovery, the trial court dismissed Plaintiff's complaint on the ground that Plaintiff was required to show that he suffers emotional distress as a result of his inability to procreate a child in order to recover for such malpractice and that Plaintiff did not claim such emotional distress in a deposition taken when he was nineteen years old."[1] The New Jersey Appellate Court reversed

---

[1] *Brodsky v. Osunkwo*, New Jersey Appellate Division. A-4195-10T1. April 10, 2012, unpublished data.

Fertility Preservation in Male Cancer Patients, ed. John P. Mulhall, Linda D. Applegarth, Robert D. Oates and Peter N. Schlegel. Published by Cambridge University Press. © Cambridge University Press 2013.

the trial court and stated that the patient has a claim, and that it is not necessary for him to prove that he is emotionally distressed by his infertility. The Appellate Court found that infertility is a *physical disability* and that the patient can bring a malpractice action against the oncologist. The outcome of the case will, of course, depend on how well each side presents their argument; however, it is an important lesson to oncologists that they must be prepared to give cancer patients and their parents, if the patient is a minor, this important life altering information.

A patient's fertility options depend upon that patient's age and circumstances. The most common method for preserving a male cancer patient's fertility is the collection and cryopreservation of his sperm prior to him undergoing any cancer treatment. The method of obtaining the sperm will depend primarily on the patient's age. A patient of sufficient maturity can usually make a deposit through ejaculation. If that is not possible, a sexually mature male cancer patient can undergo epididymal aspiration or a testicular biopsy in order to retrieve sperm for cryopreservation. Postpubertal patients who are not capable of ejaculation can undergo epididymal sperm aspiration and testicular sperm extraction in order to retrieve their sperm for cryopreservation and later use. Although the science is not fully developed yet, testicular tissue cryopreservation for prepubertal males is on the horizon [1].

Creation of embryos for cryopreservation is another option for male patients who are married or in a relationship and wish to create embryos with their partner or spouse. For reasons which will be discussed later in this chapter, this option carries more legal risk to the patient than the cryopreservation of his sperm alone. Nevertheless, this is also a scientifically established option for many male cancer patients.

In a recent survey of male cancer patients, 30–40% of patients reported that their physicians did not discuss their future fertility or the option of cryopreservation with them [1]. Adolescent patients report physicians raising the issue of their fertility with them in uncomfortable circumstances, i.e., in the presence of their parents [1] (note that physicians should keep informed on state law requirements regarding parental involvement in the medical treatment of a minor; discussions with minors outside the presence of parents could run foul of such laws). These survey results indicate that there is clear room for improvement in

this area. This need for improvement has spawned an entirely new medical field christened "oncofertility" – a medical field focused on both oncology and fertility preservation. Practitioners of oncofertility argue that, especially in the treatment of younger cancer patients, fertility should be a factor in determining the appropriate treatment plan. The goal is to coordinate both fertility and cancer treatment to best meet the needs, both immediate and future, of the patient.

Legal and ethical issues surrounding the fundamental procreative right of a minor male cancer patient

Annually, the United States spends over $200 billion on cancer treatment and research [2]. Presumably as a result of the billions of dollars dedicated to cancer research over the years, the five-year survival rate for cancer has increased from 35% between 1950 and 1954 to 67% between 1996 and 2004 [2]. This is an incredible achievement. However, this achievement creates new legal and ethical issues for medical professionals, especially with respect to the very youngest cancer patients and the preservation of their fertility.

An analysis of legal and ethical issues involving fertility must begin with a discussion of the fundamental right to procreate. This fundamental right is the underpinning of both US and international law addressing ethical and legal issues involving fertility. International law, expressed in various international declarations and conventions, recognizes and protects each individual's fundamental right to reproduce. The United Nations Universal Declaration of Human Rights and the European Convention on Human Rights state that men and women "have the right to marry and to found a family" [3,4]. Similarly, the United Nations International Covenant on Civil and Political Rights proclaims "the right … to found a family shall be recognized" [5]. The Cairo Declaration on Human Rights in Islam recognizes that "the family is the foundation of society" [6]. In addition, both the European Court of Human Rights and the Supreme Court of Israel have held that the right to become a parent is a fundamental human right [7]. Taken together, these declarations, conventions, and judicial decisions illustrate universal recognition of the fundamental right to reproduce.

In the United States, a series of decisions by the US Supreme Court establish a US citizen's right to reproduce as well. As early as 1942, in a case entitled *Skinner v. Oklahoma*, the Supreme Court described the right to procreate as a "basic liberty" [8]. In *Skinner*, the Supreme Court determined that an Oklahoma statute giving the state the power to sterilize certain prisoners was unconstitutional because sterilization would prevent the prisoners from ever having children, thus infringing upon their right to procreate [8]. Although still subject to some debate, later Supreme Court decisions recognize that the Constitution and Bill of Rights establish a right to privacy that encompasses an individual's decisions regarding procreation, marriage, and parenting [9].

This right applies to both adults and minors. However, several Supreme Court decisions have specifically addressed the procreative rights of minors [10]. In *Ohio v. Akron Center for Reproductive Health*, the Supreme Court held that a female minor exhibiting sufficient maturity can decide on her own whether to undergo an abortion [11]. This case involved a state law requiring a female minor to obtain parental consent prior to undergoing an abortion [12]. Subsequent Supreme Court decisions dealing with this same or a similar issue have established that such parental consent laws are only constitutionally permissible if they provide a judicial bypass by which a minor can demonstrate her maturity, making parental consent unnecessary [13]. The Supreme Court has also established that, as part of this right to privacy, minors cannot be prohibited access to contraception [14].

While minors have a fundamental right to procreate, their ability to exercise this right is often limited by their lack of capacity to make critical decisions. It is therefore the responsibility of adults, usually parents or guardians, to assist a minor in protecting or exercising his or her rights. In the context of a young male cancer patient, ethical and legal questions arise involving the appropriate role of parents in assisting their minor children in making decisions regarding the children's present and future fertility, and specifically in providing consent to medical procedures.

An adult patient must freely and voluntarily consent to any medical procedure that could affect his or her reproductive capabilities. An adult male cancer patient who is unable to produce a sperm specimen for cryopreservation through ejaculation must consent to an invasive procedure to extract the sperm. The physician's responsibility is to counsel the patient on whether such a procedure poses a significant risk to the patient's health or complicates the cancer treatment. Consent becomes more complicated when the patient is a minor.

When a minor is not of sufficient maturity to make decisions regarding the exercise of his procreative right, the minor's parents must choose whether and how to exercise this right on his behalf. The parental decision-making authority is circumscribed by a general requirement that the parents make decisions that are in the best interests of the child, but what does a physician do if he or she believes the parents are not acting in their child's best interests – specifically, where the parents' decision would result in the child losing his ability to procreate? Consider a situation where a young but postpubertal male is diagnosed with cancer. The treating physician, concerned with the quality of life of this young patient, advises his parents to consider taking action to preserve their son's fertility for a potential future family. The parents respond that, due to strongly held religious beliefs, they cannot consent to any medical procedure involving assisted reproductive technologies (ART). An argument can be made here that the parents are infringing upon their child's right to procreate and the child is too young to weigh in on the decision or give his consent. The physician has done all he or she can by bringing the issue of fertility to the parents' attention. What more can the physician do?

If the parents were refusing treatment for their son which could result in the child's death, the physician has sufficient legal remedies. The courts can act to appoint a temporary legal guardian to advocate for the child's best interests or take other actions to protect the interests of the child. In the spring of 1999, Minnesota parents and their 13-year-old son garnered national attention when they opposed life-saving chemotherapy treatments for the son, who was diagnosed with Hodgkin's lymphoma [15]. The boy, Danny Hauser, and his parents, Colleen and Anthony Hauser, cited religious reasons as the basis for choosing alternative medical treatment over chemotherapy. When Danny Hauser and his parents failed to show up for his second chemotherapy treatment, the hospital contacted authorities who filed a petition alleging that Colleen and Anthony were medically neglecting their son [15]. After the judge reviewed records describing Danny's medical condition, the judge found that chemotherapy and radiation would be in the child's best interests and ordered the Hausers to select an oncologist

[15]. Although the Hausers initially resisted the judge's decision, Danny did eventually complete chemotherapy and radiation and was in remission by the fall of 2009 [16]. Here is an example of how physicians can access and utilize the legal system if they feel that parents' decisions are not in the best interests of their child.

Significantly, however, parents' refusal to preserve their child's future ability to have his own biological children does not present the same kind of urgent, life-threatening circumstances as a refusal to provide cancer treatment. It is not yet known whether a court would interfere in such a situation.

A parent's authority to make medical decisions on behalf of a minor child is limited in cases where a minor is of sufficient maturity to weigh in on his own medical treatment. What if the child is 16 years of age and of sufficient maturity to make his own decisions regarding his procreative future? The physician discusses the patient's fertility with him and the patient states that he does not desire to cryopreserve his sperm [4]. He does not intend to be a father. The physician should speak to the patient's parents. Technically, the patient is still a minor and the parents still have authority to make medical decisions on their son's behalf. The physician's best option is to make the parents aware of the issue so that the patient and his parents can determine the appropriate course of action. If the parents want the patient to cryopreserve his sperm and the patient stands firmly against it, the physician cannot force the patient to make a sperm deposit. However, if the parents succeed in obtaining a court order requiring the patient to make a sperm deposit for cryopreservation, the physician is required to comply with the court order.

As discussed earlier, the Supreme Court has recognized a mature female minor's right to make decisions regarding her right to procreate. One can certainly draw a parallel from females making decisions regarding abortion to male cancer patients making decisions regarding the cryopreservation of their sperm. Therefore, a decision to cryopreserve sperm (or not to cryopreserve sperm) by a mature minor male cancer patient may be honored by a court of law in the event of a dispute between him and his parents over the exercise of his procreative right.

To date, there does not appear to be any case of parents being prosecuted for failing to preserve the procreative right of their child or infringing upon a child's decision not to exercise his procreative right. However, advances in reproductive technology make it increasingly likely that such situations will become the subject of future Supreme Court decisions.

Even as courts wrestle with these complex legal issues, medical practitioners will have to deal with more practical and procedural questions that present potential legal and ethical dilemmas. These questions include: how to discuss future disposition of cryopreserved sperm with a minor; whether a minor can sign clinic forms indicating future disposition of cryopreserved sperm; and whether clinics should honor parents' wishes concerning the future disposition of their son's sperm.

In cases where physicians are treating minors, specifically minors who require medical treatment for cancer, physicians can find themselves faced with any number of ethical dilemmas that do not have easy solutions. Perhaps the most troublesome ethical questions arise when the patient and his parents disagree over treatment. Consider the situation described above, where a minor male cancer patient expresses opposition to any procedure necessary to retrieve, collect, and cryopreserve his sperm. His parents, however, desire to preserve their son's fertility and express this desire to the physician. The parents are willing to sign any consent forms necessary. In this type of situation, the physician is faced with a difficult ethical dilemma – his patient's wishes are in conflict with the wishes of the individuals with the legal authority to make medical decisions on his behalf. The physician may also feel that the patient's opposition to preservation of his fertility is not in his own best interests. What is the physician's ethical obligation to the patient?

If harm to the patient is a relevant factor in considering this issue, the potential for harm appears to be less if the physician ignores the patient's wishes. The sperm is simply being gathered and frozen – not used (at least at this point) to conceive a child against the patient's wishes. Therefore, the practical effect of the act of preserving the patient's sperm does not seem to cause significant harm to the patient. On the other hand, failing to preserve the patient's sperm could cause significant harm in the event the patient experiences a change of heart at a later date.

Another potential factor to discuss in considering the physician's ethical obligation is whether the physician is acting in the patient's "best interests." Here, both the physician and the patient's parents may feel that the patient's decision is ill-advised and short-sighted. The physician has the support and consent of the patient's parents and is authorized to act in what he considers to be the patient's "best interests" by the individuals with legal decision-making authority. However, it should be noted, even with the parent's consent, the physician is collaborating in an effort to usurp the decision-making power of his patient, and such action could take that physician down a slippery ethical slope. Although a physician may never consider acting against the wishes of an adult patient, even when the physician disagrees with the adult patient's decision, where the patient is a minor and the physician is acting under the authority of a legal parent or guardian, the ethical path may seem to be unclear.

Finally, consider a similar scenario except that the patient is consenting to any procedures necessary to preserve his fertility against the wishes of his parents. Under these facts, if the physician does not follow the wishes of his patient, the patient's future ability to have his own biological children would be lost permanently. Now, failure to follow a minor patient's express wishes could create significant harm to the patient and would not appear to be in the child's "best interests." The difficulty in finding answers to these ethical questions is underscored by how changing one fact can radically impact the analysis of the physician's ethical obligation.

How a male cancer patient can effectively preserve his right to procreate

Rule number 1: Male cancer patients should strongly consider cryopreserving their sperm rather than embryos created from their sperm

As already discussed, US and international law recognize that each individual has a fundamental and protected right to procreate. When a man and a woman decide to create embryos together, they are exercising their right to procreate simultaneously, and both share rights over the resulting embryos. This situation does not infringe upon either partner's right to procreate as long as both gamete providers share a mutual desire to conceive a pregnancy together with the embryos. However, substantial difficulties present

themselves when gamete providers with existing cryopreserved embryos no longer agree over the embryos' use and disposition. Therefore, a male cancer patient can best protect his individual right to procreate by cryopreserving his sperm alone.

There is no existing US case law specifically dealing with a male cancer patient's right to use embryos he cryopreserves with a spouse or partner; however, recently a Pennsylvania court has decided that a female cancer patient has the right to use embryos that were cryopreserved during the marriage despite the objection of her ex-husband.[2] However, a few US courts have been confronted with a divorcing husband and wife who created embryos during their marriage and now dispute the embryos' future use. The facts and legal arguments vary somewhat from case to case but the practical result of most all court decisions is to protect an individual's right not to become a parent if that is the individual's wish.

The courts that have adjudicated these types of disputes have generally applied one of three approaches in their analyses. First, the approach that has been applied most often is the contractual approach. In this approach, the court determines the proper disposition of the cryopreserved embryos based on the terms of any agreement entered into by the disputing parties, unless the disposition identified in the agreement violates public policy [17]. A married couple is unlikely to have entered into an agreement between themselves specifically addressing disposition of the embryos. The documents that the court is more likely to examine are the documents provided to the couple by the clinic in which the clinic asks the couple to designate how they would like the embryos disposed of in the event of their separation or divorce or the death of either or both parties. If the couple has addressed the disposition of the embryos in their wills, that would also be evidence that the court would find relevant. These documents evidence the parties' intent at the time of the disputed embryos' creation.

The second approach is the balancing test. In this approach, the procreative right of each disputing party is balanced against that of the other. This type of test is necessarily extremely case-specific [18]. The third approach is the contemporaneous mutual consent approach. This is similar to the first approach, the contractual approach, in that the court first looks

---

[2] *Reber vs. Reiss*, 2012 Pa Super 8.

to whether the disputing parties have an agreement in place expressing their intentions as to the disposition of the embryos. However, under this approach, the court will disregard consent expressed in documents signed at the time of cryopreservation if the gamete provider has since changed his or her mind, and has expressly withdrawn his or her consent to the other party's use [19].

Until recently, there were no cases decided by a US court involving a cancer survivor in which the disputed embryos were clearly the cancer survivor's only opportunity to become a biological parent.[2] In at least four of the six cases decided by US courts to date it is clear that the parties wishing to use the embryos either already had existing biological children (*A.Z. v. B.Z.*), had the potential to conceive future biological children irrespective of the embryos (*J.B. v. M.B.*), wanted to donate the embryos (*Davis v. Davis*), or were not biologically related to the embryos (*Litowitz*). Only *Reber vs. Reiss* discussed below confronted this issue and one another US court considered such a situation in dicta and stated that the court's decision would be more difficult if the party seeking to use the disputed embryos "could not achieve parenthood by any other reasonable means" [20].

However, the European Court of Human Rights adjudicated this exact question in 2002. In *Evans v. the United Kingdom*, a 34-year-old British woman, Natalie Evans, sought access to embryos she created with a former partner, identified as J. [21]. In July of 2000, Ms. Evans and her partner started fertility treatment at the Bath Assisted Conception Clinic in the UK. In October of that year, Ms. Evans was diagnosed with a precancerous condition requiring the surgical removal of her ovaries. The clinic informed both Ms. Evans and J. that, should they choose to cryopreserve embryos prior to Ms. Evans' procedure, each would have to sign a form consenting to the in-vitro fertilization (IVF). They were also informed that, pursuant to UK law, each of them would be able to withdraw their consent at any time prior to an embryo transfer. Ms. Evans considered exploring other means of preserving her ova but J. provided reassurance that it would not be necessary [21].

Ms. Evans underwent one cycle of IVF to create and cryopreserve six embryos composed of her ova and her partner's sperm. After the removal of her ovaries, Ms. Evans was instructed to wait for two years before undergoing an embryo transfer. During that two-year period, her relationship with J. ended. J. subsequently

withdrew his consent to the continued storage of the embryos and Ms. Evans' use of the embryos. Ms. Evans petitioned the United Kingdom's High Court seeking an injunction to prevent the destruction of the embryos and requiring J. to restore his consent. The High Court denied her requested relief in October of 2003. On appeal, the Court of Appeal upheld the High Court's decision [21].

Ms. Evans appealed to the European Court of Human Rights. The European Court of Human Rights requested that the government of the United Kingdom prevent the destruction of the embryos until the European Court had an opportunity to decide the case. The embryos were not destroyed and the clinic acknowledged that it would treat Ms. Evans if J. would consent [21].

Before the European Court on Human Rights, Ms. Evans argued that requiring the father's consent for the continued storage and implantation of the embryos breached several provisions of the European Convention on Human Rights, namely Article 2 (the right to life), Article 9 (the right to respect for privacy and family life), and Article 14 (the prohibition on discrimination). The European Court on Human Rights rejected all three arguments. The court stated that English law must govern its determination of when life begins and English law does not recognize embryos as having independent rights or interests. Therefore, Article 2 did not apply. Next, the court found that the United Kingdom had strong public-policy justifications for its "bright-line" rule that parties to fertility treatments may withdraw consent at any time prior to transfer and that this rule did not violate Articles 8 or 14.

Rather than a "bright-line" rule, Ms. Evans advocated for a balancing of her procreative rights against those of J. Even though these embryos represented Ms. Evans' only means of conceiving her own biological child, the court stated that "it would be difficult for a court to judge whether the effect on [Ms. Evans] of J.'s withdrawal of consent would be greater than the impact of the invalidation of that withdrawal of consent would have on J." [21]. This statement squarely addresses a fundamental issue for cancer patients in the United States: whether the balancing of interests in this type of case would result in a different outcome had the disputed embryos been an individual's only means of having his or her own biological child.

Fast forward to 2012. The US addressed this in a recent case, Bret Howard Reber vs. Andrea Lynn Reiss.[2] In this case Mr. Reber and Ms. Reiss married in 2002. A year later, Ms. Reiss, who was then 36 years old, developed breast cancer. Ms. Reiss delayed chemotherapy treatment so that she and her husband could undergo IVF treatment to preserve her ability to have a biological child of her own. Luckily 13 embryos were created. In 2006, Ms. Reiss has finished her chemotherapy treatment, but Mr. Reber wants a divorce because he has developed a relationship with another woman, who gave birth to his biological son.

Ms. Reiss is now 44 years old, has a no children, and soon will no longer have a husband. Ms. Reiss seeks custody of the 13 embryos so she can have a child but Mr. Reber wants the embryos destroyed. In this case, there was no written agreement about what to do with the embryos in the event of a divorce. The lower court acknowledged that ordinarily the spouse who doesn't want to procreate prevails, but since this was a unique situation, it balanced the competing interests of the spouses. In doing so, it found that Ms. Reiss's inability to achieve biological parenthood without the use of the embryos outweighted Mr. Reber's desire to avoid procreation, and granted Ms. Reiss custody of the embryos to do as she pleased. On appeal to the Superior Court, Mr. Reber argued that there are other ways Ms. Reiss could become a parent. She could adopt or she could become a foster parent. The Superior Court disagreed, and stated that an adoption "occupies a different place for a woman than the opportunity to be pregnant and/or have biological child."[3] The Superior Court also noted that adoption is a complicated process and that placement is less likely for an older, single woman with a medical history. Mr. Reber tried another approach and expressed concerns that under the circumstances, any child born to Ms. Reiss would not know him as the father. Mr. Reber was adopted, and would want the child to know his father. Ms. Reiss countered by saying that she would not have any problem if Mr. Reber wanted communication and involvement with the child. Finally, Mr. Reber raised the issue of child support and that any child born as a result of the embryos would be a financial burden to him. Ms. Reiss "vowed" not to seek Mr. Reber's financial support, and even though both courts were unwilling to rely on this "vow," they felt it appropriate to leave the issue open to be decided at a later date if and when necessary. So, in the end, the Superior Court ruled such that Ms. Reiss keeps the embryos and, if she chooses, can build a family of her own. In the end this is a

significant victory for cancer patients; however, it only applies in the state of Pennsylvania and the Superior Court is not the highest court in Pennsylvania.

As a result, and based on the majority of existing case law, a male cancer patient cryopreserving embryos he creates with a partner runs a real risk that the partner could refuse him access to those embryos in the future. If the patient's partner revokes her consent to the use of the embryos, under either the contemporaneous mutual consent (contractual) or the balancing test approaches described earlier, a court is likely to honor the partner's right to avoid parenthood. Even if, under the contractual approach, the patient and his partner clearly indicate an intent at the time of cryopreservation that the patient will have the right to use the embryos in the future and application of the contractual approach calls for the adjudicating court to honor the executed documents and the intent expressed in them, a court may not require anyone to become a biological parent against his or her will. It is for these reasons that cancer patients are advised to cryopreserve their sperm rather than the embryos they create with someone else. In this way, a cancer patient's procreative right does not come into conflict with any other individual's procreative right, and the cancer patient is the only person with authority to make decisions regarding his own gametes.

The cases involving disputes over use or ownership of cryopreserved embryos raise some compelling ethical questions. Perhaps the most ethically troublesome scenario is the situation described in the *Evans* case – where the embryos in dispute are one gamete provider's only means of having a biological child and the other gamete provider is refusing consent to the embryos' use. If courts refuse to allow the opposing gamete provider to become a biological parent against his or her will, then the courts are effectively preventing one gamete provider from ever exercising his or her right to become a biological parent. In balancing the procreative rights of these two gamete providers, is a decision that permanently prevents an individual from ever becoming a biological parent ethical? Many neutral third parties would argue that such a result is entirely unjust and unethical because no one individual should have the power to revoke their consent and permanently prevent another from becoming a biological parent. Nevertheless, at least in most instances, with the exception of the Reiss case described above, this appears to be the current state of the law.

---

[3] *Reber vs. Reiss*, 2012 Pa Super 86.

There are additional benefits to cryopreserving sperm rather than embryos which warrant mentioning. If this chapter focused on female cancer patients as well as male cancer patients, it would necessarily discuss how science has not yet advanced to the point where the cryopreservation of ova is an established option. In order to maximize her future fertility, a female's best option is to cryopreserve embryos, because the pregnancy rate from thawed embryos is so much higher than from thawed ova. This discrepancy does not exist between the pregnancy rates from thawed sperm and thawed embryos, so males who elect to cryopreserve their sperm rather than embryos are not disadvantaged from a fertility perspective. In addition, should a male cancer patient fail to survive his cancer treatments, there are significantly fewer ethical and emotional issues surrounding destruction of sperm in comparison to destruction of embryos. This means there is less potential for conflict and an increased likelihood that the patient's wishes with regard to destruction of his sperm will be honored. This is not to say that there are no advantages for a male cancer patient to cryopreserve embryos rather than sperm. In particular, and as will be discussed in more detail below, the cryopreservation of embryos could increase a widow's ability to obtain social security benefits for the child and allow the child to obtain any inheritance(s) left by the deceased. In these situations, a practitioner's job is to educate the patient so that any decision he makes is an informed decision. If the patient decides to freeze embryos rather than sperm, that is acceptable as long as the patient was presented with all of his options.

Rule number 2: One's intentions should be clearly and unequivocally stated

When a male cancer patient elects to cryopreserve his sperm or embryos created from his sperm for future use, he should clearly indicate his desired disposition of the sperm should he fail to survive his cancer treatments. There are several different ways that a cancer patient can establish his intentions with regard to the future use and custody of his sperm or embryos. First and foremost, a cancer patient should indicate his preferences with regard to future use and custody of his sperm or embryos in his will. Second, a cancer patient should clearly indicate his preferences with regard to disposition in the paperwork provided to him by the sperm bank or clinic. Third, if cryo-

preserving embryos, the cancer patient can also enter into an agreement with his partner or spouse indicating how the embryos should be disposed of in the event of his death. All of these documents should be consistent and, as a whole, provide clear evidence of the patient's intentions. Taking these actions creates the highest likelihood that a court would uphold the patient's wishes in the event a dispute arises over the custody or use of the patient's sperm or embryos after his death.

The importance of a male cancer patient stating his intentions clearly and unequivocally is greatest should the cancer patient fail to survive his cancer treatments. In such a situation, there are two types of disputes that are most likely to arise. First, if the patient was married or had a girlfriend, a dispute could arise between the widow and the patient's family. Another common type of dispute could arise between a widow and entities providing benefits to her or any resulting children (social security, life insurance companies, etc.). Because the cancer patient is no longer able to appear in court or speak on his own behalf, having a will or similar documentation clearly expressing his intentions with regard to the posthumous use of his cryopreserved sperm or embryos is valuable and potentially persuasive.

In the majority of cases dealing with these types of disputes, evidence of the sperm provider's intent plays a significant role in the court's adjudication. In one decision in the California Court of Appeals, a widow was denied access to her husband's sperm because, in the agreement with the sperm bank, the husband indicated that his sperm should be discarded in the event of his death. The court stated: "In determining the disposition of gamete material, to which no other party had contributed and thus as to which another party's right to procreational autonomy was not implicated, the intent of the donor controlled" [22]. The court was not convinced by the widow's argument that her procreational rights were being violated by her inability to use her deceased husband's cryopreserved sperm [23].

There are several cases in which widows have sought social security benefits for their children who were conceived either from their husband's sperm or from embryos created with their husband's sperm, after the husbands lost their battles with cancer. In all three cases, the Social Security Administration disputed the widow's claim because the children were conceived and born posthumously. Widows who have been able to demonstrate clear intent on their husband's part to parent children posthumously are more likely to prevail. In one case, the husband was diagnosed with cancer while he and his wife were trying to have a child [24]. The husband delayed his cancer treatments so that he could cryopreserve his sperm for his wife's use [24]. His wife conceived their biological children after his death [25]. The court concluded that the children were entitled to the benefits [26]. In another case, a widow sought to have her husband's children, conceived and born after his death, recognized as his legal heirs under New Jersey law to strengthen her claim to benefits from the Social Security Administration [27]. The husband was only 26 when he was diagnosed with leukemia. He was advised to start chemotherapy immediately. He cryopreserved two separate sperm samples, one prior to his first treatment and the second one month into his chemotherapy. The New Jersey court concluded that the twin girls born to his widow were the husband's heirs, citing his "intentional conduct" which "created the possibility of having long-delayed after born children" [27]. In a third case, a married couple discovered that the husband had leukemia and the husband cryopreserved his sperm [28]. The husband underwent an unsuccessful bone marrow transplant and passed away. The widow conceived and gave birth to her husband's biological children, twin girls, after her husband's death. The court concluded that the children would be entitled to benefits through their biological father if the widow could demonstrate the biological link between her deceased husband and the children and if she could demonstrate that her husband consented to reproduce posthumously and support any resulting children [29].

Unlike the *Evans* decision discussed earlier, which some might view as an unjust and unethical result, these decisions seem more ethically appropriate. When considering whether posthumous use of an individual's sperm or embryos itself is ethical, the answer depends to some extent on whether the individual would have consented or did consent to the use. If there is consent, the use seems ethical. In these cases, the courts focused on the intent and consent of the patient to determine whether it was appropriate for the spouse to use her husband's sperm or embryos to conceive a child after his death. The courts consented to such use where the evidence suggested the husband intended to parent a child after his death. Similarly, the courts denied such use where the evidence suggested the husband would not have consented.

Is it just and/or ethical, however, to deny a wife the ability to use embryos she created with her husband if, although there is no evidence of his consent to such use, these embryos represent the wife's only means of having her own biological child? This factual scenario is distinguishable from the *Evans* case because there is no living individual actively withdrawing his consent to the use of the embryos. Instead, the second gamete provider is deceased and can voice neither his objection nor his consent. In *Evans*, the court would not force a living individual to become a parent against his will, but is the same result just and ethical where a deceased individual may be made a parent? There is no direct harm to the deceased individual himself, but there may be negative consequences for the individual's family or existing children with regard to inheritance rights and other benefits. Perhaps this harm is outweighed by the spouse's right to procreate.

Children born from posthumously retrieved sperm are considered differently than children conceived from sperm retrieved during a patient's lifetime. This is due in large part to the focus on the intentions of a patient. It is significantly easier to convince a court that an individual consented to posthumous conception of his biological child when the individual took steps to cryopreserve his sperm during his lifetime. There is a Ninth Circuit Court of Appeals decision from 2009 in which the court denied social security benefits to a child born to a widow when that child was conceived from her deceased husband's posthumously retrieved sperm [30]. In its decision, the Court noted that the married couple here had been married five years, had no children, and there was "no evidence to suggest that [the husband] consented to the [posthumous extraction] procedure, or had ever contemplated having a child postmortem." In fairness, the husband in this case was killed in an accident, so unlike a man diagnosed with cancer, there were limited reasons for this man to preserve his sperm in anticipation of his possible death. While there are many anecdotal cases of sperm being extracted postmortem and used either by wives, girlfriends, or parents (to create a grandchild), these cases are not as relevant for the male cancer patient.

A recent case has shed some light on the right of a widow to obtain social security benefits for a posthumous conception and birth for a cancer patient. Karen and Robert Capato married in 1999. Robert died of cancer less than 3 years later. With the help of in vitro fertilization, Karen gave birth to twins

18 months after her husband's death. Karen's application for Social Security survivors benefits for the twins, which the Social Security Administration (SSA) denied, prompted this litigation.[4] Since the twins were conceived and born after the death of their father, the case before the United States Supreme Court questioned whether the twins were entitled to social security benefits. The Supreme Court held that the children were not entitled to benefits since Florida state law did not provide for the twins in this instance. The District Court observed that Fla. Stat. Ann. §732.106 (West 2010) defines "afterborn heirs" as "heirs of the decedent *conceived before his or her death*, but born thereafter." App. to Pet. for Cert. 27a (emphasis added by District Court). The court also referred to §742.17(4), which provides that a posthumously conceived child "shall not be eligible for a claim against the decedent's estate unless the child has been provided for by the decedent's will." *Id.*, at 28a. The Supreme Court of the United States concluded that the courts should use the state's intestacy law, where the deceased lived at his time of death, to determine whether a child is entitled to benefits. If the child could inherit from the deceased under the state's law at the time of death then the resulting child could get social security benefits. Unfortunately, each state has a different intestacy law and whether posthumous children will be entitled to benefits will now be dependent on whether, at the time of the parent's death, the child qualified as an heir. It is worth noting that many states depend on the intent of the descendent to father a child posthumously when deciving who is an heir.

A physician who receives a request to extract sperm from a patient postmortem has a number of ethical questions to consider. First, is it ethical to perform a postmortem sperm extraction? As is the case with each of the ethical questions raised in this chapter, there is no bright-line rule. Instead, the correct answer will depend on the specific circumstances of the case. Take the 2009 decision by the Ninth Circuit described above as an example [30]. This was a case where the Ninth Circuit upheld a denial of social security benefits to a widow who applied for the benefits on behalf of her child who was conceived from sperm extracted from her husband posthumously. The facts of the case strongly suggest that the husband did not intend, and did not consent to, the postmortem extraction of his sperm. Was it therefore ethically appropriate for a physician to perform the postmortem extraction?

There was no harm to the patient in performing the procedure, as the patient was deceased. The best interests of the patient are also not a particularly relevant factor. On the other hand, to many people it may seem unjust and unethical to perform a medical procedure on a patient where the evidence suggests the patient would not have consented. A parallel may be drawn here to organ donation – it seems unlikely that a physician would extract organs from a body if that individual did not consent to being an organ donor during his or her lifetime. Is it not then similarly inappropriate and unethical to extract an individual's sperm where that individual did not consent to such extraction during his lifetime?

Continuing the parallel to organ donation, would the ethical issue be different if the family members of the deceased individual consented to the organ donation? For instance, if the parents of a deceased individual consented to the donation of their son's healthy heart, it would then seem ethically appropriate to extract that heart and donate it to someone in medical need. Similarly, if a wife or parents of a deceased patient request that the physician perform a sperm extraction so that they may have an opportunity to bring that patient's child into the world, does it now seem more ethically acceptable? This answer does not seem quite so clear, especially if the spouse and parents are in a dispute over whether the extraction is appropriate, and/or over the use of the extracted sperm.

The ethical questions appear less murky when the patient consented to the sperm extraction or made a sperm donation during his lifetime. Once again, it is useful to underscore the importance of a patient clearly stating his intentions with regard to the posthumous use or extraction of his sperm in order to assist physicians in navigating these complicated legal and ethical waters.

Rule number 3: Recognize the patient's right not to reproduce

Physicians may start with the general assumption that their patient will have an interest in creating a family some day. This may not be the case. It is important to inform each patient of his options, but remain aware that some patients will not have an interest in preserving their fertility. Information is power, and so is a patient's right to individual autonomy.

---

[4] *Astrue vs. Capato*, No. 11-159, Supreme Court of the United States 2012.

Rule number 4: Be aware of storage costs and time limitations

Most clinics that offer storage of frozen gametes offer discounts or plans for the costs associated with storing frozen gametes for cancer patients. Patients should discuss these options with their fertility clinic or sperm banking facility. There are also organizations that can provide financial assistance for fertility preservation. Patients will be required to sign consent forms with the clinics where they freeze specimens as well as any other potential long-term storage facilities to which they might transfer their specimens if they are not planning on using them in the short-term future. These consent forms will likely contain an agreement to pay for the storage costs. In the event that storage fees are not paid, the facility may continue to pursue payment directly or may employ a collections agency in an effort to collect payment. It is highly unlikely that the facility would ever discard the frozen gametes or embryos due to non-payment of storage fees; however, this is a possibility. In the event of the death of the patient providing the sperm specimen, their next of kin and/or estate will likely become responsible for the storage fees. The patient should be aware of this, and should have allocated sufficient funds for these fees.

Some facilities put time limits for the storage of the gametes or embryos on the consent form and state that the specimen will be discarded when that time limit is reached if no action is taken by the progenitor or their next of kin/estate. It remains unclear whether or not an agreement such as this one is enforceable. In at least one case, a US court has acknowledged the possibility that disputed embryos could be discarded in accordance with consents signed by the couple who created the embryos. This seems to suggest that time limitations established by sperm banking facilities are enforceable, but this specific issue has not yet been tested in the courts [31].

A court in Iowa found a divorcing couple to remain responsible for the cryopreservation fees for the storage of their frozen embryos throughout the litigation attempting to decide whether the embryos could be used over one party's objection. Furthermore, the court ruled that the party voicing the objection to the disposition of the embryos should be responsible for the costs of their continued cryopreservation [32]. Although this case is not binding across the country, it suggests that a party objecting to the disposition of gametes or sperm should be prepared to continue paying storage costs until the dispute is resolved.

Conclusion

The legal landscape surrounding sperm and tissue cryopreservation is ever-changing. Nevertheless, the information presented above reflects the current state of the law and provides physicians with a basis on which to assist their male cancer patients in securing their future fertility. As technology advances, there is little doubt that new ethical and legal questions will continue to arise. The best advice for physicians is to treat the preservation of a patient's fertility in the same manner that they treat a patient's fight against cancer – by informing the patient of all the options available so that the patient can choose the path that best fits his preferences and desires.

References

1. Practice Committee of the American Society for Reproductive Medicine; Practice Committee of the Society for Assisted Reproductive Technology. Ovarian tissue and oocyte cryopreservation. *Fertil Steril* 2006; 86 (5 Suppl 1): S142–7.

2. Dolin G *et al*. Medical hope, legal pitfalls: potential legal issues in the emerging field of oncofertility, 49 *Santa Clara Law Rev* 673, 673 (2009).

3. European Convention for the Protection of Human Rights and Fundamental Freedoms, art 12, 213 U.N,T.S. 222 (Nov. 4, 1950).

4. Universal Declaration of Human Rights, G.A. Res. 217A(III), art. 16(1), U.N. GAOR, 3d Sess., U.N. Doc. A/810 (Dec. 10, 1948).

5. International Convention on Civil and Political Rights, art 23(2), 999 U.N.T.S. 179 (Dec. 16, 1966).

6. The Cairo Declaration on Human Rights in Islam, Aug. 5, 1990, World Conference on Human Rights, U.N. Doc. A/CONF.157/PC/62/Add.18 (June 9, 1993). www1.umn.edu/humanrts/instree/cairodeclaration. html.

7. CA 2401/95 Nahmani v. Nahmani, [1996] IsrSC 50(4) 661 (opinion of Dorner, J. (English translation available at elyon1.court.gov.il/Files ENG/95/010/024/z01/950240 10.z01.pdf)); *Evans v. The United Kingdom*, at 4 (App. No. 6339/05) (Eur. Ct. H.R. Apr. 10, 2007). www.echr.coe.int/eng.

8. *Skinner v. Oklahoma ex rel. Williamson*, 316 U.S. 535, 541 (1942).

9. *Carey v. Population Services*, 431 U.S. 678, 684–85 (1977); *Eisenstadt v. Baird*, 405 U.S. 438, 453 (1972);

Wash. v. Glucksberg, 521 U.S. 702, 726–27 (1997); *Stanley v. Illinois*, 405 U.S. 645 (1972).

10. *Carey*, 431 U.S. at 693; *Planned Parenthood of Central Missouri v. Danforth*, 428 U.S. 52, 74 (1976).

11. *Ohio v. Akron Center for Reproductive Health et al.*, 497 U.S. 502, 510–11 (1990).

12. *Ohio v. Akron Center for Reproductive Health et al.*, 497 U.S. 506 (1990).

13. *Planned Parenthood of Southeastern Pennsylvania et al. v. Casey et al.*, 505 U.S. 833, 899 (1992); *Ayotte v. Planned Parenthood*, 546 U.S. 320, 324 (2006).

14. *Carey*, 431 U.S. at 693–94.

15. Stachura S. Family lands in court over son's cancer treatment. *Minnesota Public Radio* (May 8, 2009). www.minnesota.publicradio.org; Minnesota judge rules teen must see cancer doctor (May 15, 2009). wcco.com/local/chemo.therapy.ordered.2.1010319.html.

16. Wolfe W. Danny Hauser finishes his cancer treatment. *Star Tribune* November 6, 2009. www.startribune.com/projects.45440392.html.

17. *Roman v. Roman*, 193 S.W. 3d 40, 52–53 (Tex. App. 2006); *In re Marriage of Litowitz*, 48 P. 3d, 261, 268–69 (Wash. 2002) *cert. denied* 537 U.S. 1191 (2003); *Kass v. Kass*, 91 N.E. 2d 174, 180 (N.Y. 1998).

18. *Davis v. Davis*, 842 S.W. 2d 588, 603–4 (Tenn. 1992) *cert. denied sub nom Stower v. Davis*, 507 U.S. 911.

19. *AZ v. BZ*, 725 N.E. 2d 1051, 1054 (Mass. 2000); *In re Marriage of Arthur Witten III*, 672 N.W. 2d 768, 782–83 (Iowa Sup. 2003).

20. *Davis*, 842 S.W. 2d at 604.

21. *Evans v. the United Kingdom*, at 4 (App. No. 6339/05) (Eur. Ct. H.R. Apr. 10, 2007). www.echr.coe.int/eng.

22. *Estate of Kievernagel*, 166 Cal. App. 4th 1024 (Cal. App. 2008).

23. *Estate of Kievernagel* 166 Cal. App 4th 1032–33 (Cal. App. 2008).

24. *Gillett-Netting v. Barnhart*, 371 F. 3d 593, 594 (9th Cir. 2004).

25. *Gillett-Netting v. Barnhart*, 371 F. 3d 596 (9th Cir. 2004).

26. *Gillett-Netting v. Barnhart*, 371 F. 3d 599 (9th Cir. 2004).

27. *In re Estate of Kolacy*, 332 A. 2d 1257, 1264 (N.J. Super. 2000).

28. *Woodward v. Commissioner of Social Security*, 760 N.E. 2d 257, 260 (Mass. 2000).

29. *Woodward v. Commissioner of Social Security*, 760 N.E. 2d 272 (Mass. 2000).

30. *Vernoff v. Astrue*, 568 F. 3d 1102, 1111–1112 (9th Cir. 2009).

31. *Litowitz*, 48 P. 3d at 269.

32. *Witten*, 672 N.W. 2d at 783.

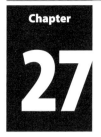

The use of ejaculation induction procedures in cancer patients

Dana A. Ohl, Mikkel Fode, Nancy L. Brackett, Charles M. Lynne, Susanne A. Quallich, and Jens Sønksen

Introduction

Of the many causes of male infertility, ejaculatory dysfunction is relatively uncommon. Likewise, in cancer patients, it accounts for a small number of the total visits to practitioners. Nevertheless, there are certain situations in which the inability to ejaculate prevents fertility preservation or restoration in men before and after cancer treatment. This chapter will review the causes of ejaculation difficulties among this patient population, and potential treatments to circumvent the problem.

Physiology of ejaculation

During ejaculation sperm travel distally via the vasa deferentia, which join the seminal vesicles to form the ejaculatory ducts. These then enter the prostatic urethra just lateral to the verumontanum. The site of entry into the prostatic urethra is distal to the bladder neck and proximal to the external urethral sphincter, and this location is relevant in preventing retrograde ejaculation into the bladder, as the bladder neck contracts during ejaculation. The ejaculate that emerges from the urethra is a mixture of secretions from these various organs, with the majority coming from the seminal vesicles (approximately two-thirds) and the prostate. Sperm from the testes and mucoid bulbourethral gland secretions account for 1–2% of the volume [1]. After initial coagulation of the ejaculate, liquefaction is achieved by the proteolytic enzyme, prostate-specific antigen (PSA).

There are several neural components that control sexual function. Sensory input arising from genital stimulation is carried by the dorsal nerves of the penis, which arise from spinal cord levels S2–S4. Penile erection is initiated by parasympathetic fibers arising from the same spinal level. Seminal emission and bladder neck closure are under sympathetic nerve control arising from spinal levels T10–L2 and coursing through the sympathetic chains, the inferior mesenteric plexus, and the pelvic nerves. Periurethral muscle contraction is controlled by pudendal nerves, also originating from S2–S4 [2].

During initial sexual stimulation, skeletal muscle contraction compresses the bulbourethral glands, leading to meatal extrusion of a mucoid "pre-ejaculate." Just prior to ejaculation, these muscles tonically contract to very high pressure, and without this high-pressure contraction, ejaculation threshold is not reached [3]. After skeletal muscle contraction peaks, seminal emission into the prostatic urethra ensues and the bladder neck tightly contracts, preventing retrograde flow of semen [4]. Finally, the external sphincter relaxes and rhythmic contractions of the periurethral muscles lead to antegrade projectile ejaculation.

Etiologies of ejaculatory dysfunction and relationship to cancer

Abnormalities of any of the above-mentioned events can lead to ejaculatory dysfunction.

Premature ejaculation (PE) is a very common sexual dysfunction, with an incidence as high as 31% in a large cross-sectional study [5]. It is characterized by ejaculation occurring prior to or immediately after intromission, sooner than the man wishes and causing distress to the man and/or his partner. Stopwatch studies suggest that an ejaculatory latency time of less than 1.5 minutes predicts self-identification of PE [6]. PE may be lifelong or acquired. There are no published reports of which the authors are aware that acquired PE is related to the diagnosis or treatment of cancer.

Fertility Preservation in Male Cancer Patients, ed. John P. Mulhall, Linda D. Applegarth, Robert D. Oates and Peter N. Schlegel. Published by Cambridge University Press. © Cambridge University Press 2013.

Idiopathic anejaculation/anorgasmia is characterized by the inability of the man to reach climax and ejaculate during sexual activity and/or masturbation. Many will have intermittent nocturnal emissions, suggesting normal ejaculation reflex components [7]. Most researchers in this area believe that this condition is psychogenic [8].

A variation of idiopathic anorgasmia is situational anorgasmia, in which the stress of a situation prevents the ability to climax. This is seen occasionally in a man under pressure to produce a semen specimen for in-vitro fertilization (IVF) [9]. A cancer patient, struggling with the recent diagnosis and upcoming treatment, may have enough stress to prevent obtaining a specimen for cryopreservation, as well [10,11].

Retrograde ejaculation is caused by failure of bladder neck closure during seminal emission, allowing the semen to flow backwards into the bladder. A man with retrograde ejaculation usually has a normal sense of climax, but no fluid is emitted from the urethra. The patient may notice cloudiness of the post-orgasm urine due to the presence of ejaculate. Retrograde ejaculation may be due to sympatholytic medications (such as alpha-blockers) [12], bladder neck surgery (transurethral prostatectomy) [13], and neurogenic dysfunction.

Often, the causes of neurogenic retrograde ejaculation may also cause total absence of ejaculation. The difference is only a matter of degree. If the sympathetic dysfunction is mild, there may still be seminal emission, but a weak contraction of the bladder neck may allow retrograde flow of semen. When the sympathetic dysfunction is more complete, neurogenic anejaculation may be the result. In testicular cancer patients who undergo retroperitoneal lymph node dissection (RPLND), there may be an insult to the neural structures that control ejaculation. If the neural insult is mild, retrograde ejaculation may occur, but the resultant dysfunction is usually total loss of seminal emission [14]. More complete neurogenic dysfunction, resulting in total loss of seminal emission, is discussed next.

Neurogenic anejaculation is caused by a variety of conditions, and therefore there may be varied presentations. In some cases, there may be complete inability to initiate an ejaculatory reflex. In other situations, an ejaculatory reflex may be possible, but there may be total loss of seminal emission because of end-nerve adrenergic dysfunction.

Etiologies of anejaculation not related to cancer include spinal cord injury (SCI) [15], diabetic neuropathy [16,17], spina bifida, multiple sclerosis, transverse myelitis, and vascular spine injuries. Medications, such as alpha-blockers, usually cause retrograde ejaculation, but in some individuals the response might be anemission. Antidepressants commonly cause anorgasmia and resultant inability to ejaculate [18].

Men with testicular cancer suffer from three potential insults to their fertility. **Pre-treatment subfertility** is a situation where the semen quality is compromised after orchiectomy, but before additional treatments [19]. This can compromise cryopreservation attempts. The reason for pre-treatment subfertility is not known. **Treatment-related subfertility** is the result of suppression of spermatogenesis due to radiation and/or chemotherapy damage to the germ cells. Ejaculatory dysfunction due to **retroperitoneal lymph node dissection (RPLND)** is the third possible insult to male fertility due to testis cancer treatment.

RPLND is an integral part of the treatment plan for many men with testicular cancer. Since the region where testicular cancer tends to spread, the lymph nodes just inferior to the renal veins surrounding the great vessels, is the location of the sympathetic components controlling ejaculation, the ejaculatory control mechanism is at risk in this type of operation. Nerve-sparing procedures have been devised to prevent ejaculatory dysfunction from this operation [20], but in cases of large tumor volume, and in post-chemotherapy situations, ejaculatory dysfunction remains common. It is strongly recommended that men cryopreserve semen prior to RPLND.

Procedures to induce ejaculation

Penile vibratory stimulation (PVS)

This is a method of inducing ejaculation in men via hyperstimulation of the sensory afferents of the penis. PVS has its greatest utility in inducing a response in men with spinal cord injury in whom the reflex arc is intact.

Stimulation is performed with a FertiCare vibrator, which has been FDA-approved for this purpose (Fig. 27.1). The vibrator is placed on the penile frenulum, with the goal of overstimulating the penile dorsal nerves (Fig. 27.2). This vibrator has optimized

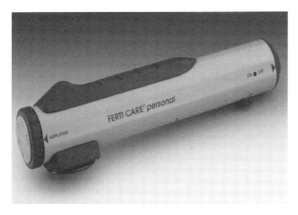

Figure 27.1. FertiCare Personal penile vibrator (Multicept A/S, Copenhagen, Denmark).

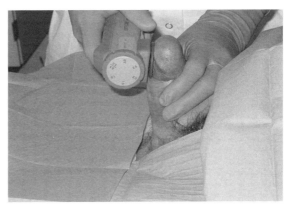

Figure 27.2. Penile vibrator in proper position, stimulating the penile frenulum.

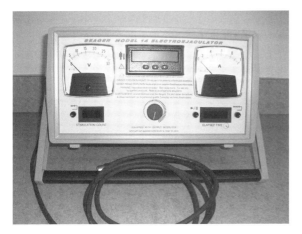

Figure 27.3. Seager Electroejaculator unit (Dalzell Medical Systems, The Plains, GA, USA).

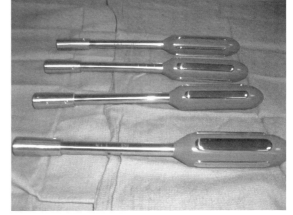

Figure 27.4. Seager Electroejaculator probes (Dalzell Medical Systems, The Plains, GA, USA).

vibration parameters, as defined by Sønksen *et al.* [20]. Simulation is carried out for three minutes, with rest periods of one minute between stimulation cycles. Repeated cycles are performed until ejaculation occurs, or six unsuccessful cycles have passed.

In performing PVS, the intention is to induce a reflex response, initiating the ejaculatory reflex. Response rates in upper motor neuron spinal cord injury are as high as 92% [21]. The procedure is less successful in men with missing portions of the local ejaculatory reflex. This includes lower motor neuron SCI, post-radical prostatectomy, diabetic neuropathy, and men who have undergone RPLND.

Electroejaculation (EEJ)

This is a method of inducing ejaculation that can work with, or without, an intact ejaculatory reflex arc. The

Seager Electroejaculator device is used for the procedures (Figs. 27.3 and 27.4). A rectal probe is inserted and cyclic electrical stimulation given to the pelvic floor and ejaculatory organs to induce an ejaculatory response (Fig. 27.5). Since the procedure is more invasive, there is an increased potential for complications, such as rectal injury. Furthermore, in men with normal sensation, unlike the SCI population, the EEJ procedure must be performed under general anesthesia. The procedure is nearly universally successful in inducing an ejaculate in all types of ejaculatory dysfunction. Early observations suggested that the response with EEJ was substantially different than that seen with PVS, but physiological measurements of the two procedures suggest that they are not so different [3].

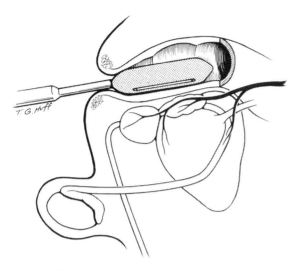

Figure 27.5. Anatomic positioning of the electroejaculation probe.

The greatest experience with EEJ, similar to PVS, has been in the SCI population [22], but the technique has proven efficacious in other etiologies as well. Successful ejaculation induced by EEJ has been seen in men with SCI, diabetic neuropathy, multiple sclerosis, idiopathic anejaculation, post-rectal cancer surgery, and post-RPLND for testicular cancer (see further discussion of RPLND patients below).

Ejaculation induction procedures for semen cryopreservation

Adults

In men who are presented with a new diagnosis of cancer, there is a great deal of stress. There is uncertainty about their own survival, and anxiety over what the treatment plan will be like and how much suffering is in the future as a result. Therefore, a situational anejaculation problem may arise.

There have been anecdotes of the use of penile vibratory stimulation in men who are unable to obtain a semen specimen when presented with the pressure of doing so for an IVF procedure [9]. PVS may allow such men to be successful. The same concept may be applied to those who feel the pressure to produce a specimen for cryopreservation after cancer diagnosis, but the practice is certainly not well established and/or documented in this patient population.

Adolescents

The adolescent patient with cancer represents a challenge in fertility preservation. There is an inherent discomfort in discussing the procurement of a specimen by masturbation, and in many cases it cannot be obtained [23]. Parents may overrule the idea of masturbation for their children, and the boys themselves may not admit to having masturbated in the past. Furthermore, an adolescent is clearly not mature enough to fully grasp the impact of current decision making on his future parenting potential. In situations where obtaining a semen specimen is problematic in this patient population, electroejaculation may have a role.

There have been two small series of the use of EEJ to obtain semen specimens from adolescents prior to chemotherapy. Muller *et al.* offered semen preservation to 45 boys aged 13–18 [24]. Ejaculation induction was unnecessary in 21, as they were successful in producing a specimen by masturbation. Two underwent successful EEJ under anesthesia. Sperm yields were variable. In the entire group (masturbation and EEJ), the total number of spermatozoa ranged from 0 to 210 million and sperm motility from 9% to 86%. One 13-year-old boy had a successful procedure with EEJ, and this success suggests that common thought on the age limit for attempts at cryopreservation may need to be extended, as this boy produced 75 million sperm with 38% motility via EEJ [24]. The same group reported success in one adolescent with the use of PVS [25].

Hovav *et al.* performed EEJ in six young male cancer patients (average age 18 years) prior to treatment. Average sperm concentrations were 16 million (range 0–45 million) and motility averaged 14% (range 0–53%) [26].

Fertility restoration after RPLND

Medical management

In men who suffer from either retrograde ejaculation or anejaculation due to RPLND, medical management may have a role. Since the problem is sympathetic denervation of the ejaculatory organs, sympathomimetic agents, such as ephedrine and imipramine, can be tried [27–29]. Efficacy rates remain well under 50% for these interventions, but since they are quite non-invasive, a trial of medical management cannot be criticized. If medical management is not enough to reverse retrograde ejaculation, post-ejaculation bladder harvest of sperm can be performed. This is done by first emptying the bladder and installing a sperm-friendly medium, and then, when ejaculation has taken place, collecting the sperm by catheterization. After processing, the sperm can be used for assisted reproductive technologies (ART).

Electroejaculation following RPLND

Because the dysfunction following RPLND affects sympathetic nerves arising from the spinal cord and coursing through the sympathetic chain, the reflex arc is not intact, since it lacks the outflow to effect the response. Therefore, PVS has no utility in the treatment of post-RPLND ejaculatory dysfunction. EEJ, on the other hand, does not depend on an intact reflex arc, and thus may be utilized for this purpose.

Electroejaculation in RPLND patients was first reported by Bennett et al. in 1987 [30]. The University of Michigan series was extended from this in a subsequent publication of results of 24 RPLND patients who underwent EEJ under general anesthesia. Twenty-one of the 24 men had total motile sperm counts in excess of 10 million. The average sperm count and motilities obtained were 289 million and 18%, respectively, for the antegrade fractions, and 2051 million and 13%, respectively, for the retrograde fractions. Three patients who underwent EEJ, with successful ejaculation induction, had no sperm present in the ejaculate. Two had experienced chemotherapy injury and one had carcinoma in situ in the remaining testis, obviously impairing fertility. With intrauterine insemination (IUI), 36.8% of the couples attempting fertility conceived a pregnancy, with a cycle fecundity of 9% per cycle [31].

Cost–benefit analysis

There are costs associated with ART in the United States, which are normally paid by the patients themselves. EEJ is no exception. Most testicular cancer survivors suffering from infertility following treatment who wish to have children will have to pay for such services. Therefore, cost-effectiveness must be considered in making recommendations for such patients.

A cost–benefit analysis published in 2001 suggested some guidelines for decision making in this area [32]. In this report, it was clear that EEJ coupled with IUI is cost-effective for men with SCI, in whom the EEJ procedure can be performed in the clinic setting without the need for an anesthetic. The analysis suggested that even though the cycle fecundity was relatively low,

the additional cost of moving to IVF increased the cost of care to unacceptably high levels. Therefore, for SCI men, repeated cycles of EEJ with IUI was determined to be the most cost-effective approach.

With non-SCI men, the analysis was not so straightforward. Since non-SCI men, including those who have had an RPLND, require an anesthetic to undergo EEJ, the increased cost of the anesthetic made EEJ/IUI *not* cost-effective for most couples. The recommendation for those individuals, as a group, was to bypass insemination altogether, and go directly to IVF. Since IVF with intracytoplasmic sperm injection (ICSI) can be performed with testicular aspirates, the need for EEJ was questioned.

An exception to this guideline can be envisioned when the total motile sperm count is in excess of 40 million with EEJ. In this subset of the case series, the cycle fecundity of EEJ coupled with IUI was 17.6%. This efficiency in achieving pregnancy made EEJ/IUI cost-effective. Therefore, if one examines a man who had had an RPLND, without prior chemotherapy, and finds normal testis size and a normal follicle-stimulating hormone (FSH) level, consideration can be given to an initial attempt with EEJ under anesthesia and IUI. If the total motile sperm count after processing is less than 40 million, future attempts at pregnancy should employ testis sperm aspiration and IVF. However, if the total motile sperm count exceeds 40 million after laboratory processing, continued attempts with EEJ and insemination may proceed.

Conclusion

Ejaculatory dysfunction, while an uncommon cause of infertility in cancer patients, needs to be considered in men having difficulty producing a specimen for cryopreservation or in men who are post-RPLND. In those individuals, after consideration of cost-effectiveness, penile vibratory stimulation and/or electroejaculation may have some benefit in the treatment plan.

References

1. Chughtai B, Sawas A, O'Malley RL, et al. A neglected gland: a review of Cowper's gland. *Int J Androl* 2005; 28: 74–7.

2. Thomas AJ. Ejaculatory dysfunction. *Fertil Steril* 1983; 39: 445–54.

3. Sønksen J, Ohl DA, Wedemeyer G. Sphincteric effects during penile vibratory ejaculation and

electroejaculation in men with spinal cord injuries, *J Urol* 2001; 165: 426–9.

4. Bohlen D, Hugonnet CL, Mills RD, *et al.* Five meters of H2O: the pressure at the urinary bladder neck during human ejaculation. *Prostate* 2000; 44: 339–41.

5. Laumann EO, Paik A, Rosen RC. Sexual dysfunction in the United States: prevalence and predictors. *JAMA* 1999; 281: 537–44.

6. Waldinger MD, Zwinderman AH, Olivier B, *et al.* Proposal for a definition of lifelong premature ejaculation based on epidemiological stopwatch data. *J Sex Med* 2005; 2: 498–507.

7. Hovav Y, Dan-Goor M, Yaffe H, *et al.* Nocturnal sperm emission in men with psychogenic anejaculation. *Fertil Steril* 1999; 72: 364–5.

8. Geboes K, Steeno O, De Moor P. Primary anejaculation: diagnosis and therapy. *Fertil Steril* 1975; 26: 1018–20.

9. Emery M, Senn A, Wisard M, *et al.* Ejaculation failure on the day of oocyte retrieval for IVF: case report. *Hum Reprod* 2004; 19: 2088–90.

10. Roopnarinesingh R, Keane D, Harrison R. Detecting mood disorders in men diagnosed with cancer who seek semen cryopreservation: a chance to improve service. *Ir Med J* 2003; 96: 104–7.

11. Bashore L. Semen preservation in male adolescents and young adults with cancer: one institution's experience. *Clin J Oncol Nurs* 2007; 11: 381–6.

12. Hellstrom WJ, Sikka SC. Effects of acute treatment with tamsulosin versus alfuzosin on ejaculatory function in normal volunteers. *J Urol* 2006; 176: 1529–33.

13. Thorpe AC, Cleary R, Coles J, *et al.* Written consent about sexual function in men undergoing transurethral prostatectomy. *Br J Urol* 1994; 74: 479–84.

14. Kedia KR, Markland C, Fraley EE. Sexual function following high retroperitoneal lymphadenectomy. *J Urol* 1975; 114: 237–9.

15. Sønksen J, Biering-Sørensen F. Fertility in men with spinal cord or cauda equina lesions. *Sem Neurol* 1992; 12: 106–14.

16. Genuth S. Insights from the diabetes control and complications trial/epidemiology of diabetes interventions and complications study on the use of intensive glycemic treatment to reduce the risk of complications of type 1 diabetes. *Endocrine Pract* 2006; 12 (Suppl 1): 34–41.

17. Sexton WJ, Jarow JP. Effect of diabetes mellitus upon male reproductive function. *Urology* 1997; 49: 508–13.

18. Montejo AL, Llorca G, Izquierdo JA, *et al.* Incidence of sexual dysfunction associated with antidepressant agents: a prospective multicenter study of 1022 outpatients. *J Clin Psychiatry* 2001; 62 (Suppl 3): 10–21.

19. Fossa SD, Aabyholm T, Vespestad S, *et al.* Semen quality after treatment for testicular cancer. *Eur Urol* 1993; 23: 172–6.

20. Donohue JP, Foster RS, Rowland RG, *et al.* Nerve-sparing retroperitoneal lymphadenectomy with preservation of ejaculation. *J Urol* 1990; 144: 287–91.

21. Sønksen J, Biering-Sørensen F, Kristensen JK. Ejaculation induced by penile vibratory stimulation in men with spinal cord lesion. The importance of the vibratory amplitude. *Paraplegia* 1994; 32: 651–60.

22. Ohl DA, Quallich SA, Sønksen J, Brackett NL, Lynne CM. Anejaculation: an electrifying approach. *Semin Reprod Med* 2009; 27: 179–85.

23. Edge B, Holmes D, Makin G. Sperm banking in adolescent cancer patients. *Arch Dis Child* 2006; 91: 149–52.

24. Muller J, Sønksen J, Sommer P, *et al.* Cryopreservation of semen from pubertal boys with cancer. *Med Pediatr Oncol* 2000; 34: 191–4.

25. Schmiegelow ML, Sommer P, Carlsen E, *et al.* Penile vibratory stimulation and electroejaculation before anticancer therapy in two pubertal boys. *J Pediatr Hematol Oncol* 1998; 20: 429–30.

26. Hovav Y, Dan-Goor M, Yaffe H, *et al.* Electroejaculation before chemotherapy in adolescents and young men with cancer. *Fertil Steril* 2001; 75: 811–13.

27. Gilja I, Parazajder J, Cvitkovic P, *et al.* Retrograde ejaculation and loss of emission: possibilities of conservative treatment. *Eur Urol* 1994; 25: 256–8.

28. Narayan P, Lange P, Fraley E. Ejaculation and fertility after extended retroperitoneal lymph node dissection for testicular cancer. *J Urol* 1982; 127: 685–8.

29. Yuanhui X. Treatment of functional retrograde ejaculation with acupuncture and TCM herbal drugs. *J Trad Chinese Med* 2002; 22: 286–7.

30. Bennett CJ, Seager SW, McGuire EJ. Electroejaculation for recovery of semen after retroperitoneal lymph node dissection: case report. *J Urol* 1987; 137: 513–15.

31. Ohl DA, Denil J, Bennett CJ, *et al.* Electroejaculation following retroperitoneal lymphadenectomy. *J Urol* 1991; 145: 980–3.

32. Ohl DA, Wolf LJ, Menge AC, *et al.* Electroejaculation and assisted reproductive technologies in the treatment of anejaculatory infertility. *Fertil Steril* 2001; 76: 1249–55.

Sperm extraction in the pre-therapy patient

Wayland Hsiao and Peter N. Schlegel

Introduction

Advances in cancer treatment have led to greater longevity and an increased recognition that quality of life, including paternity, is a significant issue. Sperm cryopreservation prior to treatment is the preferred management to preserve fertility for men planning treatment that may affect future fertility. This chapter will discuss the options for fertility preservation in a man with cancer, and will specifically focus on the treatment options available to the cancer patient who is found to be azoospermic at the time of cancer diagnosis. At the end of the chapter we propose a treatment algorithm that may simplify the approach to the cancer patient desiring to preserve fertility and may help avoid unnecessary procedures.

Cryopreservation of sperm remains the cornerstone of fertility preservation in the man with cancer. While a man with normal or even low sperm counts in his ejaculate can relatively easily present a sample for cryopreservation, there are a number of reasons that cancer patients may be azoospermic at the time of their diagnosis. One possibility is that the cancer itself may disrupt fertility even prior to the initiation of antineoplastic treatment, and suboptimal semen analysis parameters have been seen even before systemic treatment in patients with leukemia, lymphoma, and testicular cancer [1–6]. Studies have shown that up to 13.8% of all patients who attempt to bank sperm prior to cancer treatment are azoospermic [7,8]. It remains controversial, however, whether the type of malignancy predicts lower sperm quality or affects assisted reproduction outcomes [5,7,9,10]. Therefore, even if it is not a cancer of the reproductive tract itself (testis, seminal vesicles, prostate, or urethra), cancer may affect the reproductive tract.

In the era before the introduction of intracystoplasmic sperm injection (ICSI), successful in-vitro fertilization required many millions of motile sperm that were capable of undergoing the acrosome reaction. Therefore, the use of surgically retrieved sperm was limited in the assisted reproduction laboratory of that era. With the advent of ICSI [11] it became possible to use exceedingly low numbers of surgically retrieved sperm (even non-motile testicular sperm) for successful assisted reproduction. Therefore, in the modern era of widespread application of ICSI, the ability to preserve fertility has been expanded even to those men who lack sperm in the ejaculate. With surgically retrieved sperm, we are able to preserve fertility potential as long as we are able to find sperm in the reproductive tract.

The challenges for the azoospermic cancer patient are unique because the urgency of getting necessary chemotherapy must be balanced with the need to undergo procedures to successfully preserve sperm. Any fertility treatment offered must be of minimal morbidity while not significantly delaying needed chemotherapeutic treatment. For azoospermic patients, fertility preservation options include cryopreservation of testicular spermatozoa from the normal testis, cryopreservation of spermatozoa from the diseased testis (in cases of testicular cancer), or cryopreservation of epididymal or vasal sperm.

We will now discuss the various methods available to retrieve sperm for cryopreservation. The indications for a procedure and the available data will be reviewed.

Fertility Preservation in Male Cancer Patients, ed. John P. Mulhall, Linda D. Applegarth, Robert D. Oates and Peter N. Schlegel. Published by Cambridge University Press. © Cambridge University Press 2013.

Percutaneous testicular and epididymal aspiration

For patients who both have normal levels of sperm production and are either azoospermic (obstructive azoospermia) or anejaculate, percutaneous testicular or epididymal aspiration can be performed under local anesthesia. Percutaneous techniques for sperm retrieval include fine-needle testicular sperm aspiration (TESA), percutaneous epididymal sperm aspiration (PESA), and percutaneous biopsy of the testis. Anesthesia can be achieved with a local skin block and a spermatic cord nerve block. Again, these procedures should not be performed on patients with nonobstructive azoospermia because of the potentially low yield due to poor sperm production. Patients who fall into this category would include cancer patients who have a history of vasectomy or other inguinopelvic surgery that can potentially cause vasal obstruction. Also, patients with congenital absence of the vas deferens would be good candidates. Finally, patients with any malignancy that may cause vasal obstruction or would preclude masturbation or electroejaculation may be good candidates for these procedures, assuming adequate levels of sperm production.

Fine-needle TESA is the easiest of these procedures to perform, but yields much lower numbers of sperm than open surgical retrieval [12]. After local anesthesia is given to the scrotal skin, as well as a spermatic cord block, the testis is stabilized and a needle is inserted deep into the testis along its long axis. The needle is withdrawn slightly and redirected in order to disrupt the testicular architecture while aspiration is performed. The procedure can be repeated to increase the yield of testicular tissue.

PESA can also be performed under local anesthesia. For this procedure, we use a 21-gauge butterfly needle attached to a 20 mL syringe. The needle is inserted into the caput epididymis and then slowly withdrawn until fluid can be seen in the tubing. The tubing is then clamped and the fluid flushed out with medium. Difficulties in the procedure include being unable to palpate and stabilize the epididymis effectively, failure to retrieve sperm, and admixture of degenerating sperm with better-quality sperm samples.

The final percutaneous procedure is biopsy of the testicle using a 15-gauge biopsy gun with a short (1 cm) excursion, again under local anesthesia with a spermatic cord block to provide anesthesia. We usually start by making a small nick in the inferior aspect of

the scrotal skin overlying the trapped testis or use a larger-bore needle to make a small hole in the scrotal skin. The biopsy gun is then advanced along that same tract right up to the tunica albugina of the testis and the biopsy gun fired. Multiple biopsies can be obtained through a single entry site. It is best to avoid performing the biopsy along the midline longitudinal plane, and we angle our biopsies towards the contralateral shoulder because of the large longitudinal vessel that is commonly on the midline of the anterior testis. This procedure can provide higher sperm yield than needle aspiration, but it provides fewer sperm with lower motility than microsurgical epididymal sperm aspiration [13].

Surgical retrieval of vasal or epididymal sperm

Patients with epididymal obstruction but with normal sperm production are candidates for surgical retrieval of epididymal sperm. Our preferred approach is a microsurgical epididymal sperm aspiration (MESA), the technique by which the epididymis is exposed microsurgically and punctured with a pulled glass pipette and epididymal fluid is aspirated. Using the microsurgical approach we are able to retrieve many millions of sperm that can be subsequently cryopreserved. While theoretically sperm can also be aspirated and preserved from the vas by performing a hemivasotomy, aspiration of the epididymis is our preferred approach because any vasal obstruction would also cause epididymal dilation, and sperm quality (motility) is generally better closer to the testis in obstructed patients. In cancer patients, there are very limited data on these procedures. Baniel and Sella reported on three testicular cancer patients in whom vasal and epididymal sperm were successfully aspirated from the cancer-bearing testis and cryopreserved at the time of orchiectomy [14]. In this series two pregnancies were achieved using the cryopreserved sperm.

Surgical retrieval of testicular sperm

In those patients who have primary testicular failure (non-obstructive azoospermia) surgical retrieval of testicular sperm coupled with IVF-ICSI may represent the only hope of fertility preservation. The traditional approach to testicular sperm extraction (TESE) involved a random testicular biopsy followed by evaluation for sperm in the andrology laboratory. The

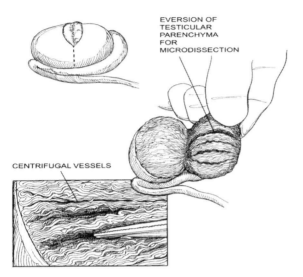

Figure 28.1. MicroTESE: a transverse incision is made in the testis and the testicular tissue is everted and microdissected for thorough inspection of all tubules. (© Brady Urology Foundation, 2011.)

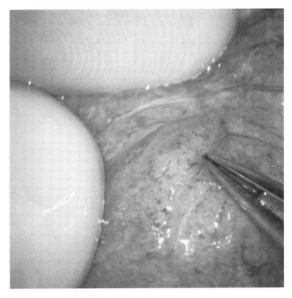

Figure 28.2. MicroTESE: intraoperative picture of tubules more likely to harbor spermatogenesis, indicated by forceps.

risk of testicular injury along with low spermatozoa yields in conventional TESE led to the development of microsurgical TESE (microTESE). The technique involves placing a wide incision in the tunica albuginea in an avascular region and eversion of the testicular parenchyma, allowing for microscopic inspection of the testicular parenchyma and identification of sperm-producing tubules (Fig. 28.1). Under high-power (25×) magnification, tubules with spermatozoa appear larger and more opaque than the fibrotic Sertoli-cell-only tubules (Fig. 28.2). Subtunical vessels as well as intratesticular vessels can also be identified and better preserved using the operating microscope. Overall, microTESE has been shown to result in an increased chance of retrieving sperm, higher numbers of sperm harvested, and decreased testicular tissue removed [15,16].

Testicular cancer patients: special considerations

Testicular cancer patients have a unique set of problems from a fertility preservation perspective because at least one testis will typically be removed during cancer treatment. However, there remain a variety of options available to these patients for preservation of spermatozoa. Sperm retrieval is possible at the time of orchiectomy from either the contralateral normal testis or the normal parenchyma of the affected testis (such retrieval is done on a sterile "back-table" after extirpation of the testis from the patient to avoid spillage and contamination). Vasal or epididymal sperm can also be retrieved from the orchiectomy specimen. In cases of partial orchiectomy, the surrounding normal testicular parenchyma can be examined and specimens collected for cryopreservation as well.

A number of case reports have shown that testicular sperm from the testicle harboring the cancer can result in successful live birth [17–19], but more research with larger numbers of patients is needed before this becomes routine practice. However, it is also possible to obtain sperm from the epididymis or vas in these patients. In a fascinating study, Delouya *et al.* reviewed pathologic specimens of 39 radical orchiectomy specimens with an emphasis on the extent of spermatogenesis present in the normal surrounding parenchyma [20]. In this study, 50% of evaluable epididymal sections contained sperm. When the testicular parenchyma was examined, 40% of the specimens had full spermatogenesis as the dominant histological pattern, and nearly 80% of the testes revealed evidence of focally complete spermatogenesis. This study is important because it suggests that in up to 50% of orchiectomy specimens, epididymal or vasal sperm can be successfully retrieved and cryopreserved. For those patients whose production is so low that there

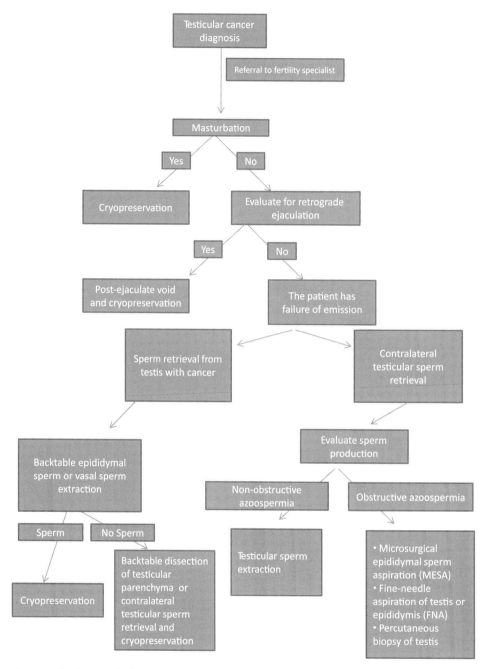

Figure 28.3. Algorithm for fertility preservation in the newly diagnosed testicular cancer patient.

are no sperm in the epididymis, sperm should be found in about 40% of patients with random biopsy while, theoretically, sperm can be found in up to 80% of specimens with a testicular microdissection approach in a sterile field after removal of the radical orchiectomy specimen from the patient. Interestingly, these numbers agree with data generated by Schrader *et al.* in one of the largest studies of preoperative sperm retrieval outcomes, which reported on 31 azoospermic men with either testicular cancer or lymphoma prior to chemotherapy [21]. In testicular cancer patients, standard testicular sperm extraction was performed

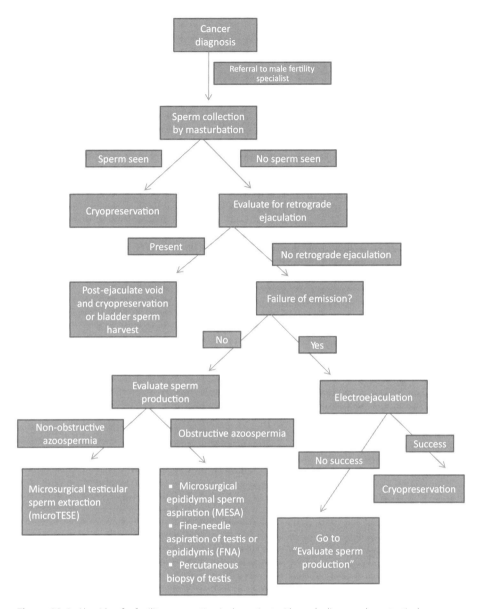

Figure 28.4. Algorithm for fertility preservation in the patient with newly diagnosed non-testicular cancer.

on the contralateral testicle. Lymphoma patients underwent bilateral standard testicular sperm extraction prior to chemotherapy. The sperm retrieval rate was 43% (6/14) in testicular cancer and 47% (8/17) in patients with Hodgkin's or non-Hodgkin's lymphoma.

Routine testicular sperm extraction after orchiectomy, however, would not be without its disadvantages. As Delouya *et al.* wisely note, the violation of the tunica albuginea for testis dissection for sperm

retrieval may affect pathologic staging [20]. Therefore, cryopreservation of vasal or epididymal sperm on a backtable may be the preferred first-line approach in this setting because of higher sperm yields, providing sperm which are more likely to survive cryopreservation, with better preservation of pathologic staging. With all this in mind, we propose an algorithm for fertility preservation in the newly diagnosed testicular cancer patient (Fig. 28.3).

Conclusion

Cancer patients interested in future fertility face a number of unique challenges, including balancing timing of treatment for cancer with possible treatments for fertility preservation. While cryopreservation is the current cornerstone of male fertility preservation, there are numerous ways in which sperm can be obtained for cryopreservation. In order to simplify the approach to the patient with newly diagnosed non-testicular cancer who desires to preserve fertility, we propose a second algorithm (Fig. 28.4). We hope that this algorithm will make the approach much more straightforward and avoid unnecessary procedures.

Acknowledgments

Dr. Hsiao is supported by a grant from the Frederick J. and Theresa Dow Wallace Fund of the New York Community Trust.

References

1. Spermon JR, Ramos L, Wetzels AM, et al. Sperm integrity pre- and post-chemotherapy in men with testicular germ cell cancer. *Hum Reprod* 2006; 21: 1781–6.

2. Berthelsen JG, Skakkebaek NE. Gonadal function in men with testis cancer. *Fertil Steril* 1983; 39: 68–75.

3. Sanger WG, Armitage JO, Schmidt MA. Feasibility of semen cryopreservation in patients with malignant disease. *JAMA* 1980; 244: 789–90.

4. Viviani S, Ragni G, Santoro A, et al. Testicular dysfunction in Hodgkin's disease before and after treatment. *Eur J Cancer* 1991; 27: 1389–92.

5. Williams DH 4th, Karpman E, Sander JC, et al. Pretreatment semen parameters in men with cancer. *J Urol* 2009; 181: 736–40.

6. van Casteren NJ, Boellaard WP, Romijn JC, Dohle GR. Gonadal dysfunction in male cancer patients before cytotoxic treatment. *Int J Androl*; 33: 73–9.

7. Lass A, Akagbosu F, Abusheikha N, et al. A programme of semen cryopreservation for patients with malignant disease in a tertiary infertility centre: lessons from 8 years' experience. *Hum Reprod* 1998; 13: 3256–61.

8. Ragni G, Somigliana E, Restelli L, et al. Sperm banking and rate of assisted reproduction treatment: insights from a 15-year cryopreservation program for male cancer patients. *Cancer* 2003; 97: 1624–9.

9. Khalifa E, Oehninger S, Acosta AA, et al. Successful fertilization and pregnancy outcome in in-vitro fertilization using cryopreserved/thawed spermatozoa from patients with malignant diseases. *Hum Reprod* 1992; 7: 105–8.

10. Padron OF, Sharma RK, Thomas AJ, Agarwal A. Effects of cancer on spermatozoa quality after cryopreservation: a 12-year experience. *Fertil Steril* 1997; 67: 326–31.

11. Palermo G, Joris H, Devroey P, Van Steirteghem AC. Pregnancies after intracytoplasmic injection of single spermatozoon into an oocyte. *Lancet* 1992; 340: 17–18.

12. Friedler S, Raziel A, Strassburger D, et al. Testicular sperm retrieval by percutaneous fine needle sperm aspiration compared with testicular sperm extraction by open biopsy in men with non-obstructive azoospermia. *Hum Reprod* 1997; 12: 1488–93.

13. Sheynkin YR, Ye Z, Menendez S, et al. Controlled comparison of percutaneous and microsurgical sperm retrieval in men with obstructive azoospermia. *Hum Reprod* 1998; 13: 3086–9.

14. Baniel J, Sella A. Sperm extraction at orchiectomy for testis cancer. *Fertil Steril* 2001; 75: 260–2.

15. Schlegel PN. Testicular sperm extraction: microdissection improves sperm yield with minimal tissue excision. *Hum Reprod* 1999; 14: 131–5.

16. Tsujimura A, Matsumiya K, Miyagawa Y, et al. Conventional multiple or microdissection testicular sperm extraction: a comparative study. *Hum Reprod* 2002; 17: 2924–9.

17. Carmignani L, Gadda F, Gazzano G, et al. Testicular sperm extraction in cancerous testicle in patients with azoospermia: a case report. *Hum Reprod* 2007; 22: 1068–72.

18. Descombe L, Chauleur C, Gentil-Perret A, et al. Testicular sperm extraction in a single cancerous testicle in patients with azoospermia: a case report. *Fertil Steril* 2008; 90: 443.e1–4.

19. Kohn FM, Schroeder-Printzen I, Weidner W, et al. Testicular sperm extraction in a patient with metachronous bilateral testicular cancer. *Hum Reprod* 2001; 16: 2343–6.

20. Delouya G, Baazeem A, Boman JM, et al. Identification of spermatozoa in archived testicular cancer specimens: implications for bench side sperm retrieval at orchiectomy. *Urology* 2010; 75: 1436–40.

21. Schrader M, Muller M, Sofikitis N, et al. "Onco-tese": testicular sperm extraction in azoospermic cancer patients before chemotherapy-new guidelines? *Urology* 2003; 61: 421–5.

Chapter

29

Fertility preservation in the pediatric population: germ cell culture and transplantation

Kate H. Kraft and Thomas F. Kolon

Childhood cancer

Approximately 10 700 new cases of childhood cancer were diagnosed among children aged 0–14 years in 2010. Although childhood cancers are rare, comprising less than 1% of all new cancer diagnoses, cancer is the second leading cause of death in children [1]. According to the International Classification of Childhood Cancer, the most common childhood cancers include leukemia (31%), brain and other nervous system (21%), neuroblastoma (7%), Wilms' tumor (5%), non-Hodgkin's lymphoma (4%), Hodgkin's lymphoma (4%), rhabdomyosarcoma (3%), retinoblastoma (3%), osteosarcoma (2.5%), and Ewing sarcoma (2%) [1]. The survival rate of most childhood cancers has grown progressively more favorable over the past several decades, with five-year relative survival rates less than 50% before the 1970s rising to 80% today. The increased success of therapy in young boys with cancer has shifted the emphasis toward long-term quality-of-life issues [1].

While improved treatments such as chemotherapy and radiation have prolonged cancer survival in boys, they can produce significant complications such as infertility that may not be apparent until adulthood. A multicenter study of five-year childhood cancer survivors of solid tumor malignancies and Hodgkin's lymphoma diagnosed before 20 years of age revealed a 15% incidence of compromised fertility, seen more commonly in boys than in girls [2]. Many young cancer survivors have an increased desire for children and feel the cancer survival experience would potentially make them better parents [3]. In 2006, the American Society of Clinical Oncology (ASCO) recommended that oncologists discuss fertility preservation with all newly diagnosed cancer patients at the earliest

opportunity [4]. Smaller studies have shown that infertility can result in significant stress among this population [5,6].

Cancer treatment: radiation and chemotherapy

The most common treatment options available to pediatric cancer patients include surgical resection when indicated, chemotherapy, and radiation. The risk of infertility can be stratified based on the type of malignancy and the associated treatment [7] (Table 29.1). Chemotherapy and radiation may be well tolerated by the patient in the short term but can inflict dose-dependent toxicity on the gonads, severely damaging the germinal epithelium of the testis and permanently impeding fertility [8,9]. One of the most common long-term adverse side effects of chemotherapy in men is treatment-induced gonadal failure. Depending on the type and dose of a chemotherapeutic agent, rates of azoospermia in male patients undergoing chemotherapy range between 33% and 90% [10]. The germinal epithelium is particularly susceptible to injury from cytotoxic agents because of its high mitotic rate. The extent of injury to spermatogenesis depends on patient age, type of chemotherapeutic agent, dose, and schedule. Both prepubertal and postpubertal testes are at risk of injury from chemotherapeutic agents [8,11,12]. Spermatogenesis may take up to two years to recover from cytotoxic impairment, although sperm counts are typically at their lowest during the first six months after completion of therapy [13]. A delay in recuperation of spermatogenesis as long as 14 years has been reported

Fertility Preservation in Male Cancer Patients, ed. John P. Mulhall, Linda D. Applegarth, Robert D. Oates and Peter N. Schlegel.
Published by Cambridge University Press. © Cambridge University Press 2013.

Table 29.1. Risk of subfertility after treatment for common cancers in childhood and adolescence

Low risk (<20%)

Acute lymphoblastic leukemia
Wilms' tumor
Soft tissue sarcoma: stage I
Germ cell tumors (wish gonadal preservation and no
    radiotherapy)
Retinoblastoma
Brain tumor: surgery only, cranial irradiation
    <24 Gy

Medium risk (20–80%)

Acute myeloblastic leukemia (difficult to quantify)
Hepatoblastoma
Osteosarcoma
Ewing sarcoma: non-metastatic
Soft tissue sarcoma: stage II or III
Neuroblastoma
Non-Hodgkin's lymphoma
Hodgkin's lymphoma: alternating treatment
Brain tumor: craniospinal radiotherapy, cranial irradiation
    >24 Gy

High risk (>80%)

Total-body irradiation
Localized radiotherapy: pelvic or testicular
Chemotherapy conditioning for bone marrow transplantation
Hodgkin's lymphoma: treatment with alkylating drugs
Soft tissue sarcoma: stage IV (metastatic)
Ewing sarcoma: metastatic

previously [14,15]. Semen analysis following completion of therapy in postpubertal patients, with focus on sperm concentration, motility, and morphology, may help assess future reproductive potential. Compared to the germinal epithelium, Leydig cells are comparatively resistant to the effects of chemotherapy [16].

The effects of radiation, even in low doses, result in significant disturbances of testicular tissue at the cellular level, thereby compromising spermatogenesis [17]. These treatment methods can destroy sperm counts, motility, morphology, or even the integrity of genetic material. Testes are usually not subject to direct radiation, except in rare cases, but body scatter can distribute radiation to the testes indirectly, depending on the proximity of the radiation field to the target, the field size and shape, the x-ray energy, and the depth of the target. Scatter dose is increased particularly when the treated field extends into the pelvis. Additionally, young boys may be at greater risk for scatter because of their short trunk length [18]. In the adult literature, recovery from azoospermia after radiation may take as long as six years [19]. A gonadal shield can lower the radiation dose to the testes between 3- and 10-fold

[20], and this reduction can significantly impact fertility potential by decreasing the period without spermatozoa in semen following discontinuation of radiation therapy [19]. Hormone therapy has also been considered for gonadal protection, with the thought that if the proliferation of germ cells could be hormonally halted, they would be less vulnerable to cytotoxic therapy. Attempts to develop a successful hormonal regimen to protect the gonads have failed to date [21].

Ash evaluated testicular function following incremental doses of radiation in cancer patients and reported that oligospermia may occur at doses starting at 10 cGy. Azoospermia can occur around 35 cGy, and permanent sterilization can occur with doses as low as 100 cGy [9]. In stem cell transplant patients, total-body irradiation can expose the testes to radiation doses sufficient for permanent infertility [22]. As with chemotherapy, Leydig cells are more resistant to the effects of radiation than germinal epithelial cells, but studies have shown functional changes in Leydig cells following testicular irradiation. The effect on Leydig cells worsens in younger patients, but prepubertal boys who undergo radiation therapy in childhood proceed through puberty normally, indicating a subclinical impact on Leydig cell function [23]. Cranial radiation may impair male fertility not by direct insult to the testes but rather by disruption of the hypothalamic–pituitary–gonadal (HPG) axis [24]. Additionally, the primary malignancy itself, such as Hodgkin's lymphoma or testicular cancer, may render the patient azoospermic even before initiation of treatment [25,26].

Options for fertility preservation

Sperm acquisition

Infertility may be a long-term adverse consequence of childhood cancer treatment, particularly since limited means for preserving fertility in prepubertal boys are currently available. Options for male fertility preservation include sperm banking for postpubertal boys and cryopreservation and transplantation of spermatogonia and testicular tissue for prepubertal boys (Table 29.2). Hormone suppression has been discussed as an alternative option, but little evidence supports the efficacy of this option either in reducing the risk of infertility or in facilitating recovery of spermatogenesis after treatment [27].

Table 29.2. Fertility preservation options for males

	Sperm banking (masturbation)	Sperm banking (alternative collection methods)	Radiation shielding of gonads	Testicular tissue freezing	Testicular sperm extraction	Donor sperm	Adoption
Medical Status	Standard	Experimental	Standard	Experimental	Standard	Standard	Standard
Definition	Sperm obtained through masturbation and then frozen	Sperm obtained through testicular extraction or electroejaculation under sedation	Use of shielding to reduce the dose of radiation delivered to the testes	Tissue obtained through biopsy and frozen for future use	Use of biopsy to obtain individual sperm from testicular tissue	Sperm donated by a man for artificial insemination or IVF	Process that creates a legal parent–child relationship
Pubertal status	After puberty	After puberty	Before or after puberty	Before or after puberty	After puberty	After puberty	After puberty
Time requirement	Outpatient procedure	Outpatient procedure	In conjunction with radiation treatments	Outpatient procedure	Outpatient procedure	Readily available for purchase	Varies depending on type of adoption
Success rates	Generally high; the most established technique for men	If sperm is obtained, similar to standard sperm banking	Possible with select radiation fields and anatomy	No available human success rates	30–70% in postpubertal patients	50–80%	N/A

Cryopreservation of sperm before onset of oncologic therapy is the most reliable method of preserving future fertility in adolescent boys. Banking sperm prior to initiation of therapy is essential, as quantity and condition of sperm acquired after starting treatment may be diminished [27]. Instructions for collection should include practicing abstinence for at least 48 hours and submission of multiple semen samples to maximize the amount of sperm available for cryopreservation [28]. Patients may be unable to submit semen samples acquired by masturbation, because of age, embarrassment, cultural or religious beliefs [29]. Sperm banking may also be limited by time constraints surrounding treatment, which limit focus on fertility and promote expedient initiation of therapy.

More invasive alternatives for semen collection are available if masturbation is not possible or if the patient has obstructive azoospermia [28]. These options include microsurgical epididymal sperm aspiration, testicular sperm extraction, or electroejaculation [30]. Assisted reproductive techniques such as intracytoplasmic sperm injection (ICSI) require only minimal numbers of viable sperm to complete fertilization successfully, which may allow azoospermic patients to achieve paternity despite reduced sperm counts [28]. Penile vibratory stimulation is an alternative method that generates a potent sensory effect on the ejaculatory reflex center, thereby inducing antegrade ejaculation. Due to its non-invasive and relatively simple technology, penile vibratory stimulation may be considered a first-line choice for future fertility. However, young boys may have difficulty grasping this concept or executing the procedure [31].

Performed under general anesthesia, electroejaculation involves manual expression of seminal fluid from the perineal and penile urethra as well as bladder catheterization for retrograde emission. Alternatively, a testicular biopsy for sperm extraction may also be conducted under general anesthesia. These are less desirable techniques for sperm harvesting because of the need for a general anesthetic, and studies on young cancer patients suggest poor motility among sperm obtained using these methods [32].

Stem cell autotransplantation

All options for fertility preservation in prepubertal boys remain experimental and should probably be pursued only under the auspices of a clinical trial approved by the institutional review board. Principles behind fertility preservation in this age group include collecting testicular tissue sampled prior to chemotherapy and/or radiation and subsequently autotransplanting spermatogonial stem cells (SSC) harvested from the stored tissue after successful cancer treatment [33]. The open biopsy of testicular tissue has proven safe with no evidence of long-term adverse effects in cryptorchid patients undergoing orchiopexy. SSC transplant was first achieved in a murine model [34], and since then additional spermatogonial autotransplantation endeavors with bovine, goat, and primate stem cells have proven successful [35–37]. Recent reports show that embryonic primordial germ cells isolated from mice have the potential to function as germ-line stem cells, colonizing the testis and generating male germ cells [38]. This suggests that the testicular microenviroment is unique in that it permits germ-line stem cells to enter differentiation [39].

Transplantation may be achieved by grafting tissue to an ectopic site where sperm can be generated once revascularization of the graft takes place, or SSCs can be transplanted directly back into the testis to recolonize the seminiferous tubules [34,35]. Three different methods to introduce donor cells into recipient tubules have been described in the rodent model. First, cells are injected directly into seminiferous tubules, flowing to the rete testis. Second, cells are injected directly into the rete testis. Third, donor cells are injected into an efferent ductule, also leading to the rete testis [40]. Additionally, spermatogonial cells from a variety of species, including human, can colonize the basal membrane of seminiferous tubules of mice after transplantation.

Stem cell culture

Spermatogonial cells taken from prepubertal individuals in bovine, mouse, rat, and hamster models have been successfully propagated in in-vitro culture [41–45]. Such experimentation permits in-vitro functional testing of spermatogonial stem cells in a preclinical setting [46–50]. Small testicular tissue samples are insufficient for complete recolonization of the testis following cancer treatment, and therefore in-vitro proliferation of human spermatogonial stem cells is required to achieve a sufficient number of cells for successful autotransplantation.

The first successful long-term culture and propagation of human spermatogonial cells was recently reported by Sadri-Ardekani et al., who colonized mouse seminiferous tubules with human spermatogonial stem cells from long-term cultured testicular

cells, indicating stem cell capability of these cells after long-term culture [51]. Their culture system resulted in a more than 18 000-fold increase in spermatogonial stem cells. Their calculations suggest that at least a 1300-fold increase in spermatogonial stem cells is needed for sufficient transplantation, based on the fact that a biopsy size of 0.2 mL from a prepubertal testis needs to increase 65-fold to colonize an adult testis of approximately 13 mL [51,52]. The 18 000-fold increase in human spermatogonial stem cells proves more than sufficient for adequate transplantation [51]. Other factors such as discerning an ideal culture medium for SSC proliferation are being refined in the animal model and require mastering before such techniques are clinically applicable [53].

Only recently have prepubertal human spermatogonia successfully been harvested and cultured in a murine model [54]. Wu et al. isolated pure populations of prepubertal human spermatogonia using protein markers, and stem cell potential of the prepubertal germ cells was demonstrated by transplantation to mouse testes. These human germ cells subsequently migrated to the basement membrane of the murine seminiferous tubule and were maintained as SSCs. The migration of human spermatogonia to the mouse tubules indicates a conservation of the "homing" mechanism in these prepubertal germ cells despite the divergence in species [54]. The ability to maintain prepubertal human SSCs in vitro lends hope to future efforts to preserve fertility in prepubertal boys undergoing cancer treatment.

Although cryopreservation of testicular tissue in the prepubertal population remains experimental, a majority of parents wish to proceed with tissue banking when it is offered at the time of their child's diagnosis. A recent survey of parents demonstrated a 76% rate of acceptance toward testicular tissue cryopreservation for patients with stage IV sarcomas whose therapy would be highly gonadotoxic. Among those, 68% felt that proceeding with tissue banking for possible future fertility preservation was "a great idea for my son" [55]. The same series has reported no acute adverse effects of the testicular biopsy, suggesting that this procedure is well tolerated and carries low morbidity [55]. Therefore, families interested in fertility preservation for their young sons should be encouraged to proceed with testicular tissue cryopreservation but informed explicitly of its experimental nature.

To date, no human pregnancy utilizing SSC transplantation has been reported. Live births using grafted testicular tissue to generate spermatozoa have been reported only in rodents [39]. Essential steps for successful recolonization of germ cells include safe retrieval of sufficient testicular tissue before cytotoxic therapy, cryopreservation and thawing of cell suspensions or tissue, enrichment of SSCs, and efficient non-invasive transfer of germ cell suspensions into the rete testis [39]. Concerns regarding spermatogonial auto-transplantation include achieving an adequate biopsy of gonadal tissue without damaging the testis and avoiding reintroduction of tumor cells from the transplanted stem cells. Risk of malignancy relapse may be even higher with the isolation of gonadal tissue, given the blood–testis barrier and the potential for harboring contaminated cells. Flow cytometry has been shown to eliminate leukemic cell contamination from testicular samples [56]. Additional methods for eradicating malignant cells prior to autotransplantation, particularly in the case of non-solid tumors, are currently in development [56,57].

If the patient or his family does not wish to pursue cryopreservation of sperm or testicular tissue, alternative options for reproduction in pediatric cancer survivors include use of donor oocytes, donor sperm, and adoption.

Future directions and ethical issues

Studies to date addressing the attitudes of pediatric patients toward reproductive potential have been limited by pooling young boys and adolescents with adults. The male pediatric cancer patient population spans a wide age range and has varying levels of maturity and concern about future fertility [30]. The possibility of infertility usually takes young cancer survivors by surprise. Surveys of these patients reveal that 30–60% do not recall receiving any information regarding the risk of infertility from their healthcare providers at the time of their cancer diagnosis [58–61]. Survivors of adolescent cancer recall discussions of possible infertility occurring more often after initiation of therapy rather than at the time of their diagnosis [62].

Fertility remains an important concern for young survivors of pediatric cancer, and they are particularly interested in producing their own offspring rather than choosing a third-party option or adoption [60,62]. As many as 76% of young male cancer survivors have expressed a desire to have children after completion of their cancer treatment [58], and many cancer patients have articulated that their cancer experience would actually make them better parents [58,60]. Qualitative studies have also shown that infertility may cause long-term distress and anxiety in male cancer patients [6,58]. Male cancer patients who have banked sperm have reaped psychological benefit, as it provided hope for life after therapy and served as a positive factor in coping with their diagnosis [63]. For those whose prognosis is poor, some patients and their families consider the possibility of posthumous reproduction, which the American Society for Reproductive Medicine recommends physicians encourage should the family desire this form of fertility preservation [64]. However, this decision is fraught with numerous ethical quandaries. Human conception is possibly the most responsible action in the range of human life, and therefore these authors (TFK and KHK) cannot morally recommend this form of "conception without consent."

Although describing the risks for infertility to newly diagnosed cancer patients is considered important among oncologists, such discussions rarely take place [65]. According to providers in a recent survey, only 63.3% discuss infertility as a possible side effect with all of their oncology patients at risk [66]. A number of obstacles prevent candid discussion between healthcare providers and cancer patients concerning the prospect of infertility, including lack of knowledge regarding fertility preservation techniques and appropriate referral sites, concern about potential delay in initiation of cancer therapy, overestimation of the financial expense involved in fertility preservation, lack of time for addressing the issue, and the investigational nature of many fertility preservation methods offered [4,30].

Vadaparampil et al. performed a qualitative analysis of four major categories influencing pediatric oncologists' discussion of fertility preservation with their patients: (1) physician factors, (2) parent factors, (3) patient factors, and (4) institutional factors [67]. ASCO formulated a consensus statement to develop guidance to practicing oncologists about available fertility preservation methods. They cited the following as essential to the role of the oncologist in advising patients about fertility preservation options: to discuss infertility as a potential risk of therapy, to answer basic questions about whether fertility preservation options decrease the chance of successful cancer treatment or compromise the health of offspring, and to refer patients as needed to reproductive specialists and psychosocial providers [4]. An oncologist's recommendation to pursue fertility preservation options strongly predicts whether a male patient will choose to bank sperm and suggests that physician support affects a patient's interest in fertility preservation [60].

A new diagnosis of cancer requires a multidisciplinary approach, including access to reproductive specialists to discuss future fertility preservation and facilitate timely implementation of fertility preservation techniques. Only one-third of pediatric oncologists were aware of sperm banking facilities when asked whether they knew of fertility preservation resources within the healthcare system [68]. When available, psychological counseling should be offered to oncology patients as well to minimize the distress surrounding potential fertility. While resources in this regard may be limited, the onus is on the oncology team, including nursing staff and social workers, to educate patients about fertility preservation and expedite referrals when indicated [30]. Healthcare providers need more formal practice guidelines or training programs to enhance productive communication with patients when facing the challenges of a cancer diagnosis and loss of fertility [69].

Despite ASCO's recommendations that all oncologists discuss fertility preservation with all patients of childbearing age, most practitioners have not adopted this concept when counseling patients. In a review of qualitative interviews with both pediatric and adult oncologists, the majority cited little or no training in fertility preservation as significantly impacting their conversation with patients about fertility and leaving them feeling they did not have the requisite skills to discuss fertility preservation [69]. Approximately half of pediatric oncologists report they need to learn more about fertility preservation in their patient population [67], and only a third seek the assistance of a reproductive endocrinologist or other specialists with respect to their patients' fertility issues [66]. Additionally, practitioners stated that speaking about fertility to patients who did not speak English or for whom English was a second language made them uncomfortable, as they felt that the need for interpretation, different cultural backgrounds, and religious preferences created an awkward environment for frank discussion [69].

Studies also suggest that oncologists are uncomfortable addressing fertility preservation with their patients if the cancer prognosis is poor [65,69]. The thought of fertility may not seem appropriate and creates emotional discomfort for some specialists when they prioritize the survival of their patients [65]. Pediatric patients may be quite ill when they initially present with their cancer diagnosis, and discussing fertility or pursuing fertility preservation techniques may thwart initiation of therapy. No literature to date, however, suggests any hindrance to a cancer patient's survival secondary to participation in fertility preservation techniques [4]. Approximately half of pediatric oncologists state that their male patients could delay treatment for 1–2 days to bank sperm, and many claim that mentioning the need for fertility preservation is perceived as a sign of hope for both patients and their families [67]. If feasible, arrangements for semen preservation should be expedited before treatment, as even a single cancer therapy session can disturb sperm quality [70].

Even if the prognosis is relatively good for their patients, pediatric oncologists find that parents are so emotional upon learning their child's diagnosis of cancer that they do not want to burden them further with information about possible sterility [67,69]. About half of pediatric oncologists believe parents and adolescent patients would like to hear about fertility preservation, but the practitioners are uncomfortable discussing it or do not have sufficient knowledge to initiate the dialog [67]. Particularly, conversations about fertility are related to issues of sexuality, which pediatric oncologists often perceive as a humiliating topic for both patients and parents [68]. Physicians should consider having private discussions about fertility separately with both the parents and the patient [68].

Male pediatric cancer patients maintain a dichotomous estimation of infertility. Physicians describe half of their patients having an open mind when engaging in a fertility preservation discussion, while the other half feels embarrassed and does not want to consider fertility preservation or future children [67]. Approximately one in five patients refuses to pursue sperm banking despite his parents' desires, and in all cases the patient's preferences are respected [67]. Although a patient may be reproductively mature and capable of banking sperm, his developmental level may prohibit him from comprehending fertility preservation options and their implications [67].

Additional barriers to fertility preservation include lack of institutional support. Almost half of pediatric oncologists have not established a relationship with a fertility clinic or specialist or are unaware of such resources in their region [67]. Approximately 10% of providers believe the success rates of male sperm banking are too low to justify pursuing this option [66]. The high costs incurred with reproductive technology are also prohibitive. Cryopreservation of sperm involves not only initial payments but also annual fees that accumulate over time. In 2006, the cost of sperm banking was estimated at $1500 for three samples stored for three years, and costs continue to rise for patients who may need sperm extraction by methods other than masturbation or for prolonged storage of sperm [4]. For patients who may not be interested in fathering children for the next 10–15 years, this option can remain quite costly. At the time the patient desires to have children, the cost of subsequent thawing, culture, fertilization, embryo transfer, and pregnancy blood test can reach over $3000 [4]. Oncologists frequently refer to the high costs associated with fertility preservation techniques and uncertainty about their success as impediments to their discussion of fertility with patients [69]. In a survey of pediatric oncologists, the most commonly reported barriers to discussion of fertility preservation were issues surrounding insurance and expense, and another study found that 7.1% of oncologists surveyed felt that the cost of infertility treatment for males is too high to justify [66,67]. One review cited that 51% of oncologists thought most men could not afford sperm banking due to out-of-pocket costs [65], but in a separate survey of young men seeking fertility preservation, only 7% claimed that financial reasons prohibited banking sperm [60].

Obtaining informed consent from patients less than 18 years of age further complicates fertility preservation in children. This issue is particularly difficult in prepubertal boys, for whom only experimental techniques are available. An additional ethical aspect is the issue of legal ownership of the banked testicular material. At one institution, 6.25% of patients desired to bank sperm, but their parents refused to have their sons take part in semen preservation [71]. The question remains whether parents have a right to refuse their children the opportunity to consider their future reproductive potential and participate in fertility preservation. The American Academy of Pediatrics recommends obtaining the assent of the patient when making decisions regarding the health care of older children and adolescents. By recognizing the importance of assent, physicians empower their pediatric patients to the extent of their capacity [72]. The issue of obtaining assent is complicated by the fact that parents may decide against pursuing treatment despite what the child may desire when he is old enough to make

an informed decision. Deferring fertility preservation techniques against the patient's ultimate wishes could eradicate any opportunity for future fertility.

Conclusion

The steady rise in survival rates among children with cancer has allowed these patients to live a healthy life into adulthood. The aggressive treatment options responsible for this increase in survival unfortunately may negatively impact them in the future, particularly when considering fertility. Treatment options for fertility preservation in the postpubertal boy include semen cryopreservation and may make future parenthood a realistic option for these patients. While methods for preserving fertility, such as testicular tissue banking, remain experimental for prepubertal boys, families should be encouraged to consider them and may find a sense of comfort in knowing that fertility in the future may be possible. The focus on survival can dominate when a family first receives their son's oncologic diagnosis, but addressing fertility and expediting techniques for fertility preservation is essential for maintaining long-term quality of life in pediatric cancer survivors.

Acknowledgments

Special thanks to Ralph L. Brinster, VMD, PhD, for his invaluable review of the chapter.

References

1. American Cancer Society. *Cancer Facts and Figures 2010*. Atlanta, GA: American Cancer Society, 2010.

2. Byrne J, Mulvihill JJ, Myers MH, *et al*. Effects of treatment on fertility in long-term survivors of childhood or adolescent cancer. *N Engl J Med* 1987; 317: 1315–21.

3. Schover LR, Rybicki LA, Martin BA, Bringelsen KA. Having children after cancer. A pilot survey of survivors' attitudes and experiences. *Cancer* 1999; 86: 697–709.

4. Lee SJ, Schover LR, Partridge AH, *et al*. American Society of Clinical Oncology recommendations on fertility preservation in cancer patients. *J Clin Oncol* 2006; 24: 2917–31.

5. Rieker PP, Fitzgerald EM, Kalish LA. Adaptive behavioral responses to potential infertility among survivors of testis cancer. *J Clin Oncol* 1990; 8: 347–55.

6. Green D, Galvin H, Horne B. The psycho-social impact of infertility on young male cancer survivors: a

qualitative investigation. *Psychooncology* 2003; 12: 141–52.

7. Wallace WH, Anderson RA, Irvine DS. Fertility preservation for young patients with cancer: who is at risk and what can be offered? *Lancet Oncol* 2005; 6: 209–18.

8. Howell SJ, Shalet SM. Testicular function following chemotherapy. *Hum Reprod Update* 2001; 7: 363–9.

9. Ash P. The influence of radiation on fertility in man. *Br J Radiol* 1980; 53: 271–8.

10. Fallat ME, Hutter J. Preservation of fertility in pediatric and adolescent patients with cancer. *Pediatrics* 2008; 121: e1461–9.

11. Aubier F, Flamant F, Brauner R, *et al*. Male gonadal function after chemotherapy for solid tumors in childhood. *J Clin Oncol* 1989; 7: 304–9.

12. Ben Arush MW, Solt I, Lightman A, Linn S, Kuten A. Male gonadal function in survivors of childhood Hodgkin and non-Hodgkin lymphoma. *Pediatr Hematol Oncol* 2000; 17: 239–45.

13. Hart R. Preservation of fertility in adults and children diagnosed with cancer. *BMJ* 2008; 337: a2045.

14. Buchanan JD, Fairley KF, Barrie JU. Return of spermatogenesis after stopping cyclophosphamide therapy. *Lancet* 1975; 2: 156–7.

15. Watson AR, Rance CP, Bain J. Long term effects of cyclophosphamide on testicular function. *Br Med J* 1985; 291: 1457–60.

16. Shalet SM, Tsatsoulis A, Whitehead E, Read G. Vulnerability of the human Leydig cell to radiation damage is dependent upon age. *J Endocrinol* 1989; 120: 161–5.

17. Rowley MJ, Leach DR, Warner GA, Heller CG. Effect of graded doses of ionizing radiation on the human testis. *Radiat Res* 1974; 59: 665–78.

18. Gracia CR, Ginsberg JP. Fertility risk in pediatric and adolescent cancers. *Cancer Treat Res* 2007; 138: 57–72.

19. Hansen PV, Trykker H, Svennekjaer IL, Hvolby J. Long-term recovery of spermatogenesis after radiotherapy in patients with testicular cancer. *Radiother Oncol* 1990; 18: 117–25.

20. Fraass BA, Kinsella TJ, Harrington FS, Glatstein E. Peripheral dose to the testes: the design and clinical use of a practical and effective gonadal shield. *Int J Radiat Oncol Biol Phys* 1985; 11: 609–15.

21. Shetty G, Meistrich ML. Hormonal approaches to preservation and restoration of male fertility after cancer treatment. *J Natl Cancer Inst Monogr* 2005; 34: 36–9.

22. Socie G, Salooja N, Cohen A, *et al*. Nonmalignant late effects after allogeneic stem cell transplantation. *Blood* 2003; 101: 3373–85.

23. Castillo LA, Craft AW, Kernahan J, Evans RG, Aynsley-Green A. Gonadal function after 12-Gy testicular irradiation in childhood acute lymphoblastic leukaemia. *Med Pediatr Oncol* 1990; 18: 185–9.

24. Littley MD, Shalet SM, Beardwell CG, *et al*. Hypopituitarism following external radiotherapy for pituitary tumours in adults. *Q J Med* 1989; 70: 145–60.

25. Vigersky RA, Chapman RM, Berenberg J, Glass AR. Testicular dysfunction in untreated Hodgkin's disease. *Am J Med* 1982; 73: 482–6.

26. Petersen PM, Skakkebaek NE, Vistisen K, Rorth M, Giwercman A. Semen quality and reproductive hormones before orchiectomy in men with testicular cancer. *J Clin Oncol* 1999; 17: 941–7.

27. Chung K, Irani J, Knee G, *et al*. Sperm cryopreservation for male patients with cancer: an epidemiological analysis at the University of Pennsylvania. *Eur J Obstet Gynecol Reprod Biol* 2004; 113 (Suppl 1): S7–11.

28. Shin D, Lo KC, Lipshultz LI. Treatment options for the infertile male with cancer. *J Natl Cancer Inst Monogr* 2005; 34: 48–50.

29. Pacey AA. Fertility issues in survivors from adolescent cancers. *Cancer Treat Rev* 2007; 33: 646–55.

30. Levine J, Canada A, Stern CJ. Fertility preservation in adolescents and young adults with cancer. *J Clin Oncol* 2010; 28: 4831–41.

31. Schmiegelow ML, Sommer P, Carlsen E, *et al*. Penile vibratory stimulation and electroejaculation before anticancer therapy in two pubertal boys. *J Pediatr Hematol Oncol* 1998; 20: 429–30.

32. Hovav Y, Dan-Goor M, Yaffe H, Almagor M. Electroejaculation before chemotherapy in adolescents and young men with cancer. *Fertil Steril* 2001; 75: 811–13.

33. Brinster RL. Male germline stem cells: from mice to men. *Science* 2007; 316: 404–5.

34. Brinster RL, Avarbock MR. Germline transmission of donor haplotype following spermatogonial transplantation. *Proc Natl Acad Sci U S A* 1994; 91: 11303–7.

35. Schlatt S, Foppiani L, Rolf C, Weinbauer GF, Nieschlag E. Germ cell transplantation into X-irradiated monkey testes. *Hum Reprod* 2002; 17: 55–62.

36. Honaramooz A, Behboodi E, Blash S, Megee SO, Dobrinski I. Germ cell transplantation in goats. *Mol Reprod Dev* 2003; 64: 422–8.

37. Izadyar F, Den Ouden K, Stout TA, *et al*. Autologous and homologous transplantation of bovine spermatogonial stem cells. *Reproduction* 2003; 126: 765–74.

38. Chuma S, Kanatsu-Shinohara M, Inoue K, *et al.* Spermatogenesis from epiblast and primordial germ cells following transplantation into postnatal mouse testis. *Development* 2005; 132: 117–22.

39. Jahnukainen K, Ehmcke J, Soder O, Schlatt S. Clinical potential and putative risks of fertility preservation in children utilizing gonadal tissue or germline stem cells. *Pediatr Res* 2006; 59: 40R–47R.

40. Ogawa T, Arechaga JM, Avarbock MR, Brinster RL. Transplantation of testis germinal cells into mouse seminiferous tubules. *Int J Dev Biol* 1997; 41: 111–22.

41. Aponte PM, Soda T, Teerds KJ, *et al.* Propagation of bovine spermatogonial stem cells in vitro. *Reproduction* 2008; 136: 543–57.

42. Kanatsu-Shinohara M, Muneto T, Lee J, *et al.* Long-term culture of male germline stem cells from hamster testes. *Biol Reprod* 2008; 78(4): 611–7.

43. Hamra FK, Chapman KM, Nguyen DM. Self renewal, expansion, and transfection of rat spermatogonial stem cells in culture. *Proc Natl Acad Sci U S A* 2005; 102: 17430–5.

44. Kanatsu-Shinohara M, Ogonuki N, Inoue K, *et al.* Long-term proliferation in culture and germline transmission of mouse male germline stem cells. *Biol Reprod* 2003; 69: 612–16.

45. Kubota H, Avarbock MR, Brinster RL. Growth factors essential for self-renewal and expansion of mouse spermatogonial stem cells. *Proc Natl Acad Sci U S A* 2004; 101: 16489–94.

46. Nagano M, McCarrey JR, Brinster RL. Primate spermatogonial stem cells colonize mouse testes. *Biol Reprod* 2001; 64: 1409–16.

47. Creemers LB, Meng X, den Ouden K, *et al.* Transplantation of germ cells from glial cell line-derived neurotrophic factor-overexpressing mice to host testes depleted of endogenous spermatogenesis by fractionated irradiation. *Biol Reprod* 2002; 66: 1579–84.

48. Izadyar F, Spierenberg GT, Creemers LB, den Ouden K, de Rooij DG. Isolation and purification of type A spermatogonia from the bovine testis. *Reproduction* 2002; 124: 85–94.

49. van Pelt AM, Roepers-Gajadien HL, Gademan IS, *et al.* Establishment of cell lines with rat spermatogonial stem cell characteristics. *Endocrinology* 2002; 143: 1845–50.

50. Nagano M, Patrizio P, Brinster RL. Long-term survival of human spermatogonial stem cells in mouse testes. *Fertil Steril* 2002; 78: 1225–33.

51. Sadri-Ardekani H, Mizrak SC, van Daalen SK, *et al.* Propagation of human spermatogonial stem cells in vitro. *JAMA* 2009; 302: 2127–34.

52. Beres J, Papp G, Pazonyi I, Czeizel E. Testicular volume variations from 0 to 28 years of age. *Int Urol Nephrol* 1989; 21: 159–67.

53. Shen F, Zhang C, Zheng H, *et al.* Long-term culture and transplantation of spermatogonial stem cells from BALB/c mice. *Cells Tissues Organs* 2010; 191: 372–81.

54. Wu X, Schmidt JA, Avarbock MR, *et al.* Prepubertal human spermatogonia and mouse gonocytes share conserved gene expression of germline stem cell regulatory molecules. *Proc Natl Acad Sci U S A* 2009; 106: 21672–7.

55. Ginsberg JP, Carlson CA, Lin K, *et al.* An experimental protocol for fertility preservation in prepubertal boys recently diagnosed with cancer: a report of acceptability and safety. *Hum Reprod* 2010; 25: 37–41.

56. Fujita K, Tsujimura A, Miyagawa Y, *et al.* Isolation of germ cells from leukemia and lymphoma cells in a human in vitro model: potential clinical application for restoring human fertility after anticancer therapy. *Cancer Res* 2006; 66: 11166–71.

57. Geens M, Van de Velde H, De Block G, *et al.* The efficiency of magnetic-activated cell sorting and fluorescence-activated cell sorting in the decontamination of testicular cell suspensions in cancer patients. *Hum Reprod* 2007; 22: 733–42.

58. Schover LR. Psychosocial aspects of infertility and decisions about reproduction in young cancer survivors: a review. *Med Pediatr Oncol* 1999; 33: 53–9.

59. Ginsberg JP, Ogle SK, Tuchman LK, *et al.* Sperm banking for adolescent and young adult cancer patients: sperm quality, patient, and parent perspectives. *Pediatr Blood Cancer* 2008; 50: 594–8.

60. Schover LR, Brey K, Lichtin A, Lipshultz LI, Jeha S. Knowledge and experience regarding cancer, infertility, and sperm banking in younger male survivors. *J Clin Oncol* 2002; 20: 1880–9.

61. Burns KC, Boudreau C, Panepinto JA. Attitudes regarding fertility preservation in female adolescent cancer patients. *J Pediatr Hematol Oncol* 2006; 28: 350–4.

62. Nieman CL, Kinahan KE, Yount SE, *et al.* Fertility preservation and adolescent cancer patients: lessons from adult survivors of childhood cancer and their parents. *Cancer Treat Res* 2007; 138: 201–17.

63. Saito K, Suzuki K, Iwasaki A, Yumura Y, Kubota Y. Sperm cryopreservation before cancer chemotherapy helps in the emotional battle against cancer. *Cancer* 2005; 104: 521–4.

64. Ethics Committee of the American Society for Reproductive Medicine. Fertility preservation and reproduction in cancer patients. *Fertil Steril* 2005; 83: 1622–8.

65. Schover LR, Brey K, Lichtin A, Lipshultz LI, Jeha S. Oncologists' attitudes and practices regarding banking sperm before cancer treatment. *J Clin Oncol* 2002; 20: 1890–7.

66. Goodwin T, Elizabeth Oosterhuis B, Kiernan M, Hudson MM, Dahl GV. Attitudes and practices of pediatric oncology providers regarding fertility issues. *Pediatr Blood Cancer* 2007; 48: 80–5.

67. Vadaparampil S, Quinn G, King L, Wilson C, Nieder M. Barriers to fertility preservation among pediatric oncologists. *Patient Educ Couns* 2008; 72: 402–10.

68. Quinn GP, Vadaparampil ST. Fertility preservation and adolescent/young adult cancer patients: physician communication challenges. *J Adolesc Health* 2009; 44: 394–400.

69. Quinn GP, Vadaparampil ST, King L, *et al.* Impact of physicians' personal discomfort and patient prognosis on discussion of fertility preservation with young cancer patients. *Patient Educ Couns* 2009; 77: 338–43.

70. Lass A, Akagbosu F, Abusheikha N, *et al.* A programme of semen cryopreservation for patients with malignant disease in a tertiary infertility centre: lessons from 8 years' experience. *Hum Reprod* 1998; 13: 3256–61.

71. Bashore L. Semen preservation in male adolescents and young adults with cancer: one institution's experience. *Clin J Oncol Nurs* 2007; 11: 381–6.

72. Informed consent, parental permission, and assent in pediatric practice. Committee on Bioethics, American Academy of Pediatrics. *Pediatrics* 1995; 95: 314–17.

Chapter

30

Exogenous androgens: effect on spermatogenesis

Mohit Khera

Introduction

Androgens play an important role in the development of male sexual organs, such as the penis, prostate, epididymis, vas deferens, and seminal vesicles. Moreover, intratesticular testosterone levels are crucial for the maintenance of spermatogenesis and inhibition of germ cell apoptosis. The use of exogenous testosterone has been increasing over the last several decades. Many testosterone users/abusers and clinicians are unaware of the fact that the use of exogenous testosterone has been shown to suppress the hypothalamic–pituitary–gonadal (HPG) axis and result in infertility. It is important that clinicians understand the effects of exogenous testosterone on spermatogenesis and educate their patients about its potential effects on fertility. Indeed, several studies are currently under way to develop the use of exogenous testosterone as a natural male contraceptive [1].

Testosterone production and secretion

In order to understand the effects of exogenous testosterone on spermatogenesis, one must know how the HPG axis functions (Fig. 30.1). The production of testosterone is regulated by luteinizing hormone (LH) from the anterior pituitary. In turn, LH secretion is regulated by gonadotropin-releasing hormone (GnRH), which is secreted from the hypothalamus. GnRH is secreted in a pulsatile fashion and is significantly elevated at the time a boy enters puberty. This elevation in GnRH, and subsequent increase in LH, results in a surge in testosterone levels and thus the development of male sexual characteristics and spermatogenesis.

Testosterone is synthesized by the Leydig cells within the testicles. The testes are not able to store

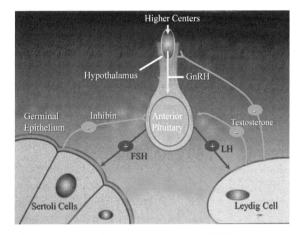

Figure 30.1. Hypothalamic–pituitary–gonadal (HPG) axis.

testosterone adequately on their own or convert testosterone into its more potent form, dihydrotestosterone (DHT). This is because the testes lack the enzyme, 5-alpha-reductase, which converts testosterone into DHT. To compensate for this, the testes have high levels of androgen-binding protein (ABP), which is made by the Sertoli cells and helps to maintain high intratesticular levels of testosterone [2].

Testosterone levels vary on the basis of a diurnal rhythm, with the highest levels of circulating testosterone occurring in the early morning hours. In a study of the effect of normal aging on the circadian rhythm in serum total testosterone levels, hourly blood samples were obtained for 24 hours from 17 young men (mean age 25.2 years) and 12 older, healthy men (mean age 71 years) [3]. The diurnal rhythm of total testosterone observed in young men was markedly attenuated or absent in older yet otherwise healthy men, suggesting that these altered diurnal patterns may be a consequence of normal aging (Fig. 30.2).

Fertility Preservation in Male Cancer Patients, ed. John P. Mulhall, Linda D. Applegarth, Robert D. Oates and Peter N. Schlegel. Published by Cambridge University Press. © Cambridge University Press 2013.

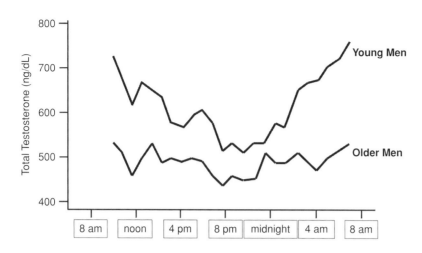

Figure 30.2. Diurnal variation in serum total testosterone levels in young men (mean age 25.2 years) and older men (mean age 71 years). (Reproduced with permission from Bremner *et al.* Loss of circadian rhythmicity in blood testosterone levels with aging in normal men. *J Clin Endocrinol Metab* 1983; 56: 1278–81 [3].)

In the blood, testosterone circulates mostly in a bound form; approximately 60% of testosterone is bound to sex-hormone binding globulin (SHBG) and 38% is bound to serum albumin [4]. The binding between testosterone and SHBG is very tight, and when bound in this fashion testosterone is not considered to be biologically available [4,5]. Conversely, testosterone is weakly bound to albumin and can readily dissociate from the complex and thus become bioavailable [4,5].

Approximately 2% of the circulating testosterone within the blood is unbound and free to enter cells to exert its metabolic effects [4,5]. Thus, the amount of bioavailable testosterone is the sum of the free testosterone and the albumin-bound testosterone [4]. The distinction between bioavailable testosterone and total testosterone (bioavailable plus SHBG-bound) may be important when levels of testosterone are measured in the hypogonadal male. SHBG is synthesized in the liver, and its levels can be increased by hyperthyroidism and cirrhosis and decreased by hypothyroidism, acromegaly, and obesity [4,5]. SHBG levels also increase as men age, and these increases can lead to variability in testosterone levels and their impact on biological function [4,5].

Testosterone and male sexual development

Between the 7th and 12th week of gestation, the male gonads begin to differentiate. The undifferentiated gonad develops into a testis through the expression and action of the SRY gene, located on the short arm of the Y chromosome. The testis in turn produces anti-Müllerian hormone (AMH) and testosterone. AMH causes regression of Müllerian structures, and testosterone causes the development of Wolffian structures such as the seminal vesicles, vas deferens, and epididymis. Thus, all embryos will develop into females unless testosterone and AMH are expressed. Finally, increased intratesticular testosterone will result in an increase in the number of gonocytes per tubule.

Requirements for spermatogenesis

Both follicle-stimulating hormone (FSH) and LH secretion from the anterior pituitary induce spermatogenesis. FSH binds to receptors within the Sertoli cells and induces spermatogenesis. LH induces testosterone production, which is needed for the maintenance of spermatogenesis and inhibition of germ cell apoptosis [6]. The seminiferous tubules are exposed to levels of testosterone up to 100 times greater than those present in circulating serum. There are data to indicate that as the testis matures, the Sertoli cells become less responsive to FSH and more dependent on testosterone for spermatogenesis [7]. Finally, epididymal function also has been shown to be dependent on testosterone. Studies have demonstrated that during androgen deprivation the epididymis eventually loses its ability to allow for sperm maturation [8].

Hypogonadism and male infertility

Androgen deficiency is a serious problem in the older male population, thought to affect approximately 1 in 200 men [9]. Mulligan *et al.* observed that roughly 39%

of men over the age of 45 years had low serum testosterone levels, defined as less than 300 ng/dL. Approximately 20–30% of infertile males will be found to have low testosterone or increased LH levels [10].

We know now that beginning at approximately 20–30 years of age, men experience a decline in testosterone and free testosterone levels by 0.4% and 1.3% per year, respectively [11]. The common symptoms of this decline in androgens have not been fully defined, as have those associated with declining estrogen levels in women. Signs and symptoms of hypogonadism include changes in bone mineral density [12,13], muscle strength [14,15], cognition [16], body composition [17], and sexual function [18].

When a patient is diagnosed with hypogonadism, it is important to determine whether the cause is primary or secondary hypogonadism. While primary hypogonadism usually is due to testicular failure, secondary hypogonadism results from an impairment of LH secretion from the anterior pituitary. One study found that roughly 3.4% of infertility patients will present with secondary infertility [19]. When secondary infertility is suspected, as in the presence of severely depressed testosterone levels and either elevated prolactin or low gonadotropin levels, it is prudent to obtain an MRI of the pituitary to rule out any macroadenomas or secreting tumors.

Anabolic steroid use and infertility

The use of testosterone supplementation dates back as far as 2000 BC, when the ancient Aryuvendic manuscripts describe the ingestion of testicular tissue for the treatment of impotence. In 1889 Brown-Sequard reported self-administered injections of testicular extract. He reported reversal of the aging process. In 1935 the first reports of testosterone derivation from cholesterol appeared, and in 1938 testosterone propionate for strength enhancement was first described in the literature. In 1939 Ruzicka and Butenandt won the Nobel Prize for the synthesis of testosterone.

Testosterone has been associated with athletic performance and with "doping." Doping is defined as the use of a drug or blood product to improve athletic performance. In 1936 the German Olympic athletes were first rumored to be using testosterone. In 1950, the Soviet weightlifters began the first systemic use of anabolic steroids, but it was not until 1976 that

Table 30.1. Anabolic : androgenic ratio for selected anabolic steroids

Anabolic-androgenic steroid	Anabolic : androgenic ratio
Testosterone (TC, TE, T gels)	1
Methyltestosterone (Halotestin)	1
Methandrostenolone (Dianabol)	2–5
Oxymetholone (Anandrol)	9
Oxandrolone (Oxandrin)	10
Nandrolone (Deca-durbolin)	10
Stanozol (Winstrol)	30

Adapted from Kuhn CM. Anabolic steroids. *Recent Prog Horm Res* 2002; 57: 411–34.

the first Olympic drug testing program was initiated. It is estimated that 3–12% of male athletes in high school in the United States have used steroids [20]. In addition, it is reported that 14% of college athletes use/abuse anabolic steroids, and approximately 30–75% of professional athletes and bodybuilders have abused anabolic steroids [21].

Traditionally athletes have been known to use anabolic-androgenic steroids (AAS). AAS are synthetic derivatives of testosterone. The anabolic component promotes nitrogen storage for protein synthesis, and the androgenic component, mediated by the androgen receptor, produces virilization. Athletes usually desire AAS that have a high anabolic-to-androgenic ratio (Table 30.1).

Exogenous administration of synthetic testosterone results in negative feedback on the HPG axis and thus inhibition of the secretion of both FSH and LH. Despite normal-to-high serum androgen concentrations achieved with anabolic steroid use, those concentrations may not produce the testicular concentrations necessary to maintain spermatogenesis, and many male users of anabolic steroids develop hypogonadotropic hypogonadism with subsequent testicular atrophy and azoospermia. Anabolic steroid use commonly results in oligospermia or azoospermia along with abnormalities of sperm motility and morphology [22,23].

Testosterone inhibits both GnRH and gonadotropin secretion. Suppression of gonadotropins results in hypospermatogenesis and a reduction in the number of spermatozoa in the ejaculate [24]. Complete inhibition of intratesticular testosterone can result in azoospermia [25,26].

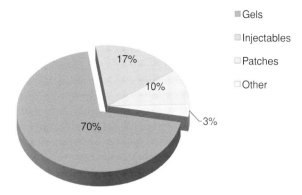

Figure 30.3. Testosterone replacement therapy (TRT): gels are the most commonly prescribed form of testosterone replacement.

Different types of testosterone supplementation

Numerous forms of testosterone supplementation are available and each may have a different effect on the degree and rate of spermatogenic suppression. Currently most testosterone replacement therapy (TRT) users in the United States are receiving some form of transdermal gel therapy (Fig. 30.3). In 2006, roughly 70% of the TRT users were using transdermal gel therapy, 17% were using testosterone injections, 10% were using transdermal testosterone patches, and 3% were using some other form of testosterone supplementation, such as an oral formulation. Injectable testosterone tends to result in peak supraphysiologic serum levels three days after injection and then in subtherapeutic levels at day 14 to 21. This subsequent decline in testosterone is known as "testosterone crash." Transdermal testosterone gels and patches tend to cause a more constant release of testosterone and result in less fluctuation in serum testosterone levels. Bodybuilders and professional athletes tend to use illicit steroids that have a higher anabolic-to-androgenic ratio (Table 30.1). For example, testosterone enanthate has an anabolic-to-androgenic ratio of 1 : 1, while stanozolol (Winstrol) has an anabolic-to-androgenic ratio of 30 : 1. Thus, stanozolol appears to be a more popular choice of testosterone supplementation than testosterone enanthate for most bodybuilders and professional athletes. Patients with a history of exogenous androgen use usually can be identified by evaluating their testosterone and gonadotropin levels. The use of anabolic steroids suppresses gonadotropic secretion from the pituitary as well as endogenous testosterone production from Leydig cells.

Rebound therapy for idiopathic oligo/asthenospermia

In the 1960s androgens were used in the treatment of idiopathic oligospermia. The belief was that the administration of high doses of testosterone would cause an initial suppression of gonadotropins and spermatogenesis and that abrupt cessation of the androgens would then cause a rebound effect resulting in an overall net increase in gonadotropins and spermatogenesis. Numerous trials concluded that androgens had little to no effect on endocrine outcomes and sperm parameters [27]. In a Cochrane review the authors found that there is not enough evidence to evaluate the use of androgens for male subfertility [28]. Randomized controlled trials including 930 patients were unable to show any beneficial rebound effects in men with idiopathic oligospermia.

Recovery of spermatogenesis after exogenous testosterone use

Several studies have assessed the recovery of spermatogenesis after exogenous testosterone usage. Liu and colleagues conducted a meta-analysis of 30 studies that investigated the rate, extent, and predictors of reversibility of hormonal male contraception [29]. The primary outcome was the time required for the sperm concentration to reach 20 million/mL. They evaluated 1549 men who were treated with either androgens or androgens plus progestagen for at least three months. The median times for sperm to recover to thresholds of 20, 10, and 3 million/mL were 3.4 months (95% CI 3.2–3.5), 3.0 months (2.9–3.1), and 2.5 months (2.4–2.7), respectively. There were higher rates of recovery with older age, Asian origin, shorter treatment duration, shorter-acting testosterone preparations, higher sperm concentrations at baseline, faster suppression of spermatogenesis, and lower blood concentrations of LH at baseline. The probability of recovery to 20 million/mL was 67% (61–72) within 6 months, 90% (85–93) within 12 months, 96% (92–98) within 16 months, and 100% within 24 months.

Another study by a WHO task force evaluated 271 men who received 200 mg of testosterone enanthate weekly [30]. After 6 months, 157 (65%) of the men were azoospermic. The mean time to azoospermia was 120 days. After six months of treatment, the patients entered the recovery phase. While 84% of men were able to achieve a sperm density > 20 million/mL after a median of 3.7 months, only 46% of patients were able to achieve their baseline sperm density.

Finally, a study by Mills and associates also evaluated the recovery of spermatogenesis after exogenous testosterone administration [31]. They retrospectively reviewed 22 men who had sought treatment for infertility and had a recent history of AAS usage. The duration of testosterone use, the delivery method, and the initial hormone profile were recorded. In addition, the time to recovery of sperm in the ejaculate and post-treatment hormone profiles were documented. All men were required to discontinue exogenous testosterone usage and were treated with human chorionic gonadotropin (hCG) 3000 units intramuscularly every other day for a minimum of three months and until recovery of spermatogenesis. Semen analyses and hormone assays were checked at four weeks and then every month. All except two men recovered sperm in the ejaculate. Of the two men without sperm, one had insufficient follow-up and the other was suspected of continuing to use multiple anabolic steroids and was lost to follow-up. The study found that those patients who were using intramuscular testosterone at the time of presentation recovered spermatogenesis in an average of 3.1 months. However, those patients who were receiving transdermal testosterone supplementation at the time of presentation recovered spermatogenesis in an average of 7.4 months [31]. The authors concluded that impairment of fertility following TRT suppression is reversible, and that the rate of sperm return appears to be related to the delivery system.

Success rates of recovering spermatogenesis after exogenous testosterone use are generally quite good. In one study, men with idiopathic hypogonadotropic hypogonadism were treated with hCG alone or in combination with human menopausal gonadotropin (hMG), resulting in 40 pregnancies among 22 patients (92%), with a mean conception time of 7.6 months after sperm were first noted in the ejaculate [32]. Mean sperm concentration at conception was 16 million sperm per mL with a mean motile fraction of 38% [32,33]. However, it is known that not all men recover spermatogenesis after TRT. In one study, abnormally low testosterone and gonadotropin levels were documented 2.5 years after steroid use was discontinued [33].

Wang *et al.* found that oligospermia induced by exogenous testosterone was associated with normally functioning residual spermatozoa [34]. In this prospective study, 12 healthy men were studied while participating in a multicenter testosterone enanthate contraceptive efficacy study. Data were analyzed from only eight subjects, whose sperm concentrations were between 1.3 and 10 million/mL at the suppression phase. Testosterone enanthate (200 mg) was administered intramuscularly weekly during the suppression and testosterone treatment (efficacy) phases (total 15 months). Sperm function tests were performed during the pre-treatment, during suppression (usually after 6–10 weeks of treatment, when sperm concentration was anticipated to decrease to < 10 million/mL), and during the recovery phase. Investigators found that sperm concentration was reduced, but sperm motility, motility characteristics, and morphology were not affected by testosterone enanthate treatment. The residual spermatozoa in the ejaculate exhibited normal hyperactivation, could acrosome react, and maintained the capacity to penetrate and fuse with the oocyte. They concluded that suppression of spermatogenesis to moderate oligospermia (< 10 million/mL) with exogenous testosterone enanthate administration was not associated with impaired sperm function of the residual spermatozoa.

Raising testosterone levels and preserving fertility

Many young men with a diagnosis of hypogonadism desire testosterone supplementation. However, they are equally concerned about protecting their fertility. It is clear that for those hypogonadal patients who desire to protect their future fertility, exogenous testosterone should be discouraged. A more appropriate approach in these patients is to increase their own endogenous testosterone. There are several ways to accomplish this. However, all of these methods, except for hCG injections, are considered off-label use.

One option is to initiate use of clomiphene (Clomid) 50 mg every other day or 25 mg every day. Because Clomid is an estrogen receptor blocker and raises serum FSH and LH levels, it is not as effective in raising serum testosterone levels when the patient's LH and FSH levels are already elevated, as seen in primary testis failure. Other methods of increasing endogenous testosterone include the use of anastrazole (Arimidex). Arimidex is an aromatase inhibitor and blocks the conversion from testosterone to estradiol. This is especially useful in obese patients, who tend to have an increased amount of aromatization. In adults, there is concern that long-standing suppression of estradiol may increase the risk of osteoporosis and osteopenia, and lead to joint pain.

hCG injections can also be used to increase endogenous serum testosterone levels. hCG is an LH analog that stimulates Leydig cell production of testosterone. Intramuscular injections can vary from two to three times per week, and from 1500 to 3000 units and higher. Note that high doses of hCG are not needed to stimulate and maintain spermatogenesis. Roth *et al.* induced experimental gonadotropin deficiency in 37 normal men with the GnRH antagonists and randomized them to receive one of four low doses of hCG: 0, 15, 60, or 125 IU subcutaneously every other day or 7.5 g daily testosterone gel for 10 days [35]. Testicular fluid was obtained by percutaneous aspiration for steroid measurements at baseline, and after 10 days of treatment. Intratesticular testosterone (IT-T) concentrations increased in a dose-dependent manner with very low-dosage hCG administration from 77 nmol/L (40, 122 nmol/L) to 923 nmol/L (894, 1017 nmol/L) in the 0 and 125 IU groups, respectively ($p < 0.001$). Moreover, serum hCG was significantly correlated with both IT-T and serum testosterone ($p < 0.01$). The authors concluded that doses of hCG, far lower than those used clinically, increase IT-T concentrations in a dose-dependent manner in normal men with experimental gonadotropin deficiency. While hCG injections may be beneficial in raising serum testosterone levels and preserving fertility, hCG injections can be costly, and the invasive nature of this medication can also be a deterrent to many patients.

Testosterone as a male contraceptive

Many companies have tried to develop hormonal contraceptives. The goal is to cause a withdrawal of the gonadotropin support to the testis, which results in suppression of spermatogenesis and intratesticular testosterone [36]. Although several companies have tried testosterone alone, others have used testosterone in combination with progestagens [36]. Studies have also demonstrated that there are ethnic variations in spermatogenic response to exogenous testosterone, with a lesser suppression among Caucasians than in Asians. In addition, high doses of testosterone, such as testosterone enanthate, have been shown to be associated with a decline in high-density lipoprotein cholesterol (HDL-C) concentration [37]. Progestagen has been shown to act synergistically with testosterone,

thus necessitating the use of less testosterone and resulting in fewer side effects. Promising results have been obtained using oral desogestrel, with high rates of azoospermia achieved in men from several ethnic backgrounds.

A study by Brady and associates investigated the effect of subcutaneous etonogestrel with depot testosterone on spermatogenesis in normal men over a period of 48 weeks [38]. Nine healthy men completed the study and received three subcutaneous 68 mg etonogestrel implants. These men also received testosterone pellets (400 mg) at weekly intervals for 12 weeks. They found that sperm concentrations of less then 1 million/mL were achieved in all men within 16 weeks of treatment. All men became azoospermic, although the time to achieve this state varied from 8 to 28 weeks. Azoospermia was maintained in eight of the nine men treated for 48 weeks, one subject showing partial recovery after 40 weeks. While testosterone levels remained in the physiological range throughout, no adverse effects such as weight gain, change in body composition, or decline in HDL-C concentrations were noted. The study concluded that the combination of three etonogestrel implants with depot testosterone results in rapid and consistent suppression of spermatogenesis that can be maintained for up to one year and may be an approach for a long-acting male hormonal contraceptive.

Conclusion

Exogenous testosterone use and abuse has been present in our society for many years. However, many patients and clinicians are unaware that exogenous testosterone is a natural contraceptive that can lead to impaired semen parameters and infertility. Provision of exogenous testosterone to a hypogonadal man in his reproductive years should be approached with caution, and treatment should be focused mainly on raising his own endogenous testosterone level. Clinicians and patients should be aware of the potential for irreversible suppression of spermatogenesis in a limited number of patients.

References

1. Page ST, Amory JK, Anawalt BD, *et al.* Testosterone gel combined with depomedroxyprogesterone acetate is an effective male hormonal contraceptive regimen and is not enhanced by the addition of a GnRH antagonist. *J Clin Endocrinol Metab* 2006; 91: 4374–80.

2. van Roijen JH, Ooms MP, Weber RF, *et al.* Comparison of the response of rat testis and accessory sex organs to treatment with testosterone and the synthetic androgen methyltrienolone (R1881). *J Androl* 1997; 18: 51–61.

3. Bremner WJ, Vitiello MV, Prinz PN. Loss of circadian rhythmicity in blood testosterone levels with aging in normal men. *J Clin Endocrinol Metab* 1983; 56: 1278–81.

4. Braunstein GD. Testes. In eds. *Basic and Clinical Endocrinology*, 5th edn. Samford, CT: Appleton and Lange, 1997; pp. 422–52.

5. Petak SM, Nankin HR, Spark RF, *et al.* American Association of Clinical Endocrinologists Medical Guidelines for clinical practice for the evaluation and treatment of hypogonadism in adult male patients: 2002 update. *Endocr Pract* 2002; 8: 440–56.

6. Singh J, O'Neill C, Handelsman DJ. Induction of spermatogenesis by androgens in gonadotropin-deficient (hpg) mice. *Endocrinology* 1995; 136: 5311–21.

7. Sharpe RM, Kerr JB, McKinnell C, Millar M. Temporal relationship between androgen-dependent changes in the volume of seminiferous tubule fluid, lumen size and seminiferous tubule protein secretion in rats. *J Reprod Fertil* 1994; 101: 193–8.

8. Cooper TG. Epididymis and sperm function. *Andrologia* 1996; 28 (Suppl 1): 57–9.

9. Morales A, Tenover JL. Androgen deficiency in the aging male: when, who, and how to investigate and treat. *Urol Clin North Am* 2002; 29: 975–82, x.

10. Handelsman DJ. Testicular dysfunction in systemic disease. *Endocrinol Metab Clin North Am* 1994; 23: 839–56.

11. Wu FC, Tajar A, Pye SR, *et al.* Hypothalamic-pituitary-testicular axis disruptions in older men are differentially linked to age and modifiable risk factors: the European Male Aging Study. *J Clin Endocrinol Metab* 2008; 93: 2737–45.

12. Kiratli BJ, Srinivas S, Perkash I, Terris MK. Progressive decrease in bone density over 10 years of androgen deprivation therapy in patients with prostate cancer. *Urology* 2001; 57: 127–32.

13. Stoch SA, Parker RA, Chen L, *et al.* Bone loss in men with prostate cancer treated with gonadotropin-releasing hormone agonists. *J Clin Endocrinol Metab* 2001; 86: 2787–91.

14. Bhasin S, Storer TW, Berman N, *et al.* Testosterone replacement increases fat-free mass and muscle size in hypogonadal men. *J Clin Endocrinol Metab* 1997; 82: 407–13.

15. Murray MP, Gardner GM, Mollinger LA, Sepic SB. Strength of isometric and isokinetic contractions: knee muscles of men aged 20 to 86. *Phys Ther* 1980; 60: 412–19.

16. Moffat SD, Zonderman AB, Metter EJ, *et al.* Longitudinal assessment of serum free testosterone concentration predicts memory performance and cognitive status in elderly men. *J Clin Endocrinol Metab* 2002; 87: 5001–7.

17. Katznelson L, Finkelstein JS, Schoenfeld DA, *et al.* Increase in bone density and lean body mass during testosterone administration in men with acquired hypogonadism. *J Clin Endocrinol Metab* 1996; 81: 4358–65.

18. Davidson JM, Chen JJ, Crapo L, *et al.* Hormonal changes and sexual function in aging men. *J Clin Endocrinol Metab* 1983; 57: 71–7.

19. Pierik FH, Van Ginneken AM, Dohle GR, *et al.* The advantages of standardized evaluation of male infertility. *Int J Androl* 2000; 23: 340–6.

20. Lukas SE. Current perspectives on anabolic-androgenic steroid abuse. *Trends Pharmacol Sci* 1993; 14: 61–68.

21. Yesalis CE, Kennedy NJ, Kopstein AN, Bahrke MS. Anabolic-androgenic steroid use in the United States. *JAMA* 1993; 270: 1217–21.

22. Holma PK. Effects of an anabolic steroid (metandienone) on spermatogenesis. *Contraception* 1977; 15: 151–62.

23. Kilshaw BH, Harkness RA, Hobson BM, Smith AW. The effects of large doses of the anabolic steroid, methandrostenolone, on an athlete. *Clin Endocrinol (Oxf)* 1975; 4: 537–41.

24. Sun YT, Irby DC, Robertson DM, de Kretser DM. The effects of exogenously administered testosterone on spermatogenesis in intact and hypophysectomized rats. *Endocrinology* 1989; 125: 1000–10.

25. McLachlan RI, O'Donnell L, Meachem SJ, *et al.* Hormonal regulation of spermatogenesis in primates and man: insights for development of the male hormonal contraceptive. *J Androl* 2002; 23: 149–62.

26. Weinbauer GF, Nieschlag E. Gonadotrophin-releasing hormone analogue-induced manipulation of testicular function in the monkey. *Hum Reprod* 1993; 8 (Suppl 2): 45–50.

27. De Kretser DM, Burger HG, Fortune D, *et al.* Hormonal, histological and chromosomal studies in adult males with testicular disorders. *J Clin Endocrinol Metab* 1972; 35: 392–401.

28. Vandekerckhove P, Lilford R, Vail A, Hughes E. Androgens versus placebo or no treatment for

idiopathic oligo/asthenospermia. *Cochrane Database Syst Rev* 2000; (2): CD000150.

29. Liu PY, Swerdloff RS, Christenson PD, *et al.* Rate, extent, and modifiers of spermatogenic recovery after hormonal male contraception: an integrated analysis. *Lancet* 2006; 367: 1412–20.

30. Contraceptive efficacy of testosterone-induced azoospermia in normal men. World Health Organization Task Force on methods for the regulation of male fertility. *Lancet* 1990; 336: 955–9.

31. Mills JN, Grober ED, Khera M, *et al.* Recovery of spermatogenesis after exogenous testosterone administration. *J Urol* 2008; 179 (4 Suppl): 656–7. Abstract #1910.

32. Burris AS, Clark RV, Vantman DJ, Sherins RJ. A low sperm concentration does not preclude fertility in men with isolated hypogonadotropic hypogonadism after gonadotropin therapy. *Fertil Steril* 1988; 50: 343–7.

33. Jarow JP, Lipshultz LI. Anabolic steroid-induced hypogonadotropic hypogonadism. *Am J Sports Med* 1990; 18: 429–31.

34. Wang C, Leung A, Superlano L, *et al.* Oligozoospermia induced by exogenous testosterone is associated with normal functioning residual spermatozoa. *Fertil Steril* 1997; 68: 149–53.

35. Roth MY, Page ST, Lin K, *et al.* Dose-dependent increase in intratesticular testosterone by very low-dose human chorionic gonadotropin in normal men with experimental gonadotropin deficiency. *J Clin Endocrinol Metab* 95: 3806–13.

36. Anderson RA, Wallace AM, Kicman AT, Wu FC. Comparison between testosterone enanthate-induced azoospermia and oligozoospermia in a male contraceptive study. IV. Suppression of endogenous testicular and adrenal androgens. *Hum Reprod* 1997; 12: 1657–62.

37. Anderson RA, Wallace AM, Wu FC. Comparison between testosterone enanthate-induced azoospermia and oligozoospermia in a male contraceptive study. III. Higher 5 alpha-reductase activity in oligozoospermic men administered supraphysiological doses of testosterone. *J Clin Endocrinol Metab* 1996; 81: 902–8.

38. Brady BM, Walton M, Hollow N, *et al.* Depot testosterone with etonogestrel implants result in induction of azoospermia in all men for long-term contraception. *Hum Reprod* 2004; 19: 2658–67.

Chapter

31

Fertility preservation in the female with cancer

Kenny A. Rodriguez-Wallberg and Kutluk Oktay

Introduction

The loss of fertility resulting from cancer treatment has a recognized negative impact on the quality of life of cancer survivors [1]. In women, infertility may be regarded as an essential loss of femininity, and infertility after cancer is often associated with psychosocial distress [2,3]. Since the incidence of most cancers increases with age, delayed childbearing, as is the trend in Western societies, results in more female cancer survivors interested in fertility preservation.

In 2006, an expert panel commissioned by the American Society of Clinical Oncology (ASCO) published guidelines for fertility preservation for male and female patients [1]. The only established fertility preservation methods recognized at that time were sperm cryopreservation and embryo cryopreservation, for male and female patients respectively, and all other options were considered experimental. By this date, technical improvements in methods for cryopreservation of oocytes have resulted in an increasing number of pregnancies and children born worldwide after fertilization of frozen–thawed oocytes, leading thus to the current acceptance of oocyte freezing as a new established method for female fertility preservation [4]. The remaining options, still experimental, include the freezing of ovarian tissue for future retransplantation or for in-vitro culture and maturation of ovarian follicles. Those experimental methods are also the only options that can be offered to prepubertal girls.

The most common cancer diagnoses in females are summarized in Table 31.1. According to the SEER Cancer Statistics Review, for the year 2010 over 700 000

Table 31.1. Cancer incidence in females estimated for year 2010 in the USA

Primary site	Estimated new cancer cases for 2010
All sites	739 940
Breast	207 090
Digestive system	125 790
Colon	53 430
Rectum	17 050
Pancreas	21 770
Respiratory system	110 010
Lung and bronchus	105 770
Genital organs	83 750
Endometrium	43 470
Ovary	21 880
Cervix	12 200
Urinary system	41 640
Urinary bladder	17 770
Kidney and renal/pelvis	22 870
Endocrine system	35 040
Thyroid	33 980
Lymphoma	33 980
Skin	31 400
Melanoma	29 260
Leukemia	18 360

Adapted from: Cancer Facts & Figures – 2010, American Cancer Society (ACS), Atlanta, Georgia, 2010. Incidence projections are based on rates from the North American Association of Central Cancer Registries (NAACCR) 1995–2006, representing about 89% of the US population.
SEER Cancer Statistics Review 1975–2007, National Cancer Institute, updated January 7, 2011 [5].

Fertility Preservation in Male Cancer Patients, ed. John P. Mulhall, Linda D. Applegarth, Robert D. Oates and Peter N. Schlegel. Published by Cambridge University Press. © Cambridge University Press 2013.

new cases of cancer in females were estimated in the USA [5].

Early counseling to preserve fertility

To prevent damage to fertility potential, fertility preservation options should be offered and performed before patients start their gonadotoxic treatments. However, despite the fact that fertility issues are recognized in young women with cancer, timely and effective communication between cancer care specialists and young patients is not always achieved [3]. In a recent survey in the USA, nearly half of healthcare professionals at one large academic center reported never referring cancer patients of reproductive age to a reproductive endocrinologist for fertility preservation [6], which contrasts with data indicating that approximately three out of four cancer patients younger than 35 years and childless at the time of cancer treatment may be interested in having children in the future [2].

Oncologists should thus be prepared to discuss the negative impact of cancer therapy on reproductive potential in the same way as any other risks of cancer treatment are discussed. Furthermore, patients interested in fertility preservation should be promptly referred to a reproductive medicine expert to improve success of fertility preservation measures [7], and close collaboration between the oncology team and the reproductive medicine unit is needed.

To preserve fertility after receiving a cancer diagnosis requires that decisions have to be made. Time constraints to process the diagnosis of cancer and its treatment and to make informed decisions with long-lasting consequences can further increase emotional distress. However, information empowers patients to ask pertinent questions and may avoid emotional distress by providing realistic expectations [3]. Patients who receive more detailed information tend to report greater satisfaction with their medical care. Informed patients may be involved in treatment decisions as well, which improves the patient's long-term quality of life [8]. Counseling of female patients should also cover the option of deciding not to take fertility preserving measures, and should include information on alternative treatments to become a parent, such as egg donation and adoption [3].

Table 31.2. Chemotherapy agents and their risk for ovarian failure in women

High risk	Cyclophosphamide
	Ifosphamide
	Melphalan
	Busulfan
	Nitrogen mustard
	Procarbazine
	Chlorambucil
Intermediate risk	Cisplatin
	Adriamycin
Low risk	Bleomycin
	Actinomycin D
	Vincristine
	Methotrexate
	5-Fluorouracil

Gonadal damage induced by cancer treatment

Chemotherapy

Knowledge of the risk of gonadal damage caused by cancer treatment is essential to recognize patients at risk of gonadal failure [9]. Table 31.2 summarizes the gonadotoxic impact of chemotherapy agents on the female ovary. The primordial oocytes, which constitute the female follicle pool, are at maximum number at approximately five months of gestation (approximately 6–7 million). Primordial oocytes are non-renewable and are reduced through apoptotic loss to 1–2 million at the time of birth, and thereafter the pool continues to decrease throughout the female life span, until complete depletion occurs during menopause. Of note, women's undeveloped oocytes and pre-granulosa cells of primordial follicles are particularly sensitive to alkylating agents, and ovarian failure is common after such treatment [10].

Because of a reduction of the primordial follicle pool with aging, older women have a higher risk of developing ovarian failure and permanent infertility after a cancer treatment than younger women [11]. Some female patients will recover a certain degree of ovarian function following chemotherapy or radiotherapy treatments, and they should be recommended not to delay childbearing for too many years [10]. In the clinical setting, gynecological examination by ultrasound, including estimation of antral follicle counts and the determination of hormones such as follicle-stimulating hormone (FSH), inhibin, and anti-Müllerian hormone (AMH) may help the clinician in evaluating the patient's remaining ovarian reserve after a cancer treatment and counseling her on the

Table 31.3. Radiotherapy protocols with high or intermediate impact on ovarian function [9]

High risk of amenorrhea
Total-body irradiation (TBI) for bone marrow transplant/stem cell transplant
Pelvic or whole abdominal radiation dose ≥ 6 Gy in adult women
Pelvic or whole abdominal radiation dose ≥ 10 Gy in postpubertal girls
Pelvic radiation or whole abdominal dose ≥ 15 Gy in prepubertal girls

Intermediate risk of amenorrhea
Pelvic or whole abdominal radiation dose 5–10 Gy in postpubertal girls
Pelvic or whole abdominal radiation dose 10–15 Gy in prepubertal girls
Craniospinal radiotherapy dose ≥ 25 Gy

chances of achieving a pregnancy. However, patients should be advised to avoid conception in the 6–12-month period immediately following completion of treatment, because of the toxicity of cancer treatments on growing oocytes [12]. This is due to the higher risk of teratogenesis during or immediately following chemotherapy. Nevertheless, DNA integrity has been shown to return over time after a cancer treatment [13], and no increase in childhood malignancies or genetic malformations was shown in a large follow-up study of more than 4000 children of cancer survivors [14].

Radiotherapy

For the treatment of cancer in the female, radiotherapy can be administered as external beam (teletherapy) or intracavitary (brachytherapy). The damage to female reproductive organs by radiotherapy is dose-dependent. The ovaries, uterus, and vagina may be compromised and damaged whenever they receive direct irradiation, but they can also be damaged through scattered radiation [15]. The ovarian primordial follicles are very sensitive to radiation, and the extent of the damage depends on the dose and fractionation schedule when the ovaries are located in the irradiation field [16]. Age at the time of ovarian exposure to radiotherapy is also an important factor, as younger women have a greater reserve of primordial follicles than older women and may thus have a higher remaining primordial pool after a cancer treatment [11]. Table 31.3 presents a compilation of current knowledge on the impact of radiation on ovarian function in women. In pediatric patients, failure in

pubertal development may be the first sign of gonadal failure.

The effects of uterine irradiation on fertility and pregnancy have been investigated in cohorts of adult and childhood cancer survivors [17,18]. Radiotherapy of the uterus seems to induce restricted uterine capacity, restricted blood flow, and impaired uterine growth during pregnancy. As a consequence, radiotherapy-treated female patients present with a high risk of spontaneous abortion, premature labor, and low-birthweight offspring [17,18]. The uterine damage seems to be more pronounced in the patients who are youngest at the time of radiotherapy [19]. Irradiation of the vagina is associated with loss of lubrication and in some cases stenosis, anatomical impairments to fertility, and sexual issues [15].

Fertility preservation options for local treatment of cancer

Shielding to reduce radiation damage and ovarian transposition

Shielding to reduce radiation to the reproductive organs, when possible, is the standard medical procedure currently offered to female patients. When shielding of the gonadal area is not possible, the surgical fixation of the ovaries far from the radiation field by oophoropexy (ovarian transposition) may be considered. This procedure may be carried out laparoscopically and it has been performed particularly in cases of gynecological cancer and Hodgkin's lymphoma. By incising the utero-ovarian ligaments and the peritoneum parallel to the infundibulopelvic ligaments, it is possible to mobilize the ovaries out of the pelvis. Lateral transposition seems to be more protective than median transposition of the ovaries [20].

Ovarian transposition reduces the risk of ovarian failure by about 50%, and such patients may retain some menstrual function and fertility [1]. Failure of this procedure may be related to scattered radiation and damage of the blood vessels that supply the ovaries [1].

Fertility-sparing surgery

Fertility-sparing surgery may be an option for selected patients. Conservative surgery aimed at preserving

Table 31.4. Fertility-sparing interventions in female patients [10]

Diagnosis	Type of surgery	Description	Obstetric outcome	Oncologic outcome
Cervical cancer stage IA1, IA2, IB1	Radical vaginal trachelectomy	Laparoscopic pelvic lymphadenectomy. Vaginal resection of the cervix and surrounding parametria keeping the corpus of the uterus and the ovaries intact	Spontaneous pregnancies described in up to 70%. Risk of second trimester pregnancy loss and preterm delivery	Rates of recurrence and mortality are comparable to those described for similar cases treated by means of radical hysterectomy or radiation therapy
Borderline ovarian tumors FIGO stage I	Unilateral oophorectomy	Removal of the affected ovary only, keeping in place the unaffected one and the uterus	Pregnancies have been reported, and favorable obstetric outcome	Oncologic outcome is comparable with the more radical approach of removing both ovaries and the uterus. Recurrence 0–20% vs. 12–58% when only cystectomy was performed
Ovarian epithelial cancer stage I, grade 1	Unilateral oophorectomy	Removal of the affected ovary only, keeping in place the unaffected one and the uterus	Pregnancies have been reported, and favorable obstetric outcome	7% recurrence of the ovarian malignancy and 5% mortality
Malignant ovarian germ cell tumors/sex cord stromal tumors	Unilateral oophorectomy	Removal of the affected ovary only	Pregnancies have been reported, and favorable obstetric outcome	Risk of recurrence similar to historical controls
Endometrial adenocarcinoma grade 1, stage 1A (without myometrial or cervical invasion)	Hormonal treatment with progestational agents for 6 months	Follow-up with endometrial biopsies every 3 months	Pregnancies have been reported	Recurrence rate 30–40%. Five percent recurrence during progesterone treatment

reproductive organs offers the opportunity to achieve pregnancy naturally in some cases. However, it offers no guarantee of pregnancy or live birth. Causes of subfertility unrelated to cancer diagnosis or surgery type may preexist in the patients, and some such patients may require assisted reproduction treatments [21]. Indications for fertility-sparing surgery often include a well-differentiated, low-grade tumor in its early stages or with low malignant potential.

The most established fertility preservation procedure for women in this group is the radical trachelectomy, offered to women with early-stage cervical cancer. Over 300 cases have been reported from the USA, Canada, and Europe [22]. The classical treatment of cervix cancer otherwise includes radical hysterectomy with bilateral pelvic lymphadenectomy in early-stage disease, or chemotherapy and radiotherapy for advanced-stage disease. Table 31.4 summarizes current indications for fertility-sparing interventions among women of fertile age [10].

Fertility preservation methods for systemic gonadotoxic treatment

Cryopreservation of embryos or oocytes after controlled ovarian stimulation

Adult women wishing to preserve fertility may undergo a hormonal stimulation treatment, currently known as controlled ovulation stimulation, for retrieval of matured oocytes and egg freezing, or, if the woman wishes, for in-vitro fertilization (IVF) of the retrieved eggs and embryo freezing. Oocyte retrieval is an outpatient procedure undertaken usually by vaginal ultrasound assistance under sedation or general anesthesia. Fertilization of the oocytes for embryo cryopreservation has traditionally been offered to women who have a partner. Single women may consider using a sperm donor, or otherwise freezing the oocytes unfertilized.

An IVF cycle may require 2–6 weeks, depending on the women's menstrual cycle phase at the time of planning the treatment. Transfer of frozen–thawed embryos today is a clinical routine in conventional IVF programs worldwide and it has been used for nearly 25 years. Intact embryos after thawing have the same implantation potential as fresh embryos, and this can lead to a 59% pregnancy rate and a 26% live birth rate [23].

The recent development of cryopreservation techniques, including vitrification of oocytes, has improved success rates in survival of oocytes, fertilization rates, and pregnancy rates, approaching that of fresh oocytes [4,24]. Today, both oocyte and embryo cryopreservation are well-established procedures, and both may be offered at many IVF clinics worldwide.

Stimulation protocols for women with breast cancer

Breast cancer is the most frequent cancer diagnosis in women of reproductive age. With current treatments, more than 80% of patients younger than 40 years of age are successfully treated today. Although breast cancers are usually diagnosed at an early stage, there is a high prevalence of ductal infiltration in this age group, and most of these patients are likely to undergo adjuvant systemic chemotherapy, and in some cases adjuvant endocrine therapy as well. The adjuvant endocrine therapy with tamoxifen, usually recommended for at least five years for patients with endocrine-sensitive tumors, will further delay the possibility of pregnancy for young breast cancer patients, as they would be recommended not to conceive during their most fertile years. If the female patient is 35 years old at the time of cancer diagnosis, she will be 40 years of age at the end of tamoxifen therapy, and her chances of conceiving then will be greatly reduced because of her advanced age.

Because of the elevation of circulating estradiol levels during conventional ovulation stimulation treatments for IVF, alternative and potentially safer protocols, including natural-cycle IVF or the use of tamoxifen and aromatase inhibitors to reduce estrogen exposure, have been introduced [25]. Natural-cycle IVF gives only one oocyte or embryo per cycle, and this treatment protocol has a high rate of cycle cancellation. Stimulation protocols with letrozole, an aromatase inhibitor, seem to offer a better fertility outcome with regard to the number of oocytes and embryos obtained, when compared to tamoxifen stimulation protocols [25]. Short-term

follow-up after stimulation treatments with letrozole for fertility preservation have not shown any detrimental effects on survival in women with breast cancer [26]. Further improvements in letrozole stimulation protocols combined with gonadotropins for breast cancer patients have been recently reported. Triggering of oocyte maturation with gonadotropin-releasing hormone (GnRH) agonists instead of human chorionic gonadotropin (hCG) further decreases estradiol exposure post-triggering and reduces the risk of ovarian hyperstimulation syndrome in breast cancer patients [27]. In-vitro maturation (IVM) of immature yielded oocytes has been shown to increase the number of oocytes and embryos cryopreserved for these patients [28].

Although aromatase inhibitors are contraindicated during pregnancy, data indicate that fertility treatments with letrozole are safe and the use of letrozole before conception does not induce any increased risks for the fetus [29].

Cryopreservation of immature oocytes

Freezing immature oocytes, although still experimental, is an option for female fertility preservation that can be offered to women who may not have enough time to complete a cycle for ovarian stimulation, and for patients who have a contraindication for hormonal stimulation. The oocytes are retrieved in the natural cycle and frozen at an immature stage or after IVM. Immature oocytes survive cryopreservation better than mature metaphase II oocytes [30]. After thawing they can be matured in vitro and fertilized. IVM of oocytes is at an experimental stage and needs further development [31]. Only a few fertility centers worldwide offer this technique.

Ovarian tissue freezing

The vast majority of eggs exist in the ovarian cortex within primordial follicles. Ovarian cortical tissue can be harvested immediately after the diagnosis of malignant disease by an outpatient laparoscopy or, if an operation is imminent, via laparotomy. Although the timing of ovarian biopsy is crucial and it is important to carry out cryopreservation before high-risk gonadotoxic therapy, young women, adolescents, and girls normally have an abundant number of primordial follicles, and attempts to cryopreserve ovarian tissue may still be worthwhile after the first courses of chemotherapy if the procedure was not possible before. This procedure does not require ovarian stimulation and does not cause any significant delay to initiation of cancer treatment.

Methods for cryopreservation of human ovarian tissue have been reported since the end of the 1990s, with functioning tissue after thawing [32]. Follicles in slices of cryopreserved–thawed tissue are able to survive long-term in in-vitro organ culture and have been transplanted to immunodeficient mice with development of mature oocytes in the xenografts [33,34]. Slow programmed freezing is the current protocol for cryopreservation of ovarian tissue, but poor survival of ovarian stroma is the main limitation of this method. Vitrification techniques for freezing of ovarian tissue have been developed, and they seem to improve the viability of all compartments of the tissue, with a survival rate of follicles similar to that after slow freezing, much better integrity of ovarian stroma, and undamaged morphology of blood vessels [35].

Sexual maturity is not required for ovarian tissue freezing, and this is the only viable option in prepubertal girls.

Ovarian tissue transplantation

Transplantation of frozen–thawed ovarian cortex is a new and promising method for recovery of fertility [36,37]. There have been hundreds of patients undergoing ovarian tissue freezing, but only a small percentage of these have returned for ovarian transplantation.

Ovarian tissue can be transplanted orthotopically, i.e., at the anatomical intrapelvic ovarian site [38], or heterotopically, i.e., at other places including extrapelvic sites [39].

Autotransplantation is only possible if absence of malignant cells in the graft is confirmed. Methods for the detection of cancer cells in the ovarian tissue of patients who have suffered from hematological malignancies are under development, including immunohistochemistry or the polymerase chain reaction (PCR) applied to the tissue. The investigation of residual malignant cells in the ovarian tissue may also be performed by xenotransplantation to immunodeficient mice [40]. To date, autotransplantation of ovarian tissue in patients who have suffered from systemic hematological malignancies is not recommended, because of the high risk of retransmission of malignancy, and only patients with cancer cases associated with a very low risk of ovarian compromise, such as squamous cell carcinoma of the

cervix, Wilms' tumor, Hodgkin's and non-Hodgkin's lymphoma, should be considered for future autotransplantation [15].

In-vitro culture of ovarian follicles

Studies on in-vitro culture and maturation of human ovarian follicles aiming to obtain mature oocytes for fertilization started over a decade ago [41]. In-vitro culture and maturation of isolated follicles or within a piece of thawed tissue will be the option for patients with hematological and ovarian malignancies. Although many improvements have been reported, this method is at present still at the developmental stage [42–44].

Cryopreservation of ovarian tissue offers hope to prepubertal cancer patients and their families, but it also raises several medical questions. The normality of imprinted genes of cryobanked oocytes matured in vitro has yet to be verified experimentally. Ovarian tissue cryopreservation and transplantation has been shown not to interfere with proper genomic imprinting in mouse pups [45], but additional studies in other animal models are needed. Fig. 31.1 illustrates current fertility preservation options for both female and male patients.

Gonadal protection by drugs

Data collected from observational studies have encouraged the empirical use of GnRH agonists or antagonists during chemotherapy [46]. However, the fact that prepubertal children with cancer still develop ovarian failure after chemotherapy suggests that this treatment is of limited benefit [47], and the bulk of the data from experimental studies is still inconclusive. Primordial follicles, which constitute the ovarian reserve pool, do not express gonadotropin receptors, and hence hormonal manipulation is not likely to affect them [48].

The few clinical trials performed to date do not support a beneficial effect of suppressing ovarian cycling by GnRH agonists. Three out of four published randomized studies have reported no effect of concurrent GnRH therapy during chemotherapy on ovarian reserve and hormonal ovarian markers [49,50] or menstrual history and clinical fertility outcomes [51] in female patients with Hodgkin's lymphoma and breast cancer. The only randomized study that reported benefit from this therapy reported a short follow-up and included young breast cancer

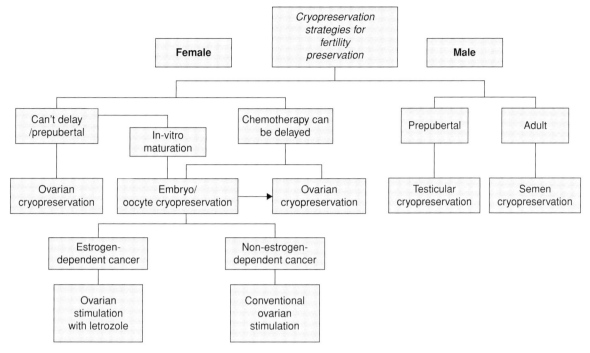

Figure 31.1. Fertility preservation in both sexes involves various assisted reproduction techniques, almost all being experimental. Depending on the patients' age, the type of cancer, the time available, and whether the female patient has a partner or not, a different strategy may be needed. (Partially modified from Sonmezer M, Oktay K. Fertility preservation in female patients. *Hum Reprod Update* 2004; 10: 251–66.)

patients [52]. The administration of the sphingosine-1-phosphate (S1P) receptor agonist FTY720 to rhesus monkey ovaries has been shown to prevent chemotherapy- and radiotherapy-induced germ cell death, and this agent seems promising for the development of drugs for ovarian protection [53].

References

1. Lee SJ, Schover LR, Partridge AH, *et al.* American Society of Clinical Oncology recommendations on fertility preservation in cancer patients. *J Clin Oncol* 2006; 24: 2917–31.

2. Schover LR, Rybicki LA, Martin BA, Bringelsen KA. Having children after cancer. A pilot survey of survivors' attitudes and experiences. *Cancer* 1999; 86: 697–709.

3. Rosen A, Rodriguez-Wallberg KA, Rosenzweig L. Psychosocial distress in young cancer survivors. *Seminars in Oncology Nursing* 2009; 25: 268–77.

4. Grifo JA, Noyes N. Delivery rate using cryopreserved oocytes is comparable to conventional in vitro fertilization using fresh oocytes: potential fertility preservation for female cancer patients. *Fertil Steril* 2010; 93: 391–6.

5. Altekruse SF, Kosary CL, Krapcho M, *et al. SEER Cancer Statistics Review, 1975–2007.* Bethesda, MD: National Cancer Institute. seer.cancer.gov/csr/1975_2007, based on November 2009 SEER data submission, posted to the SEER website, 2010 (accessed January 2012).

6. Forman EJ, Anders CK, Behera MA. Pilot survey of oncologists regarding treatment-related infertility and fertility preservation in female cancer patients. *J Reprod Med* 2009; 54: 203–7.

7. Lee S, Ozkavukcu S, Heytens E, Moy F, Oktay K. Value of early referral to fertility preservation in young women with breast cancer. *J Clin Oncol* 2010; 28: 4683–6.

8. Wang X, Cosby LG, Harris MG, *et al.* Major concerns and needs of breast cancer patients. *Cancer Nurs* 1999; 22: 157–63.

9. Rodriguez-Wallberg KA, Oktay K. Fertility preservation medicine: options for young adults and children with cancer. *J Pediatr Hematol Oncol* 2010; 32: 390–6.

10. Rodriguez-Macias Wallberg KA, Keros V, Hovatta O. Clinical aspects of fertility preservation in female patients. *Pediatr Blood Cancer* 2009; 53: 254–60.

11. Wallace WH, Anderson RA, Irvine DS. Fertility preservation for young patients with cancer: who is at risk and what can be offered? *Lancet Oncol* 2005; 6: 209–18.

12. Meirow D, Epstein M, Lewis H, Nugent D, Gosden RG. Administration of cyclophosphamide at different stages of follicular maturation in mice: effects on reproductive performance and fetal malformations. *Hum Reprod* 2001; 16: 632–7.

13. Simon B, Lee SJ, Partridge AH, Runowicz CD. Preserving fertility after cancer. *CA Cancer J Clin* 2005; 55: 211–28.

14. Hawkins MM. Pregnancy outcome and offspring after childhood cancer. *BMJ* 1994; 309: 1034.

15. Ajala T, Rafi J, Larsen-Disney P, Howell R. Fertility preservation for cancer patients: a review. *Obstet Gynecol Int* 2010; 2010: 160386.

16. Gosden RG, Wade JC, Fraser HM, Sandow J, Faddy MJ. Impact of congenital or experimental hypogonadotrophism on the radiation sensitivity of the mouse ovary. *Hum Reprod* 1997; 12: 2483–8.

17. Wo JY, Viswanathan AN. Impact of radiotherapy on fertility, pregnancy, and neonatal outcomes in female cancer patients. *Int J Radiat Oncol Biol Phys* 2009; 73: 1304–12.

18. Green DM, Sklar CA, Boice JD, *et al.* Ovarian failure and reproductive outcomes after childhood cancer treatment: results from the Childhood Cancer Survivor Study. *J Clin Oncol* 2009; 27: 2374–81.

19. Larsen EC, Schmiegelow K, Rechnitzer C, *et al.* Radiotherapy at a young age reduces uterine volume of childhood cancer survivors. *Acta Obstet Gynecol Scand* 2004; 83: 96–102.

20. Huang KG, Lee, CL, Tsai CS, Han CM, Hwang LL. A new approach for laparoscopic ovarian transposition before pelvic irradiation. *Gynecol Oncol* 2007; 105: 234–7.

21. Wong I, Justin W, Gangooly S, *et al.* Assisted conception following radical trachelectomy. *Hum Reprod* 2009; 24: 876–9.

22. Liou WS, Yap OW, Chan JK, Westphal LM. Innovations in fertility preservation for patients with gynecologic cancers. *Fertil Steril* 2005; 84: 1561–73.

23. Marrs RP, Greene J, Stone BA. Potential factors affecting embryo survival and clinical outcome with cryopreserved pronuclear human embryos. *Am J Obstet Gynecol* 2004; 190: 1766–71.

24. Oktay K, Cil AP, Bang H. Efficiency of oocyte cryopreservation: a meta-analysis. *Fertil Steril* 2006; 86: 70–80.

25. Oktay K, Buyuk E, Libertella N, Akar M, Rosenwaks Z. Fertility preservation in breast cancer patients: a prospective controlled comparison of ovarian stimulation with tamoxifen and letrozole for embryo cryopreservation. *J Clin Oncol* 2005; 23: 4347–53.

26. Azim AA, Costantini-Ferrando M, Oktay K. Safety of fertility preservation by ovarian stimulation with letrozole and gonadotropins in patients with breast cancer: a prospective controlled study. *J Clin Oncol* 2008; 26: 2630–5.

27. Oktay K, Türkçüoğlu I, Rodriguez-Wallberg KA. GnRH agonist trigger for women with breast cancer undergoing fertility preservation by aromatase inhibitor/FSH stimulation. *Reprod Biomed Online* 2010; 20: 783–8.

28. Oktay K, Buyuk E, Rodriguez-Wallberg KA, Sahin G. In vitro maturation improves oocyte or embryo cryopreservation outcome in breast cancer patients undergoing ovarian stimulation for fertility preservation. *Reprod Biomed Online* 2010; 20: 634–8.

29. Tulandi T, Martin J, Al-Fadhli R, *et al.* Congenital malformations among 911 newborns conceived after infertility treatment with letrozole or clomiphene citrate. *Fertil Steril* 2006; 85: 1761–5.

30. Boiso I, Martí M, Santaló J, *et al.* A confocal microscopy analysis of the spindle and chromosome configurations of human oocytes cryopreserved at the germinal vesicle and metaphase II stage. *Hum Reprod* 2002; 17: 1885–91.

31. Oktay K, Demirtas E, Son WY, *et al.* In vitro maturation of germinal vesicle oocytes recovered after premature luteinizing hormone surge: description of a novel approach to fertility preservation. *Fertil Steril* 2008; 89: 228.e19–22.

32. Hovatta O, Silye R, Abir R, Krausz T, Winston RM. Extracellular matrix improves survival of both stored and fresh human primordial and primary ovarian follicles in long-term culture. *Hum Reprod* 1997; 12: 1032–6.

33. Hovatta O, Silye R, Krausz T, *et al.* Cryopreservation of human ovarian tissue using dimethylsulphoxide and propanediol-sucrose as cryoprotectants. *Hum Reprod* 1996; 11: 1268–72.

34. Van den Broecke R, Liu J, Handyside A, *et al.* Follicular growth in fresh and cryopreserved human ovarian cortical grafts transplanted to immunodeficient mice. *Eur J Obstet Gynecol Reprod Biol* 2001; 97: 193–201.

35. Keros V, Xella S, Hultenby K, *et al.* Vitrification versus controlled-rate freezing in cryopreservation of human ovarian tissue. *Hum Reprod* 2009; 24: 1670–83.

36. Oktay K, Oktem O. Ovarian cryopreservation and transplantation for fertility preservation for medical indications: report of an ongoing experience. *Fertil Steril* 2010; 93: 762–8.

37. von Wolff M, Donnez J, Hovatta O, *et al.* Cryopreservation and autotransplantation of human ovarian tissue prior to cytotoxic therapy – a technique in its infancy but already successful in fertility preservation. *Eur J Cancer* 2009; 45: 1547–53.

38. Oktay K, Karlikaya G. Ovarian function after transplantation of frozen, banked autologous ovarian tissue. *N Engl J Med* 2000; 342: 1919.

39. Oktay K, Buyuk E, Veeck L, *et al.* Embryo development after heterotopic transplantation of cryopreserved ovarian tissue. *Lancet* 2004; 363: 837–40.

40. Meirow D, Hardan I, Dor J, *et al.* Searching for evidence of disease and malignant cell contamination in ovarian tissue stored from hematologic cancer patients. *Hum Reprod* 2008; 23: 1007–13.

41. Hovatta O, Silye R, Abir R, Krausz T, Winston RM. Extracellular matrix improves survival of both stored and fresh human primordial and primary ovarian follicles in long-term culture. *Hum Reprod* 1997; 12: 1032–6.

42. Telfer EE, McLaughlin M, Ding C, Thong KJ. A two-step serum-free culture system supports development of human oocytes from primordial follicles in the presence of activin. *Hum Reprod* 2008; 23: 1151–8.

43. Xu M, Kreeger PK, Shea LD, Woodruff TK. Tissue-engineered follicles produce live, fertile offspring. *Tissue Eng* 2006; 12: 2739–46.

44. Xu M, Barrett SL, West-Farrell E, *et al.* In vitro grown human ovarian follicles from cancer patients support oocyte growth. *Hum Reprod* 2009; 24: 2531–40.

45. Sauvat F, Capito C, Sarnacki S, *et al.* Immature cryopreserved ovary restores puberty and fertility in mice without alteration of epigenetic marks. *PLoS One* 2008; 3(4): e1972.

46. Blumenfeld Z, Avivi I, Eckman A, *et al.* Gonadotropin-releasing hormone agonist decreases chemotherapy-induced gonadotoxicity and premature ovarian failure in young female patients with Hodgkin lymphoma. *Fertil Steril* 2008; 89: 166–73.

47. Yap JK, Davies M. Fertility preservation in female cancer survivors. *J Obstet Gynaecol* 2007; 27: 390–400.

48. Oktay K, Briggs D, Gosden RG. Ontogeny of follicle-stimulating hormone receptor gene expression in isolated human ovarian follicles. *J Clin Endocrinol Metab* 1997; 82: 3748–51.

49. Behringer K, Wildt L, Mueller H, *et al.* No protection of the ovarian follicle pool with the use of GnRH-analogues or oral contraceptives in young women treated with escalated BEACOPP for advanced-stage Hodgkin lymphoma. Final results of a phase II trial from the German Hodgkin Study Group. *Ann Oncol* 2010; 21: 2052–60.

50. Waxman JH, Ahmed R, Smith D, *et al.* Failure to preserve fertility in patients with Hodgkin's disease. *Cancer Chemother Pharmacol* 1987; 19: 159–62.

51. Ismail-Khan R, Minton S, Cox C, *et al.* Preservation of ovarian function in young women treated with neoadjuvant chemotherapy for breast cancer: a randomized trial using the GnRH agonist (triptorelin) during chemotherapy. *J Clin Oncol* 2008; 26 (Suppl): Abstract 524.

52. Badawy A, Elnashar A, El-Ashry M, Shahat M. Gonadotropin-releasing hormone agonists for prevention of chemotherapy-induced ovarian damage: prospective randomized study. *Fertil Steril* 2009; 91: 694–7.

53. Zelinski MB, Murphy M, Lawson M, *et al.* Intraovarian delivery of a sphingosine-1-phosphate (S1P) agonist, FTY720, prior to ovarian X-irradiation yields fertilization, embryonic development and pregnancy in rhesus monkeys. *Fertil Steril* 2008; 90 (Suppl 1): S1.

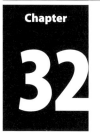

Chapter

32

Psychosocial issues surrounding the use of sperm donation

Allison B. Rosen and Lisa Rosenzweig

Introduction

The increasing availability and use of fertility preservation measures has allowed long-term survivors of cancer to hope that they will be able to create their families using their own genes. However, despite the existence of advanced technology in cancer treatment and reproductive medicine, some male survivors will experience infertility and must, if they are to have a family, rely upon donor insemination or adoption. Although both donor insemination and adoption will be discussed in this chapter, donor insemination, which brings unique challenges, will be emphasized. In both cases, survivors can benefit from psycho-educational counseling to prepare them for common issues that arise from these methods of creating a family. This chapter will focus on the needs of male cancer patients during two critical times: the time of diagnosis and the time when they intend to create their families. In addition, common obstacles to providing comprehensive care will be outlined, with suggestions for improving medical and psychological treatment.

Background

Improvements in the medical treatment of cancer have resulted in an increased number of long-term cancer survivors who will need information about reproductive issues, as they shift focus from preserving life to living it [1–3]. Fertility can be impaired by the disease itself, or it can be damaged as a result of aggressive chemotherapy and/or radiation therapy, bone marrow transplantation, or other treatment regimens. This damage may be temporary or permanent. There is general consensus among oncologists, reproductive specialists, and allied professionals that all patients

affected by cancer during or prior to their reproductive years should be informed about possible fertility impairment due to treatment for cancer, as well as possible fertility preservation measures [4–8].

Despite this consensus, there are several barriers to effective communication about fertility-sparing options. In addition, information about fertility-sparing options and alternative family building is not routinely offered to all patients needing it [9–16], despite the fact that we know such information is important to patients [17–25].

Barriers to communication

Several investigations have clarified the communication problems physicians encounter when caring for their patients. In an early study, Schover et al. found that while physicians agreed that fertility preservation options should be provided to patients at risk of infertility, 48% reported that they either never brought it up or mentioned it to less than a quarter of men at risk [12]. The physicians overestimated the costs of sperm banking, thought it would be too expensive for their patients, and did not know the location of convenient facilities. Similarly, Zapzalka et al. found that physicians lacked knowledge of specialized reproductive options; only 26% of oncologists knew about intracytoplasmic sperm injection (ICSI) at the time of their study [26]. Without knowledge of ICSI, physicians may refrain from suggesting sperm banking because they are not aware of the fact that an individual sperm can be injected directly into an egg for fertilization, thus providing a solution to problems concerning sperm morphology, count, and mobility.

More recently, Quinn et al. found that, while most physicians in their investigation discussed the possibility of infertility or fertility impairment with their patients, few provided specific information [9,10]. The reasons the physicians cited for their difficulties in discussing these issues were a lack of knowledge of options for fertility preservation, a lack of time for the discussions, challenges specific to their medical settings, and lack of training in how to discuss fertility preservation. Practices, services, and interdisciplinary exchange vary widely between programs and institutions. For instance, Goodwin *et al.*, investigating pediatric health professionals' knowledge and attitudes about fertility preservation, showed information deficits with regard to advanced fertility preservation techniques [16]. The investigators cited limited interdisciplinary interchange, and 64.3% reported difficulties with access to centers providing fertility preservation. Anderson *et al.* prospectively followed 1030 children at risk for fertility problems, finding that oncologists provided information to 83% of the postpubertal boys and 39% of the boys in early puberty [13].

How to discuss fertility preservation

Patients' age and life context are important factors in individualizing discussions about fertility preservation. The needs of children (and their parents), adolescents (and their parents), adults (unmarried, married, with children, and without children) are different. However, some of the commonly cited barriers to providing information (e.g., lack of time, lack of knowledge of convenient resources, difficulty discussing sensitive topics) can be addressed as general issues.

A team approach

The most effective approach for cancer care providers is within the context of a *team*. Team members, working from their respective professional perspectives and areas of expertise, best address the complex emotional, legal, medical, and ethical issues of the cancer patient. In addition to the physician, the team should have mental health providers, nurses, genetic counselors, attorneys, and ethicists (if necessary). The involvement of multiple disciplines allows for common patient concerns to be addressed amongst various members of the team, leaving more time for more medical aspects of care to be addressed by the physician.

In addition, there are many educational resources that can be recommended to patients. Two excellent books have been written for cancer patients that

discuss cancer, infertility, and sperm banking [27,28]. The Internet can also be a valuable resource for patient information and support. For instance, the American Cancer Society has helpful books and booklets on its website [29]. The website provides information about a variety of topics such as understanding chemotherapy, sexuality after cancer, addressing depression and anxiety, and fertility preservation. It also lists several links to informative non-profit organizations. In addition to saving time in the physician's office, written resources allow patients to clarify questions to ask of their providers when they are less overwhelmed by the initial diagnosis.

Finding sperm banks

Sperm banks are easy to locate via the Internet. The website www.spermbankdirectory.com provides a list of sperm banks in the United States. Many large banks allow the patient to collect sperm at home and mail it to the bank [30]. In contrast to physician perceptions, patients do not typically refrain from banking because of the expense [12]. Cryopreservation of three ejaculates for a five-year period is under $2000, and many sperm banks offer cancer patients payment plans to defer expenses.

Discussing sensitive topics

The mental health providers on the cancer team are trained to recognize preexisting psychological problems, as well as those that may arise in reaction to the cancer diagnosis. Although estimates vary, research suggests that between 10% and 50% of adult cancer patients experience high levels of distress from the cancer diagnosis alone [31–33]. Psychologists and social workers can effectively address patient anxiety and depression, identify couple conflict, and clarify patient misperceptions. They can discuss sensitive issues such as the disposition of sperm samples in the event of patient death. They are able to elaborate the pros and cons of banking, especially if the patient is an adolescent who might find such discussions uncomfortable in front of his parents, and they can intervene in the event the adolescent disagrees with his parents about the value of banking [12,33]. Patients may have unrealistic fears about the health of their future children [21], and psychologists, social workers, nurses, and genetic counselors can discuss the source of these fears, as well as the short- and long-term effects of cancer on physical health, identity formation, and sexuality. They can present realistic expectations about the probability of success of procedures, and provide help finding institutional review board (IRB)-approved programs, if parents are attempting to preserve the fertility of their prepubertal child [18,19].

In general, a knowledgeable team approach to patient care provides the best service and is valued by patients. Banking sperm (regardless of whether or not it is used) provides hope to the patient and helps in the psychological fight against cancer [18,22,33]. Correspondingly, Green et al. found that patients denied such opportunities have reported such intense reactions as depression and anger when recalling the time when they were initially diagnosed [25]. Similar reactions have been found in a number of investigations: resentment at having been denied a significant life choice, a sense of frustrated rage at the injustice of human suffering, and irritation about not having been provided with information about the possibility of infertility [11,17–19,21–25].

Psychological reactions to infertility

Patients who are involuntarily childless because they did not bank sperm, or who are childless due to a combination of male-factor and female-factor infertility, may experience a number of losses. We know that infertility itself affects not just the ability to father a child, but also a number of psychological domains. Natchtigall and his colleagues found that men suffered lowered self-esteem, stigmatization, role failure, and loss of potency [34]. Mason interviewed 18 men diagnosed with male-factor infertility, and found that they described such reactions as guilt, shame, anger, isolation, loss, and a sense of personal failure [35]. A number of other investigators have found similar reactions [36–39]. Further, infertility may cause stress in the marital relationship and can affect men's sexuality [40–42]. While infertility does not affect all men the same way, and many men manage it without it affecting their overall psychological well-being [43], men who are infertile due to male-factor infertility may suffer more distress than do women when infertility is due to female factors [43,44]. Men typically respond to their infertility with coping styles that involve denial, distancing from their feelings, and avoidance [39,45]. They may engage in cognitive distraction, regulate their own emotions (rather than turning to others), and view infertility in a problem-solving manner [46].

Donor sperm is not typically the preferred path to parenthood for most cancer survivors, but it allows patients to become parents and create a family. Schover et al. found that cancer survivors tended to believe that the cancer experience enhanced their parenting skills and increased the value of family life [21]. If they were infertile and did not have the option of having a biological child, Schover et al. found that 61% of the men surveyed would be willing to consider creating their families through adoption and 23% through donor insemination [21]. In addition, one might speculate that surviving cancer, with its emotional and physical difficulties, has the potential to augment personal resiliency in some individuals, allowing cancer patients to "see the bigger picture" and pursue family building regardless of the manner of conception.

History of sperm donation

Artificial insemination has been used for centuries. However, it has been shrouded in secrecy and stigmatized until relatively recently. In 1870, Dr. John Hunter, a Scottish physician, reported that he had successfully inseminated the wife of a linen draper using her husband's sperm. In 1885, a French physician, Dehault, published a booklet about artificial insemination [47]. In 1884 professor William Pencoast of Philadelphia's Jefferson Medical College performed an insemination on an unconscious Quaker woman using the sperm of one of his medical students [48]. Neither husband nor wife was informed about the physician's use of donor sperm until the couple achieved a pregnancy. At this point, the husband was told about the method of conception. He decided not to tell his wife about the use of another man's sperm.

During this period, few doctors performed donor inseminations [49]. Insemination was considered private, and records that could identify paternity were infrequent. Only fresh sperm was used. The secrecy protected parents and offspring, since donor insemination was considered adultery on the mother's part. Religious leaders condemned the process, considering it to be a sin, and many recommended that those using it be put in prison. These attitudes continued into the 1950s in the United States [49]. In 1954, the Supreme Court of Cook County ruled that artificial insemination was "contrary to public policy and good morals, and considered adultery on the mother's part." They continued, "A child so conceived, was born out of wedlock and therefore illegitimate. As such, it is the child of the mother, and the father has no rights or interest in said child." This position continued until 1964, when Georgia became the first state to legitimize children conceived via donor insemination.

In 1973, the Uniform Parentage Act was passed, which legitimized children conceived via donor sperm, provided that a woman's husband gave permission and the procedure was performed under a doctor's supervision [49]. Legally, the child was then considered the husband's biological child. In 1993, Thomas Steel, a sperm donor, was denied paternal rights regarding his biological offspring in Manhattan's Family Court, a ruling which became a fundamental tenet of family law. Thereafter, when donating, a sperm donor is required to sign papers acknowledging that he gives up all legal and other rights over biological children conceived with his sperm.

In 1953, the first successful pregnancy was achieved using frozen sperm, and in the early 1970s the first commercial sperm bank opened. In 1990, the UK passed the Human Fertilisation and Embryology Act, which created a system for licensing fertility clinics and procedures and established a central registry of donor births to be maintained by the Human Fertilisation and Embryology Authority (HFEA). In the United States, the Food and Drug Administration (FDA), the American Society for Reproductive Medicine (ASRM), the American Association of Tissue Banks, and the Centers for Disease Control and Prevention (CDC) now govern the procedures used in sperm banks.

Medical screening

All United States sperm banks are required to screen every potential donor for genetically inheritable diseases and infectious diseases transmitted through sperm [50]. The regulations are increasingly strict, providing reassurance that genetic and infectious diseases are unlikely to be passed on to parents or offspring except in rare circumstances. Sperm donors must be fit and healthy with a high "sperm count." A sociologist studying sperm banks in the United States found that 90% of applicants are rejected for insufficient sperm count and other reasons [51]. Typically, donors are interviewed about their medical history, their children, siblings, parents, and grandparents for three to four generations back. This information is not verifiable,

since it depends on the report of the potential sperm donor.

Donors usually donate for a specified time, generally ranging from 6–24 months. One sample will be divided into 6–12 vials depending on the quantity of the sperm and the technique for preparing it. Sperm banks have different exclusion criteria, with some excluding donors who are short, homosexual, bald, or have a poor family medical history [52,53].

Sperm banks provide such basic information such as race, skin color, height, weight, eye color, and blood group to the intended parents. Some of this information is available through the Internet, and other information is available only when a couple utilizes the specific sperm bank for their treatment. Some sperm banks provide additional information for a fee; others make basic information available when the children of a donor reach the age of majority.

Payment to a sperm donor is usually relatively insignificant. In the United States, the donor may receive payment for each donation as well as for each vial that is produced. In the United Kingdom and other European countries, donors only receive money for their expenses. The typical sperm donor in the United States receives $50–75 per donation [51].

Cultural differences in sperm donation

Sperm donation is viewed very differently in different parts of the world. Turkey bans sperm donation entirely [54]. Currently, it is also a criminal offence for a woman to travel abroad to get pregnant using sperm donation. Since March 2010, the legal consequence for a mother and any Turkish doctors and medical institutions recommending or aiding in finding foreign sperm banks, is 1–3 years in prison. Italy also bans sperm donation for couples wishing to have a child [55].

Other countries, concerned with the needs and rights of children to know their origins, have passed laws providing access to information about their sperm donors [47]. In 1986, Sweden passed legislation granting children access to identifying information about their donors. Several other countries have followed this practice: Austria, Switzerland, Great Britain, and New Zealand. Since 2006, all European Community countries are required to keep documentation about sperm donors for a minimum of 30 years [47].

Research on donor insemination

Due to secrecy surrounding its use, there is a dearth of research on donor insemination [47]. Further, small sample sizes and skewed demographics limit potential generalizability to the larger population [47]. Long-term follow-up of cancer survivors employing donor insemination to create their families is even less frequently assessed. However, preliminary research in this area suggests that patients considering donor insemination may have a variety of common concerns. Will their child conceived using frozen sperm be healthy [56–59]? Will they be satisfied with the process [56,60,61]? Will their child love them? Will they love their child [60,62,63]? Should they "just adopt" [64,65]?

Children conceived through donor insemination are at no increased risk for obstetrical complications or problems in infant development [56–58]. Children conceived by donor insemination combined with in-vitro fertilization (IVF) do not differ from the general population in terms of stillbirth, chromosomal abnormalities, prematurity, birthweight, sex ratio, or birth defects when the use of hormones for ovulation induction is controlled and the number of embryos transferred is controlled [59]. Further, parental satisfaction tends to be high after children are born [56,60,61].

Several studies have investigated why couples prefer donor insemination to adoption, with reasons including dislike of the process of adoption, the desire to experience pregnancy, and the fact that one parent is genetically related to the child [64,65]. If the couple wishes to maintain privacy, they can be discreet about the use of a donor. In addition, parents can have more genetic information about the child than is usually possible with international adoption, and parents can control the prenatal environment. Typically, donor insemination is also much less expensive than adoption.

Some couples worry that the child conceived using donor sperm will love the genetic parent more than the non-genetic parent, but this concern is not borne out in the literature. Golombok *et al.* studied 94 families with children conceived using donor insemination up to 12 years of age from Great Britain, the Netherlands, Italy, and Spain [62]. The investigators concluded that the absence of a genetic link does not interfere with attachment. The psychological and social development of donor-insemination children was normal, and there were no detectable differences between children conceived with IVF and donor insemination. Later investigations also supported these results [60,65].

Adoption

According to Schover's research, some patients prefer adoption to donor insemination for a variety of reasons [21]. They may have this preference because they fear the consequences of a family that is composed of the biological mother and another man, the semen provider. For instance, they may fear that the child may love one parent more than the other, as discussed above. They may be committed to the value of adoption (e.g., "There are already so many unwanted children who need homes"). They may have religious, legal, or cultural objections to donor insemination. They may want to have more information about the child than is available with donor insemination; in the case of open domestic adoption the birth mother and the adopting parents may have contact, sometimes throughout the life of the child.

However, cancer patients may face discrimination when trying to adopt, particularly when trying to adopt internationally [66,67]. For instance, China will not place a child with an individual or family who has had a history of cancer, regardless of type of cancer, stage of cancer, or years since treatment. Currently, many countries are in the process of revising their laws to protect children from illegal adoption practices, reducing the number of overall adoptions into the United States from other countries. In developing countries, a cancer diagnosis may not be as treatable as it is in more advanced countries and, wishing to protect the best interests of the child, countries may be concerned about early parental death.

Domestic adoption in the United States involves a process in which the birth mother typically chooses the parents to whom she will relinquish her baby. The birth mother may realize the treatable nature of many cancers, and therefore it may be easier for a cancer survivor to adopt a child domestically. The birth mother may identify with the parents' struggle and courage during cancer, may know individuals who have successfully survived cancer, and may feel that the cancer experience will result in stronger adoptive parents. Adoption involves a home study, birth and marriage records, financial records, background checks, and paperwork specific to the agency and country. Adoption after a cancer history usually requires, in addition, a letter from an oncologist stating that the adopting parents are two years post-treatment and will likely survive to the child's age of majority [66].

Recipient counseling in preparation for donor insemination

Mental health providers agree that individuals and couples using donor gametes should be offered a clinical session to prepare them for the process of creating their families in this fashion [47]. Whether or not this counseling should be legally mandated is debated. Some countries require pre-treatment counseling (e.g., Canada, Australia [47,68]). Other countries recommend it, but do not require it (e.g., New Zealand, Great Britain, Germany [47,69]). In the United States, medical guidelines suggest counseling, but do not require it, and individual medical programs may proceed entirely as they see fit [70].

The reason mental health providers agree about the importance of pre-treatment counseling is the fact that couples need information about the medical, legal, and psychosocial issues involving the use of donor sperm. Traditionally, the pre-treatment counseling involves evaluation and discussion of the couple's readiness to proceed, evaluation of the couple's marital stability and communication style, discussion about the meaning of the characteristics they used to select the donor, and information and discussion about whether or not to disclose the use of donor sperm to their future child [39,47] as well as to others.

In order to assess the couple's readiness for creating a family using donor sperm, the psychologist or social worker will discuss the emotional reactions of the couple to their medical history. As discussed above, we know that individuals surviving the cancer and infertility diagnosis may be at increased risk for anger, shock, and depression [25]. They may suffer lowered self-esteem, stigmatization, role failure, guilt, isolation, and a sense of personal failure [34–36]. The counselor can determine if these reactions are still present. Will the man project his sense of "failure" onto the child [39], or will the woman fantasize about the donor [47]. Is the man concerned the child will not look anything like him and feel embarrassed about public exposure of his infertility [47]? Is he worried about the child bonding with him (as the non-biological parent) or his ability to love the child? These questions and more can be addressed through pre-treatment counseling.

The mental health provider can also assess potential conflict, the couple's communication style, and their marital stability. Of concern is whether or not both partners feel that this is an option they want. Do they agree? Is the man being coerced in any way by his wife's desire to have a child [39]? Is the female partner angry with her male partner for "doing this to them" or "making" her taking ovulation medication? Are family members or societal pressures influencing them? The mental health professional can also identify any needs for further counseling to strengthen the marital relationship during this potentially emotionally and physically taxing time.

Sperm donor selection

Donor selection involves the couple exploring the meaning of the characteristics they value in themselves and a child, and hence the qualities they use to select their donor [71]. Typically, the recipients of donor gametes rank medical history, race, personality, intelligence, and appearance as of prime importance [71]. The mental health professional usually explores the implications of a couple's choices, to ensure that the couple understands that they cannot create the "perfect child." During the interview, the mental health professional may explore how they will feel if friends comment about the child's appearance, intelligence, etc. The couple must accept that they will never find a complete replacement for the husband and that they will not be able to "even the score" for life's "injustice" (i.e., they suffered cancer and then infertility). The counselor can also explore the possibility of failure and the couple's plans in the event they cannot conceive using donor insemination.

Although many couples perceive donor recipient counseling as "gate-keeping" and fear that their parental suitability and competency is being evaluated, there are very few criteria that would interfere with a couple's desire to proceed with family building. The guidelines suggested by the ASRM identify specific reasons to deny or delay access to treatment: active substance abuse; ongoing or a history of emotional abuse, physical abuse, or neglect; or uncontrolled psychiatric diagnoses [72]. The guidelines recommend that the treatment team, rather than just the mental health provider, make the decision. Rather than denying treatment "forever," the mental health professional discusses the reasons for delaying treatment with the couple and provides resources to enable the couple to proceed with family building after treatment that addresses the reasons for the suggested delay (e.g., alcohol abuse). Treatment is deferred, not denied.

Research on the effect of disclosure to children about the use of donor sperm is limited. Klock found that until 1999 disclosure rates were relatively low [73]. Parental reasons for non-disclosure of the child's genetic origins included the wish to protect the child from distress at finding out that the individual who is his or her father is not genetically related, raising the child's curiosity about the donor and then not being able to provide information about him, protecting the father from the child's potential rejection, and lack of support in how to tell the child [74–76]. Parents may want to tell their child of his or her genetic origins, but may feel they lack the skills to do so. Parents wonder when and how they should disclose. Should they disclose when the child is young? How young? How should they address the questions a three-year-old might have? They are interested in the meaning a child might ascribe at different developmental periods to a genetically unrelated parent. Discussions and provisions of resources such as children's books individualize treatment and may facilitate focusing on the needs of the child.

Although some parents express concern about disclosing children's genetic origins, common reasons parents give for making the choice to disclose include avoiding the burden of secrecy for the lifetime of the child, avoiding the risk of disclosure by someone other than the parents, avoiding accidental discovery, avoiding inadvertent disclosure through genetic testing, the belief that a child has the ethical right to know, potential for inaccurate medical information if the child relies on his or her parent's medical history or his or her heritage, violation of trust in the event of accidental disclosure, normalizing the experience for the child by introducing the topic at a young age rather than shock if discovered during adolescence or adulthood, and the child being able to discuss issues openly rather than suffering alone won his or her fears and suspicions [74–78].

Perhaps most importantly, recipient counseling introduces intended parents to the mental health profession, demystifies psychological intervention, and allows the couple to explore issues without the stigma of "therapy." If trust is established, the mental health professional can serve as a resource if the couple desires therapy, whether in the present or in the future.

Conclusion

Providing comprehensive individualized care to cancer patients involves a number of professionals and an integrated team approach. The potentially complex medical, legal, and emotional issues can best be addressed by team members operating within their professional disciplines. Mental health providers can identify emotional distress and discuss the short- and long-term implications of fertility preservation in a sensitive, compassionate manner during the stress of the initial diagnosis and treatment.

Donor insemination may allow individuals and couples the opportunity to bear children. However, donor insemination as a method of conception involves a variety of losses for the survivor and his spouse. Parents have questions about the similarity and differences between children conceived by donor insemination and children who have a biological connection to both parents. They need information and an opportunity to discuss their present needs and concerns, and the best way to address the future needs of their child. The counselor can provide pre-treatment education and support, and can also serve as a future resource.

References

1. National Cancer Institute. Estimated US cancer prevalence. cancercontrol.cancer.gov/ocs/prevalence/prevalence.html#survivor (accessed January 2012).

2. Altekruse SF, Kosary CL, Krapcho M, *et al. SEER Cancer Statistics Review, 1975–2007.* Bethesda, MD: National Cancer Institute. seer.cancer.gov/csr/1975_2007, based on November 2009 SEER data submission, posted to the SEER website, 2010 (accessed January 2012).

3. Summary of changes in cancer mortality,1950–2007 and 5-year relative survival rates, 1950–2006 males and females, by primary cancer site. seer.cancer.gov/csr/1975_2007/browse_csr.php?section=1&page=sect_01_table.03.html (accessed January 2012).

4. Lee SJ, Schover LR, Partridge AH, *et al.* American Society of Clinical Oncology recommendations on fertility preservation in cancer patients. *J Clin Oncol* 2006; 24: 2917–31.

5. Multidisciplinary Working Group convened by the British Fertility Society. A strategy for fertility services for survivors of childhood cancer. *Hum Fertil (Camb)* 2003; 6: A1–39.

6. European Society of Human Reproduction and Embryology (ESHRE) Task Force on Fertility Preservation in Severe Diseases. www.eshre.eu/01/default.aspx?pageid=29 (accessed January 2012).

7. Ethics Committee of the American Society for Reproductive Medicine. Fertility preservation and reproduction in cancer patients. *Fertil Steril* 2005; 83: 1622–8.

8. Lass A, Akagbosu F, Brinsden P. Sperm banking and assisted reproduction treatment for couples following cancer treatment of the male partner. *Hum Reprod Update* 2001; 7: 370–7.

9. Quinn GP, Vadaparampil ST, Gwede CK, *et al.* Discussion of fertility preservation with newly diagnosed patients: oncologists views. *J Cancer Surviv* 2007; 1: 146–55.

10. Quinn GP, Vadaparampil ST, Bell-Ellison BA, Gwede CK, and Albrecht TL. Patient-physician communication barriers regarding fertility preservation among newly diagnosed cancer patients. *Soc Sci Med* 2007; 66: 784–9.

11. Schover LR. Psychosocial aspects of infertility and decisions about reproduction in young cancer survivors: a review. *Med Pediatr Oncol* 1999; 33: 53–9.

12. Schover LR, Brey K, Lichtin A, Lipshultz LI, Jeha S. Oncologists' attitudes and practices regarding banking sperm before cancer treatment. *J Clin Oncol* 2002; 20: 1890–7.

13. Anderson RA, Weddell A, Spoudeas HA, *et al.* Do doctors discuss fertility issues before they treat young patients with cancer? *Hum Reprod* 2008; 23: 2246–51.

14. Crawshaw M, Glaser A, Hale J, Sloper P. Professionals' views on the issues and challenges arising from providing a fertility preservation service through sperm banking to teenage males with cancer. *Hum Fertil* 2004; 7: 23–30.

15. Van den Berg H, Langeveld NE. Parental knowledge of fertility in male childhood cancer survivors. *Psychooncology* 2008; 17: 287–91.

16. Goodwin T, Oosterhuis EB, Kierman M, Hudson GV. Attitudes and practices of pediatric oncology providers regarding fertility issues. *Pediatric Blood Cancer* 2007; 48: 80–5.

17. Tschudin S, Bitzer J. Psychological aspects of fertility preservation in men and women affected by cancer and other life-threatening diseases. *Human Reprod Update* 2009; 15: 587–97.

18. Rosen A, Rodriguez-Wallberg K, Oktay K. Psychological issues of cancer survivors. In Donnez J, Kim SS, eds. *Principles and Practice of Fertility Preservation.* Cambridge: Cambridge University Press, 2011; pp. 473–84.

19. Rosen A, Rodriguez-Wallberg KA, Rosenzweig L. Psychosocial distress in young cancer survivors. *Semin Oncol Nurs* 2009; 25: 268–77.

20. Schover LR, Rybicki LA, Martin BA, Bringelsen KA. Having children after cancer: a pilot survey of survivors' attitudes and experiences. *Cancer* 1999; 86: 697–709.

21. Schover LR, Brey K, Lichtin A, Lipshultz LI, Jeha S. Knowledge and experience regarding cancer, infertility, and sperm banking in younger male survivors. *J Clin Oncol* 2002; 20: 1880–9.

22. Saito K, Suzuki K, Iwasaki A, Yumura Y, Kubota Y. Sperm cryopreservation before cancer chemotherapy helps in the emotional battle against cancer. *Cancer* 2005; 104: 521–4.

23. Oosterhuis EB, Goodwin T, Kiernan M, Hudson MM, Dahl GV. Concerns about infertility risks among pediatric oncology patients and their parents. *Pediatr Blood Cancer* 2008; 50: 85–9.

24. Oppenheim D, Brugieres L, Hartmann O. Adolescents treated for cancer and fertility preservation. Psychological aspects. *Gynecol Obstet Fertil* 2005; 33: 627–31.

25. Green D, Galvin H, Horne B. The psycho-social impact of infertility on young male cancer survivors: a qualitative investigation. *Psychooncology* 2003; 12: 141–52.

26. Zapzalka D, Redmon J, Pryor J. A survey of oncologists regarding sperm cryopreservation and assisted reproductive techniques for male cancer patients. *Cancer* 1999; 86: 1812–17.

27. Schover LR. *Sexuality and Fertility after Cancer.* New York, NY: Wiley, 1997.

28. Schover LR, Thomas AJ. *Overcoming Male Infertility: Understanding its Causes and Treatments.* New York, NY: Wiley, 2000.

29. American Cancer Society. Fertility and cancer: what are my options? www.cancer.org/Treatment/TreatmentsandSideEffects/PhysicalSideEffects/FertilityandCancerWhatAreMyOptions/fertility-and-cancer (accessed January 2012).

30. Live on: sperm banking by mail. www.liveonkit.com (accessed January 2012).

31. Merckaert I, Libert Y, Messin S, *et al.* Cancer patients' desire of psychological support: prevalence and implications for screening patients' psychological need. *Psychooncology* 2010; 19: 141–9.

32. Strong V, Waters R, Hibberd C, *et al.* Emotional distress in cancer patients: the Edinburgh Cancer Centre symptom study. *Br J Cancer* 2007; 96: 868–74.

33. Crawshaw MA, Glaser AW, Hale JP, Sloper P. Male and female experiences of having fertility matter raised alongside a cancer diagnosis during the teenage and young adult years. *Eur J Cancer Care* 2009; 18: 381–90.

34. Nachtigall R, Becker G, Wozny M. The effects of gender specific diagnosis on men's and women's response to infertility. *Fertil Steril* 1992; 57: 113–21.

35. Mason MC. *Male Infertility: Men Talking*. London: Routledge, 1993.

36. Leiblum S, Kennan E, Lane M. The psychological concomitants of in vitro fertilization. *J Psychosom Obstet Gynaecol* 1987; 6: 165–78.

37. Glover L, Abel P, Gannon K. Male subfertility: is pregnancy the only issue? Psychological responses matter too – and are different in men. *BMJ* 1998; 316: 405–6.

38. Berg B, Wilson J, Weingartner P. Psychological sequelae of infertility treatment: the role of gender and sex-role identification. *Soc Sci Med* 1991; 33: 1071–80.

39. Petok W. The psychology of gender-specific infertility diagnoses. In Covington S, Hammer Burns L, eds. *Infertility Counseling: A Comprehensive Handbook for Clinicians*, 2nd edn. New York, NY: Cambridge University Press, 2006; pp. 37–60.

40. Newton C. Counseling the infertile couple. In Covington S, Hammer Burns L, eds. *Infertility Counseling: A Comprehensive Handbook for Clinicians*, 2nd edn. New York, NY: Cambridge University Press, 2006; pp. 143–55.

41. Connolly K, Edelmann R, Cook I. Distress and marital problems associated with infertility. *J Reprod Infant Psychol* 1987; 5: 49–57.

42. Irvine S. Male infertility and its effect on male sexuality. *Sex Marital Ther* 1996; 11: 273–80.

43. Rieker P, Fitzgerald E, Kalish L. Adaptive behavioral responses to potential infertility among survivors of testis cancer. *J Clin Oncol* 1990; 8: 347–55.

44. Mikulincer M, Horesh N, Levy-Shiff R, *et al*. The contribution of adult attachment style to the adjustment to infertility. *Br J Med Psychol* 1998; 71: 265–80.

45. Daniluk J. Gender and infertility. In Leiblum SR, ed. *Infertility: Psychological Issues and Counseling Strategies*. New York, NY: Wiley, 1997; pp. 103–25.

46. Stanton A. Cognitive appraisals, coping processes, and adjustment to infertility. In Stanton A, Dunkel-Schetter C, eds. *Infertility: Perspectives from Stress and Coping Research*. New York, NY: Plenum, 1991; pp. 87–108.

47. Thorn P. Recipient counseling for donor insemination. In Covington S, Hammer Burns L, eds. *Infertility Counseling: A Comprehensive Handbook for Clinicians*, 2nd edn. New York, NY: Cambridge University Press, 2006; pp. 305–318.

48. Peck P. Anonymous sperm donation. www.medicinenet.com/script/main/art. asp?articlekey=50877 (accessed January 2012).

49. Sperm donation. en.wikipedia.org/wiki/Sperm_donation (accessed January 2012).

50. Sperm Bank of California. Donor screening process. www.thespermbankofca.org/content/donor-screening-process (accessed January 2012).

51. American Sociological Association. Sperm donors valued less than egg donors. www.sciencedaily.com/releases/2007/05/070525204143.htm, posted May 26, 2007 (accessed January 2012).

52. Wanjek C. The good, the bad and the ugly sperm. *LiveScience*. www.livescience.com/10462-good-bad-ugly-sperm.html (accessed January 2012).

53. Orlando L. FDA recommends barring gay men from being sperm donors. www.buzzle.com/editorials/6-7-2005-71220.asp (accessed January 2012).

54. Sperm bank ban in Turkey sparks debate. *Daily News Economic Review*. www.hurriyetdailynews.com/n.php?n=sperm-bank-ban-sparks-debate-2010-07-30, posted July 30, 2010 (accessed January 2012).

55. Boggio A. Italy enacts new law on medically assisted reproduction. *Hum Reprod* 2005; 20: 1153–7.

56. Amuzu B, Laxoca R, Shapiro S. Pregnancy outcome, health of children and family adjustment after donor insemination. *Obstet Gynecol* 1990; 75: 899–905.

57. Milson I, Bergman P. A study of parental attitudes after donor insemination (AID). *Acta Obstet Gynecol Scand* 1982; 61: 125–8.

58. Clayton C, Kovacs GT. AID offspring: initial follow-up of 50 couples. *Med J Aust* 1982; 1: 338–9.

59. Lansac J and Royère D. Follow-up studies of children born after frozen sperm donation. *Hum Reprod Update* 2001; 7: 33–7.

60. Brewaeys A. Parent–child relationships and child development in donor insemination families. *Hum Reprod Update* 2001; 7: 38–46.

61. Gillet W, Daniels K, Herbison G. Feelings of couples who have had a child by donor insemination. The degree of congruence. *J Psychsom Obstet Gynecol* 1996; 17: 135–42.

62. Golombok S, Brewaeys A, Giavazzi M, *et al*. The European study of assisted reproduction families: the transition into adolescence. *Hum Reprod* 2002; 17: 830–40.

63. Golombok S, Jadva V, Lycett E, *et al*. Families created by gamete donation. Follow-up at age 2. *Hum Reprod* 2005; 20: 286–93.

64. Daniels K. Adoption and donor insemination: factors affecting couples' choices. *Child Welfare* 1994; 73: 1473–80.

65. Baran A, Pannor R. *The Psychology of Donor Insemination*, 2nd edn. New York, NY: Amistad, 1993.

66. Rosen A. Third-party reproduction and adoption in cancer patients. *J Natl Cancer Inst Monogr* 2005; 34: 91–3.

67. Rosen A. Fertility, pregnancy and adoption: knowing your options. SHARE Adoption Program. Presented September 28, 2010. vimeo.com/17158077 (accessed January 2012).

68. Canadian Women's Health Network. Bill C-6: an Act respecting assisted human reproduction and related research, 2004. www.cwhn.ca/resources/cwhn/billc6.html (accessed January 2012).

69. Daniels K. New Zealand: from secrecy and shame to openness and acceptance. In: Blyth E, Landau R, eds. *Third-Party Assisted Conception Across Cultures: Social, Legal and Ethical Perspectives*. London: Jessica Kinsley, 2004; pp. 148–67.

70. American Society for Reproductive Medicine. Informing offspring of their conception by gamete donation. *Fertil Steril* 2004; 81: 527–31.

71. Sachs P, Burns LH. Recipient counseling for oocyte donation. In Covington S, Hammer Burns L, eds. *Infertility Counseling: A Comprehensive Handbook for Clinicians*, 2nd edn. New York, NY: Cambridge University Press, 2006; pp. 319–38.

72. Ethics Committee of the American Society for Reproductive Medicine. Child-rearing ability and the provisions for fertility services. *Fertil Steril* 2004; 82: 564–7.

73. Klock S. To tell or not to tell: the issue of privacy and disclosure. In Leiblum S, ed. *Infertility, Psychological Issues and Counselling Strategies*. New York, NY: Wiley, 1997; pp. 167–88.

74. Cook R, Golombok S, Bish A. *et al*. Disclosure of donor insemination: Parental attitudes. *Am J Orthopsychiatry* 1995; 65: 549–59.

75. Nachtigall R, Becker G, Szupinski Quigora S, *et al*. The disclosure decision: concerns and issues of parents of children conceived through donor insemination. *Am J Obstet Gynecol* 1998; 178: 1165–70.

76. Lindblad F, Gottlieb C, Lalos O. To tell or not to tell: what parents think about telling their children that they were born following donor insemination. *J Psychosom Obstet Gynecol* 2000; 21: 193–203.

77. Rumball A, Adair A. Telling the story: parents' scripts for donor offspring. *Hum Reprod* 1999; 14: 1392–9.

78. Gottlieb C, Lalos O, Lindblad R. Disclosure of donor insemination to the child: the impact of Swedish legislation on couples' attitudes. *Hum Reprod* 2000; 15: 2052–6.

Chapter

33

Medical therapy for male infertility

Loren Jones and Craig Niederberger

Introduction

Male infertility in the cancer patient has a variety of etiologies, and the medical therapy for its treatment does not differ significantly from that for the infertile male without cancer. For the purposes of this chapter, it is understood that cancer itself is an etiology, albeit a non-specific one, of male infertility. Broadly, medical treatment of male infertility can be categorized into specific and empiric therapies. Specific therapy is utilized to correct a reversible endocrinopathy or other disorder, increasing the patient's chance of conception. Empiric therapy is employed without a firm diagnosis of the specific cause of the patient's infertility in an effort to improve his semen parameters and fertility. Furthermore, empiric therapy may be implemented not only in idiopathic infertility, but also in men in whom specific therapy has failed or for whom no specific therapy exists. In order to establish a diagnosis and to direct empiric or targeted therapy, an endocrine evaluation is essential to the treating physician.

While diagnostic improvements have made the diagnosis of idiopathic infertility less common, the oligoasthenospermic or normospermic man who has been unable to conceive with a "normal" partner for more than a year is still commonly seen. Evaluating the efficacy of empiric treatment in these patients is difficult for a number of reasons. First, a "normal" value of testosterone can fall within a very broad range, it varies between patients, and its ideal level for spermatogenesis and fertility is unclear. Further, because sperm numbers in semen analyses are highly variable over time and the thresholds for abnormality are set far below averages, regression to the mean virtually guarantees improvement in semen quality in an oligospermic population with or without treatment. A significant number of these patients may be able to conceive if given more time [1]. These limitations, along with lack of standardization of controlled studies, make it difficult to evaluate the value of empiric therapies through the published literature.

This chapter reviews the endocrine evaluation of the infertile male cancer patient, and discusses the specific and empiric therapies available to treat the infertile man.

Evaluation of the infertile male cancer patient

Along with comprehensive history, physical examination, and semen analysis, the endocrine evaluation of the male infertility patient is of utmost importance in guiding medical therapy. This evaluation and endocrine workup is designed to discover any reversible cause of the infertility before empiric therapy is initiated. The most common correctable causes of infertility including varicocele, endocrinopathy, infectious or immunologic causes, and obstruction can be discovered through this initial workup. In addition, the comprehensive evaluation of the infertile man may uncover previously unknown medical pathology [2]. The cancer patient in particular may have multiple etiologies for male-factor infertility, so a careful history of radiation and chemotherapy exposure along with a comprehensive endocrine evaluation is essential.

The endocrine evaluation should assess androgen steroidogenesis and control, disorders of aromatization, markers of spermatogenic function, and investigate for extratesticular endocrine pathology. As

Fertility Preservation in Male Cancer Patients, ed. John P. Mulhall, Linda D. Applegarth, Robert D. Oates and Peter N. Schlegel. Published by Cambridge University Press. © Cambridge University Press 2013.

detailed elsewhere in this text, androgen steroidogenesis and spermatogenesis is dependent on an intact hypothalamic–pituitary–gonadal (HPG) axis. As such, the infertility endocrine workup is designed to identify any defects in the HPG axis that would cause hypoandrogenism or dysfunctional spermatogenesis.

A well-identified problem with the diagnosis of hypoandrogenism is that there is no unambiguous definition of low testosterone. Morning levels are typically referenced, although there are multiple ranges of normal in use. The most common in clinical practice is the Food and Drug Administration (FDA) range of 300–1000 ng/dL [3]. The American Association of Clinical Endocrinologists (AACE) guidelines include a range of 280–800 ng/dL [4]. A substantial problem that clinicians face is the significant variability between the different assays commonly used to measure testosterone [5]. In addition, a significant percentage of serum testosterone is bound to proteins (primarily sex-hormone binding globulin [SHBG] and albumin), making it unavailable for use [6]. In order to improve the specificity of serum testosterone, it is useful to consider this distribution of serum testosterone and to calculate the percentage of bioavailable testosterone. Commercial assays for free testosterone have proven inaccurate, while those for albumin and SHBG are relatively reliable, making a calculated bioavailable testosterone preferred in the endocrine evaluation [7].

Estradiol is utilized to evaluate for aromatase dysfunction [8] and follicle-stimulating hormone (FSH) is obtained in order to differentiate between obstructive and non-obstructive azoospermia [9]. In its negative feedback loop with the pituitary, FSH levels indirectly reflect circulating inhibin B, with higher FSH implying worsening spermatogenesis. Inhibin B is an ideal marker for spermatogenesis [10], although its relative expense makes FSH the preferred test. Finally, a prolactin is obtained if clinically indicated. The luteinizing hormone (LH) level is obtained as a measure of steroidogenesis.

In summary, a recommended endocrine workup in the infertile man consists of morning testosterone, LH, FSH, SHBG, albumin, and estradiol along with prolactin if symptoms such as visual field defects, headache, or erectile dysfunction are present. If the initial testosterone is borderline, it is repeated three times, 30 minutes apart, for an average. This battery of tests greatly assists in the selection of targeted or empiric therapy for male infertility.

Medications

Clomiphene citrate

Clomiphene citrate was originally investigated as an empiric therapy to treat idiopathic oligospermia, and it has been used as treatment for subfertile men since the late 1960s [11]. It acts as an antiestrogen that blocks estradiol's feedback inhibition of the pituitary and hypothalamus in the HPG axis, increasing both endogenous gonadotropin-releasing hormone (GnRH) from the hypothalamus, and LH secretion from the pituitary [12]. This, in turn, increases testicular testosterone production and may improve spermatogenesis in selected men. In 1969, Heller et al. first reported on the improvement of semen parameters with the use of clomiphene citrate in men [13]. In this study, clomiphene increased both serum gonadotropins and testosterone, and a dose of 50 mg each day resulted in an increased sperm count. However, this study was not performed on an infertile population. Since then, investigators have conducted nine controlled studies, with the majority showing no efficacy over placebo or vitamin C [14]. However, three of the nine studies did show an improvement in both sperm count and pregnancy rates after treatment with clomiphene citrate [15–17].

Paulson randomized 40 men with azoospermia or oligospermia to receive treatment with clomiphene or cortisone, and reported improved semen parameters and pregnancy rates in the clomiphene group [15]. It is unclear whether this effect was from a positive response to the clomiphene or a negative response to the cortisone without the inclusion of a placebo arm. Wang et al. randomized 46 men with idiopathic oligospermia to be treated with four months of a placebo, clomiphene citrate (25 or 50 mg/day), mesterolone, or pentoxifylline, or four months of testosterone enanthate [16]. Treatment with clomiphene citrate resulted in a significant increase in the mean sperm concentration and pregnancy rates, while treatment in the other arms showed no effect. This study is limited by the small number of men in each treatment arm, but is strengthened by the inclusion of a placebo. In their study, Check et al. randomized 100 men with normal semen parameters from couples with idiopathic infertility to therapy with either 25 mg of clomiphene citrate daily or 500 mg of vitamin C daily as a placebo [17]. Within 8 months, 29 of 50 couples (58%) in the clomiphene citrate treatment arm achieved a pregnancy, compared to only 8 of 50 (16%) in the ascorbic acid arm. There were no appreciable changes in sperm counts, motility, or morphology after either treatment, nor were there any significant differences in semen parameters in those conceiving versus those who did not.

Clomiphene citrate also has applicability as specific therapy in azoospermic men. In 1993, Akin first described its use to stimulate sperm production in a previously azoospermic man with incomplete androgen resistance [18]. More recently, Hussein *et al.* completed a multicenter trial of 42 patients with non-obstructive azoospermia who were treated with clomiphene citrate [19]. In this study, men underwent an initial testicular biopsy, after which clomiphene was administered and titrated to achieve and maintain serum testosterone levels between 600 and 800 ng/dL. After this therapy, 64.3% of patients demonstrated sperm in their semen ranging from 1 to 16 million sperm per mL, with 35.7% remaining azoospermic. In these patients, surgical testicular biopsy and sperm extraction were performed. Sufficient sperm for intracytoplasmic sperm injection (ICSI) were retrieved in all patients. Although there was no control arm in this study, its findings show a role of clomiphene citrate in men with non-obstructive azoospermia as empiric therapy to stimulate sperm production.

The problem with studies of clomiphene as empiric therapy is that results in the target population most likely to respond, those with low testosterone, may be diluted. Clomiphene has been studied as specific therapy for men with hypogonadotropic hypogonadism. In a 2006 study, four patients who were evaluated for infertility and found to have idiopathic adult-onset hypogonadotropic hypogonadism were treated with clomiphene citrate 50 mg, three times weekly [20]. Three of the four men responded to clomiphene alone with increases in testosterone, FSH, and LH. Semen parameters also improved, and two of the men achieved pregnancies with clomiphene alone. While small, this study demonstrated that select men with hypogonadotropic hypogonadism can be treated with clomiphene citrate alone instead of the more expensive human chorionic gonadotropin (hCG) and human menopausal gonadotropin (hMG) therapy that is discussed later in this chapter.

An initial starting dose of 25 mg daily or 50 mg every other day is most common, and titration may be required to achieve optimal hormonal response. If simple androgen replacement is the target, total testosterone levels above 300 ng/dL or bioavailable testosterone levels above 150 ng/dL are sought. For superphysiological stimulation, total testosterone levels above 600 ng/dL are the titration target. Side effects are generally self-limited and mild. Hyperaggressive behavior is the most common serious side effect, and is most often encountered when initial testosterone level is very low.

A few studies suggest that treatment with clomiphene citrate may improve semen parameters and pregnancy rates in patients with idiopathic infertility [15–17] and a recent study demonstrated improved pregnancy rates by combining clomiphene therapy with an antioxidant [21]. In addition, one study has shown the drug's benefit as specific therapy in azoospermic patients prior to surgical sperm extraction [19], another has shown its benefit in patients with incomplete androgen resistance [18], and another demonstrated specific applicability in men with idiopathic adult-onset hypogonadotropic hypogonadism [20]. Due to its low cost and high tolerability, along with some favorable results in controlled studies, clomiphene citrate remains a treatment option in selected cases. The majority of evidence, however, suggests that empiric clomiphene citrate is not an effective treatment for male infertility without a specific etiology such as hypoandrogenism [14], and its extended use should not delay more effective methods of assisted reproduction.

Tamoxifen

Like clomiphene, tamoxifen citrate is an antiestrogen that blocks estradiol's feedback inhibition in the HPG axis [12], stimulating gonadotropin release. It is most commonly used in the treatment of advanced breast cancer and was first proposed as a treatment for male infertility in the 1970s by Vermeulen and Comhaire [22]. In their work, these investigators demonstrated that treating men with idiopathic oligospermia with tamoxifen for 6–9 months resulted in a significant increase in gonadotropins, testosterone, and estradiol levels. A significant increase in sperm density was observed only in subjects with sperm counts below 20 million/mL and normal FSH levels. With no placebo group included, these findings can be explained by normal variance in sperm density over time and regression to the mean. Several other uncontrolled studies have had similar findings.

Between 1977 and 1992, four controlled studies of tamoxifen were completed, and all had negative results [23]. Adamopoulos and colleagues published a controlled trial of a combination of tamoxifen citrate and testosterone undecanoate versus placebo, hypothesizing that the tamoxifen would increase spermatogenesis and the androgen would increase sperm motility [24]. These investigators reported improvements in sperm count, motility, and morphology after six months of treatment. More importantly, the incidence of spontaneous pregnancy was 33.9% in the active treatment group compared to 10.3% in the placebo group. Despite this promising trial, the weight of the evidence is that tamoxifen does not demonstrate efficacy, and its use as empiric therapy is not recommended.

Aromatase inhibitors

Aromatase is the enzyme responsible for the conversion of testosterone and androstenedione to estradiol and estrone, respectively [25]. Peripheral conversion of testosterone by aromatase in the adipose tissue is the primary source of circulating estradiol in men. The subset of patients with infertility and a normal or decreased testosterone level along with an increased estradiol (a testosterone-to-estradiol level less than 10) may benefit from an aromatase inhibitor.

Raman and Schlegel treated 140 subfertile men found to have abnormal testosterone-to-estradiol ratios (less than 10) with 100–200 mg testolactone daily or 1 mg anastrazole daily [25]. These investigators observed that men treated with testolactone experienced increased testosterone-to-estradiol ratios during therapy and that the change was confirmed in subgroups of men with Klinefelter syndrome (5.3 pretreatment vs. 12.4 during). A total of 12 oligospermic men in this group had semen analyses before and during testolactone treatment, and an increase in sperm concentration, motility, morphology, and motility index was observed.

In the anastrazole group, similar changes in the testosterone-to-estradiol ratios were observed in all groups (7.2 pre-treatment vs. 18.1 during) except in patients with Klinefelter syndrome. A total of 25 oligospermic men with semen analysis before and during anastrozole treatment were noted to have an increase in semen volume, sperm concentration, and motility index. These changes were similar to those observed in men treated with testolactone. From this study, men with a low serum testosterone-to-estradiol ratio can rationally be treated with an aromatase inhibitor. Anastrozole and testolactone have similar effects on hormonal profiles and semen analysis and appear to have similar efficacy in all patients except those with Klinefelter syndrome, for whom testolactone appeared to have greater efficacy.

Gonadotropin-releasing hormone (GnRH)

Synthetic analogs of GnRH increase pituitary gonadotropin secretion. GnRH dosed through either frequent administration or the use of a portable pump for pulsatile infusion is an alternative therapy for some patients with hypogonadotropic hypogonadism and has been shown to produce better results in testicular size than exogenous gonadotropins in the treatment of these patients [26]. Sperm production, however, does not seem to be improved compared to using hCG and hMG. GnRH therapy is only effective in patients with intact native pituitary glands and is not indicated in patients with acquired hypogonadotropic hypogonadism due to tumors, pituitary surgery, or trauma. The therapy is inconvenient because of the need for pulsatile infusion and is generally reserved for patients who do not respond to clomiphene citrate or gonadotropin therapy.

Controlled studies have evaluated the empiric use of GnRH in men with idiopathic infertility without significant improvements reported in seminal parameters or pregnancy rate. Because of the substantial expense of GnRH and its difficulty in dosing, it is not currently recommended as first-line treatment for male infertility.

Human chorionic gonadotropin (hCG) and human menopausal gonadotropin (hMG)

FSH and LH are secreted by the anterior pituitary in response to pulsatile GnRH and are responsible for testicular production of spermatogenesis and steroidogenesis, respectively. hCG and hMG were initially isolated from the urine of pregnant and menopausal women and have been used to treat male infertility. hCG acts similarly to LH by stimulating Leydig cells in the testes to secrete testosterone, while hMG has both LH and FSH activity.

Clomiphene citrate is preferred in responders, because of its ease of administration and low cost, but hCG and hMG have been used very effectively as specific therapy for hypogonadotropic hypogonadism. In the patient with acquired pituitary failure, treatment with 2000 IU of hCG three times per week usually initiates spermatogenesis [26]. However, hCG may be administered biweekly as well, usually at an initial dose of 2500 IU twice weekly, increasing to 5000 IU as necessary, or beginning at the latter dose if the initial conditions are severe. In one strategy, after six months of therapy, non-responders and patients with congenital forms of hypogonadism are started on FSH therapy in the form of 75 IU hMG three times weekly. In men treated with hCG and hMG for hypogonadotropic hypogonadism, testicular size is an important prognostic factor in determining sperm production. In a 30-year review of 36 patients, Miyagawa and colleagues reported that long-term administration of hCG/hMG for 12–240 months resulted in sperm production in only 36% of small-testis subjects (volume 1.6 ± 0.9) but in 71% of the large-testis subjects (volume 7.5 ± 3.5) [27].

The success of hCG and hMG as specific therapy for hypogonadotropic hypogonadism has led investigators to study their effects on men with idiopathic infertility, with limited success. In 1987, Knuth *et al.* randomized 39 men to treatment with 2500 IU hCG twice a week plus 150 IU hMG 3 times a week for 13 weeks and placebo [28]. In this controlled trial, there was no reported improvement in seminal parameters, and while there was an increase in pregnancy rate, it was not significant.

Recombinant FSH

Isolated FSH deficiency is a rare disorder in which the administration of hMG has been shown to effectively stimulate spermatogenesis [14]. More recently, recombinant FSH (rFSH) has become available, giving another therapy option for this condition. In lieu of hMG, rFSH may also be used in combination therapy with hCG, although at substantially increased expense.

FSH, purified FSH, and rFSH have also been investigated as empiric treatment in men with idiopathic infertility [29]. Some studies have shown that FSH treatment may restore sperm structure, while reports on the effects of FSH on other sperm parameters and spontaneous pregnancy rates are mixed or negative [30]. Caroppo and colleagues postulated that rFSH would be of benefit as a specific therapy for infertile male partners of couples undergoing in-vitro fertilization with intracytoplasmic sperm injection (IVF-ICSI)

cycles, rather than as a blanket empiric therapy for subfertile male patients in general [29]. In these investigators' study, 33 patients with idiopathic oligoasthenoteratospermia who failed to conceive after previous ICSI attempts received either rFSH 150 IU for 3 months (23 patients) or no treatment (10 patients). The authors observed that treatment with rFSH induced a significant increase in testicular volume and sperm parameters and that the mean fertilization rate after ICSI cycles was higher in treated patients, although not at the statistical significance threshold sought. Importantly, the pregnancy rate in the treated group was 30.4%, with no pregnancies recorded in the control group. Recombinant human FSH is a promising pre-treatment for oligospermic patients undergoing ICSI, by improving sperm parameters, sperm structure, and fertilization rate.

Androgens

In patients with an intact HPG axis, exogenous androgen supplementation results in feedback inhibition of gonadotropin release. This inhibition acts to decrease the intratesticular testosterone and spermatogenesis, despite normal or increased serum testosterone [31]. Androgen supplementation has been used empirically in the treatment of idiopathic infertility as both continuous therapy and "rebound" therapy to stimulate spermatogenesis, without any positive effect. As many patients are converted to complete azoospermia, "rebound" therapy is to be condemned.

Mesterolone is the most commonly used synthetic androgen available for oral administration. Doses from 2 mg/day to 150 mg/day have been studied for the treatment of idiopathic male infertility. In 1989, the World Health Organization sponsored a randomized double-blind study in which 157 men were randomized to receive 75 mg/day of mesterolone, 150 mg/day of mesterolone, or placebo for eight months [32]. In this study, no significant difference was observed in sperm concentration or pregnancy rates between the arms. Further, four other controlled studies of androgen therapy versus placebo failed to show any positive effect on fertility [14,23].

In testosterone "rebound" therapy, high doses of exogenous androgens are administered in an effort to suppress the pituitary in the hope that once the androgen therapy is stopped the pituitary will rebound and spermatogenesis will resume within four months with improved semen parameters. In the only controlled study of this therapy, Wang *et al.* did not demonstrate any efficacy in a small group of patients [16]. Results from early uncontrolled studies were not reproduced in subsequent trials [23].

Empiric androgen therapy and testosterone rebound therapy have significant potential toxicity and no demonstrated benefit in the treatment of infertile men. In fact, it is clear from the literature that exogenous androgens have a contraceptive effect on men, and they are therefore not recommended in the treatment of the infertile male, or any man desiring fertility.

Nutraceuticals

Recently, two studies have evaluated the effect of coenzyme Q_{10} (CoQ_{10} or ubiquinone) on semen parameters and conception. CoQ_{10} is a component of the mitochondrial respiratory chain, playing a crucial role both in energy metabolism and as a liposoluble chain-breaking antioxidant for cell membranes and lipoproteins [33]. Its reduced form ubiquinol (QH_2) is present in sperm in high concentrations and has been postulated as having a protective role as an antioxidant [33]. These roles in the energy chain of the sperm and as an antioxidant have led to hypotheses that empiric treatment of idiopathic asthenospermic men with CoQ_{10} may improve sperm motility and conception rates.

Balercia *et al.* studied the effectiveness of CoQ_{10} in improving semen quality in men with idiopathic infertility in a placebo-controlled, double-blind randomized trial [33]. These investigators treated 60 infertile patients with either 200 mg/day CoQ_{10} or placebo for six months and measured the variations in semen parameters with CoQ_{10} and ubiquinol concentrations in seminal plasma and spermatazoa. The authors reported that with treatment, CoQ_{10} and ubiquinol increased significantly in both seminal plasma and sperm cells and spermatozoa motility improved. Subjects with a lower baseline value of motility and levels of CoQ_{10} had a statistically significant higher probability to be responders to the treatment. In another study, Safarinejad randomized 212 men with idiopathic oligoasthenoteratospermia to receive 300 mg CoQ_{10} orally daily or placebo for 26 weeks [34]. He reported significant improvement in sperm density, motility, and morphology with treatment, and also observed an increase in the mean acrosome reaction in the treated group.

These studies show promise that supplementation with CoQ_{10} improves certain semen parameters, with motility improvement being consistent between both investigations. Further, the biological rationale for therapy and the high tolerability of CoQ_{10} make it an empiric option for patients with idiopathic infertility. Based on the two randomized trials, treatment with 200–300 mg per day of CoQ_{10} is reasonable, particularly in men with asthenospermia. However, further investigation is needed to draw final conclusions and to evaluate the effect of CoQ_{10} supplementation on pregnancy rates.

Antioxidants

High levels of reactive oxygen species in semen have been suggested to be an independent risk factor for male-factor infertility, regardless of whether the patients have normal or abnormal semen parameters [35]. As such, supplementation with known antioxidants such as vitamins C and E, pentoxifylline, and allopurinol have been proposed as a method to reduce free-radical damage to sperm and increase fertility. Recently, Ghanem and co-investigators reported results of a placebo-controlled trial of clomiphene citrate (25 mg per day) and vitamin E (400 mg per day) of men with sperm count and motility below WHO 4th edition thresholds, hypothesizing that the antioxidant effect of vitamin E in combination with the anti-estrogen would improve pregnancy rates [21]. Sperm count, forward progressive motility, and pregnancy rate were higher in the treated group compared to placebo. This study provided the first controlled trial that showed a benefit of an antioxidant in combination with endocrine therapy. Future trials are warranted to study the underlying mechanisms of the observed improvement in sperm and pregnancy and to study the effects of other antioxidants. However, these promising results and the safety of moderate doses make antioxidant supplementation an acceptable option for the infertile man attempting to conceive.

Treatment of hyperprolactinemia

Routine screening for hyperprolactinemia in the infertile man has not been shown to be useful and is not routinely recommended. However, when symptoms such as visual field defects, headache, or erectile dysfunction are present, a serum prolactin is indicated. If hyperprolactinemia is found, workup should include a careful history and physical, a baseline testosterone, and an MRI of the brain. Most men with a prolactin-secreting adenoma will have low gonadotropin and testosterone levels, leading to erectile dysfunction and infertility. If a pituitary macroadenoma (greater than 1 cm in largest dimension) is discovered, medical therapy may be effective, but referral to a neurosurgeon for evaluation for possible transphenoidal or endoscopic excision is recommended. Two-thirds of men with hyperprolactinemia will have a microadenoma (less than 1 cm in greatest dimension) or no visible adenoma despite elevated serum prolactin [36]. In these men, medical therapy is the preferred treatment.

The secretion of prolactin is mainly regulated by dopamine inhibition [37]. Therefore, the most commonly used medications for the medical therapy of hyperprolactinemia are the dopamine agonists bromocriptine and cabergoline. Bromocriptine was the first medication introduced, but cabergoline is more popular today because of its similar efficacy and fewer side effects. In 1998, De Rosa et al. studied sexual and gonadal function along with semen parameters in men with prolactinomas treated with cabergoline and bromocriptine, and found that treatment with cabergoline normalized prolactin levels, improving gonadal and sexual function and fertility in males with prolactinoma earlier than did bromocriptine treatment, providing good tolerability and excellent patient compliance [38].

Treatment for hyperprolactinemia is initiated with cabergoline 0.5 mg once weekly and increased to 0.5 mg twice a week if necessary. After a therapeutic dose is achieved, serum prolactin and testosterone should be checked every six months, and the dose can be titrated to 1 mg twice weekly to keep serum prolactin levels less than 15 µg/L [36]. If response is suboptimal, repeat MRI should be considered.

Treatment of infectious and inflammatory infertility

Infection and inflammation in the male reproductive tract are potentially treatable causes of male infertility. Infections in the urethra, prostate, epididymus, or testicles could disrupt sperm production or function, cause obstruction, inhibit accessory gland function, or cause inflammation [39].

Infection in the urinary tract with *Chlamydia trachomatis* has long been hypothesized as a cause of male infertility. Chlamydia has a high prevalence and is a common cause of non-gonococcal urethritis

and acute epididymitis in young men. Further, it has been linked to low sperm counts and development of anti-sperm antibodies in some studies [40]. Infection with chlamydia has been reported to decrease sperm function and motility [40], although the mechanism is unclear. De Barbeyrac et al. reported a series of 270 subfertile couples studied prospectively and observed that the presence of past or current chlamydia infection was not associated with either abnormal semen parameters or IVF outcomes [41]. Regardless of whether chlamydia directly causes sperm dysfunction, it can lead to a variety of genitourinary problems including epididymitis, orchitis, ductal obstruction, and disruption of the blood–testis barrier, all of which can cause or contribute to male infertility. Men with pyospermia or symptoms of urethritis or epididymo-orchitis should be evaluated and treated for chlamydial infections. In cases of chlamydial infection, and in other infections of the urethra, empiric treatment for gonococcal and non-gonococcal organisms is indicated, as co-infection is common. For urethritis, one dose of ceftriaxone and a week of doxycycline or one 2 g dose of azithromycin are recommended therapies.

Epididymitis and bacterial orchitis may cause a temporary decline in sperm concentration and motility, and may lead to ductal obstruction [42]. Appropriate antibiotic selection requires consideration of patient characteristics. In sexually active men, *C. trachomatis* and *Neisseria gonorrhoeae* are common pathogens and must be considered, particularly with coexisting urethral symptoms. In the pediatric population, in older men, and in men with recent urinary tract instrumentation, *Escherichia coli* is the most common organism. Laboratory workup should include a Gram stain of a urethral smear and a midstream urine specimen to identify the bacteria, and treatment should be tailored appropriately. In cases where an infecting organism cannot be identified, therapy should be directed towards the most likely organism. In cases of chronic epididymitis, a 4–6-week trial of appropriate antibiotics is indicated.

Prostatitis is another genitourinary infection that may have deleterious effects on reproduction. A National Institutes of Health (NIH) study group classified prostatitis into four categories: acute bacterial (type I), chronic bacterial (type II), chronic abacterial/chronic pelvic pain (type III), and asymptomatic inflammatory (type IV) [43]. Types I and II prostatitis are readily treated with long-term courses of lipophilic antibiotics that penetrate the prostate, such as trimethoprim–sulfamethoxazole and fluoroquinolones. Patients receiving long-term fluoroquinolone therapy should be advised that their use carries an increased risk of tendonopathy and tendon rupture. Type IV prostatitis is an incidental finding at prostate biopsy and has not been investigated as a cause for infertility. Most recent research has focused on type III prostatitis or chronic pelvic pain with conflicting findings. Some authors have associated abacterial prostatitis with abnormal semen parameters, which may be the cause of infertility in some patients. Potts and Pasqualotto observed that men with chronic abacterial prostatitis had increased seminal oxidative stress, which may explain the impaired sperm motility noted in these patients [44]. Further research is necessary to define the role of type III prostatitis in male infertility, but empiric medical treatment is appropriate.

Treatment of immunological infertility

The tight junctions between Sertoli cells isolate the testes from the body's immune system, and create the blood–testis barrier. Therefore, white blood cells (WBC) in the reproductive tract and semen may indicate pathology in the infertile man. Many authors have studied WBC concentrations in fertile and infertile men, and many studies suggest that increased concentrations of leukocytes in the genital tract and semen are associated with infertility [42]. The presence of leukocytes in a semen analysis may represent a sign of antibody-mediated immunity. Anti-sperm antibodies (ASA) are found in up to 12% of men who present for an infertility evaluation, and are thought to contribute to male-factor infertility in a variety of ways [45].

Anti-sperm antibodies may impair sperm motility, passage through the cervix and female reproductive tract, and the ability of the sperm to penetrate the oocyte [46]. Further, ASA may lead to spontaneous abortion, although the evidence for this outcome is incomplete. ASA testing should be completed in the infertile patient who has increased round cells found to be WBC in the semen analysis, a history of testis injury or surgery, sperm agglutination or clumping on semen analysis, poor penetration of mucus on a postcoital test, or other unexplained infertility.

The mainstay of medical therapy for immune-mediated infertility is systemic immunosuppression with corticosteroids. Investigators have conducted two randomized controlled trials comparing corticosteroid to placebo in couples with immunologic infertility. In 1987, Haas and Manganiello enrolled 43 men to be randomized between treatment with 96 mg methylprednisolone in three divided doses for seven days followed by a two-day tapering of the drug, or placebo [47]. This study failed to show an improvement in semen parameters or pregnancy rates in the treatment group, although a significant effect was observed on sperm-associated IgG in men given methylprednisolone. In the second trial, Hendry et al. randomized 43 subfertile men with circulating antibodies to spermatozoa to receive soluble prednisolone (20 mg twice daily on days 1–10 of the female partner's menstrual cycle, followed by 5 mg on days 11 and 12) or placebo for nine months [48]. These authors found that while semen parameters between the groups did not differ, the treatment group was significantly more likely to become pregnant (9 vs. 2 pregnancies). Further, the titers of antibodies in the seminal fluid decreased significantly in the treatment arm. These two studies suggest that moderate doses of steroids over a longer period are more effective in treating immunologic infertility than high-dose steroids over a shorter time frame.

Corticosteroid therapy has also been advocated as a pre-treatment prior to assisted reproductive techniques, although this has never been shown to be effective in a controlled trial. In the senior author's practice, patients are treated with prednisone 40 mg daily for two weeks, followed by a tapering dose of 20 mg daily for one week, and 10 mg daily for a final week. Assisted reproductive techniques are performed at the two-week mark.

Side effects of corticosteroids are common, with up to 60% of patients reporting mild reactions, although major complications such as aseptic necrosis of the hip are very rare. The limited data at present seem to suggest that moderate-dose corticosteroid therapy is the treatment of choice in the infertile patient with ASA. Further, because of the relative tolerability and safety, pre-treatment in men with ASA who are participating in assisted reproduction is reasonable.

Summary

As in the man without cancer, male-factor infertility in the oncology patient has several causes, and there are multiple medical therapies, both for correctible conditions that lead to infertility, and for idiopathic infertility and oligospermia. The workup and endocrine evaluation of the subfertile man is essential in identifying any reversible disorders, as the treatment of identifiable pathology has a high rate of success. Further, the workup may identify men with severe infertility who should either be treated more aggressively with surgical options and assisted reproductive techniques or be counseled about alternative options such as adoption.

A man in whom a specific disorder is identified should be treated appropriately with targeted therapy, and then undergo repeat evaluation, including semen analysis, in order to evaluate the need for additional empiric therapy. Although the data for the efficacy of empiric treatment is mixed, multiple studies have demonstrated a benefit to treating the man with idiopathic oligospermia or idiopathic infertility. In addition, medications such as clomiphene citrate are generally safe and inexpensive, making their use popular and reasonable. Empiric therapy with antioxidants and nutraceuticals remains promising, although further research is necessary in order to fully establish their effects. As our scientific knowledge of male reproduction improves, future research should focus not only on new empiric therapies, but also on identifying the specific problems that lead to infertility and developing targeted treatments to correct those problems.

References

1. Collins JA, Wrixon W, Janes LB, Wilson EH. Treatment-independent pregnancy among infertile couples. *N Engl J Med* 1983; 309: 1201–6.

2. Honig SC, Lipshultz LI, Jarow J. Significant medical pathology uncovered by a comprehensive male infertility evaluation. *Fertil Steril* 1994; 62: 1028–34.

3. AndroGel [package insert]. Marietta, GA: Unimed Pharmaceuticals, LLC, 2007.

4. Baskin HJ, Cobin RH, Duick DS, *et al.* American Association of Clinical Endocrinologists medical guidelines for clinical practice for the evaluation and treatment of hyperthyroidism and hypothyroidism. *Endocr Pract* 2002; 8: 457–69.

5. Wang C, Catlin DH, Demers LM, Stacevic B, Swerdloff RS. Measurement of total serum testosterone in adult men: comparison of current laboratory methods versus liquid chromatography-tandem mass spectrometry. *J Clin Endocrinol Metab* 1999; 89: 534–43.

6. Bhasin S. Testicular disorders. In Kronenberg HM, Melmed S, Polonsky KS, Reed Larsen P, eds. *Williams Textbook of Endocrinology*, 11th edn. Philadelphia, PA: Saunders, 2008.

7. Vermeulen A, Vedonck L, Kaufman JM. A clinical evaluation of simple methods for the estimations of free testosterone in serum. *J Clin Endocrinol Metab* 1999; 84: 3666–72.

8. Raman JD, Schlegel PN. Aromatase inhibitors for male infertility. *J Urol* 2002; 167: 624–9.

9. Schoor RA, Elhanbly S, Niederberger CS, Ross LS. The role of testicular biopsy in the modern management of male infertility. *J Urol* 2002; 167: 197–200.

10. Kumanov P, Nandipati K, Tomova A, Agarwal A. Inhibin B is a better marker of spermatogenesis than other hormones in the evaluation of male factor infertility. *Fertil Steril* 2006; 86: 332–8.

11. Mellinger RC, Thompson RJ. The effect of clomiphene citrate in male infertility. *Fertil Steril* 1966; 17: 94–103.

12. Loose D, Stancel G. Estrogens and progestins. In Brunton LL, Lazo JS, Parker KL, eds. *Goodman & Gilman's The Pharmacological Basis of Therapeutics*, 11th edn. New York, NY: McGraw-Hill, 2006.

13. Heller CG, Rowley MJ, Heller GV. Clomiphene citrate: a correlation of its effect on sperm concentration and morphology, total gonadotropins, ICSH, estrogen and testosterone excretion, and testicular cytology in normal men. *J Clin Endocrinol Metab* 1969; 29: 638–49.

14. Sigman M, Jarow J. Male infertility. In Wein AJ, Kavoussi LR, Novick AC, Partin AW, Peters CA. *Campbell–Walsh Urology*, 9th edn. Philadelphia, PA: Saunders, 2007.

15. Paulson DF. Cortisone acetate versus clomiphene citrate in pre-germinal idiopathic oligospermia. *J Urol* 1979; 121: 432–4.

16. Wang C, Chan CW, Wong KK, Yeung KK. Comparison of the effectiveness of placebo, clomiphene citrate, mesterolone, pentoxyfylline, and testosterone rebound therapy for the treatment of idiopathic oligospermia. *Fertil Steril* 1983; 40: 358–65.

17. Check JH, Chase JS, Nowroozi K, Wu CH, Adelson HG. Empirical therapy of the male with clomiphene in couples with unexplained fertility. *Int J Fertil* 1989; 34: 120–2.

18. Akin JW. The use of clomiphene citrate in the treatment of azoospermia secondary to incomplete androgen resistance. *Fertil Steril* 1993; 59: 223–4.

19. Hussein A, Ozgok Y, Ross L, Niederberger C. Clomiphene administration for cases of

nonobstructive azoospermia: a multicenter study. *J Androl* 2005; 26: 787–91.

20. Whitten SJ, Nangia AK, Kolettis PN. Select patients with hypogonadotropic hypogonadism may respond to treatment with clomiphene citrate. *Fertil Steril* 2006; 86: 1664–8.

21. Ghanem H, Shaeer O, El-Segini A. Combination clomiphene citrate and antioxidant therapy for idiopathic male infertility: a randomized controlled trial. *Fertil Steril* 2010; 93: 2232–5.

22. Vermeulen A, Comhaire F. Hormonal effects of an antiestrogen, tamoxifen, in normal and oligospermic men. *Fertil Steril* 1978; 29: 320–7.

23. Boyle K. Nonsurgical treatment of male infertility: empiric therapy. In Lipshultz L, Howards S, Niederberger C, eds. *Infertility in the Male*, 4th edn. Cambridge: Cambridge University Press, 2009.

24. Adamopouos DA, Pappa A, Billa E, *et al.* Effectiveness of combined tamoxifen citrate and testosterone undecanoate treatment in men with idiopathic oligozoospermia. *Fertil Steril* 2003; 80: 914–20.

25. Raman J, Schlegel P. Aromatase inhibitors for male infertility. *J Urol* 2002; 167: 624–9.

26. Liu L, Chaudhari N, Corle D, Sherins RJ. Comparison of pulsatile subcutaneous gonadotropin-releasing hormone and exogenous gonadotropins in the treatment of men with isolated hypogonadotropic hypogonadism. *Fertil Steril* 1988; 49: 302–8.

27. Miyagawa Y, Tsujimura A, Matsumiya K, *et al.* Outcome of gonadotropin therapy for male hypogonadotrophic hypogonadism at university affiliated male infertility centers: a 30-year retrospective study. *J Urol* 2005; 173: 2072–5.

28. Knuth UA, Hönigl W, Bals-Pratsch M, Schleicher G, Nieschlag E. Treatment of severe oligospermia with human chorionic gonadotropin/human menopausal gonadotropin: a placebo-controlled, double blind trial. *J Clin Endocrinol Metab* 1987; 65: 1081–7.

29. Caroppo E, Niederberger C, Vizziello GM, D'Amato G. Recombinant human follicle-stimulating hormone as a pretreatment for idiopathic oligoasthenoterato-zoospermic patients undergoing intracytoplasmic sperm injection. *Fertil Steril* 2003; 80: 1398–403.

30. Foresta C, Bettella A, Garolla A, Ambrosini G, Ferlin A. Treatment of male idiopathic infertility with recombinant human follicle-stimulating hormone: a prospective, controlled, randomized clinical study. *Fertil Steril* 2005; 84: 654–61.

31. Coviello AD, Bremner WJ, Matsumoto AM, *et al.* Intratesticular testosterone concentrations comparable with serum levels are not sufficient to maintain normal sperm production in men receiving a hormonal contraceptive regimen. *J Androl* 2004; 25: 931–8.

32. World Health Organization. Mesterolone and idiopathic male infertility: a double-blind study. *Int J Androl* 1989; 12: 254–64.

33. Balercia G, Buldreghini E, Vignini A, *et al.* Coenzyme Q10 treatment in infertile men with idiopathic asthenozoospermia: a placebo-controlled, double-blind randomized trial. *Fertil Steril* 2009; 91: 1785–92.

34. Sarafinejad M. Efficacy of coenzyme Q_{10} on semen parameters, sperm function and reproductive hormones in infertile men. *J Urol* 2009; 182: 237–48.

35. Agarwal A, Sharma RK, Nallella KP, *et al.* Reactive oxygen species as an independent marker of male factor infertility. *Fertil Steril* 2006; 86: 878–85.

36. Mills J, Meacham R. Nonsurgical treatment of male infertility: specific therapy. In Lipshultz L, Howards S, Niederberger C, eds. *Infertility in the Male*, 4th edn. Cambridge: Cambridge University Press, 2009.

37. Gillam MP, Molitch ME, Lombardi G, Colao A. Advances in the treatment of prolactinomas. *Endocr Rev* 2006; 27: 485–534.

38. De Rosa M, Colao A, Di Sarno A, *et al.* Cabergoline treatment rapidly improves gonadal function in hyperprolactinemic males: a comparison with bromocriptine. *Eur J Endocrinol* 1998; 138: 286–93.

39. Bar-Chama N, Goluboff E, Fisch H. Infection and pyospermia in male infertility: is it really a problem? *Urol Clin North Am* 1994; 21: 469–75.

40. Gonzales FG, Munoz G, Sanches R, *et al.* Update on the impact of *Chlamydia trachomatis* infection on male fertility. *Andrologia* 2004; 36: 1–23.

41. de Barbeyrac B, Papaxanthos-Roche A, Mathieu C, *et al. Chlamydia trachomatis* in subfertile couples undergoing an in vitro fertilization program: a prospective study. *Eur J Obstet Gyneol Reprod Biol* 2006; 129: 46–53.

42. Kasturi S, Oserberg E, Tannir J, Brannigan R. The effect of genital tract infection and inflammation on male infertility. In Lipshultz L, Howards S, Niederberger C, eds. *Infertility in the Male*, 4th edn. Cambridge: Cambridge University Press, 2009.

43. Krieger JN, Nyberg L, Nickel JC. NIH consensus definition and classification of prostatitis. *JAMA* 1999; 282: 236–7.

44. Potts JM, Pasqualotto FF. Seminal oxidative stress in patients with chronic prostatitis. *Andrologia* 2003; 35: 304–8.

45. Turek PJ, Lipshultz LI. Immunologic infertility. *Urol Clin North Am* 1994; 21: 447–68.

46. Cropp CS, Schlaff WD. Antisperm antibodies. *Arch Immunol Ther Exp (Warsz)* 1990; 38: 31–46.

47. Haas GG, Manganiello P. A double-blind, placebo-controlled study of the use of methylprednisolone in infertile men with sperm-associated immunoglobulins. *Fertil Steril* 1987; 47: 295–301.

48. Hendry WF, Hughes L, Scammell G, Pryor JP, Hargreave TB. Comparison of prednisolone and placebo in subfertile men with antibodies to spermatozoa. *Lancet* 1990; 335: 85–8.

Chapter 34

Management of the varicocele in the treated patient

Michael L. Eisenberg and Larry I. Lipshultz

Introduction

British surgeon T. B. Curling originally coined the term varicocele in 1843 to describe the pathologic dilation of veins of the spermatic cord [1]. However, the Roman encyclopedist Celsus, who practiced from AD 25 to 35, provided the earliest descriptions of treatment for varicoceles. While early varicocelectomy was performed for pain or cosmetic improvement, it was not until 1952 that the association between varicocele and infertility was recognized. A man with testicular biopsy-proven maturation arrest in whom the sperm count improved after varicocelectomy was described by T. S. Tulloch [2]. Other reports of similar findings soon followed, and the focus of interest in varicoceles shifted from pain to subfertility [1,3]. Currently, approximately 37 000 varicocelectomies are performed annually in the USA [4].

Varicoceles result from a reversal of blood flow within the internal and external spermatic and cremasteric veins [5]. While epidemiologic studies suggest that approximately 15% of all men in the general population have a clinical varicocele, between 19% and 41% of men evaluated for infertility are found to have varicoceles [6–8]. Interestingly, the incidence of varicoceles is increased to approximately 70% in men with secondary infertility, suggesting that varicoceles may lead to a progressive decline in fertility potential [9]. As illustrated in a study from Denmark, which found no varicoceles in boys aged 6–9 years but increasing numbers in boys aged 10–14 years, varicoceles usually arise some time after puberty [10]. There is also evidence for a genetic component to the disease, as the rates of clinical varicoceles are found to be higher in first-degree relatives (i.e., brothers, fathers) of patients with varicoceles than in fertile controls [11,12].

In clinical practice, most reports of varicocele-related testicular damage show persistent abnormalities of semen analysis parameters including concentration, motility, and/or morphology [3,5,8,13,14]. Moreover, the morphologic "stress pattern," which consists of increased numbers of elongated, tapered sperm heads and amorphous cells, is commonly, though not consistently, identified within varicocele patients [15]. Men with varicoceles are found to have a lower number of morphologically normal sperm, even using the current "strict" morphology criteria [16,17]. At the cellular level, varicoceles are found to increase germ cell apoptosis, which may contribute to oligospermia in both the human and rat model [18,19].

While many varicocele patients have abnormal semen analyses, some men with a clinical varicocele are found to have normal semen morphology and concentrations but are nevertheless infertile. Such a finding caused some investigators to study whether sperm function was compromised in the varicocele patient. The acrosome reaction during zona pellucida binding has been the focus of several studies [20–22]. Indeed, investigators showed that 45% of infertile men with a varicocele had an abnormal acrosome reaction, which could be normalized for many of these men after varicocelectomy [20].

While many investigators have reported that treatment of varicocele improves semen parameters, pregnancy rates, and intrauterine insemination (IUI) pregnancy and birth rates, there is still controversy regarding the efficacy of varicocelectomy in the management of infertility [23–42]. Much of the uncertainty with regard to treatment likely stems from the heterogeneity of the entity itself, as varicoceles exist in different sizes and grades defined on the basis of physical examination and ultrasonographic characteristics. Within these grades, there are ranges of semen abnormalities. In addition, while some men with infertility have varicoceles and abnormal semen parameters, men with normal fertility and normal semen analyses can also harbor the identical spermatic cord pathology. Given the clinical variation, it is perhaps not surprising that there is some controversy as to the efficacy of repair.

Pathophysiology

In addition to the controversy surrounding the clinical benefit of varicocelectomy, another uncertain aspect of the varicocele is its pathophysiology. The primary proposed hypotheses involve hyperthermia, increased venous pressure, abnormal testicular blood flow, hormonal imbalance, toxic substances, and reactive oxygen species. While it is difficult to identify a single or dominant factor, it is likely that many of these etiological causes contribute to the infertile phenotype seen in clinical practice.

Scrotal temperature, normally maintained a few degrees below body core temperature, optimizes the environment for testicular function. The inflowing arterial blood from the testicular artery is cooled in the spermatic cord by returning venous blood in the pampiniform plexus. A dilation of the venous plexus could therefore disrupt the efficiency of this system. Experiments involving induced cryptorchidism or testicular hyperthermia as a means of contraception, as well as data from recreational wet heat exposure, indicate that testicular heating impairs semen parameters [43–46].

Another means by which a varicocele might impair testicular function is through venous pressure. While increased venous pressure could plausibly limit arterial inflow in an effort to maintain normal intratesticular pressures, the evidence supporting this hypothesis is limited [47,48].

Several studies have suggested that infertile patients with varicoceles have lower than normal serum testosterone concentrations, leading to the hypothesis that varicoceles may alter Leydig cell function. Some reports have suggested that serum testosterone levels are lower in men with varicoceles, but other reports have questioned such claims [49–54]. In 1992, the results of a World Health Organization multicenter study of varicoceles led to the conclusion that men over the age of 30 with a varicocele had lower serum testosterone levels than did men under 30 with a varicocele [55]. Because such a pattern is not seen in men without varicoceles, the WHO concluded that a varicocele represents a progressive lesion with a time-dependent effect on Leydig cell function. The true androgen-mediated effect of the varicocele on impaired fertility, however, may relate more to the intratesticular testosterone concentration than to serum levels.

Production of reactive oxygen species (ROS) is necessary for normal sperm function via intracellular signal transduction, during which it facilitates capacitation, the acrosome reaction, and attachment to the oocyte. However, pathologic conditions can lead to excess production or delayed removal of ROS. Such an accumulation of ROS can result in peroxidation of sperm membrane lipids, altering sperm morphology and motility [56,57]. While most studies show that seminal ROS levels are higher in men with varicoceles than in controls, others have questioned the association between varicoceles and ROS levels [58–60].

Diagnosis

The physical examination remains the gold standard for the diagnosis of varicoceles. Patients should be examined in a warm environment in the standing position. Most practitioners currently utilize the Dubin classification to grade varicoceles. A grade 1 varicocele is palpable only during a Valsalva maneuver. A grade 2 varicocele is easily palpable along the spermatic cord with no ancillary maneuvers. A grade 3 varicocele is large enough to be visible through the scrotal skin. An estimated 90% of varicoceles are unilateral and on the left side. Unilateral right-sided varicoceles are rare and should raise suspicions of a retroperitoneal process that warrants radiologic evaluation [61,62].

While radionuclide imaging and venography have been used to diagnose varicoceles, ultrasound remains the adjunctive radiologic modality most often used to detect varicoceles. The commonly used characterization of a varicocele by ultrasound is that it is a vein of at least 3.0 mm in diameter with reversal of flow with Valsalva maneuver. Varicoceles detected only by radiologic studies, in the absence of any suspicion on physical examination, are termed subclinical and do not impact fertility or warrant repair [63,64]. However, radiologic imaging can play an important role in the detection of recurrent or persistent varicoceles following varicocelectomy.

Management of varicocele

The Male Infertility Best Practice Policy Committee of the American Urological Association along with the Practice Committee of the American Society for Reproductive Medicine outlined criteria that should be met before varicocele treatment is considered [65]:

(1) the varicocele is palpable on physical examination of the scrotum

(2) the couple has known infertility

(3) the female partner has normal fertility or a potentially treatable cause of infertility

(4) the male partner has abnormal semen parameters

In addition, men who are not currently attempting procreation but have a palpable varicocele, abnormal semen analyses, and desire future fertility should be offered varicocelectomy. As varicoceles may lead to progressive testicular dysfunction, younger males who have a palpable varicocele with normal semen parameters should be monitored with semen analyses at one- or two-year intervals so that abnormalities in spermatogenesis can be detected.

Adolescents with clinical varicoceles and reduced testicular size should also be offered varicocele repair, because evidence suggests that catch-up growth with improved sperm production occurs [66,67]. If there is no suggestion of impaired testicular size, close follow-up with both physical examination and semen analyses are suggested for detection of early signs of testicular damage.

Surgery and percutaneous embolization are the two modalities for varicocele treatment. No randomized trials comparing treatment modalities have shown clear superiority of one or the other, and each technique has distinct advantages and disadvantages.

Surgery

Hartmann described one of the first techniques for varicocelectomy through a scrotal approach in 1904 [1]. Due to the high rate of testicular artery injury and recurrence, this technique largely has been abandoned. In the modern era, surgeons use a retroperitoneal, laparoscopic, inguinal, or subinguinal technique (Fig. 34.1).

The retroperitoneal approach was originally described by Palomo in 1948. When this technique is used, the internal spermatic vein is ligated above the internal ring with preservation of the testicular

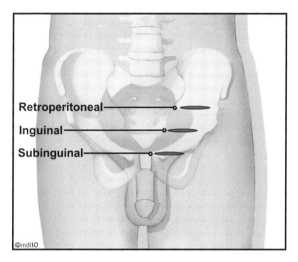

Figure 34.1. Varicocelectomy: retroperitoneal, inguinal, and subinguinal approaches.

artery [68]. A disadvantage of this approach is the relatively high recurrence rate of approximately 15%, thought to be due to the difficulties of ligating the external spermatic veins, which have been linked to recurrence [69].

The laparoscopic approach is conceptually similar to the retroperitoneal approach in that the internal spermatic vein is ligated just proximal to the internal ring. Again the rate of recurrence or persistence of the varicocele is thought to be increased because of the inability to ligate external spermatic veins [69]. In addition, isolation and sparing of the testicular artery can occasionally be difficult and can lead to its sacrifice. While collateral blood supply to the testis does come from the iliac system and usually is sufficient to prevent testicular atrophy, ligation of the testicular artery is unlikely to benefit fertility. Another caveat with regard to the laparoscopic approach is that the technique should be performed only by surgeons with extensive experience in laparoscopic surgery. Risks of intra-abdominal injury and higher equipment costs are also associated with the laparoscopic approach.

Both the inguinal and subinguinal approaches allow the use of microscopic magnification and permit more precise ligation of testicular veins with preservation of other spermatic cord structures. The microscopic technique generally is regarded as the preferred method by experts in the field of male reproductive medicine and surgery. The magnification is thought to translate into lower rates of complications such as hydrocele formation (rare with microscopic and 6–10% with macroscopic techniques) and recurrence (1–3% with microscopic technique) [69]. Some authors also suggest that the microscopic approach improves the overall efficacy of the repair [70,71].

The inguinal approach (Ivanissevich) involves a 3–4 cm incision along the inguinal canal. After the canal is opened, the spermatic cord is isolated and then inspected under the surgical microscope at approximately 15× magnification. The surgeon is then able to identify and ligate internal and external spermatic veins while preserving the testicular artery/arteries and lymphatics of the spermatic cord. A micro-tip Doppler probe may be used to aid in identification and preservation of the testicular artery. The subinguinal approach is similar in its use of the operating microscope; however, the incision lies just over the external ring. This fascia-sparing approach is thought to speed postoperative recovery. However, a disadvantage is that the number of vessels will increase as one progresses distally along the cord, and this complexity of the vascular anatomy below the external ring can lead to a more tedious dissection.

Percutaneous embolization

First described in 1978, percutaneous embolization involves occlusion of the internal spermatic vein with coils, balloons, or sclerotherapy [72]. The procedure is generally performed using local anesthesia and with an interventional radiologist gaining venous access through either the femoral or the internal jugular vein. After accounting for the initial success rate of 73% and a recurrence rate of around 5%, Pryor and Howards found an overall success rate of the technique of around 68% [73]. Cayan et al. reviewed the literature and found an overall pregnancy rate between 20% and 40% after percutaneous varicocele treatment [69]. Because complex venous anatomy can preclude access to the testicular venous system, such techniques require extensive experience and competency. Percutaneous embolization is indicated for recurrent or persistent varicoceles which have anomalous venous anatomy that can be delineated and treated in a single setting.

Efficacy of varicocelectomy

Impaired sperm production is a known complication of cancer treatment, with different chemotherapeutic regimens having varying degrees of toxic impact on spermatogenesis. While neither the impact of varicoceles nor the efficacy of their repair on impaired sperm production post-chemotherapy is precisely known, one can attempt to extrapolate from studies performed in normospermic and oligospermic men. Indeed, debate exists as to the utility of varicocelectomy. While some studies suggest no benefit, others have shown improvements in semen parameters and pregnancy rates. Goldstein et al. described their initial experience with microsurgical varicocelectomy and reported outcomes in 271 men with available data [71]. The authors reported improved sperm concentration (36.9 to 46.8 million/mL), motility (39.6% to 45.7%) and normal morphology (48.4% to 52.1%) with all comparisons significant. A postoperative pregnancy rate of 43% was also reported. Cayan et al. also reported similar improvements in sperm concentration (29.7 to 36.6 million/mL) and motility (25.6% to 43.5%) after varicocele treatment, with 46.6% of men having a more than 50% increase in their total motile sperm count [70].

In contrast, the most recent Cochrane review on varicocelectomy showed no improvement in the odds of pregnancy (OR 1.10, 95% CI 0.73–1.68) after varicocele treatment [74]. The analysis pooled results of randomized controlled trials that assessed efficacy of varicocele treatment, either surgical or radiologic. The primary outcome examined was the live birth rate, and a secondary outcome examined was pregnancy rate. Eight studies were included in the meta-analysis, examining a total of 607 men (Table 34.1). The authors did acknowledge that men with subclinical varicoceles, as well as men with normal semen analyses, were included in treatment arms of analyzed studies despite current practice discouraging the treatment of such men. When the analysis was restricted to include only the studies with men who possessed abnormal semen parameters or clinical varicoceles, only three studies remained. While the statistical power was reduced, the odds ratio did suggest a possible benefit to varicocele treatment, although the confidence interval was wide (2.08, 95% CI 0.60–4.25). It should be noted that after the Cochrane review was released, a new randomized controlled trial studying the efficacy of varicocele repair showed significantly increased odds of spontaneous pregnancy after varicocelectomy ($p < 0.01$) (Table 34.1) [31].

Many have criticized the systematic review for both its inclusion criteria and its outcome measures. The inclusion of trials that enrolled men with subclinical

Table 34.1. Summary of randomized controlled trials comparing outcomes after varicocele repair

Study	Treatment	Cases	Density[a] Pre	Post	p-value	Motility[a] Pre	Post	p-value	Pregnancy Pre	Post	p-value
Nilsson et al. 1979 [23]	Varicocelectomy	96	47 ± 41	49 ± 40	NS	32 ± 8	32 ± 7	NS	8%	18%	0.22
Breznik et al. 1993 [24]	High ligation/embolization	79	NA	NA		NA	NA		34%	54%	0.11
Madgar et al. 1995 [25]	Varicocelectomy	45	15	32	0.05	30	55	< 0.001	60%	40%	0.24
Yamamoto et al. 1996 [26]	High ligation	85	15 ± 18.1	20.9 ± 18.9	NS	21.7 ± 15.1	23.2 ± 16.7	NS	7%	10%	0.7
Nieschlag et al. 1998 [27]	High ligation/embolization	125	16	25	0.001	NA	NA		29%	25%	0.69
Grasso et al. 2000 [28]	Varicocelectomy	68	16.39	16	NS	22.1 ± 2.8	23.0 ± 2.7	NS	3%	6%	1
Unal et al. 2001 [29]	Varicocelectomy	42	47.9 ± 35.7	59.8 ± 50.1	0.038	39.0 ± 14.0	48.0 ± 14.0	0.001	10%	5%	1
Krause et al. 2002 [30]	Sclerotherapy	67	11.7 ± 21.0	10.8 ± 22.5	NS	NA	5.4 ± 22.1	NS	16%	18%	1
Abdel-Meguid et al. 2011 [31] [b]	Varicocelectomy	73	18.1 ± 5.1	32.2 ± 10.6	<0.0001	25.3 ± 12.8	41.0 ± 10	< 0.0001	33%	14%	0.01

[a] All comparisons represent treatment arm. No statistical improvement in control arm of any study.
[b] Not included in most recent Cochrane review [74].

varicoceles and with normal semen parameters – both groups which are known not to benefit from varicocele treatment – weakens any conclusions that could be reached by a meta-analysis including such studies. In addition, while conception rate remains the ultimate goal for all infertile couples, focusing solely on pregnancy as an outcome ignores the contribution of the female member of the infertile couple, as well as the benefits that improved semen parameters may play. Indeed, Cayan et al. elegantly showed that varicocelectomy can improve semen parameters sufficiently to downgrade the level of assisted reproductive technology (ART) that is required (converting couples from IVF to IUI, or from IUI to spontaneous conception) [75]. Examining semen parameters provides a more objective endpoint, as details about the female partner or use of ART were not available for all studies in the Cochrane analysis.

Agarwal et al. examined semen parameter endpoints after reviewing data from several observational and randomized trials [76]. A total of 17 studies met inclusion criteria and showed that varicocele treatment can lead to significant improvements in sperm concentration (9.7 million/mL, 95% CI 7.3–12.1), motility (9.9%, 95% CI 4.9–15.0), and WHO sperm morphology (3.2%, 95% CI 0.7–5.6). The same

investigative group also performed a systematic review of pregnancy outcomes after varicocele treatment but included only studies of men with palpable varicoceles and abnormal semen parameters. These authors found significantly increased odds of pregnancy after varicocele treatment (OR 2.87, 95% CI 1.33–6.20) [77]. Thus, using current clinical criteria for varicocele intervention, varicocele repair does appear to show benefit.

Varicocelectomy and azoospermia

The prevalence of azoospermia is estimated at 2% of all men and 10–15% of subfertile men. Azoospermia is a known complication of several chemotherapy regimens. While spontaneous recovery is possible, many men will never have motile sperm return to their ejaculate. While most men are offered pre-treatment sperm banking, for those who do not store sperm, the prognosis for future fertility is uncertain. Available literature regarding men with non-obstructive azoospermia (NOA) suggests that in men with a coexistent varicocele there does appear to be some benefit to varicocele treatment.

Varicoceles are found in 4.3–13.3% of men with azoospermia or severe oligospermia [78]. As mentioned earlier in this chapter, the first link

Table 34.2. Summary of studies examining varicocele repair in men with non-obstructive azoospermia

Study	Treatment	Cases	Success rate (%)	Mean postoperative sperm density (million/mL)
Matthews *et al.* 1998 [32]	Subinguinal	22	55	2.2
Kim *et al.* 1999 [33]	Inguinal	28	43	1.2
Kadioglu *et al.* 2001 [34]	Inguinal	24	21	0.04
Cakan and Altug 2004 [35]	Inguinal	13	23	0.7
Schlegel and Kaufman 2004 [36]	Subinguinal	31	22	NA
Esteves and Glina 2005 [37]	Subinguinal	17	47	0.8
Gat *et al.* 2005 [38]	Embolization	32	56	3.81
Poulakis *et al.* 2006 [39]	Embolization	14	59	3.1
Pasqualotto *et al.* 2006 [40]	Subinguinal	27	33	0.7
Ishikawa *et al.* 2008 [41]	Inguinal	6	33	0.2
Lee *et al.* 2007 [42]	Inguinal	19	36	0.36

between infertility and varicocele was made in 1952 by Tulloch, whose treatment of an azoospermic male led to sperm in the ejaculate and a spontaneous pregnancy [1]. Since then, other investigators have explored the role of varicocele repair in men with NOA. While no randomized trials exist, most observational studies support the role of varicocele repair in men with NOA. Kim and associates reviewed their experience with 28 NOA men who had either unilateral or bilateral varicocelectomy [33]. Of these men, 43% were found on follow-up to have developed sperm in their ejaculate. Schlegel and Kaufman reviewed their experience with 31 men with NOA and reported that 22% had sperm in their ejaculate after varicocelectomy [36].

Weedin *et al.* recently performed a meta-analysis on the utility of varicocele repair in men with NOA [79]. The authors reviewed 11 publications, which included 233 patients with a mean age of 30.1 years and 13.3 months of follow-up (Table 34.2). Nine reports included surgical varicocelectomy, and two publications reported men treated with percutaneous embolization of the internal spermatic vein. Motile sperm were reported in 91 of 233 (39.1%) of men who initiated 14 (6%) spontaneous pregnancies and 10 additional pregnancies that required ART. It is also important to note that 11 patients (4.6%) who had sperm in their ejaculate after varicocele repair were azoospermic again in 2–6 months. Thus, men should be counseled on the importance of sperm banking following recovery of motile sperm, as treatment gains may be transient.

The authors also explored the prognostic utility of a testis biopsy to predict recovery of sperm in the ejaculate following repair. Men whose biopsy showed a Sertoli-cell-only pattern had a low rate of sperm in the semen postoperatively (5/44 patients, 11%). In contrast, men with biopsy-proven hypospermatogenesis (30/55 patients, 55%) or maturation arrest (24/57 patients, 42%) had much higher rates of motile sperm in the postoperative ejaculate. It is estimated that 18% of azoospermic men will have microdeletions in the Y chromosome [80]. As varicocele repair is unlikely to improve fertility in such men with incidental varicoceles, the practitioner must assess the integrity of the Y chromosome of such men.

It is important to note that the etiology of NOA was not clearly delineated in all studies; thus, it is difficult to determine if the etiology of NOA can also predict varicocele treatment success. Whether men with genetic or idiopathic NOA respond in a similar fashion to those with gonadotoxin or chemotherapy exposure remains to be determined.

Varicocelectomy and hypogonadism

Cancer and its treatment may lead to hypogonadism. Testosterone deficiency has been linked to premature mortality and several comorbidities such as sexual and erectile dysfunction, diabetes, and metabolic syndrome; thus its treatment is necessary. It is hypothesized that a varicocele may impair Leydig cell function with subsequent impairment of testosterone production.

Table 34.3. Summary of studies examining changes in testosterone after varicocele repair

Study	Treatment	Cases	Serum testosterone concentration		p-value
			Preoperative	Postoperative	
Su *et al.* 1995 [81]	Microsurgical varicocelectomy	53	319 ± 12 ng/dL	409 ± 23 ng/dL	0.0004
Gat *et al.* 2004 [52]	Embolization	83	12.1 ± 6.1 nmol/L	17.2 ± 8.4 nmol/L	< 0.001
Ishikawa and Fujisawa 2004 [84]	Varicocelectomy	42	13.0 ± 4.2 pg/mL	13.6 ± 3.9 pg/mL	NS
Zhody *et al.* 2011 [82]	Microsurgical varicocelectomy	103	379.1 ± 205.8 ng/dL	450.1 ± 170.2 ng/dL	< 0.0001
Tanrikut *et al.* 2011 [83]	Microsurgical varicocelectomy	325	358 ± 126 ng/dL	454 ± 168 ng/dL	< 0.001

Several investigators have explored the possibility that varicocele treatment can improve serum testosterone levels (Table 34.3). Su and colleagues retrospectively reviewed the records of 53 men who underwent microscopic varicocelectomy and found that serum testosterone levels increased from a mean of 319 ng/dL to 409 ng/dL postoperatively ($p < 0.01$) [81]. In 56% of men with testosterone levels in the hypogonadal range, levels increased to normal following varicocelectomy. They also found that men who had at least one firm testis had better response to treatment. Interestingly, men with a lower grade of varicocele had greater improvements in testosterone postoperatively. Gat and colleagues reported hormonal outcomes in 83 men who underwent internal spermatic vein embolization for varicoceles [52]. Similar to surgical outcomes, serum testosterone levels increased by 43%, from 347.8 to 496.3 ng/dL ($p < 0.01$). Zohdy *et al.* also compared a group of infertile men who underwent either varicocelectomy ($n = 103$) or ART ($n = 38$) and found that the men who had varicocelectomy had significant improvements in serum testosterone levels, from 379.1 to 450.1 ng/dL ($p < 0.01$) [82]. Moreover, 75.5% of men with hypogonadism at baseline increased to the normal testosterone range following varicocele treatment. Interestingly, the authors also found significant increases in erectile function of men undergoing varicocele repair ($p < 0.01$). Tanrikut and associates examined 325 men with clinical varicoceles and found a lower serum testosterone level compared to age-matched controls [83]. Moreover, after surgical repair, there was a significant increase in serum testosterone levels from 358 to 454 ng/dL ($p < 0.001$).

Yet not all studies support varicocelectomy as a treatment for hypogonadism. Ishikawa and Fujisawa studied 42 men who underwent varicocele repair and reported no significant difference between preoperative and postoperative serum free testosterone levels

(12.97 ± 4.16 to 13.59 ± 3.93 pg/mL) [84]. While varicocele treatment may increase serum testosterone levels, it is unclear whether such treatment remains a viable alternative to testosterone replacement therapy for hypogonadal men.

Varicocele treatment in the era of advanced reproductive technology

In-vitro fertilization (IVF) and intracytoplasmic sperm injection (ICSI) have transformed the role of the andrologist and the treatment of the varicocele [85]. While technologies exist that can bypass treatment of the male patient, the risks to both members of the couple and to the child should be considered. With the use of assisted reproduction, risks of ovarian hyperstimulation or multiple gestation pregnancies exist. Indeed, 2008 Society for Assisted Reproductive Technology (SART) data estimate the risk of twin births at 15.4–33.3% and the risk of triplet or higher births at 0.6–2.0%. These multiple gestations present risks of pregnancy-related complications to the mother and prematurity to the children. Moreover, recent data from Sweden showed that children conceived with IVF had a 42% higher risk of pediatric malignancies [86]. Whether the etiology relates to the use of the technology itself or to the inherent infertility of the parents remains uncertain. Nevertheless, it is clear that a reasoned approach to the management of varicoceles and male infertility is warranted. It is also important to note that improvements in semen parameters and spontaneous pregnancy are not achieved immediately after varicocele repair, taking an average of six months after repair for pregnancies to occur [71].

Investigators have also explored cost-effectiveness considerations involving varicocelectomy in order to determine if varicocele treatment represents a better choice than assisted reproduction. Schlegel compared varicocelectomy to intracytoplasmic sperm injection (ICSI) in 1997 and found that the price per delivery for varicocelectomy was $26 268, compared to $89 091 for ICSI, and concluded that varicocele treatment remained a better option [87]. Meng and associates performed a decision analysis in 2005 to compare varicocelectomy with ART [88]. The authors included an assessment of preoperative semen parameters as well as including IUI as a viable treatment alternative. They also concluded that varicocele treatment is a better option than ART.

While spontaneous pregnancy is common after varicocelectomy in oligospermic men, the sperm counts after varicocelectomy in men with NOA often continue to warrant ART to achieve pregnancy. For this reason, Lee and colleagues explored the cost-effectiveness of varicocelectomy in men with NOA compared to testicular sperm extraction (TESE) and IVF-ICSI [89]. The authors concluded that microsurgical TESE was more cost-effective than varicocelectomy, with a lower cost per pregnancy ($69 731 vs. $79 576). The authors do note that costs of procedures and treatment success rates will vary by institution and the variations will affect the study conclusions.

In all cases, the practitioner must evaluate the couple and the reproductive capacity of both members before deciding upon treatment recommendations. Advanced maternal age or other female factors may necessitate IVF, in which case varicocelectomy is unlikely to benefit the patient in achieving the goal of procreation. However, maintenance of testicular function is also an important goal of varicocele treatment, as is the possibility and desire for more than one pregnancy.

References

1. Noske HD, Weidner W. Varicocele: a historical perspective. *World J Urol* 1999; 17: 151–7.

2. Tulloch WS. A consideration of sterility factors in light of subsequent pregnancies. *Edinburgh Med J* 1952; 59: 29–34.

3. Benoff S, Gilbert BR. Varicocele and male infertility: part I. Preface. *Hum Reprod Update* 2001; 7: 47–54.

4. Meacham RB, Joyce GF, Wise M, *et al.* Male infertility. *J Urol* 2007; 177: 2058–66.

5. Marmar JL. The pathophysiology of varicoceles in the light of current molecular and genetic information. *Hum Reprod Update* 2001; 7: 461–72.

6. Cockett AT, Takihara H, Cosentino MJ. The varicocele. *Fertil Steril* 1984; 41: 5–11.

7. Hendry WF, Sommerville IF, Hall RR, Pugh RC. Investigation and treatment of the subfertile male. *Br J Urol* 1973; 45: 684–92.

8. Naughton CK, Nangia AK, Agarwal A. Pathophysiology of varicoceles in male infertility. *Hum Reprod Update* 2001; 7: 473–81.

9. Witt MA, Lipshultz LI. Varicocele: a progressive or static lesion? *Urology* 1993; 42: 541–3.

10. Oster J. Varicocele in children and adolescents: an investigation of the incidence among Danish school children. *Scand J Urol Nephrol* 1971; 5: 27–32.

11. Raman JD, Walmsley K, Goldstein M. Inheritance of varicoceles. *Urology* 2005; 65: 1186–9.

12. Mokhtari G, Pourreza F, Falahatkar S, Kamran AN, Jamali M. Comparison of prevalence of varicocele in first-degree relatives of patients with varicocele and male kidney donors. *Urology* 2008; 71: 666–8.

13. Schoor RA, Elhanbly SM, Niederberger C. The pathophysiology of varicocele-associated male infertility. *Curr Urol Rep* 2001; 2: 432–6.

14. Jarow JP. Effects of varicocele on male fertility. *Hum Reprod Update* 2001; 7: 59–64.

15. MacLeod J. Seminal cytology in the presence of varicocele. *Fertil Steril* 1965; 16: 735–57.

16. Kruger TF, Menkveld R, Stander FS, *et al.* Sperm morphologic features as a prognostic factor in in vitro fertilization. *Fertil Steril* 1986; 46: 1118–23.

17. Vazquez-Levin MH, Friedmann P, Goldberg SI, Medley NE, Nagler HM. Response of routine semen analysis and critical assessment of sperm morphology by Kruger classification to therapeutic varicocelectomy. *J Urol* 1997; 158: 1804–7.

18. Simşek F, Türkeri L, Cevik I, Bircan K, Akdaş A. Role of apoptosis in testicular tissue damage caused by varicocele. *Arch Esp Urol* 1998; 51: 947–50.

19. Barqawi A, Caruso A, Meacham RB. Experimental varicocele induces testicular germ cell apoptosis in the rat. *J Urol* 2004; 171: 501–3.

20. Glazier DB, Marmar JL, Diamond SM, Gibbs M, Corson SL. A modified acrosome induction test. *Arch Androl* 2000; 44: 59–64.

21. Vigil P, Wöhler C, Bustos-Obregón E, Comhaire F, Morales P. Assessment of sperm function in fertile and infertile men. *Andrologia* 1994; 26: 55–60.

22. Fuse H, Iwasaki M, Mizuno I, Ikehara-Kawauchi Y. Evaluation of acrosome reactivity using the Acrobeads test in varicocele patients: findings before and after treatment. *Arch Androl* 2003; 49: 1–6.

23. Nilsson S, Edvinsson A, Nilsson B. Improvement of semen and pregnancy rate after ligation and division of the internal spermatic vein: fact or fiction? *Br J Urol* 1979; 51: 591–6.

24. Breznik R, Vlaisavljevic V, Borko E. Treatment of varicocele and male fertility. *Arch Androl* 1993; 30: 157–60.

25. Madgar I, Weissenberg R, Lunenfeld B, Karasik A, Goldwasser B. Controlled trial of high spermatic vein ligation for varicocele in infertile men. *Fertil Steril* 1995; 63: 120–4.

26. Yamamoto M, Hibi H, Hirata Y, Miyake K, Ishigaki T. Effect of varicocelectomy on sperm parameters and pregnancy rate in patients with subclinical varicocele: a randomized prospective controlled study. *J Urol* 1996; 155: 1636–8.

27. Nieschlag E, Hertle L, Fischedick A, Abshagen K, Behre HM. Update on treatment of varicocele: counselling as effective as occlusion of the vena spermatica. *Hum Reprod* 1998; 13: 2147–50.

28. Grasso M, Lania C, Castelli M, *et al*. Low-grade left varicocele in patients over 30 years old: the effect of spermatic vein ligation on fertility. *BJU Int* 2000; 85: 305–7.

29. Unal D, Yeni E, Verit A, Karatas OF. Clomiphene citrate versus varicocelectomy in treatment of subclinical varicocele: a prospective randomized study. *Int J Urol* 2001; 8: 227–30.

30. Krause W, Müller HH, Schäfer H, Weidner W. Does treatment of varicocele improve male fertility? Results of the "Deutsche Varikozelenstudie", a multicentre study of 14 collaborating centres. *Andrologia* 2002; 34: 164–71.

31. Abdel-Meguid TA, Al-Sayyad A, Tayib A, Farsi HM. Does varicocele repair improve male infertility? An evidence-based perspective from a randomized, controlled trial. *Eur Urol* 2011; 59: 455–61.

32. Matthews GJ, Matthews ED, Goldstein M. Induction of spermatogenesis and achievement of pregnancy after microsurgical varicocelectomy in men with azoospermia and severe oligoasthenospermia. *Fertil Steril* 1998; 70: 71–5.

33. Kim ED, Leibman BB, Grinblat DM, Lipshultz LI. Varicocele repair improves semen parameters in azoospermic men with spermatogenic failure. *J Urol* 1999; 162: 737–40.

34. Kadioglu A, Tefekli A, Cayan S, *et al*. Microsurgical inguinal varicocele repair in azoospermic men. *Urology* 2001; 57: 328–33.

35. Cakan M, Altug U. Induction of spermatogenesis by inguinal varicocele repair in azoospermic men. *Arch Androl* 2004; 50: 145–50.

36. Schlegel PN, Kaufmann J. Role of varicocelectomy in men with nonobstructive azoospermia. *Fertil Steril* 2004; 81: 1585–8.

37. Esteves SC, Glina S. Recovery of spermatogenesis after microsurgical subinguinal varicocele repair in azoospermic men based on testicular histology. *Int Braz J Urol* 2005; 31: 541–8.

38. Gat Y, Bachar GN, Everaert K, Levinger U, Gornish M. Induction of spermatogenesis in azoospermic men after internal spermatic vein embolization for the treatment of varicocele. *Hum Reprod* 2005; 20: 1013–17.

39. Poulakis V, Ferakis N, de Vries R, Witzsch U, Becht E. Induction of spermatogenesis in men with azoospermia or severe oligoteratoasthenospermia after antegrade internal spermatic vein sclerotherapy for the treatment of varicocele. *Asian J Androl* 2006; 8: 613–19.

40. Pasqualotto FF, Sobreiro BP, Hallak J, Pasqualotto EB, Lucon AM. Induction of spermatogenesis in azoospermic men after varicocelectomy repair: an update. *Fertil Steril* 2006; 85: 635–9.

41. Ishikawa T, Kondo Y, Yamaguchi K, Sakamoto Y, Fujisawa M. Effect of varicocelectomy on patients with unobstructive azoospermia and severe oligospermia. *BJU Int* 2008; 101: 216–18.

42. Lee JS, Park HJ, Seo JT. What is the indication of varicocelectomy in men with nonobstructive azoospermia? *Urology* 2007; 69: 352–5.

43. Mieusset R, Bujan L, Mansat A, Pontonnier F, Grandjean H. Effects of artificial cryptorchidism on sperm morphology. *Fertil Steril* 1987; 47: 150–5.

44. Mieusset R, Grandjean H, Mansat A, Pontonnier F. Inhibiting effect of artificial cryptorchidism on spermatogenesis. *Fertil Steril* 1985; 43: 589–94.

45. Liu YX. Temperature control of spermatogenesis and prospect of male contraception. *Front Biosci (Schol Ed)* 2010; 2: 730–55.

46. Shefi S, Tarapore PE, Walsh TJ, Croughan M, Turek PJ. Wet heat exposure: a potentially reversible cause of low semen quality in infertile men. *Int Braz J Urol* 2007; 33: 50–6.

47. Sweeney TE, Rozum JS, Gore RW. Alteration of testicular microvascular pressures during venous pressure elevation. *Am J Physiol* 1995; 269: H37–45.

48. Sweeney TE, Rozum JS, Desjardins C, Gore RW. Microvascular pressure distribution in the hamster testis. *Am J Physiol* 1991; 260: H1581–9.

49. Comhaire F, Vermeulen A. Plasma testosterone in patients with varicocele and sexual inadequacy. *J Clin Endocrinol Metab* 1975; 40: 824–9.

50. Hudson RW. Free sex steroid and sex hormone-binding globulin levels in oligozoospermic men with varicoceles. *Fertil Steril* 1996; 66: 299–304.

51. Younes AK. Low plasma testosterone in varicocele patients with impotence and male infertility. *Arch Androl* 2000; 45: 187–95.

52. Gat Y, Gornish M, Belenky A, Bachar GN. Elevation of serum testosterone and free testosterone after embolization of the internal spermatic vein for the treatment of varicocele in infertile men. *Hum Reprod* 2004; 19: 2303–6.

53. Pirke KM, Vogt HJ, Sintermann R, Spyra B. Testosterone in peripheral plasma, spermatic vein and in testicular tissue under basal conditions and after HCG-stimulation in patients with varicocele. *Andrologia* 1983; 15: 637–41.

54. Haans LC, Laven JS, Mali WP, te Velde ER, Wensing CJ. Testis volumes, semen quality, and hormonal patterns in adolescents with and without a varicocele. *Fertil Steril* 1991; 56: 731–6.

55. The influence of varicocele on parameters of fertility in a large group of men presenting to infertility clinics. World Health Organization. *Fertil Steril* 1992; 57: 1289–93.

56. Alvarez JG, Touchstone JC, Blasco L, Storey BT. Spontaneous lipid peroxidation and production of hydrogen peroxide and superoxide in human spermatozoa. Superoxide dismutase as major enzyme protectant against oxygen toxicity. *J Androl* 1987; 8: 338–48.

57. Aitken RJ, Clarkson JS. Cellular basis of defective sperm function and its association with the genesis of reactive oxygen species by human spermatozoa. *J Reprod Fertil* 1987; 81: 459–69.

58. Mazzilli F, Rossi T, Marchesini M, Ronconi C, Dondero F. Superoxide anion in human semen related to seminal parameters and clinical aspects. *Fertil Steril* 1994; 62: 862–8.

59. Weese DL, Peaster ML, Himsl KK, *et al.* Stimulated reactive oxygen species generation in the spermatozoa of infertile men. *J Urol* 1993; 149: 64–7.

60. Cocuzza M, Athayde KS, Agarwal A, *et al.* Impact of clinical varicocele and testis size on seminal reactive oxygen species levels in a fertile population: a prospective controlled study. *Fertil Steril* 2008; 90: 1103–8.

61. Dubin L, Amelar RD. Etiologic factors in 1294 consecutive cases of male infertility. *Fertil Steril* 1971; 22: 469–74.

62. Skoog SJ, Roberts KP, Goldstein M, Pryor JL. The adolescent varicocele: what's new with an old problem in young patients? *Pediatrics* 1997; 100: 112–21.

63. Jarow JP, Ogle, SR, Eskew LA. Seminal improvement following repair of ultrasound detected subclinical varicoceles. *J Urol* 1996; 155: 1287–90.

64. Demas BE, Hricak H, McClure RD. Varicoceles: radiologic diagnosis and treatment. *Radiol Clin North Am* 1991; 29: 619–27.

65. Practice Committee of American Society for Reproductive Medicine. Report on varicocele and infertility. *Fertil Steril* 2008; 90: S247–9.

66. Laven JS, Haans LC, Mali WP, *et al.* Effects of varicocele treatment in adolescents: a randomized study. *Fertil Steril* 1992; 58: 756–62.

67. Paduch DA, Niedzielski J. Repair versus observation in adolescent varicocele: a prospective study. *J Urol* 1997; 158: 1128–32.

68. Palomo A. Radical cure of varicocele by a new technique: preliminary report. *J Urol* 1949; 61: 604–7.

69. Cayan S, Shavakhabov S, Kadioglu A. Treatment of palpable varicocele in infertile men: a meta-analysis to define the best technique. *J Androl* 2009; 30: 33–40.

70. Cayan S, Kadioglu TC, Tefekli A, Kadioglu A, Tellaloglu S. Comparison of results and complications of high ligation surgery and microsurgical high inguinal varicocelectomy in the treatment of varicocele. *Urology* 2000; 55: 750–4.

71. Goldstein M, Gilbert BR, Dicker AP, Dwosh J, Gnecco C. Microsurgical inguinal varicocelectomy with delivery of the testis: an artery and lymphatic sparing technique. *J Urol* 1992; 148: 1808–11.

72. Lima SS, Castro MP, Costa OF. A new method for the treatment of varicocele. *Andrologia* 1978; 10: 103–6.

73. Pryor JL, Howards SS. Varicocele. *Urol Clin North Am* 1987; 14: 499–513.

74. Evers JH, Collins J, Clarke J. Surgery or embolisation for varicoceles in subfertile men. *Cochrane Database Syst Rev* 2009; 1: CD000479.

75. Cayan S, Erdemir F, Ozbey I, *et al.* Can varicocelectomy significantly change the way couples use assisted reproductive technologies? *J Urol* 2002; 167: 1749–52.

76. Agarwal A, Deepinder F, Cocuzza M, *et al.* Efficacy of varicocelectomy in improving semen parameters: new meta-analytical approach. *Urology* 2007; 70: 532–8.

77. Marmar JL, Agarwal A, Prabakaran S, *et al.* Reassessing the value of varicocelectomy as a treatment for male subfertility with a new meta-analysis. *Fertil Steril* 2007; 88: 639–48.

78. Czaplicki M, Bablok L, Janczewski Z. Varicocelectomy in patients with azoospermia. *Arch Androl* 1979; 3: 51–5.

79. Weedin JW, Khera M, Lipshultz LI. Varicocele repair in patients with nonobstructive azoospermia: a meta-analysis. *J Urol* 2010; 183: 2309–15.

80. Pagani R, Brugh VM, Lamb DJ. Y chromosome genes and male infertility. *Urol Clin North Am* 2002; 29: 745–53.

81. Su LM, Goldstein M, Schlegel PN. The effect of varicocelectomy on serum testosterone levels in infertile men with varicoceles. *J Urol* 1995; 154: 1752–5.

82. Zohdy W, Ghazi S, Arafa M. Impact of varicocelectomy on gonadal and erectile functions in men with hypogonadism and infertility. *J Sex Med* 2011; 8: 885–93.

83. Tanrikut C, Goldstein M, Rosoff JS, *et al.* Varicocele as a risk factor for androgen deficiency and effect of repair. *BJU Int* 2011; 108: 1480–4.

84. Ishikawa T, Fujisawa M. Varicocele ligation on free testosterone levels in infertile men with varicocele. *Arch Androl* 50: 2004; 443–8.

85. Cocuzza M, Cocuzza MA, Bragais FM, *et al.* The role of varicocele repair in the new era of assisted reproductive technology. *Clinics (Sao Paulo)* 2008; 63: 395–404.

86. Kallen B, Finnstrom O, Lindam A, *et al.* Cancer risk in children and young adults conceived by in vitro fertilization. *Pediatrics* 126: 2010; 270–6.

87. Schlegel PN. Is assisted reproduction the optimal treatment for varicocele-associated male infertility? A cost-effectiveness analysis. *Urology* 49: 1997; 83–90.

88. Meng MV, Greene KL, Turek PJ. Surgery or assisted reproduction? A decision analysis of treatment costs in male infertility. *J Urol* 174: 2005; 1926–31.

89. Lee R, Li PS, Goldstein M, Schattman G, Schlegel PN. A decision analysis of treatments for nonobstructive azoospermia associated with varicocele. *Fertil Steril*, 2009; 92: 188–96.

Chapter

35

Sperm extraction in the treated patient

Wayland Hsiao and Peter N. Schlegel

Introduction

With advances in in-vitro fertilization (IVF), and specifically intracytoplasmic sperm injection (ICSI), paternity is now possible for men using exceedingly small numbers of testicular sperm. Post-treatment azoospermic men who previously only had the options of donor sperm, cryopreserved sperm, or adoption now have the option of surgical sperm retrieval coupled with IVF-ICSI. This chapter will deal with the treatment options available to the cancer patient who remains persistently azoospermic after systemic therapy (whether due to chemotherapy, radiation, or surgery).

Traditionally the patient who presents with azoospermia after chemotherapy has been considered sterile if he did not bank sperm prior to chemotherapy. However, advances in sperm retrieval coupled with advanced assisted reproductive technologies (ART) have enabled even these men to successfully father children. The realization that the testicle is not uniform in terms of spermatogenesis has allowed retrieval of sperm from those men once deemed sterile. With the introduction of ICSI, we now have the ability to assist conception with very low numbers of sperm. For the man who is azoospermic after chemotherapy, there needs to be an evaluation of both ejaculatory status and levels of spermatogenesis. Patients with good sperm production who have ejaculatory dysfunction may benefit from electroejaculation (EEJ), while those men with spermatogenic compromise will most likely benefit from testicular sperm extraction (TESE). Finally, if a patient is unable or unwilling to successfully pursue any of the previous options, the use of donor sperm remains an alternative approach to fatherhood.

Use of cryopreserved sperm

Previously cryopreserved sperm greatly simplifies the algorithm for the post-chemotherapeutic azoospermic man, and the couple can go directly to IVF. While in the past there were rather strict criteria for cryopreservation of spermatozoa for subsequent use in assisted reproduction, the widespread application of ICSI has made it possible to cryopreserve even severely oligospermic samples and still achieve pregnancy and live birth. In 1992, Sanger et al. reviewed the literature and surveyed nine semen banks and identified 115 live births from the use of cryopreserved sperm from cancer survivors [1]. In addition, Agarwal et al. reported their success with the use of cryopreserved sperm in 29 men with a variety of malignancies [2]. Underlying the importance of cryopreservation prior to therapy is a study by Schmidt et al. [3]. While examining a population of testicular cancer, lymphoma, and leukemia patients reported to a Danish fertility clinic, these authors noted that 57% of their population was azoospermic after systemic treatment. Of the 35 live births in their series, 22 of them were due to the use of cryopreserved sperm. Thus, the use of cryopreserved sperm is both viable and successful, and cryopreservation should be offered to all patients prior to systemic chemotherapy or radiation treatment.

The use of ICSI with cryopreserved sperm in cancer survivors has also significantly increased the fertilization and delivery rates. Hourvitz et al. reported on 118 couples undergoing 169 IVF-ICSI cycles at Weill Cornell. From 1994 to 2005, using cryopreserved sperm and ICSI, there was a fertilization rate (per injected egg) of 77.6%, a clinical pregnancy rate of 57% (96/169), and a 50% delivery rate (85/169) [4]. As a historical control, a similar population was evaluated

Fertility Preservation in Male Cancer Patients, ed. John P. Mulhall, Linda D. Applegarth, Robert D. Oates and Peter N. Schlegel. Published by Cambridge University Press. © Cambridge University Press 2013.

from 1992 to 1994 at the same institution prior to the routine use of ICSI. Using conventional IVF, the fertilization rate was 32% and the delivery rate was 24% (13/54) [4].

While cryopreservation at present is the only proven method to preserve fertility in the pre-treatment setting, it should be noted that cryopreservation is not without its limitations. Cryopreservation can result in significant loss of sperm viability and motility [5], although the advent of ICSI has made the number of sperm needed for treatment much lower. In addition, it is controversial as to how long sperm are able to be effectively cryopreserved. In a large study by Yogev *et al.*, cryopreservation of spermatozoa in liquid nitrogen did not seem to affect the concentration of post-thaw motile sperm for storage periods of up to 14 years [6]. However, the success of these long-term stored spermatozoa in assisted reproduction remains to be seen.

Another limitation of cryopreservation is the low percentage of patients who have cryopreserved spermatozoa who actually use the sample. In a large study of 629 cancer patients who were referred for semen cryopreservation, 557 men eventually cryopreserved sperm. Of these men, only 7.5% used their banked semen within a mean follow-up period of seven years [7]. This agrees with other reports from sperm banking facilities that less than 20% of men who store sperm before cancer treatment end up using it to try to conceive [2,8–10]. Of course, this number could be artificially low because of death due to cancer, a long delay between medical therapy for cancer and attempts at childbearing, recovery of sperm production in some men, or limited access to assisted reproductive treatments.

Use of spermatozoa from men who have received chemotherapy or radiation

Men who have received chemotherapy, and even men who had non-gonadal radiation therapy, will have increased rates of sperm aneuploidy for six months or more after treatment [11]. An increase in sperm DNA fragmentation has also been observed after chemotherapy, and it may remain abnormal up to 24 months after chemotherapy [12]. In addition, studies have shown that adult male rats administered chemotherapy typical for either testicular cancer (bleomycin, etoposide, and cisplatinum) or non-Hodgkin's lymphoma (cyclophosphamide, doxorubicin, vincristine, and prednisone) have lower weight, decreased spermatogenesis, and smaller litter sizes [13,14]. Although limited in number and quality, observational studies in humans have not demonstrated an increased risk of congenital or genetic anomalies in offspring of men who have received chemotherapy or non-gonadal radiation [15–17]. Taken together, the data on sperm aneuploidy after chemotherapy and radiation may suggest a cautious approach for patients who desire to have children soon after completion of gonadotoxic therapy. However, there is a need for more research on the long-term effects of chemotherapy on the quality of sperm produced and the specific time course of chemotherapy-mediated damage caused by different chemotherapeutic regimens.

Sperm retrieval in the patient who is anejaculate following retroperitoneal or pelvic surgery

Any retroperitoneal surgery such as retroperitoneal lymph node dissection (RPLND) may affect the sympathetic chain or structurally compromise the bladder neck and may affect antegrade ejaculation. Partial ejaculatory function may be preserved, depending on the degree of nerve sparing. The preservation of ejaculatory function obviously has a tremendous impact on fertility rates. In Norwegian testicular cancer survivors who had chemotherapy, those with intact antegrade ejaculation had an 83% paternity rate, while rates for paternity were only 10% in the anejaculate group [18]. Patients who present with "anejaculation" (defined as a failure of ejaculation of semen from the urinary meatus during orgasm) may actually have retrograde ejaculation, in which all the seminal fluid flows retrograde into the bladder, or failure of emission, in which there is lack of any seminal fluid during orgasm.

For patients with retrograde ejaculation, the first-line treatment is largely medical with the use of sympathomimetics drugs. Ephedrine sulfate, imipramine hydrochloride, midodin hydrochloride, or pseudoephedrine hydrochloride have been used successfully in the treatment of retrograde ejaculation.

If attempts at medical conversion to antegrade ejaculation are unsuccessful, then sperm may be harvested by bladder sperm harvesting. Patients should alkalinize their urine with 5–10 mL of poly-citra the night before and the morning of scheduled harvest, since acidity is toxic to sperm. The patient should also stay well hydrated the day before and the day of harvest. On the day of harvest, the patient is instructed to urinate to completely empty his bladder. He is then instructed to masturbate. After orgasm, the patient should urinate into a collection cup, and this sample will contain sperm.

For patients with failure of emission, one treatment option is to undergo electroejaculation. This is a procedure generally performed under general anesthesia in the sensate patient. We do not routinely catheterize the patient prior to electroejaculation. The patient is placed in the lateral decubitus position. Anoscopy is performed to confirm that the rectum is empty and no rectal mucosal abnormalities are present. The rectal probe is inserted completely into the rectum with the electrodes oriented anteriorly, over the prostate and seminal vesicles. Stimulation is carried out with a standard electrical stimulation system. The pattern of electrical stimulation has been empirically evaluated, but it appears to work best with a gradually increasing voltage "peaked" sine wave stimulation that is abruptly ceased, with at least 5–7 second delays between stimulations. Maximal stimulation at the peak of the sine wave is increased by 1 volt for each stimulation, with a baseline of 0 volts (no electrical stimulation.) The procedure is also monitored by observation of penile tumescence and rectal temperature. Typically, penile tumescence is noted first, followed by seminal emission. When seminal emission ceases, rectal temperature of 38 °C is observed, or a maximum of 30 volts is attained, then electrostimulation is stopped. Anoscopy is performed again to ensure that there is no rectal mucosal injury, which is a potential complication of this procedure. The patient is turned supine and urethral catheterization is carried out. An initial retrograde specimen is diluted in human tubal fluid (HTF) buffered with HEPES and plasmanate, pH 7.4, and sent for immediate processing, as is the antegrade ejaculate. The bladder is then irrigated with HTF, and this second retrograde specimen is sent for immediate processing as well.

Ohl *et al.* performed electroejaculation in 24 testicular cancer patients (23 of whom had undergone RPLND) and observed seminal emission in all 24 patients. More than 10 million motile and progressive sperm were obtained in 88% (21/24) of patients. Seventeen couples underwent intrauterine insemination (IUI), and the overall cycle fecundity rate was 9% per IUI attempt [19]. Seven clinical pregnancies were established and there were five live births. Electroejaculation has also been successfully combined with IVF (obtaining a 53% fertilization rate per inseminated oocyte [20]) as well as IVF-ICSI, with a 75.5% fertilization rate per injected oocyte [21]. Rosenlund *et al.* looked at 17 couples treated for testicular cancer where most (14/17) received chemotherapy and most patients acquired sperm through electroejaculation. They employed both IVF and ICSI and had a fertilization rate of 55–57% in both groups, and the ongoing pregnancy rate for the whole cohort was 57% per cycle [22]. Finally, at Weill Cornell, we have reported a clinical pregnancy rate of 56% per retrieval and an implantation rate of 33% per embryo transferred [21]. Taken together, these studies demonstrate that treated testicular cancer patients can successfully undergo ART with electroejaculated spermatozoa.

Sperm retrieval in the patient who is azoospermic after chemotherapy

For men who are azoospermic after chemotherapy, spontaneous recovery may occur in at least a subset of patients within 2–8 years. For men treated with alkylating agents, the duration of azoospermia may be longer, so a period of observation prior to attempted TESE is recommended. For men treated with platinum-based regimens, most of those who will have sperm return to the ejaculate can have sperm detected within two years.

Those men who remain persistently azoospermic most likely have impaired spermatogenesis due to the patient's chemotherapeutic regimen, the use of radiation, the extent of surgery, the disease itself, the baseline function of the patient, or any combination of the aforementioned factors. While these men were once considered sterile, the use of advanced reproductive techniques has enabled paternity in a subset of this population. Specifically, the realization that the testis is not uniform and that there may be small pockets of spermatogenesis in these patients has enabled us to retrieve sperm in patients with non-obstructive azoospermia (NOA) using microsurgical TESE (microTESE) [23].

Table 35.1. Selected studies reporting reproductive outcomes for anejaculatory and azoospermic men after cancer treatment

Study	Sperm retrieval technique	Patient population	Patient number	Sperm retrieval	ART and birth outcomes
Hsiao et al. 2011 [29]	MicroTESE	Testicular cancer, lymphomas, leukemia, others	73	37% per patient 43% overall	Fertilization 57% Clinical pregnancy 50% Live birth 42%
Damani et al. 2002 [30]	TESE	Testicular cancer, lymphoma, others	23	65% per patient	Fertilization rate 65% Ongoing/delivered pregnancies 31%
Chan et al. 2001 [34]	TESE, microTESE	Testicular cancer, lymphoma, leukemia, others	17	45% sperm retrieval	Biochemical pregnancy 45% Live birth 33%
Rosenlund et al. 1998 [22]	EEJ, 1 TESE	Testicular cancer	15		Fertilization 57%, pregnancy 57%, per cycle Live birth 11/15
Chung et al. 1998 [21]	EEJ	Testicular cancer, spinal cord injury, psychogenic anejaculation	13		ICSI fertilization 76% Clinical pregnancy 55.6% Implantation rate 33%
Hultling et al. 1995 [20]	EEJ	Testicular cancer	10	90%	Fertilization rate 54% Pregnancy 5/6 Live birth 4/6
Ohl et al. 1991 [19]	EEJ	Testicular cancer	24	21/24 patients	Using IUI, pregnancy in 36.9% of couples

As in any patient with NOA, percutaneous aspirations or biopsies, while possible, are more likely to yield low numbers of sperm and require multiple treatments. In our view, the low yield, uncertainty of sperm retrieval, and intratesticular bleeding/scarring make these procedures less favorable, especially in this patient population with multiple insults to spermatogenesis. The risk of testicular injury, along with low spermatozoa yields, led to the development of microTESE [23]. Data from our own work, and that of others, suggest that microTESE yields the highest sperm retrieval rate in this population.

Evaluation prior to microTESE includes a through history, sexual history, chemotherapy history, physical exam, and hormonal profile. On physical exam, attention is paid to the fullness of the epididymis as well as testicular volumes. At our center, we prefer to perform microTESE in conjunction with a programmed IVF cycle to optimize the use of freshly retrieved viable sperm. The microTESE procedure involves placing a wide incision in the tunica albuginea in an avascular region to allow subsequent eversion of the testicular parenchyma for microdissection. Using high-power magnification through an operating microscope, subtunical vessels as well as intratesticular vessels can be identified and preserved. Microscopic dissection and direct examination of seminiferous tubules allow identification of the rare regions that contain sperm in men with NOA. The tubules with spermatozoa are wider and more opaque than the fibrotic Sertoli-cell-only tubules. Overall, microTESE has been shown to result in a higher number of sperm harvested, increased chance of retrieving sperm, and decreased testicular tissue removed [23,24]. The only predictor of successful treatment is the most advanced stage seen on biopsy and not the predominant stage [25]. Testicular volume, serum follicle-stimulating hormone (FSH) levels, and etiology of NOA appear to have little or no effect on the chance of sperm retrieval [25–27]. Postoperative ultrasound has demonstrated fewer acute and chronic changes after microTESE as compared to conventional TESE [28]. Of course, increased dissection may be counterbalanced by greater risk of damage to the vascularity of the testis. The overall risk of damage to testicular androgen production that is clinically significant is between 5% and 10%, depending on the number of prior interventions and the baseline level of serum testosterone. We prefer to start on the side with greater testis volume or the side with more advanced spermatogenic pattern seen on histology if a prior biopsy was done (with the most advanced being normal spermatogenesis followed by late maturation

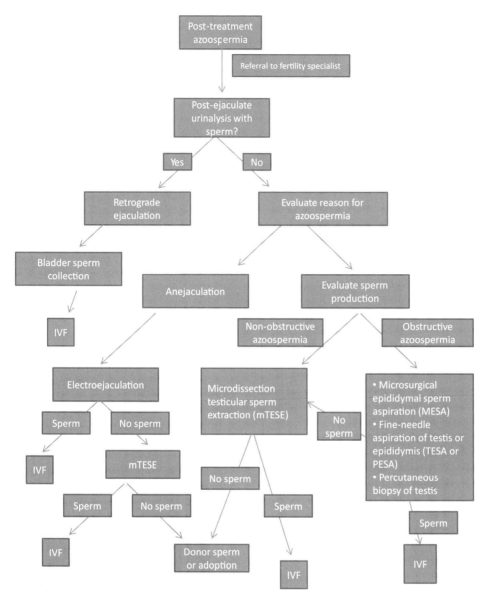

Figure 35.1. Treatment of the infertile male after cancer treatment.

arrest, early maturation arrest, and Sertoli-cell-only pattern, in that order).

At Weill Cornell Medical College we have performed 84 microTESE procedures in 73 post-chemotherapy patients. These patients presented with a history of prior treatment for malignancies, with the most common being Hodgkin's lymphoma, leukemia, testicular cancer, and non-Hodgkin's lymphoma. The mean number of years since chemotherapy was

18.6 years. Our sperm retrieval rate was 42.9% for the overall group. Fertilization rate per injected oocyte during IVF was 57%. Clinical pregnancy rate (defined as heartbeat seen on transvaginal ultrasound 32 days after embryo transfer) was 50%. The live birth rate was 42%, with 10 singleton deliveries and five twin deliveries. The sperm retrieval rate was highest in patients with a history of testicular cancer, at 85%, while patients with lymphoma had a sperm retrieval rate of 33%, and patients with sarcoma had the lowest sperm retrieval rate, at 14% [29].

Other groups have had similar results using testicular sperm. Damani *et al.* reported on 23 patients who underwent chemotherapy mostly for testicular cancer. They underwent either conventional TESE or fine-needle aspiration mapping and subsequent TESE. Sperm was successfully extracted in 65% (15/23), and a total of 26 cycles of ICSI were performed. The mean fertilization rate was 65%, with a delivery/ongoing pregnancy rate of 20.8% in 11 couples [30]. In another study, a multibiopsy approach TESE was undertaken in 12 post-chemotherapy men and sperm successfully retrieved in 29.4% (5/17) of attempts. Eight ICSI cycles were performed with a fertilization rate per injected oocyte of 68%. There was one live birth from seven embryo transfers [31]. Thus, testicular sperm extraction is an effective form of treatment for men with non-obstructive azoospermia due to oncologic or treatment-related causes.

Sperm retrieval in the patient who is azoospermic after radiation therapy

Radiation therapy is widely used for a number of malignancies, including, but not limited to, hematologic cancer, testicular cancer (with retroperitoneal exposure fields), prostate cancer, bladder cancer, and rectal cancer. Both treatment fields and scatter radiation can reach the testis, though the level will be lower with scatter. The testes are exquisitely radiosensitive, and sperm production can be affected by even very low doses of radiation, with permanent damage to spermatogenesis caused by doses over 2 Gy [32]. In testicular cancer patients, there seems to be a higher risk of infertility in those patients who received radiation therapy to the retroperitoneum (for seminoma) when compared to those that were treated with only chemotherapy (for non-seminomatous tumors) [33].

There is scant literature regarding outcomes of treatments of infertility specifically due to radiation-induced azoospermia. Most studies combine chemotherapy and radiation therapy patients, and do not give specific success rates for radiation patients [3]. In our practice, radiation to any other site including the abdomen and mediastinum does not preclude attempts at sperm retrieval with microTESE, and we have been able to successfully retrieve sperm in these patients. However, in cases where the testis itself has been irradiated, or in patients receiving total-body irradiation for bone marrow transplant, to date we have been unable to find sperm even with microTESE.

Conclusion

The challenges of sperm retrieval are unique in a cancer population. This group of patients faces the challenge of balancing the temporal rush to get to essential chemotherapy and the need to undergo sperm preservation procedures. A number of treatment options are open for the post-treatment male seeking fertility treatment. A summary of selected studies is presented in Table 35.1. For those anejaculatory males, electroejaculation represents a viable and effective treatment, especially when coupled with IVF-ICSI. For the post-chemotherapeutic man who remains persistently azoospermic, microTESE, coupled with ICSI, is also an effective treatment option. We propose an algorithm to help guide the treatment of the infertile male after cancer treatment (Fig. 35.1).

Acknowledgments

Dr. Hsiao is supported by a grant from the Frederick J. and Theresa Dow Wallace Fund of the New York Community Trust.

References

1. Sanger WG, Olson JH, Sherman JK. Semen cryobanking for men with cancer: criteria change. *Fertil Steril* 1992; 58: 1024–7.

2. Agarwal A, Ranganathan P, Kattal N, *et al.* Fertility after cancer: a prospective review of assisted reproductive outcome with banked semen specimens. *Fertil Steril* 2004; 81: 342–8.

3. Schmidt KL, Larsen E, Bangsboll S, *et al.* Assisted reproduction in male cancer survivors: fertility treatment and outcome in 67 couples. *Hum Reprod* 2004; 19: 2806–10.

4. Hourvitz A, Goldschlag DE, Davis OK, *et al.* Intracytoplasmic sperm injection (ICSI) using cryopreserved sperm from men with malignant neoplasm yields high pregnancy rates. *Fertil Steril* 2008; 90: 557–63.

5. McLaughlin EA, Ford WC, Hull MG. Motility characteristics and membrane integrity of cryopreserved human spermatozoa. *J Reprod Fertil* 1992; 95: 527–34.

6. Yogev L, Kleiman SE, Shabtai E, *et al.* Long-term cryostorage of sperm in a human sperm bank does not damage progressive motility concentration. *Hum Reprod* 2010; 25: 1097–103.

7. van Casteren NJ, van Santbrink EJ, van Inzen W, Romijn JC, Dohle GR. Use rate and assisted reproduction technologies outcome of cryopreserved semen from 629 cancer patients. *Fertil Steril* 2008; 90: 2245–50.

8. Kelleher S, Wishart SM, Liu PY, *et al.* Long-term outcomes of elective human sperm cryostorage. *Hum Reprod* 2001; 16: 2632–9.

9. Blackhall FH, Atkinson AD, Maaya MB, *et al.* Semen cryopreservation, utilisation and reproductive outcome in men treated for Hodgkin's disease. *Br J Cancer* 2002; 87: 381–4.

10. Ragni G, Somigliana E, Restelli L, *et al.* Sperm banking and rate of assisted reproduction treatment: insights from a 15-year cryopreservation program for male cancer patients. *Cancer* 2003; 97: 1624–9.

11. Burrello N, Vicari E, La Vignera S, *et al.* Effects of anti-neoplastic treatment on sperm aneuploidy rate in patients with testicular tumor: a longitudinal study. *J Endocrinol Invest* 2011; 34: e121–5.

12. O'Flaherty C, Hales BF, Chan P, Robaire B. Impact of chemotherapeutics and advanced testicular cancer or Hodgkin lymphoma on sperm deoxyribonucleic acid integrity. *Fertil Steril* 2010; 94: 1374–9.

13. Bieber AM, Marcon L, Hales BF, Robaire B. Effects of chemotherapeutic agents for testicular cancer on the male rat reproductive system, spermatozoa, and fertility. *J Androl* 2006; 27: 189–200.

14. Vaisheva F, Delbes G, Hales BF, Robaire B. Effects of the chemotherapeutic agents for non-Hodgkin lymphoma, cyclophosphamide, doxorubicin, vincristine, and prednisone (CHOP), on the male rat reproductive system and progeny outcome. *J Androl* 2007; 28: 578–87.

15. Byrne J, Rasmussen SA, Steinhorn SC, *et al.* Genetic disease in offspring of long-term survivors of childhood and adolescent cancer. *Am J Hum Genet* 1998; 62: 45–52.

16. Boice JD, Jr., Tawn EJ, Winther JF, *et al.* Genetic effects of radiotherapy for childhood cancer. *Health Phys* 2003; 85: 65–80.

17. Winther JF, Boice JD, Mulvihill JJ, *et al.* Chromosomal abnormalities among offspring of childhood-cancer survivors in Denmark: a population-based study. *Am J Hum Genet* 2004; 74: 1282–5.

18. Brydoy M, Fossa SD, Klepp O, *et al.* Paternity following treatment for testicular cancer. *J Natl Cancer Inst* 2005; 97: 1580–8.

19. Ohl DA, Denil J, Bennett CJ, *et al.* Electroejaculation following retroperitoneal lymphadenectomy. *J Urol* 1991; 145: 980–3.

20. Hultling C, Rosenlund B, Tornblom M, *et al.* Transrectal electroejaculation in combination with in-vitro fertilization: an effective treatment of anejaculatory infertility after testicular cancer. *Hum Reprod* 1995; 10: 847–50.

21. Chung PH, Palermo G, Schlegel PN, *et al.* The use of intracytoplasmic sperm injection with electroejaculates from anejaculatory men. *Hum Reprod* 1998; 13: 1854–8.

22. Rosenlund B, Sjoblom P, Tornblom M, Hultling C, Hillensjo T. In-vitro fertilization and intracytoplasmic sperm injection in the treatment of infertility after testicular cancer. *Hum Reprod* 1998; 13: 414–18.

23. Schlegel PN. Testicular sperm extraction: microdissection improves sperm yield with minimal tissue excision. *Hum Reprod* 1999; 14: 131–5.

24. Tsujimura A, Matsumiya K, Miyagawa Y, *et al.* Conventional multiple or microdissection testicular sperm extraction: a comparative study. *Hum Reprod* 2002; 17: 2924–9.

25. Su LM, Palermo GD, Goldstein M, *et al.* Testicular sperm extraction with intracytoplasmic sperm injection for nonobstructive azoospermia: testicular histology can predict success of sperm retrieval. *J Urol* 1999; 161: 112–16.

26. Ramasamy R, Lin K, Gosden LV, *et al.* High serum FSH levels in men with nonobstructive azoospermia does not affect success of microdissection testicular sperm extraction. *Fertil Steril* 2009; 92: 590–3.

27. Ramasamy R, Schlegel PN. Microdissection testicular sperm extraction: effect of prior biopsy on success of sperm retrieval. *J Urol* 2007; 177: 1447–9.

28. Ramasamy R, Yagan N, Schlegel PN. Structural and functional changes to the testis after conventional versus microdissection testicular sperm extraction. *Urology* 2005; 65: 1190–4.

29. Hsiao W, Stahl PJ, Osterberg EC, *et al.* Successful treatment of postchemotherapy azoospermia with microsurgical testicular sperm extraction: the Weill Cornell experience. *J Clin Oncol* 2011; 29: 1607–11.

30. Damani MN, Master V, Meng MV, *et al.* Postchemotherapy ejaculatory azoospermia: fatherhood with sperm from testis tissue with intracytoplasmic sperm injection. *J Clin Oncol* 2002; 20: 930–6.

31. Meseguer M, Garrido N, Remohi J, *et al.* Testicular sperm extraction (TESE) and ICSI in patients with permanent azoospermia after chemotherapy. *Hum Reprod* 2003; 18: 1281–5.

32. Shalet SM. Effect of irradiation treatment on gonadal function in men treated for germ cell cancer. *Eur Urol* 1993; 23: 148–51.

33. Huyghe E, Matsuda T, Daudin M, *et al.* Fertility after testicular cancer treatments: results of a large multicenter study. *Cancer* 2004; 100: 732–7.

34. Chan PT, Palermo GD, Veeck LL, Rosenwaks Z, Schlegel PN. Testicular sperm extraction combined with intracytoplasmic sperm injection in the treatment of men with persistent azoospermia postchemotherapy. *Cancer* 2001; 92: 1632–7.

Chapter

36

Postmortem sperm extraction

Andrew C. Kramer and Ellen R. Goldmark

Introduction

Sperm extraction from the terminally ill is a function of putting many complex issues together. Add on the expanding but still relatively scarce number of cases as precedent, with no real legal or published standard of care, and the level of controversy magnifies. Today, as in-vitro fertilization (IVF) continues to improve and gain traction, and the ability of intensive care physicians to keep terminally ill patients alive grows, the number of requests for sperm harvests from terminally ill or recently deceased patients will swell.

In examining this issue, both clinicians and family members need to compartmentalize the different issues within this debate. In this chapter, we review and organize the important facets of the discussion, including context and significance, issues of consent, ethical concerns, logistical issues, and legal matters. Our goal is to add clarity to a topic that for many years was non-existent in the literature. Still, work needs to be done to facilitate this discussion, which will undoubtedly increase in prevalence throughout the next several years.

Background and context

With the introduction, then the widespread use and acceptance, of IVF and intracytoplasmic sperm injection (ICSI), several clinical scenarios are present today that historically never existed. The first documented case of retrieval of spermatozoa from a brain-dead patient occurred in 1980, when the family of a 30-year-old man who was in a vegetative state after a motor vehicle accident requested sperm preservation [1]. Assisted reproductive technologies (ART) have been inherently fraught with debate and a certain degree of controversy. Some of this is due to ethical

considerations relating to if and for whom this technology should be applied. As we will discuss, this spirited debate has many perspectives, whether religious, ethical, or simply arising from difference of opinion. Concomitantly, tremendous strides have continued to be made in the fields of caring for critically ill patients. Indeed, it is possible to keep some patients alive for extended periods of time on life-support measures despite zero chance for any reasonable cognitive recovery.

Several cases have been sensationalized in the lay press, sparking national dialog. Two such examples include the Terri Schiavo case and the matter involving Jack Kevorkian. In the Schiavo case, an eight-year legal battle dragged on over whether a woman in a vegetative state should be kept alive [2]. Kevorkian long argued that the right to death is as important as the right to life [3]. An overarching theme that lends some degree of difficulty to the subject matter is the lack of written protocol and consensus [4]. When one combines the polarizing topic of a terminally ill patient on life support with the prospect of an assisted reproductive technique such as IVF, there is little doubt that there will be a challenging scenario.

Issues of consent

The American Medical Association (AMA) defines informed consent as "communication between a patient and a physician that results in the patient's authorization or agreement to undergo a specific medical intervention" [5]. The AMA goes on to state that the patient should "have an opportunity to ask questions to elicit a better understanding of the treatment or procedure so that he or she can make an informed decision to proceed or to refuse a particular

Fertility Preservation in Male Cancer Patients, ed. John P. Mulhall, Linda D. Applegarth, Robert D. Oates and Peter N. Schlegel. Published by Cambridge University Press. © Cambridge University Press 2013.

course of medical intervention" [5]. A cancer patient may have insight that he is about to undergo a life-threatening procedure and could consent for the use of his sperm upon death. Conversely, patients who die suddenly or become comatose may not anticipate the need to have such a discussion. The result is a problem whereby this relatively new technology leaves a blank where specific regulations would otherwise be in place. The European Society of Human Reproduction and Endocrinology (ESHRE) provided guidelines in 2006 stating that postmortem sperm retrieval should be offered if the deceased had provided a written consent [6]. According to these guidelines, extensive counseling and one year needs to pass from the time of death before the sperm could be used [6]. In 2004, the American Society for Reproductive Medicine (ASRM) suggested that postmortem sperm extraction should only be offered if the deceased had been given prior consent or his wishes to retrieve sperm were known [7].

In Canada, the Assisted Human Reproduction Regulations (AHRR) states that "Before a person removes human reproductive material from a donor's body after the donor's death for the purpose of creating an embryo, the person shall have a document signed by the donor stating that, before consenting to the removal, the donor was informed in writing that the human reproductive material will be removed in accordance with the donor's consent to create an embryo." These guidelines provide a statement of what is allowed under Canadian law [6]. Without written informed consent from the deceased, postmortem sperm extraction is prohibited, due to lack of consent based on this description.

It is clear that local regulations vary greatly on this issue. The underlying issue is that no rule can be universally applied. Instead, there should be principles for consideration of requests, rather than reliance on laws that may not be applicable to the specific patient, or the involved practitioner. Some of these principles are outlined in Table 36.1.

An interesting and potentially relevant comparison can be drawn with organ donation. According to the Uniform Anatomical Gift Act, competent adults make decisions about organ donation prior to their death [8]. Even if a patient declares that he wishes to be a donor, and documents this on a donor registration card, organ procurement organizations will still ask the family of the deceased for consent, despite the stipulation in the Uniform Anatomical Gift Act that

Table 36.1. Principles to consider when weighing a new case

Amount of formal measures taken to achieve pregnancy prior to incident
Level of consent
Mindset of parties involved
Accessibility of an IVF group
Ability to assemble a team to perform the tissue extraction
Insight of the involved parties about the many legal and ethical concerns
Reasonable ability for all parties to manage the upfront costs

the decedent's wishes be honored. The family of the decedent may ultimately decide to go against the wishes of the patient at the time of death. In contrast, in most of continental Europe, cadaveric organ procurement is based on the principle of presumed consent [9]. Under presumed consent, a deceased individual is considered a potential donor in the absence of explicit opposition to donation before death. In this scenario, the deceased would-be organ donor is not truly providing informed consent as detailed by the AMA. Using presumed consent, people could argue that sperm extraction, without explicit instruction against this specifically, is acceptable [9]. In the United States, postmortem sperm extraction has neither the leniency of organ harvest consent in Europe, nor the rigidity of the Canadian system for sperm extraction. It is and remains a black box.

In his 2006 article, Strong presents six different levels of implied or obtained consent for sperm retrieval [10]. These scenarios range from specifically documented informed consent on behalf of the postmortem patient to the issue of sperm extraction never having been discussed with the deceased at all. The first scenario, and the one with the least ambiguity, is where the patient and the surgeon performing the gamete extraction have had a direct conversation regarding the procedure, its risks, and its implications, and there is documentation of the consent after this conversation takes place. This scenario would certainly be possible in a situation where a patient is suffering from a chronic malignancy or other disease, leaving him with doubts as to his long-term mortality. This case represents true informed consent. The second scenario involves consent being obtained by a physician other than the surgeon. The patient demonstrates that he understands the risks and wishes to proceed with sperm extraction. In this situation, if a document is signed, one may argue that it can be compared to a resident consenting for a procedure. The clinician is not the primary surgeon, yet he/she explains the risks and benefits and obtains the legal documentation. The third scenario involves a signed and notarized statement from the deceased, detailing his wishes for sperm extraction. In this situation, the patient's wishes are clear, but no physician or counselor was present to fully discuss the future implications with the patient. The fourth situation involves the wife of the deceased and several family members, all able to corroborate each other regarding the patient's wishes without any documented consent. The fifth scenario involves only the patient's wife reporting that she and her husband discussed postmortem sperm retrieval without support from other family members. Finally, in the sixth example, the deceased's wife admits that the issue of postmortem sperm extraction was never explicitly discussed, but she feels certain that he would have wanted it [10].

Many would agree that in the first two scenarios the patient did provide informed consent, assuming that the physician explained the implications of the procedure and the patient had an opportunity to ask questions [11]. The four other scenarios are not consistent with the AMA's definition of informed consent, as the patient does not have an opportunity to have a discussion with a physician, nor is he able to ask questions. In the scenarios where the deceased's family and partner are stating the patient's wishes without any documentation, this could be considered by many not to be true informed consent [11]. As we will see, in the United States a physician does have a right to impose his sense of what he feels is appropriate consent for the procedure.

Ethical considerations

Some highly debated issues surrounding sperm extraction from terminally ill or newly deceased patients revolve around ethical issues. Unless the man in the relationship has an extraordinarily risky profession, he would likely have never conjured up life after his death or what would happen should catastrophe strike and he had a premature death. The couple hardly ever has a documented contingency plan for children in emergency situations [12]. It may be evident in some cases that a man did in fact take steps that illustrate his desire for children. For example, his partner may have ceased birth control pills, or even visited an IVF clinic. What is not so clear is whether the man would still want to have that child if he were not alive to serve as the father to the child. Therefore, it is not a logical conclusion to

draw that since the couple wanted children before the sentinel event, the man was making the statement that he wanted children in his absence. While many couples do desire to have children, very rarely have they discussed their desire for biological children should they not be alive to personally raise them.

The very meaning of parenthood is a term that is at the core of the debate. A common argument made by a woman dealing with her terminally ill spouse is that they always wanted to be parents but simply never reached that time in their lives, and this is their final hope to that end [13]. In this context, parenthood would be defined as simply the biological propagation of genetic material from parent to offspring. Yet a different perspective is that parenthood is not so much the passing down of genetic material into offspring, but rather the raising and nurturing of a child and playing a leading role in the child's upbringing [14]. True to this concept is that adoptive parents feel every bit as much the parents of their adopted children as their counterparts raising their own biological children [15]. In this context, parenthood is defined as the experience of raising and caring for children.

It is necessary to discern from the surviving spouse which parenthood definition best matches the patient's wishes. It is important for her to respect his wishes. When she claims that he wanted to be a parent prior to his incapacitation, does that mean he wanted to pass down his biologic genes, or to experience raising a child? Both likely played a role, but to what degree? It is difficult for surviving spouses to understand that what a man wanted while alive may be different than what he would have wanted if deceased.

Next, the vagaries of IVF must be introduced to the surviving partner prior to going forward with any discussion of sperm extraction. Many are unaware that sperm harvested from the testicle must be used in conjunction with IVF or ICSI. Unless the spouse is very medically savvy, the natural tendency might be to believe that once the sperm is harvested, it is very easy to proceed directly to pregnancy and childbirth. This is clearly far from the truth. Natural conception and intrauterine insemination (IUI) are not options with testicular sperm [16]. Therefore, the technical and ethical considerations surrounding ART must be explored early in the process.

Some oppose IVF for ethical and religious reasons. Historically, modern Jewish law has condoned posthumous sperm extraction, but Catholicism has not [17,18]. Protestant churches have held a favorable stance toward IVF, differing from their Catholic counterparts. The Islamic faith does encourage couples to seek treatment in cases of infertility, but this apparent support of fertility through medical means applies only to living, married couples [19].

As ARTs have increased in popularity, anecdotal accounts of IVF have reached the lay press, and its long-term results have been thoroughly examined in scientific publications [20]. Some oppose IVF because of reports of an increased risk of birth defects in children conceived through this process. Some studies have even pointed to twice the risk of certain birth defects in babies born after IVF and ICSI [21]. Multiple gestation, hypospadias, and Beckwith–Wiedemann syndrome are just a few of the conditions linked to IVF in certain reports [22,23]. If this is true, a potential psychological burden could be placed on a mother if she felt responsible for creating a baby through means that have clear and documented risks. Therefore, prior to choosing to make the decision to extract sperm from a critically ill man, the surviving spouse must recognize the ethical concerns inherent in the process of IVF and ICSI, realizing also that natural conception is not possible with sperm acquired this way.

Logistical issues

Just as sperm extraction cannot be undertaken without exploring the ethical considerations, so too must the technical issues fundamental to IVF be explored. One such issue is cost. Along with the shock of medical bills, loss of work, and perhaps even the terrifying and grim funeral costs, there would likely be enormous and unexpected costs associated with trying to conceive via postmortem sperm extraction. Some of these costs include sperm extraction, tissue processing, sperm storage, and finally the cost of IVF or ICSI [24]. Often, most of these costs will not be covered by insurance [25]. If it becomes evident that the cost of IVF is prohibitively high, the entire process should be ruled out immediately, long before the planning stage where families become mentally tied to the concept.

Another issue that has to be considered before fully plunging into the process is how the specimen will be obtained and where it will go once extracted. The burden of finding a fertility center all too often falls on the physician, and a center must be contracted that agrees in principle to process a specimen obtained in such circumstances. Some fertility groups may oppose

Table 36.2. Summary of logistical hurdles for postmortem ICSI

Finding a suitable IVF group
Cost of sperm banking
Cost of IVF
Identifying a surgeon to perform extraction
Getting the yolk buffer solution
Transport of tissue to the IVF center in a timely fashion
Infectious disease testing in donor
Overcoming moral/ethical concerns among all participants

due to the grounds of the situation. Often, the healthcare providers at the fertility center share the concerns of patient consent described previously and refuse to work with this sample. Once all of these pieces are in place, a surgeon, typically a urologist, must agree to perform the procedure. While many are technically capable, as with all steps in this long process, the urologist may oppose performing the procedure due to personal opinions.

Lastly, this relatively straightforward procedure still has to be executed smoothly and efficiently. It can be done either in an operating room or at the bedside, since anesthesia is rarely an issue [26]. The surgeon needs the tools and equipment available to perform the operation. A scrotal incision is made, the tunica albuginea of the testicle is exposed, and samples of the healthiest-appearing seminiferous tubules are extracted and blotted to remove blood. Then they are placed in a yolk buffer solution, which may be unique to each particular IVF group. Then the tissue, in the buffered solution, must be efficiently shipped off to the fertility center for processing. Closure of the wound is then carried out, often as the simultaneous transportation of the tissue to the fertility center is done. Without these logistical considerations, the endeavor is not possible. Further complicating matters is that the patient donating banked sperm must be tested for hepatitis and sexually transmitted diseases, and while HIV testing is also required, this is typically not possible at short notice. The logistical hurdles are listed in Table 36.2.

Legal issues

While the medical profession has often tried to shield itself from the intrusion of legal proceedings, there exist very few legal precedents to guide practitioners, and which families can consult when issues arise in this particular scenario. The few cases which have existed send confusing signals as to what our legal system says about posthumous sperm extraction and children born by this method. One such legal consideration would be delineating inheritance for children who are products of this process. In 1984, survival benefits were given in two cases in California [27]. In both, social security survivor benefits were given to children born from posthumous conception. This was contradicted in 2002, when the Massachusetts Supreme Court argued that social security survival benefits should not be granted to children of posthumous conception, instead favoring the interests of the other heirs [11,28,29]. In these cases from California and Massachusetts, sperm were used posthumously, but the sperm was extracted while the donors were alive and healthy. Therefore, the legal system has never been tested to explore the rights of offspring from sperm obtained from a deceased donor.

When it comes to the more general issues surrounding postmortem sperm extraction and IVF, the legal systems of many countries outside of the United States have been tested. A country's approach toward the issue can be classified in three broad groups: a full ban, necessity of written consent, or requirement for implied consent. France, Germany, Sweden, Canada, and parts of Australia are considered full ban. In 1984, the Parpalaix case in France tested the French legal system when the widow of a deceased cancer patient Alain Parpalaix was able to gain permission to retrieve and ultimately become inseminated with her husband's testicular sperm using IVF [30]. The full ban was executed after the Centre d'Etude et de Conservation du Sperme Humain (Center for the Study and Preservation of Human Sperm) fought in the court system to ban future such endeavors, in accordance with the country's ban at that time on IVF for post-menopausal women [30].

The United Kingdom requires written consent in order to proceed with postmortem sperm extraction and IVF. These guidelines broadly exist in the Human Fertilisation and Embryology Act of 1990 [31]. In 1997, the case of *Regina v. Human Fertilisation and Embryology Authority* expanded these guidelines to extend the terms of required written consent to patients in a vegetative state [32]. In theory, this implied that assault charges could be brought against physicians performing sperm extraction on comatose patients without written consent, in line with the concept that this was a requirement for this procedure just as it would be for any other invasive procedure [32].

There are also locations where implied consent is the rule. In Israel, there are published guidelines

written in 2003 by Attorney General Elyakim Rubenstein [33]. These did allow cases of postmortem sperm extraction for later insemination by a surviving partner. It was determined that the allowance for IVF and sperm extraction would be settled case by case, but that these requests could only be made by the female partner, never by other members of the donor's family [33].

Lastly, Belgium and the United States are examples of countries where there is no legislation on this topic. The decision is left to the opinions of the practitioners involved, including the medical personnel involved in the patient's ICU care, the urologist performing the sperm extraction, and those at the IVF group. This lack of specific legislation has made this process even more complex and vague. One consideration might be a quarantine period if sperm is taken for posthumous reproduction. This would allow the raw emotions surrounding the immediate event to decrease. As noted by Anger *et al.*, frequently the sperm extracted from postmortem patients is not used [34]. This lends support to the discussion of a delay or cooling-off period so that all parties can consider the situation more objectively.

Discussion

Sperm procurement requested for the terminally ill cancer patient mirrors the issues seen surrounding posthumous sperm extraction. These requests will continue to be pursued by families, questioned by practitioners, and challenged in the legal system. While ARTs have led to tremendous strides and created many lives, new challenges will be exposed. Patients who suffer from cancer, in some cases deemed incurable, will be given hopes of paternity through the technology afforded by IVF. While the outlook of being alive for their offspring may seem bleak, some cancer patients maintain a strong reproductive drive due to a multitude of factors, some driven by family members and spouses. The consent issues for living but terminally ill cancer patients may not be as central as they are in cases of posthumous sperm extraction, but the moral and ethical concerns still remain. This leaves practitioners to wonder what the best course of action is for the patient, family, and society.

In assessing the outcome and past success in extracting sperm from terminally ill cancer patients, we can look at the parallel population of trauma patients in whom families requested posthumous sperm retrieval. In one specific high-volume trauma center, the University of Maryland Shock Trauma Center, 5 years of data were studied and 13 requests for posthumous sperm extraction were uncovered. These were largely made by families and spouses of critically ill patients. Due to the very complexities outlined in this chapter, only four resulted in the completion of a sperm harvest. As expected, the arduous and expensive process of obtaining consent and a realization of the costs involved discouraged many from taking definitive steps toward carrying out the procedure. It has been observed that for critically ill patients who face long and uncertain recovery periods, spouses and other family members often lose their enthusiasm as the shock of the traumatic event fades. Perhaps the initial shock of the accident elicits a reaction to act definitively and do something dramatic. Over time, however, this response decreases.

To date, no pregnancies have resulted from sperm harvested from terminally ill patients at the University of Maryland Shock Trauma Center. All too often, the consent that existed was only a private, undocumented conversation between a husband and wife, or a boyfriend and girlfriend. This sparse documentation was hardly enough to get the long and arduous process of IVF off the ground.

The ASRM Ethics Committee upholds the physician's right to refuse to participate in posthumous sperm extraction when consent is unclear [7]. Confusion seems to be a central theme whenever this scenario presents itself. At busy trauma centers, protocols should be put into place so a team can be efficiently assembled to explain the ethical and technical considerations to affected families considering posthumous sperm extraction. The levels of valid consent should be circulated and easily referenced for physicians and families who need this information quickly and at a devastating crossroads in life surrounded already by loss and confusion. A team of practitioners should be efficiently assembled, including someone able to counsel families against making an emotional and impulsive decision rather than one that is well thought out. Future legal cases will likely ensue that may also guide clinicians as they grapple with counseling patients and families during a time of crisis.

In cases of cancer patients, there may be less of an impulse reaction by the family to harvest sperm, simply because they have had more time to process the diagnosis and deal with the situation. Despite this difference, we propose that medical centers create protocols dictating the stepwise measures to be taken when a request for terminally ill or posthumous sperm extraction requests are made. Consent issues and the myriad of logistical issues surrounding sperm extraction and IVF must be carefully weighed and understood both by the healthcare practitioners and by the families who either encounter or make such requests. To alleviate some of these difficulties, there could be some value in men about to get married or enter into a similar relationship to document their wishes for sperm retrieval, as scary and morbid as that situation may be. This would serve as a valuable protective measure should a tragic scenario arise. This procedure could be done in the same way that they might prepare a living will. While no couple would ever want to have to execute the wishes written in the will, it would offer peace of mind that if such a situation did arise, their wishes would be legally recorded. As the medical community continues to evolve, and as science and technology advance, it is possible that women will also seek to preserve ova in a similar manner as their male counterparts, which will undoubtedly spark debate [35]. If and when this topic becomes feasible, and ultimately discussed in a public forum, is anyone's guess.

References

1. Rothman CM. A method for obtaining viable sperm in the postmortem state. *Fertil Steril* 1980; 34: 512–14.

2. Annas G. Culture of life politics at the bedside: the case of Terry Schiavo. *N Engl J Med* 2005; 352: 1710–15.

3. Emanuel EJ, Daniels ER, Fairclough DL, Claridge BR. The practice of euthanasia and physician-assisted suicide in the United States: adherence to proposed safeguards and effects on physicians. *JAMA* 1998; 280: 507–13.

4. Swinn M, Emberton M, Ralph D, Smith M, Serhal P. Retrieving semen from a dead patient: utilitarianism in the absence of definitive guidelines. *BMJ* 1998; 317: 1583.

5. American Medical Association. Patient physician relationship topics: informed consent, 2010. www.ama-assn.org/ama/pub/physician-resources/legal-topics/patient-physician-relationship-topics/informed-consent.shtml (accessed January 2012).

6. Weber B, Kodama R, Jarvi K. Postmortem sperm retrieval: the Canadian perspective. *J Androl* 2009; 30: 407–9.

7. Ethics Committee of the American Society for Reproductive Medicine. Ethical considerations of assisted reproductive technologies. *Fertil Steril* 1999; 67 (5 Suppl 1): 1S–9S.

8. Revised Uniform Anatomical Gift Act, 2006. www.anatomicalgiftact.org (accessed January 2012).

9. Gimbel RW, Strosberg MA, Lehrman SE, Gefenas E, Taft F. Presumed consent and other predictors of cadaveric organ consent in Europe. *Prog Transplant* 2003; 13: 17–23.

10. Strong C. Gamete retrieval after death or irreversible unconsciousness: what counts as informed consent? *Camb Q Healthc Ethics* 2006; 15: 161–71.

11. Kramer AC. Sperm retrieval from terminally ill or recently deceased patients: a review. *Can J Urol* 2009; 16: 4627–31.

12. Mohta M, Sethi A, Tyagi A, Mohta A. Psychological care in trauma patients. *Injury* 2003; 34: 17–25.

13. Orr RD, Siegler M. Is posthumous semen retrieval ethically permissible? *J Med Ethics* 2002; 28: 299–302.

14. Strong C, Gingrich JR, Kutteh WH. Ethics of sperm retrieval after death or persistent vegetative state. *Hum Reprod* 2000; 15: 739–45.

15. Batzer F, Hurwitz J, Caplan A. Postmortem parenthood and the need for a protocol with posthumous sperm procurement. *Fertil Steril* 2003; 79: 1263–9.

16. Donoso A, Tournaye E, Devroey A. *Hum Repr Update* 2007; 13: 539–47.

17. Grazi RV, Wolowelsky JB. The use of cryopreserved sperm and pre-embryos in contemporary Jewish law and ethics. *Assist Reprod Technol Androl* 1995; 8: 53–61.

18. Haas J. Begotten not made: a catholic view of reproductive technology. United States Conference of Catholic Bishops. www.usccb.org/profile/programs/rlp/98rlphaa.shtml (accessed August 2010).

19. Serour GI, Dickens BM. Assisted reproductive developments in the Islamic world. *Int J Gynaecol Obstet* 2000; 70: 77–86.

20. Van Voorhis B. In vitro fertilization. *New Engl J Med* 2007; 356: 379–86.

21. Hansen M, Kurinczuk J, Bower C, Webb S. The risk of major birth defects after intracytoplasmic sperm injection and in-vitro fertilization. *N Engl J Med* 2002; 346: 725–30.

22. Ericson A, Kaillen B. Congenital malformations in infants born after IVF: a population based study. *Hum Reprod* 2001; 16: 504–9.

23. Halliday J, Oke K, Algar E, Amor D. Beckwith–Wiedemann syndrome and IVF: a case control study. *Am J Hum Genet* 2004; 75: 526–8.

24. Neumann P, Gharib S, Weinstein M. The cost of a successful delivery with in-vitro fertilization. *N Engl J Med* 1994; 331: 239–43.

25. Collins J. An international survey of the health economics of IVF and ICSI. *Hum Reprod Update* 2002; 8: 265–77.

26. Issa M, Hsaio K, Bassel Y, *et al.* Spermatic cord anesthesia block for scrotal procedures in outpatient care setting. *J Urol* 2004; 172: 2358–61.

27. Cal Super Ct, Los Angeles County, Nos. P680682 and P680683 (1984).

28. Woodward v. Commissioner of Social Security. 760 N.E.2d 257, 435 Mass. 536 (2002).

29. Crockin SL. Legally speaking. *Amer Soc Reprod Med News* 2002; Spring: 36.

30. Bahadur, G. Death and conception. *Hum Reprod* 2002; 17: 2769–75.

31. Human Fertilisation and Embryology Act 1990. http://www.legislation.gov.uk/ukpga/1990/37 (accessed January 2012).

32. Cohen P. Life after death: New York state moves to keep dead men's sperm in the family. *New Sci* 1998; 157: 23.

33. Landau, R. Posthumous sperm retrieval for the purpose of later insemination or IVF in Israel: an ethical and psychosocial critique. *Hum Reprod* 2004; 19: 1952–6.

34. Anger J, Gilbert B, Goldstein M. Cryopreservation of sperm: indications, methods, and results. *J Urol* 2003; 170: 1079–84.

35. Blumenfeld Z. How to preserve fertility in young women exposed to chemotherapy? The role of GnRH agonist cotreatment in addition to cryopreservation of embrya, oocytes, or ovaries. *Oncologist* 2007; 12: 1067–9.

Chapter 3

Fertility following antineoplastic therapy in the male: intrauterine insemination and the assisted reproductive technologies

Hey-Joo Kang, Jack Huang, and Owen K. Davis

Introduction

Improved survival rates in men with cancer have naturally given rise to consideration of life beyond cancer therapy. To this end, maintenance of reproductive potential in men with cancer should always be included in pre-treatment counseling, due to the gonadotoxicity of antineoplastic therapy. Cryopreservation of semen prior to cancer treatment is the only effective fertility preservation strategy recognized by the American Society of Clinical Oncology (ASCO) and the American Society for Reproductive Medicine (ASRM) [1,2]. If initiation of treatment is urgent, or if the decision to preserve sperm is made following commencement of treatment, sperm may still be banked in the first three months, before the development of oligospermia or azoospermia [3]. However, the cryopreservation of even a single sample prior to treatment is preferred, because of the potentially mutagenic effects of radiation and chemotherapy. There is no evidence of increased chromosomal abnormalities in offspring fathered by men exposed to chemotherapeutic agents [4].

Before the development of assisted reproductive technologies (ART), the concentration of sperm acceptable for cryopreservation was based on its intended use for intrauterine insemination (IUI). Thus, when sperm density was found to be < 10 million/mL or motility < 40%, the sample might not be cryopreserved owing to the limited potential for successful future use [5]. With the advent of in-vitro fertilization (IVF) in 1978 and the subsequent introduction of intracytoplasmic injection (ICSI) in 1992, the presence of any motile sperm merits consideration for storage [6].

In this chapter, we will review the scope of treatment options available for the couple with cryopreserved sperm or impaired spermatogenesis from cancer therapy. Evaluation of the female partner is a critical element in deciding the optimal treatment of the infertile couple and will also be discussed in detail. Lastly, we will review current laboratory techniques used in gamete micromanipulation as well as potential complications of ART.

Assisted reproductive technologies (ART)

The term ART encompasses any treatment involving retrieval of oocytes. The first live birth resulting from ART was reported by Patrick Steptoe and Robert Edwards in 1978, following laparoscopic retrieval of a single oocyte from an unstimulated ovary [7,8]. The most frequently practiced ART procedure is in-vitro fertilization, or IVF, which entails a sequence of events including controlled ovarian hyperstimulation of the ovaries to induce multifolliclular recruitment, harvesting of oocytes, fertilization of the oocytes, culture of the developing embryos and subsequent transfer to the uterus. Other assisted reproductive techniques include laparoscopic tubal transfer of gametes (gamete intrafallopian transfer, GIFT), zygotes (zygote intrafallopian transfer, ZIFT), and embryos (tubal embryo transfer, TET); it should be noted that these techniques have been largely supplanted by IVF in light of the requirement for laparoscopy and general anesthesia, and the refinements in laboratory technology.

Fertility Preservation in Male Cancer Patients, ed. John P. Mulhall, Linda D. Applegarth, Robert D. Oates and Peter N. Schlegel. Published by Cambridge University Press. © Cambridge University Press 2013.

Etiologies of female infertility

IVF was originally intended as a definitive treatment option for women with severe, irreparable tubal disease [7,8]. With improvements in laboratory techniques and success rates, the indications have expanded to include severe male-factor infertility, endometriosis, ovulatory dysfunction, diminished ovarian reserve, and unexplained infertility.

Tubal factor

Worldwide, tubal-factor infertility accounts for an estimated 30% of cases of female infertility and 9% of diagnoses among couples who undergo ART treatments in the USA [9]. Tubal obstruction can either result from acute and chronic salpingitis (e.g., *Chlamydia trachomatis*, gonorrhea), or be due to voluntary surgical sterilization, endometriosis, or peritonitis.

Tubal patency can be assessed via hysterosalpingography (HSG). A contrast agent is injected into the uterine cavity and tubal anatomy is visualized with concurrent fluoroscopy. The luminal diameter should be < 1 mm at the isthmic portion of the fallopian tube, and typically increases to 2–3 mm at the ampullary end. Free intraperitoneal spill of contract should be visualized to confirm tubal patency.

For women with tubal-factor infertility, treatment options are limited to surgical tubal reconstruction or IVF. The highest surgical success rates are obtained following reversal of tubal sterilization without coexistent infertility factors. Conception rates ranging from 45% to 82% and ectopic pregnancy rates of 7% have been reported. Fecundity rates are subject to patient selection, surgeon experience, and technical skill as well as the final length of the fallopian tube.

Current success rates following IVF in general exceed those with tubal surgery. However, tubal reconstructive surgery is a reasonable treatment option for young women with mild tubal disease and for those with ethical, religious, or financial restrictions that preclude IVF [10].

Endometriosis

Endometriosis is defined as the growth of ectopic endometrial tissue outside the uterus. This tissue is responsive to the hormonal milieu and can be a significant cause of morbidity. Clinical manifestations include dysmenorrhea, chronic pelvic pain, and dyspareunia.

The precise pathophysiology of endometriosis and its actual impact on natural conception remains elusive. Impairment of fertility may arise from distortion of pelvic anatomy due to adhesive disease and a "toxic" peritoneal environment characterized by increased inflammatory cytokines and oxidative stress [11,12], which may impede follicular development, ovum pick-up, fertilization, and embryo development.

Although somewhat controversial, there is some evidence that laparoscopic excision or ablation of endometriosis may improve pregnancy rates in patients with minimal or mild (stage I–II) endometriosis [13,14]. Asymptomatic patients with known or suspected stage I–II endometriosis may be treated empirically with clomiphene citrate (CC) or gonadotropins and IUI [15]. Patients with known or suspected moderate and severe endometriosis (stage III–IV) may be treated with either surgery or IVF. Surgical treatment is preferred in patients who are symptomatic or require pathologic confirmation.

Polycystic ovary syndrome (PCOS)

Ovulatory dysfunction is one of the most common causes of female infertility, accounting for 25% of cases [9]. Most of these patients present with either oligomenorrhea – menstruation at intervals exceeding 35 days – or amenorrhea, the absence of menstruation. In many patients, ovulatory dysfunction can be successfully treated with an ovulation inducing (OI) agent combined with timed intercourse or IUI.

Pharmacologic agents used to induce ovulation include CC, exogenous gonadotropins, aromatase inhibitors (anastrazole, letrozole), or selective estrogen receptor modulators (tamoxifen) [16]. It should be noted that patients with polycystic ovaries seen on ultrasound have an increased risk of multiple gestation [17,18] as well as a higher potential for ovarian hyperstimulation syndrome (OHSS), particularly following treatment with exogenous gonadotropins. In selected cases, those who over-respond to controlled ovarian stimulation with gonadotropins (excessive follicular response) may benefit from conversion to oocyte retrieval and IVF. This represents a safer alternative to proceeding with intercourse or IUI and can avoid cycle cancellation [19]. IVF is also indicated in patients who do not conceive following a trial of conventional OI treatment, and in couples with coexisting infertility factors.

Unexplained infertility

A diagnosis of unexplained infertility requires the absence of an identifiable cause of infertility despite a thorough investigation demonstrating tubal patency, normal semen parameters, cyclic ovulation, adequate ovarian reserve, and normal uterine anatomy. The incidence of unexplained infertility ranges from 10% to 30% [20]. Treatment options include expectant management, IUI, empiric treatment with an OI agent, or ART.

Prognostic factors: female partner

Ovarian reserve testing

Ovarian reserve refers to the endowment of female germ cells or primordial follicles. In IVF patients, advancing maternal age is associated with a decline in the number of oocytes retrieved, embryos available for transfer, and oocyte/embryo quality [21–23]. In addition to the decline in fertility, the incidence of spontaneous miscarriage also increases with advanced maternal age [24]. The increased miscarriage rate is due primarily to a higher prevalence of aneuploidy in aging oocytes secondary to meiotic non-disjunction events [25]. In addition to age alone, other biomarkers of ovarian reserve have proven clinically useful.

Ultrasonographic markers: antral follicle count

The total number of 2–5 mm diameter follicles seen on transvaginal ultrasound on menstrual cycle day 2–3 is a reliable predictor of ART yield [26]. The antral follicle count (AFC) is complementary to other markers of ovarian reserve including total ovarian volume, basal levels of follicle-stimulating hormone (FSH), estradiol, and inhibin B in predicting an individual's response to ovarian stimulation [27].

Hormonal assays

FSH

As a consequence of the ongoing depletion of primordial follicles, there is a decline in inhibin B production from the investing granulosa cells. The declining negative feedback by inhibin B results in an increase in the pituitary production of FSH [28]. FSH levels suggestive of diminished ovarian reserve (DOR) exceed 12–15 mIU/L on day 2–3 of the menstrual cycle [29,30].

Elevated serum FSH levels have been associated with poor IVF outcomes and pregnancy rates, an effect most pronounced in women over 40 years of age. It should be cautioned that a single abnormal measurement may be inaccurate, owing to inter-cycle fluctuations in FSH levels, and that a normal value does not exclude DOR.

Anti-Müllerian hormone

Anti-Müllerian hormone (AMH) is produced by the granulosa cells surrounding preantral and early antral follicles [31]. AMH levels are reliably measured independent of cycle day and are therefore a more convenient and consistent test of ovarian reserve. AMH results have been shown to correlate with FSH levels, AFC, and numbers of oocytes retrieved in an IVF cycle [32,33].

There is no universally accepted AMH level predicting diminished ovarian response. Using a cutoff of AMH level $\leq$ 1.26 ng/mL, Gnoth *et al.* reported a sensitivity of 97% and a specificity of 41% in detecting poor response [34]. Another study found a cutoff of AMH < 0.1 ng/mL to be associated with 76% sensitivity and 88% specificity in predicting poor response, and 22% sensitivity and 89% specificity in predicting non-pregnancy [35].

Clomiphene citrate challenge test

The clomiphene citrate challenge test (CCCT) involves measurement of baseline FSH level on cycle day 3, followed by administration of 100 mg CC on cycle day 5 to 9, and repeat FSH measurement on cycle day 10 [36]. An elevated FSH value greater than two standard deviations above the mean is considered to be abnormal. However, the cost-effectiveness of the CCCT in the evaluation of infertile patients has been questioned, as the majority of studies do not confirm superiority to basal FSH in predicting clinical response of women undergoing fertility treatment [37,38].

Cryopreservation

The concept of sperm cryopreservation dates back to 1776, when the Italian scientist Lazzaro Spallanzani observed that sperm became motionless when cooled by snow. Further experiments in sperm preservation were driven by the desire to help mortally wounded soldiers achieve posthumous paternity. Survival rates of frozen sperm in the early twentieth century were poor before the introduction of cryoprotectants to improve the viability of post-thawed sperm [39]. Currently, glycerol and albumin (egg yolk or human albumin) are the most commonly used cryoprotectants to maintain the structural integrity of the spermatozoa during cooling and thawing. Each component can be maintained as a separate stock solution and frozen separately until needed for use. Commercial media are also available with equally reliable survival rates.

Sperm is collected by masturbation into a sterile plastic jar. The sample should be prepared just after liquefaction of the seminal plasma. In cases of azoospermia, retrieval of viable sperm can be accomplished from several sites in the genital tract through needle aspiration or biopsy [40]. The diminished quality of surgically retrieved sperm mandates density-gradient centrifugation or washing and re-suspension prior to freezing. After combining the cryoprotectant and semen sample, the resultant solution is aliquoted into 1.5 mL vials and gradually frozen by suspension in liquid nitrogen vapor and stored in liquid nitrogen [41].

IUI versus IVF

There are no precise guidelines in deciding between IUI and IVF. In the 1950s when normative values were being established, the sperm concentrations in thousands of fertile men were compared to infertile males [42]. The investigators observed that in large cohorts of fertile men, over 70% were found to have concentrations exceeding 40 million/mL, whereas only 5–7% had counts less than 20 million/mL. Infertile men were more likely to have counts < 20 million/mL when compared to fertile men (16% vs. 5%, respectively) [43]. Sperm motility should also be considered when establishing male-factor infertility. A total motile sperm count of > 5 million has been correlated with a higher likelihood of conception. It should also be noted that there are no sperm concentrations that absolutely preclude conception except in cases of absolute azoospermia. Men with extremely low concentrations of sperm have produced viable offspring without the need for intervention, albeit the time to conceive correlates inversely with sperm concentrations.

When making a decision between IUI and IVF, one should always be cognizant of the concentration of sperm and the amount available. In cases involving a finite number of cryopreserved vials, IVF with assisted fertilization is generally the best

course of treatment to preserve the couple's ongoing reproductive potential. For fresh samples containing concentrations < 10–20 million sperm per mL, or for those with low motility or morphology, IVF-ICSI should be strongly considered, given the diminished fertilization potential [44]. In cases involving fresh or frozen testicular sperm, markedly impaired concentration and motility necessitate IVF-ICSI. Additionally, advanced age of the female partner may direct treatment toward IVF, independent of sperm quality.

Intrauterine insemination (IUI)

For patients with adequate sperm, the clinician may choose IUI. In this process, the female partner is monitored for ovulation in a medicated (OI) or natural cycle. In young ovulatory women, the typical menstrual cycle length is 26–32 days, with ovulation occurring between cycle days 12 and 18. CC or exogenous gonadotropins may benefit selected women by increasing the number of ovulated oocytes. These agents are also particularly useful for women with infrequent or irregular menses due to ovulatory dysfunction. Women who are of advanced maternal age may also benefit from controlled ovarian stimulation with IUI in selected cases. When using ovarian stimulating agents, the patients should always be counseled regarding the increased risk of multiple gestation as well as OHSS. Exogenous gonadotropin cycles are closely monitored with serial estradiol (E_2) levels and transvaginal ultrasound follicular measurements in an effort to mitigate these risks. The female partner can have ovulation triggered with a human chorionic gonadotropin (hCG) injection (CC or gonadotropins), or may monitor for her endogenous luteinizing hormone (LH) surge using urinary ovulation predictor kits (CC cycles). Ovulation is predicted to occur 24–36 hours after the induced or natural LH surge, and IUI is performed just prior to ovulation.

For the IUI procedure, the identity of the washed sperm sample is re-confirmed with the patient. The female partner is placed in the dorsal lithotomy position and a speculum is used to visualize the cervix. The sample is loaded into a flexible catheter which is then carefully inserted through the cervical canal, with injection of the processed sperm into the uterine cavity. Pregnancy can be reliably documented two weeks following the IUI.

Sperm preparation techniques for IUI and IVF

The purpose of the sperm wash is to remove debris, white blood cells, and prostaglandins from a semen sample intended for direct placement into the uterine cavity. Because an IUI will bypass the cervix – a natural barrier to infection – the wash also reduces the risk of endometritis while increasing the overall motile cohort of sperm available for fertilization. There are three methods of sperm preparation – swim-up, density-gradient centrifugation, and simple centrifugation wash.

The swim-up method is best suited for samples with normal count and motility and minimal debris. In this process, medium is gently placed over the semen in a conical tube. The specimen is transferred to a 37 °C incubator for 60 minutes to allow the sperm to swim up into the layer of media. This allows the motile sperm to separate from the debris and non-motile sperm in the underlying seminal plasma. The supernatant is collected and centrifuged twice with sperm washing media. The final pellet is collected and re-suspended in 0.5 mL of media.

Density-gradient centrifugation is preferred over swim-up in cases with low sperm counts or in instances where a high degree of debris or viscosity is encountered. It has the advantage of a shorter preparation time, requiring only a 20-minute centrifugation. In this method, colloidal silica particles of discontinuous densities are placed in a conical tube and overlaid with the semen sample. The sample is centrifuged for 15–20 minutes at 200–400 g to allow the specimen to proceed through the gradient. The non-motile sperm and debris are retained within the gradient and the motile sperm are recovered in the pellet. The pellet is re-suspended in medium and washed twice, to a final volume of 0.5 mL.

A simple wash is the addition of culture medium supplemented with protein, followed by centrifugation and re-suspension of the pellet. Use of this technique should be limited to samples with little to no debris. It has been suggested that simple washes may result in oxidative damage to the sperm by free oxygen radicals [45]. This method is rarely utilized, given the widespread availability of colloidal silica and comparable prep time of density gradients.

The optimal preparation of a sperm sample varies according to its intended use and original sperm concentration. In traditional IVF, approximately 50 000–100 000 sperm per mL are placed around each oocyte. In this case, density gradients have been suggested to improve fertilization rates, possibly due to more effective removal of inhibitory components in the seminal plasma. If the sperm concentration or motility is poor the sample should be prepared for ICSI. In these instances, there is no difference in fertilization rates between swim-up verses density-gradient techniques.

Ovarian stimulation

The neonatal ovary contains 6–7 million oogonia at 16–20 weeks of gestation, 1–2 million at birth, and 300 000–500 000 by the age of menarche [46]. As a consequence, the reproductive potential of the female partner progressively declines from age 30 until menopause. Additionally, it has been shown that embryonic aneuploidy rates rise with advancing maternal age. Thus, the optimal treatment choice for a male with cryopreserved sperm is dependent upon the age of the female partner. If the sperm concentration is < 20 million/mL and/or in cases of poor motility, IVF is indicated regardless of female age.

The goal of ovarian stimulation is the induction of maturation of multiple follicles within a single menstrual cycle. This is accomplished by daily subcutaneous injections of gonadotropins with concurrent monitoring of E_2 levels and ovarian ultrasound over a period of 10–14 days.

"Long" agonist protocols

In this approach, a gonadotropin-releasing hormone (GnRH) agonist is administered in the preceding luteal phase to suppress pituitary secretion of FSH and LH, thereby preventing early selection of the dominant follicle (Fig. 37.1). Controlled ovarian stimulation is initiated using a combination of gonadotropins (human menopausal gonadotropin [hMG] or FSH). The GnRH agonist is continued for the purpose of preventing an endogenous LH surge prior to oocyte harvest. The daily gonadotropin dose can be tapered during follicular recruitment – referred to as the step-down approach – without impairment of oocyte quality [47]. The goal of the step-down strategy is to reduce the risk of OHSS and possibly improve synchronization of follicular development. hCG is administered once the lead follicles achieve a mean diameter of 17 mm.

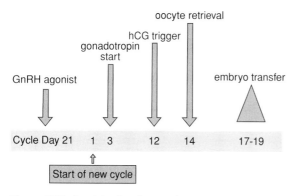

Figure 37.1. Agonist or "long" protocol.

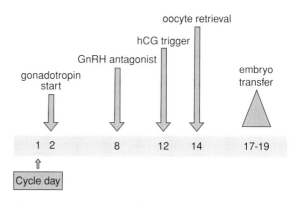

Figure 37.2. Antagonist or "short" protocol.

"Short" antagonist protocols

In the short protocol, GnRH agonist is not used in the preceding cycle. Treatment commences with administration of gonadotropins on day 2–3 of menses (Fig. 37.2). In order to prevent the physiologic surge, a GnRH antagonist is typically added when follicles reach an average diameter ≥ 13mm and/or the serum E_2 level is > 300 pg/mL (flexible protocol). The GnRH antagonist can also be started on a fixed day of the IVF cycle (day 6–8) without compromising oocyte or embryo quality [48]. As with GnRH agonist protocols, hCG is administered when at least two lead follicles reach 17 mm in mean diameter.

For the patient with diminished ovarian reserve (as evidenced by elevated FSH levels, low AFC or AMH levels), care should be taken to avoid early selection of a dominant follicle. Modification of the short protocol by the addition of estrogen patches, oral contraceptive pills, or oral estrogen in the luteal phase of the preceding cycle prevents an early rise in FSH without suppressing the subsequent ovarian response to exogenous gonadotropins.

Short protocols have traditionally been used in women predicted to be poor responders to gonadotropin stimulation. Recently, this protocol has been extended to include younger women at risk of developing OHSS. OHSS is associated with hCG-induced expression of hyperpermeability factors, principally vascular endothelial growth factor (VEGF) [49]. The long half-life of hCG (48–72 hours) potentiates this risk. The antagonist protocol allows for the ovulation trigger to be effected using a GnRH agonist, which induces an initial flare of LH secretion from the pituitary before the ensuing suppression.

Physiologic LH has a shorter half-life of 12 hours, thereby decreasing the risk of OHSS.

Ovarian stimulation for the hyper-responding patient

For the young female partner with robust ovarian reserve, and particularly in the event of polycystic ovaries, care should be taken to minimize the risk of OHSS. One option is to combine oral contraceptive pills with administration of a GnRH agonist for dual pituitary suppression prior to initiation of gonadotropin therapy. If an exaggerated response to exogenous gonadotropins occurs despite using the step-down approach, gonadotropins can be withheld, while continuing the agonist, in a process termed "coasting." This is indicated in hyper-responders with E_2 levels > 3000 pg/mL or more than 20 follicles, in an effort to inhibit the continued development of intermediate-sized follicles while allowing growth of the larger follicles.

Alternative agents may also be used to induce multifollicular recruitment while mitigating the risk of OHSS. CC is a selective estrogen receptor modulator that competes with estrogen at the level of the pituitary. This increases the level of endogenous FSH secretion in the early follicular phase, and can be used alone or in combination with low-dose supplemental gonadotropins in patients at risk for hyper-response. hCG is generally utilized to induce oocyte maturation. CC alone typically yields 1–3 oocytes, and its benefit in reducing OHSS risk should be balanced against lower pregnancy rates (10–15%) and potentially higher cancellation rates (25–40%).

In "natural-cycle" IVF, monofollicular recruitment with retrieval of a single oocyte is the intended outcome. This method was historically used prior to the availability of exogenous gonadotropins. It offers the advantages of avoiding multiple gestations and reducing medication costs, and the risk of OHSS is eliminated. However, the pregnancy rate per initiated natural cycle is only 4% and cancellation rates are extremely high (35–40%). Natural-cycle IVF is rarely used today for young, good responders. Currently, it can be used in extremely poor responders who only achieve monofollicular recruitment despite high doses of exogenous gonadotropins, or in patients for whom ovarian stimulation is contraindicated.

Alternative ovarian stimulation for the poorly responding patient

A dilute concentration of GnRH agonist can be used to exploit its initial "flare" effect, stimulating endogenous gonadotropin release from the pituitary. This "microflare" protocol is used in women with low ovarian response despite high doses of gonadotropins. Typically, 40 μg of the GnRH agonist leuprolide acetate is initiated twice daily, following administration of a short course of oral contraceptive pills, and is continued while gonadotropins are initiated on cycle day 4, concurrently or preceding gonadotropin treatment for a similar effect.

Oocyte retrieval

Physiologic ovulation is induced by a surge of LH released from the pituitary 36 hours prior to extrusion of the oocyte from the follicle. In ART, the LH homolog hCG is administered to the female partner 34–36 hours prior to harvest, allowing for in-vivo maturation of the oocytes. The patient receives intravenous sedation and is placed in the dorsal lithotomy position. The vagina and perineum are washed and prepped with an antiseptic solution to minimize the risk of iatrogenic pelvic infection, followed by copious irrigation with sterile saline. A high-frequency vaginal ultrasound transducer is used to visualize the ovary, and retrieval of the oocytes is accomplished through ultrasound-guided aspiration with a needle. A consistent vacuum pressure of 80–100 mmHg assists in the collection of follicular fluid, which is immediately transported to the embryology lab for evaluation.

Transitional media is used during collection, enumeration, and grading of oocytes. It acts as a buffer, maintaining physiologic pH and temperatures within a narrow window of 34–37 °C. Care is taken to maintain temperatures ≤ 37 °C, as higher temperatures will increase the metabolic rate of the oocyte and may adversely affect embryogenesis.

Assessment of oocyte maturity

During fetal life, the oocytes are arrested in the diplotene stage of the first meiotic prophase. At menarche, each oocyte selected for ovulation completes the first round of meiosis, signified by extrusion of the first polar body, and arrests again at metaphase of the second meiotic division. The matured oocyte is surrounded by specialized granulosa cells (the cumulus) and can be penetrated by the spermatozoon. The oocyte completes the second and final stage of meiosis only after successful fertilization [50].

In the embryology lab, the cumulus–coronal complexes are identified in the follicular aspirates, and oocyte maturity is assessed. Because the cumulus–coronal complex limits the ability to visualize the extruded polar body, oocyte maturity is estimated by the overall appearance of the cumulus–oocyte complex. Immature oocytes (germinal vesicle/MI) have tightly packed cumulus–coronal complexes and dense coronal layers, while mature (MII) oocytes have highly dispersed cumulus cells and a radiating coronal layer. Oocytes of intermediate maturity may undergo in-vitro maturation for 12–24 hours prior to fertilization, although pregnancy rates of embryos from in-vitro matured oocytes are suboptimal.

Preparation of the oocyte for fertilization and ICSI

Oocytes are inseminated 4–6 hours after harvest. Based on the available post-wash total motile sperm, a decision to fertilize by insemination or ICSI is made. In traditional IVF, 50 000–150 000 sperm per mL are incubated with each mature oocyte for 12–18 hours. Fertilization is deemed successful when two pronuclei (2 pn) are observed and the second polar body is extruded. Oocytes with three pronuclei indicate polyspermic fertilization and should be identified and removed from the cohort designated for potential embryo transfer. Screening out triploid embryos is critical, because of their ability to divide normally

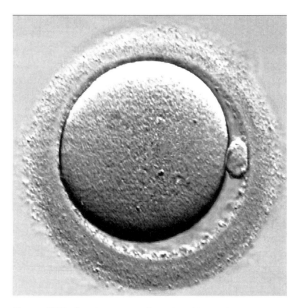

Figure 37.3. A mature oocyte. *See color plate section.*

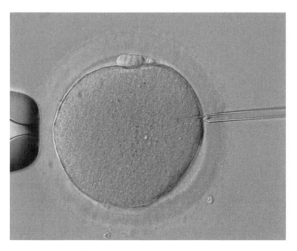

Figure 37.4. Performing ICSI.

and appear identical to 2 pn embryos on the day of transfer. The inevitable fate of transferred triploid embryos would include implantation failure or miscarriage [51].

In cases of low sperm count, motility, or morphology, the oocytes are prepared for ICSI. Mature cumulus cells are removed using hyaluronidase to allow confirmation of maturity (nuclear grading) and enhance the visualization of the oocyte during the injection procedure. Care is taken when aspirating the hyaluronidase-treated cumulus cells with hand-drawn pipettes, as contact with the oocyte membrane can induce parthenogenetic activation. The denuded oocyte is then assessed for maturity by observation of the extruded polar body. ICSI is performed only on mature oocytes (Fig. 37.3).

An individual motile and morphologically normal spermatozoon is identified for injection. A micropipette is used to mechanically immobilize the sperm's flagellum, releasing cytosolic factors that activate the oocyte. A holding pipette gently maintains oocyte position with the polar body oriented to the 12 o'clock position. The injection pipette containing the spermatozoon is introduced first through the zona pellucida and then the oolema at the 3 o'clock position until a break in the oolema is observed. The sperm is released and the pipette slowly removed (Fig. 37.4).

Fertilization rates following ICSI average 70–75% of total MII oocytes. When triploid fertilization is found following ICSI, these represent digynic embryos. Retention of the second polar body during meiosis II is the most common cause of digynic triploid embryos but may less frequently result from retention of the first polar body during meiosis I. As with dispermic fertilization following conventional IVF, these embryos should be identified and removed from the cohort of embryos for transfer.

Additional laboratory procedures

Assisted hatching (AH)

Mammalian implantation occurs 5–7 days following ovulation. Over this time period, the fertilized oocyte is transported from the fallopian tube to the uterine cavity. The zona pellucida (ZP) promotes monospermic fertilization and protects the developing embryo from the surrounding female genital tract during transport. Upon entry to the uterine cavity, the blastocyst must hatch from the ZP to allow trophectoderm cells to interact directly with endometrial cells, thus permitting implantation.

The goal of assisted hatching (AH) is to facilitate release of the blastocyst by creating an artificial breach in the ZP. AH is performed three days post insemination to permit adequate blastomere adherence, just before compaction. Several techniques have been described in performing AH; in all, care should be taken to avoid damage to the underlying blastomeres.

Partial zona dissection (PZD) involves a tangential piercing of the ZP from the 11 to the 1 o'clock position.

This segment is then rubbed with the holding pipette until a slit is made in the zona. Acid Tyrode's solution can also be used for chemical ZP drilling, and this also allows for increasing the size of the breach as needed to avoid embryo trapping. With this technique, a micropipette containing acid Tyrode's is positioned close to the zona and the solution is gently delivered. In zona thinning, the zona is attenuated without creating an actual gap in the zona. Finally, laser-assisted hatching can be used with both contact and non-contact delivery systems.

The benefit of assisted hatching is controversial. In a recent Cochrane review of 23 randomized controlled trials, there was insufficient evidence to determine any benefit of AH on live birth rates [52]. Current evidence does not support AH in first-time IVF cycles; however, some individual studies have suggested AH as beneficial in patients with repeated implantation failure. One possible benefit of AH is that it permits the aspiration and removal of extracellular fragments that may inhibit cell compaction.

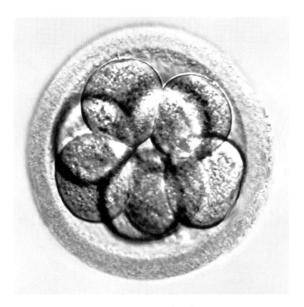

Figure 37.5. A day 3 embryo. *See color plate section.*

Autologous endometrial co-culture (AECC)

Autologous endometrial systems for embryonic culture are intended to closely mimic the uterine environment. Endometrial cells are retrieved 5–12 days after ovulation in a preceding cycle and the stromal and glandular cells are isolated and cryopreserved. The cells are thawed on the day of hCG administration in preparation for culture. Fertilized oocytes (zygotes) are placed on this reconstituted layer of endometrial cells and are cultured until post-retrieval day 3. Appropriately selected patients with a history of poor embryo quality and/or repeated implantation failure may benefit from AECC [53–56].

Pre-implantation genetic diagnosis (PGD) and screening (PGS)

Pre-implantation genetic diagnosis (PGD) for couples who carry heritable diseases reduces the potential need for therapeutic pregnancy termination following prenatal testing, or delivery of an affected child. In this process, the ZP of a 6–8-cell, day 3 embryo (Fig. 37.5) is penetrated using one of the techniques described for AH. A single blastomere is removed and polymerase chain reaction (PCR) is used to amplify the DNA fragment of interest. Only unaffected embryos or heterozygous normal embryos (in cases of autosomal

recessive disorders) are transferred. The error rate in selecting an affected embryo for transfer is 1–2% [57], and couples should be advised of this before deciding on invasive prenatal testing. Only heritable diseases with identified genetic loci are candidates for PGD.

Advanced maternal age increases errors (non-disjunction) of the first meiotic division in the oocyte, leading to increased chromosomal aneuploidy. Recurrent implantation failure and miscarriages are due in large part to aneuploidy. Single (or double) blastomere biopsy combined with fluorescent in-situ hybridization (FISH) can be used to screen embryos for chromosomal imbalances. Different colored, chromosome-specific fluorochromes hybridize with DNA after the blastomere has been fixed to a slide and the results are then analyzed. Embryos that display a pair of each fluoresced chromosome are available for transfer. Candidates for pre-implantation genetic screening (PGS) include couples with recurrent miscarriage, recurrent implantation failure, and advanced age of the female partner.

As with any treatment, the attendant risks and benefits must be considered. One drawback of PGS is the limited spectrum of fluorochromes that can be used for analysis. As a result, only the most commonly occurring aneuploidies in humans are targeted: chromosomes 13, 16, 18, 21, 22, X, and Y. By washing the probes and rehybridizing the nuclei with fluorochromes for additional chromosomes, the panel can be expanded, typically to 11 chromosomes. Aneuploidies involving the remaining, untested autosomes, as well as gene deletions, will not be detected (false negatives). Furthermore, the error rate in interpreting results has been reported to be 8–15%, due in part to overlapping and split signals [58,59]. The frequent occurrence of mosaicism within eight-cell embryos may lead to the discarding of embryos that could self-correct to euploid blastocyts (false positives) or to transfer of aneuploid embryos. Finally, the blastomere biopsy procedure itself may decrease the implantation potential of a euploid embryo following transfer. Current evidence does not demonstrate an improvement in live birth rates following PGS.

Embryo transfer

The goal of embryo transfer is delivery of a viable embryo with high implantation potential to the uterine cavity. A speculum is used to visualize the cervix, which is cleansed with saline or culture media to decrease bacterial contamination and remove excess mucus. Mucus in the cervical canal may be aspirated using a syringe. A trial transfer, avoiding contact with the uterine fundus, ensures atraumatic passage through the cervical canal. The transfer catheter is then loaded with the patient's embryo(s) and is handed to the clinician, who inserts the catheter through the cervix, with release of the embryos into the uterus. The catheter is carefully withdrawn, flushed, and microscopically inspected for possible retained embryos.

Several variables potentially affecting the outcome of embryo transfer have been studied. The specific catheter chosen should optimize navigation through the endocervical canal, yet be soft enough to avoid trauma to the endometrium and minimize the risk of inducing uterine contractility or bleeding. Several catheters are commercially available, and they are categorized as either "soft" (Cook – Cook Medical, Bloomington, IN; Wallace – Marlow Technologies, Wiloughby, OH) or "firm" (Tomcat and Tefcat – Kendell Health Care, Hampshire, MA; TDT and Frydman – Laboratoire CCD, Paris, France). Independent randomized controlled trials have demonstrated the superiority of soft catheters in routine embryo transfers; however, firm catheters may be necessary for patients with a tortuous cervical canal. Care should always be taken to avoid prostaglandin release initiated by disruption of the endometrium. Pregnancy rates have also been shown to be improved with increasing operator experience.

Ultrasound guidance allows the clinician to visualize catheter depth at the time of transfer and helps to avoid contact with the uterine fundus. Disadvantages include patient discomfort in maintaining a full bladder compounded with abdominal compression with an ultrasound probe. In a 2010 Cochrane review comparing ultrasound guidance versus clinical "touch," there was no evidence of a significant difference in the live birth outcome (OR 1.14, $p = 0.02$). When ongoing pregnancies were studied, women randomized to ultrasound guidance did have higher pregnancy rates (OR 1.38, $p < 0.0003$); however, the authors encouraged caution when interpreting the results, because of heterogeneity between studies [60].

Evidence also supports improved pregnancy rates with transfers deemed to be "easy" versus "difficult," supporting a role for trial or practice transfers prior to the actual embryo transfer. There are also preliminary studies suggesting improvement in pregnancy rates with transfer media containing hyaluronan, a glycosaminoglycan found in the female genital tract [61]. Lastly, an improvement in pregnancy rates with removal of cervical mucus has been reported. In all transfer procedures, care should be taken to minimize the interval between removal of the embryos from the incubator and placement in the uterus.

IVF outcomes

Pregnancy outcomes are dependent upon the female partner's age, ovarian reserve, quality of sperm available for fertilization, and the development of a receptive endometrium. Extrinsic factors that also influence the success of a cycle include appropriate assignment and management of the ovarian stimulation protocol, experience and quality of the embryology lab, and technical expertise of the clinicians.

National statistics are collected annually to provide information to prospective patients as well as feedback to practicing clinics. The 2009 US national data from the Society for Assisted Reproductive Technology (SART) database reports pregnancy rates for fresh and frozen non-donor embryos (Table 37.1).

Pregnancy rates using pre-treatment cryopreserved sperm in conjunction with IVF-ICSI have been equally successful. Clinical pregnancy rates and live born delivery rates of $\geq 50\%$ can be achieved with

Table 37.1. US national statistics for pregnancy and live birth rates for the year 2009 (Society for Assisted Reproductive Technology database: www.sart.org.)

	Female age <35	Female age 35–37	Female age 38–40	Female age 41–42
Fresh embryos from non-donor oocytes				
Total # of cycles	39 465	20 545	20 911	9389
% resulting in pregnancies	47.6	38.9	30.1	20.5
% resulting in live birth	41.4	31.7	22.3	12.6
Thawed embryos from non-donor oocytes				
Total # of transfers	10 757	5519	4065	1305
% resulting in live birth	35.6	30.9	26.1	22.1

cryopreserved sperm when the mean age of the female partner is 34 years [62].

Complications of ART

Ovarian hyperstimulation syndrome (OHSS)

A complication that uniquely occurs following gonadotropin ovarian stimulation is ovarian hyperstimulation syndrome (OHSS). The overall incidence of OHSS is estimated to be in the range of 0.4–10% [63], and it is dependent upon the patient population and IVF clinic. Risk factors include young age of the female partner, low body mass index (BMI), and preexisting polycystic ovarian syndrome.

The fundamental physiologic events observed in OHSS relate to vascular hyperpermeability secondary to the release of factors from the overstimulated ovaries. The resulting transudation of protein-rich fluid from the intravascular to the extravascular compartment can lead to hemoconcentration, electrolyte imbalance, and hepatic and renal dysfunction.

Several approaches have been proposed for preventing OHSS. Primary prevention involves identification of risk factors, judicious administration of the lowest effective dose of gonadotropins, and careful monitoring of follicular development and serum E_2 levels [64]. One useful strategy to prevent OHSS includes withholding gonadotropins, or "coasting," in the presence of a high serum E_2 level (> 3000 pg/mL), with delay of hCG injection until the E_2 level decreases to 2000–2500 pg/mL; alternatively, the dose of hCG

can be withheld and the cycle cancelled [64]. Reducing the dose of hCG for triggering ovulation from the standard 10 000 IU to 3000–5000 IU in patients with serum E_2 levels exceeding 2000 pg/mL is another useful strategy in mitigating the occurrence and severity of OHSS [64]. The use of a GnRH agonist for triggering ovulation in antagonist stimulation cycles is also beneficial due to the reduced half-life of the endogenous LH surge compared to hCG [65,66]. Other strategies include cryopreservation of all embryos with transfer in a non-stimulated cycle. Some have advocated the use of a dopamine agonist (cabergoline) to decrease the severity of OHSS, although evidence to support this practice is limited [67–69].

Multiple gestations

ART is associated with an increase in the incidence of multiple gestations. According to the 2007 report from the CDC/SART, the overall incidence of multiple pregnancy was 32.5% among patients treated with ART [9], the majority of which are twin gestations (29%). The incidence of triplets and higher-order gestations was 4%.

In an effort to reduce the incidence of multiple pregnancy, ASRM and SART have promulgated guidelines regarding the appropriate number of embryos to transfer [70]. These recommendations are based on the patient's age and the presence of favorable characteristics, including first cycle of IVF, good-quality embryos, and excess embryos for cryopreservation. In patients under the age of 35 with favorable characteristics, consideration should be given to transferring a single embryo. Although the risk of multiple pregnancy is significantly reduced, this risk is not completely eliminated, because of the increased incidence of monozygotic twinning in IVF cycles.

Ectopic pregnancy

ART is associated with an increased risk of ectopic pregnancy. The reported incidence of ectopic pregnancy following IVF and embryo transfer ranges from 2% to 11% [71,72], compared to a baseline of 1.2–1.4% [73]. ART also increases the risk of heterotopic pregnancy, defined as a combined intrauterine and extrauterine gestation. The occurrence of heterotopic pregnancy is extremely rare in spontaneous pregnancies, with an incidence of 1 in 30 000, but it increases to approximately 1 in 500 following IVF [74,75]. The higher incidence of ectopic and heterotopic pregnancy may be related to preexisting tubal dysfunction or uterine abnormalities in patients undergoing ART.

Perinatal outcomes from ART

To date, over 3 million babies have been born following ART worldwide [11]. Numerous studies have focused on the obstetrical and perinatal outcomes following IVF and ICSI [76–79]. Women with a history of infertility, regardless of mode of conception, have an increased risk of adverse obstetrical and perinatal outcomes. After adjusting for age and parity, subfertile women have nearly a twofold increased risk of preeclampsia and placental abruption and a threefold increase in abnormal placentation [80].

Long-term follow-up of children conceived following IVF and ICSI has been generally reassuring [81–84]. Clearly, the principal risks are those associated with multiple gestations. There are no differences in psychomotor, cognitive, intellectual, or psychological development between IVF, IVF-ICSI, and spontaneously conceived children [82–84]. Congenital abnormality rates in offspring from IVF and IVF-ICSI appear to be comparable to those in the general population.

Conclusion

Early cancer detection, combined with improved treatment protocols, has dramatically increased the survival rates for men with cancer. In recent years, a greater awareness has emerged among healthcare providers and patients of the impact of cancer treatment on future fertility, and therefore on options for fertility preservation. Cryopreservation and banking of sperm should be offered to any oncology patient interested in fertility preservation. The ultimate decision whether to utilize cryobanked sperm in the context of IUI or IVF-ICSI should be based upon several factors, including the quantity and quality of stored sperm (number of vials and post-thaw semen parameters), the age of the female partner, and an anatomic evaluation of the female genital tract. With improvements in treatment and increased survival rates, future fertility in men with cancer should be part of initial and ongoing counseling. Continued advances in reproductive medicine will assist even more couples in realizing their dream of completing their families.

References

1. Lee SJ, Schover LR, Partridge AH, *et al*. American Society of Clinical Oncology recommendations on fertility preservation in cancer patients. *J Clin Oncol* 2006; 24: 2917–31.

2. Ethics Committee of the American Society for Reproductive Medicine. Fertility preservation and reproduction in cancer patients. *Fertil Steril* 2005; 83: 1622–8.

3. Schrader M, Müller M, Straub B, Miller K. The impact of chemotherapy on male fertility: a survey of the biologic basis and clinical aspects. *Reproductive Toxicology* 2001; 15: 611–17.

4. Pont J, Albrecht W. Fertility after chemotherapy for testicular germ cell cancer. *Fertil Steril* 1997; 68: 1–5.

5. Naysmith TE, Blake DA, Harvey VJ, Johnson NP. Do men undergoing sterilizing cancer treatments have a fertile future? *Hum Reprod* 1998; 13: 3250–5.

6. Palermo G, Joris H, Devroey P, Van Steirteghem AC. Pregnancies after intracytoplasmic injection of single spermatozoon into an oocyte. *Lancet* 1992; 340: 17–18.

7. Steptoe PC, Edwards RG. Reimplantation of a human embryo with subsequent tubal pregnancy. *Lancet* 1976; 307: 880–2.

8. Steptoe PC, Edwards RG. Birth after reimplantation of a human embryo. *Lancet* 1978; 312: 366.

9. Centers for Disease Control and Prevention. *2007 Assisted Reproductive Technology Report*. www.cdc.gov/ART/ART2007 (accessed January 2012).

10. Practice Committee of American Society for Reproductive Medicine. The role of tubal reconstructive surgery in the era of assisted reproductive technologies. *Fertil Steril* 2008; 90: S250–3.

11. International Committee for Monitoring Assisted Reproductive Technology. World collaborative report on assisted reproductive technology, 2002. *Hum Reprod* 2009 24: 2310–20.

12. Toya M, Saito H, Ohta N, *et al*. Moderate and severe endometriosis is associated with alterations in the cell cycle of granulosa cells in patients undergoing in vitro fertilization and embryo transfer. *Fertil Steril* 2000; 73: 344–50.

13. Marcoux S, Maheux R, Bérubé S. Laparoscopic surgery in infertile women with minimal or mild endometriosis. *N Engl J Med* 1997; 337: 217–22.

14. Jacobson TZ, Duffy JM, Barlow D, *et al*. Laparoscopic surgery for subfertility associated with endometriosis. *Cochrane Database Syst Rev* 2010; 1: CD001398.

15. Tummon IS, Asher LJ, Martin JSB, Tulandi T. Randomized controlled trial of superovulation and

insemination for infertility associated with minimal or mild endometriosis. *Fertil Steril* 1997; 68: 8–12.

16. Messinis IE, Nillius SJ. Comparison between tamoxifen and clomiphene for induction of ovulation. *Acta Obstet Gynecol Scand* 1982; 61: 377–9.

17. MacDougall MJ, Tan SL, Jacobs HS. In vitro fertilization and the ovarian hyperstimulation syndrome. *Hum Reprod* 1992; 7: 597–600.

18. Agrawal R, Conway G, Sladkevicius P, *et al.* Serum vascular endothelial growth factor and Doppler blood flow velocities in in vitro fertilization: relevance to ovarian hyperstimulation syndrome and polycystic ovaries. *Fertil Steril* 1998; 70: 651–8.

19. Nisker J, Tummon I, Daniel S, Kaplan B, Yuzpe A. Conversion of cycles involving ovarian hyperstimulation with intra-uterine insemination to in-vitro fertilization. *Hum Reprod* 1994; 9: 406–8.

20. Templeton AA, Penney GC. The incidence, characteristics, and prognosis of patients whose infertility is unexplained. *Fertil Steril* 1982; 37: 175–82.

21. Ziebe S, Loft A, Petersen JH, *et al.* Embryo quality and developmental potential is compromised by age. *Acta Obstet Gynecol Scand* 2001; 80: 169–74.

22. Hull MG, Fleming CF, Hughes AO, McDermott A. The age-related decline in female fecundity: a quantitative controlled study of implanting capacity and survival of individual embryos after in vitro fertilization. *Fertil Steril* 1996; 65: 783–90.

23. Spandorfer SD, Chung PH, Kligman I, *et al.* An analysis of the effect of age on implantation rates. *J Assist Reprod Genet* 2000; 17: 303–6.

24. Liu H-C, Rosenwaks Z. Early pregnancy wastage in IVF (in vitro fertilization) patients. *J Assist Reprod Genet* 1991; 8: 65–72.

25. Spandorfer SD, Davis OK, Barmat LI, Chung PH, Rosenwaks Z. Relationship between maternal age and aneuploidy in in vitro fertilization pregnancy loss. *Fertil Steril* 2004; 81: 1265–9.

26. Chang M-Y, Chiang C-H, Hsieh Ts-Ta, Soong Y-K, Hsu K-H. Use of the antral follicle count to predict the outcome of assisted reproductive technologies. *Fertil Steril* 1998; 69: 505–10.

27. Bancsi LF, Broekmans FJ, Eijkemans MJ, *et al.* Predictors of poor ovarian response in in vitro fertilization: a prospective study comparing basal markers of ovarian reserve. *Fertil Steril* 2002; 77: 328–36.

28. Burger H, Cahir N, Robertson D, *et al.* Serum inhibins A and B fall differentially as FSH rises in perimenopausal women. *Clin Endocrinol* 1998; 48: 809–13.

29. Cameron TT, O'Shea FC, Rolland JM, *et al.* Occult ovarian failure: a syndrome of infertility, regular menses, and elevated follicle-stimulating hormone concentrations. *J Clin Endocrinol Metab* 1988 67: 1190–4.

30. Toner JP, Philput CB, Jones GS, Muasher S. Basal follicle-stimulating hormone level is a better predictor of in vitro fertilization performance than age. *Fertil Steril* 1991; 55: 784–91.

31. Visser JA, Themmen APN. Anti-Müllerian hormone and folliculogenesis. *Mol Cell Endocrinol* 2005; 234: 81–6.

32. Broer SL, Mol BW, Hendriks D, Broekmans FJ. The role of antimullerian hormone in prediction of outcome after IVF: comparison with the antral follicle count. *Fertil Steril* 2009; 91: 705–14.

33. Nelson SM, Yates RW, Lyall H, *et al.* Anti-Mullerian hormone-based approach to controlled ovarian stimulation for assisted conception. *Hum Reprod* 2009; 24: 867–75.

34. Gnoth C, Schuring AN, Friol K, *et al.* Relevance of anti-Mullerian hormone measurement in a routine IVF program. *Hum Reprod* 2008; 23: 1359–65.

35. Muttukrishna S, Suharjono H, McGarrigle H, Sathanandan M. Inhibin B and anti-Mullerian hormone: markers of ovarian response in IVF/ICSI patients? *BJOG* 2004; 111: 1248–53.

36. Navot D, Rosenwaks Z, Margalioth EJ. Prognostic assessment of female fecundity. *Lancet* 1987; 2: 645–7.

37. Jain T, Soules MR, Collins JA. Comparison of basal follicle-stimulating hormone versus the clomiphene citrate challenge test for ovarian reserve screening. *Fertil Steril* 2004; 82: 180–5.

38. Hendriks DJ, Mol B-WJ, Bancsi LFJMM, te Velde ER, Broekmans FJM. The clomiphene citrate challenge test for the prediction of poor ovarian response and nonpregnancy in patients undergoing in vitro fertilization: a systematic review. *Fertil Steril* 2006; 86: 807–18.

39. Shufaro Y, Schenker JG. Cryopreservation of human genetic material. *Ann N Y Acad Sci* 2010; 1205: 220–4.

40. Schlegel P. Nonobstructive azoospermia: a revolutionary surgical approach and results. *Sem Reprod Med* 2009; 27: 165–70.

41. Garner DK, Weissman A, Howles CM, Shoham , eds. *Textbook of Assisted Reproductive Technologies: Laboratory and Clinical Perspectives*, 3rd edn. London: Informa Healthcare, 2009.

42. MacLeod JGR. The male factor in fertility and infertility. II. Spermatozoon counts in 1000 men of known fertility and in 1000 cases of infertile marriage. *J Urol* 1951; 66: 436–49.

43. Smith KD R-RL, Steinberger E. Relation between indices of semen analysis and pregnancy rate in infertile couples. *Fertil Steril* 1977; 25: 503.

44. Aitken RJ, Baker HWG, Irvine DS. On the nature of semen quality and infertility. *Hum Reprod* 1995; 10: 248–9.

45. Mortimer D. Sperm recovery techniques to maximize fertilizing capacity. *Reprod Fertil Dev* 1994; 6: 25–31.

46. Baker TG. A quantitative and cytological study of germ cells in human ovaries. *Proc R Soc Lond B Biol Sci* 1963; 158: 417–33.

47. Van Voorhis BJ, Thomas M, Surrey ES, Sparks A. What do consistently high-performing in vitro fertilization programs in the U.S. do? *Fertil Steril* 2010; 94: 1346–9.

48. Tarlatzis BC, Fauser BC, Kolibianakis EM, Diedrich K, Devroey P. GnRH antagonists in ovarian stimulation for IVF. *Hum Reprod Update* 2006; 12: 333–40.

49. Agrawal R, Tan SL, Wild S, *et al.* Serum vascular endothelial growth factor concentrations in in vitro fertilization cycles predict the risk of ovarian hyperstimulation syndrome. *Fertil Steril* 1999; 71: 287–93.

50. Dekel NAE, Goren S, Feldman B, Shalgi R. Mechanism of action of GnRH-induced oocyte maturation. *J Reprod Fertil Suppl* 1989; 37: 319–27.

51. Kang HJ, Rosenwaks Z. Triploidy: the breakdown of monogamy between sperm and egg. *Int J Dev Biol* 2008; 52: 449–54.

52. Das S, Blake D, Farquhar C, Seif MM. Assisted hatching on assisted conception (IVF and ICSI). *Cochrane Database Syst Rev*. 2009; 2: CD001894.

53. Barmat LI, Liu HC, Spandorfer SD, *et al.* Autologous endometrial co-culture in patients with repeated failures of implantation after in vitro fertilization–embryo transfer. *J Assist Reprod Genet* 1999; 16: 121–7.

54. Spandorfer SD, Barmat L, Navarro J, *et al.* Autologous endometrial coculture in patients with a previous history of poor quality embryos. *J Assist Reprod Genet* 2002; 19: 309–12.

55. Spandorfer SD, Pascal P, Parks J, *et al.* Autologous endometrial coculture in patients with IVF failure: outcome of the first 1,030 cases. *J Reprod Med* 2004; 49: 463–7.

56. Spandorfer S, Soslow R, Clark R, *et al.* Histologic characteristics of the endometrium predicts success when utilizing autologous endometrial coculture in patients with IVF failure. *J Assist Reprod Genet* 2006; 23: 185–9.

57. Ray PF, Ao A, Taylor DM, Winston RML, Handyside AH. Assessment of the reliability of single blastomere analysis for preimplantation diagnosis of the Δ F508 deletion causing cystic fibrosis in clinical practice. *Prenat Diagn* 1998; 18: 1402–12.

58. Staessen C, Platteau P, Van Assche E, *et al.* Comparison of blastocyst transfer with or without preimplantation genetic diagnosis for aneuploidy screening in couples with advanced maternal age: a prospective randomized controlled trial. *Hum Reprod* 2004; 19: 2849–58.

59. Mastenbroek S, Twisk M, van Echten-Arends J, *et al.* In vitro fertilization with preimplantation genetic screening. *N Engl J Med* 2007; 357: 9–17.

60. Brown J, Buckingham K, Abou-Setta AM, Buckett W. Ultrasound versus "clinical touch" for catheter guidance during embryo transfer in women. *Cochrane Database Syst Rev* 2010; 1: CD006107.

61. Urman B, Yakin K, Ata B, Isiklar A, Balaban B. Effect of hyaluronan-enriched transfer medium on implantation and pregnancy rates after day 3 and day 5 embryo transfers: a prospective randomized study. *Fertil Steril* 2008; 90: 604–12.

62. Hourvitz A, Goldschlag DE, Davis OK, *et al.* Intracytoplasmic sperm injection (ICSI) using cryopreserved sperm from men with malignant neoplasm yields high pregnancy rates. *Fertil Steril* 2008; 90: 557–63.

63. MacDougall MJ, Tan SL, Balen A, Jacobs HS. A controlled study comparing patients with and without polycystic ovaries undergoing in-vitro fertilization. *Hum Reprod* 1993; 8: 233–7.

64. Chen D, Burmeister L, Goldschlag D, Rosenwaks Z. Ovarian hyperstimulation syndrome: strategies for prevention. *Reprod Biomed Online* 2003; 7: 43–9.

65. European Recombinant LH Study Group. Human recombinant luteinizing hormone is as effective as, but safer than, urinary human chorionic gonadotropin in inducing final follicular maturation and ovulation in in vitro fertilization procedures: results of a multicenter double-blind study. *J Clin Endocrinol Metab* 2001; 86: 2607–18.

66. Ludwig M, Felberbaum RE, Devroey P, *et al.* Significant reduction of the incidence of ovarian hyperstimulation syndrome (OHSS) by using the LHRH antagonist Cetrorelix (Cetrotide®) in controlled ovarian stimulation for assisted reproduction. *Arch Gynecol Obstet* 2000; 264: 29–32.

67. Gomez R, Gonzalez-Izquierdo M, Zimmermann RC, *et al.* Low-dose dopamine agonist administration blocks vascular endothelial growth factor (VEGF)-mediated vascular hyperpermeability without altering VEGF receptor 2-dependent luteal angiogenesis in a rat ovarian hyperstimulation model. *Endocrinology* 2006; 147: 5400–11.

68. Alvarez C, Marti-Bonmati L, Novella-Maestre E, *et al.* Dopamine agonist cabergoline reduces hemoconcentration and ascites in hyperstimulated women undergoing assisted reproduction. *J Clin Endocrinol Metab* 2007; 92: 2931–7.

69. Carizza C, Abdelmassih V, Abdelmassih S, *et al.* Cabergoline reduces the early onset of ovarian hyperstimulation syndrome: a prospective randomized study. *Reprod Biomed Online* 2008; 17: 751–5.

70. The Practice Committee of the American Society for Reproductive Medicine and the Practice Committee of the Society for Assisted Reproductive Technology. Guidelines on number of embryos transferred. *Fertil Steril* 2009; 92: 1518–19.

71. Roest J, Mous H, Zeilmaker G, Verhoeff A. The incidence of major clinical complications in a Dutch transport IVF programme. *Hum Reprod Update* 1996; 2: 345–53.

72. Azem F, Yaron Y, Botchan A, *et al.* Ectopic pregnancy after in vitro fertilization-embryo transfer (IVF-ET): the possible role of the ET technique. *J Assist Reprod Genet* 1993; 10: 302–4.

73. Chow WH, Daling JR, Cates W, Greenberg RS. Epidemiology of ectopic pregnancy. *Epidemiol Rev* 1987; 9: 70–94.

74. Marcus SF, Macnamee M, Brinsden P. Pregnancy: heterotopic pregnancies after in-vitro fertilization and embryo transfer. *Hum Reprod* 1995; 10: 1232–6.

75. Rizk B, Tan SL, Morcos S, *et al.* Heterotopic pregnancies after in vitro fertilization and embryo transfer. *Am J Obstet Gynecol* 1991; 164: 161–4.

76. Ochsenkühn R, Strowitzki T, Gurtner M, *et al.* Pregnancy complications, obstetric risks, and neonatal outcome in singleton and twin pregnancies after GIFT and IVF. *Arch Gynecol Obstet* 2003; 268: 256–61.

77. Jackson RA, Gibson KA, Wu YW, Croughan MS. Perinatal outcomes in singletons following in vitro fertilization: a meta-analysis. *Obstet Gynecol* 2004; 103: 551–63.

78. Katalinic A, Rösch C, Ludwig M. Pregnancy course and outcome after intracytoplasmic sperm injection: a controlled, prospective cohort study. *Fertil Steril* 2004; 81: 1604–16.

79. Allen VM, Wilson RD, Cheung A, Genetics Committee of the Society of Obstetricians and Gynaecologists of Canada (SOGC), Reproductive Endocrinology Infertility Committee of the Society of Obstetricians and Gynaecologists of Canada (SOGC). Pregnancy outcomes after assisted reproductive technology. *J Obstet Gynaecol Can* 2006; 28: 220–50.

80. Thomson F, Shanbhag S, Templeton A, Bhattacharya S. Obstetric outcome in women with subfertility. *BJOG* 2005; 112: 632–7.

81. Knoester M, Helmerhorst FM, Vandenbroucke JP, *et al.* Perinatal outcome, health, growth, and medical care utilization of 5- to 8-year-old intracytoplasmic sperm injection singletons. *Fertil Steril* 2008; 89: 1133–46.

82. Place I, Englert Y. A prospective longitudinal study of the physical, psychomotor, and intellectual development of singleton children up to 5 years who were conceived by intracytoplasmic sperm injection compared with children conceived spontaneously and by in vitro fertilization. *Fertil Steril* 2003; 80: 1388–97.

83. Bonduelle M, Ponjaert I, Steirteghem AV, *et al.* Developmental outcome at 2 years of age for children born after ICSI compared with children born after IVF. *Hum Reprod* 2003; 18: 342–50.

84. Ponjaert-Kristoffersen I, Tjus T, Nekkebroeck J, *et al.* Psychological follow-up study of 5-year-old ICSI children. *Hum Reprod* 2004; 19: 2791–7.

Index